## Peptide and protein hormones

| Hormone | Abbreviation | Source | Major biological action |
| --- | --- | --- | --- |
| **Adrenal glands** | | | |
| Met-enkephalin | | Adrenal medulla | Analgesic actions in CNS |
| Leu-enkephalin | | Adrenal medulla | Analgesic actions in CNS |
| **Gut** | | | |
| Bombesin | | Neurons and endocrine cells of gut | Hypothermic hormone; increases gastrin secretion |
| Cholecystokinin (Pancreozymin) | CCK | Duodenum and CNS | Stimulates gallbladder contraction and bile flow; affects memory, eating behavior |
| Gastric inhibitory polypeptide | GIP | Duodenum | Inhibits gastric acid secretion |
| Gastrin | | G-cells of midpyloric glands in stomach antrum | Increases secretion of gastric acid and pepsin |
| Motilin | | Duodenum, pineal gland | Alters motility of GI tract |
| Secretin | | Duodenum | Stimulates pancreatic acinar cells to release bicarbonate and water |
| Vasoactive intestinal polypeptide | VIP | GI tract, hypothalamus | Increases secretion of water and electrolytes from pancreas and gut; acts as neurotransmitter in autonomic nervous system |
| **Hypothalamus** | | | |
| Arg-vasotocin | AVT | Hypothalamus and pineal gland | Regulates reproductive organs |
| Corticotropin-releasing hormone | CRH | Paraventricular nuclei, anterior periventricular nuclei | Stimulates release of ACTH and β-endorphin from anterior pituitary |
| Gonadotropin-releasing hormone (Luteinizing hormone–releasing hormone) | GnRH (LHRH) | Preoptic area; anterior hypothalamus; suprachiasmatic nuclei; medial basal hypothalamus (rodents and primates); arcuate nuclei (primates) | Stimulates release of FSH and LH from anterior pituitary |
| Somatostatin (Growth hormone–inhibiting hormone) | | Anterior periventricular nuclei | Inhibits release of GH and TSH from anterior pituitary inhibits release of insulin and glucagon from pancreas |
| Somatocrinin (Growth hormone–releasing hormone) | GHRH | Medial basal hypothalamus; arcuate nuclei | Stimulates release of GH from anterior pituitary |
| Melanotropin-release inhibitory factor (Dopamine) | MIF (DA) | Arcuate nuclei | Inhibits the release of MSH (no evidence of this peptide in humans) |
| Melanotropin-releasing factor | MRF | Paraventricular nuclei | Stimulates the release of MSH from anterior pituitary (no evidence of this peptide in humans) |
| Neurotensin | | Hypothalamus; intestinal mucosa | May act as a neurohormone |
| Prolactin-inhibitory factor (Dopamine) | PIF (DA) | Arcuate nuclei | Inhibits PRL secretion |
| Prolactin-releasing hormone | | Paraventricular nuclei | Stimulates release of PRL from anterior pituitary |
| Substance P | SP | Hypothalamus, CNS, intestine | Transmits pain; increases smooth muscle contractions of GI tract |
| Thyrotropin-releasing hormone | TRH | Paraventricular nuclei | Stimulates release of TSH and PRL from anterior pituitary |
| **Liver** | | | |
| Somatomedins | | Liver, kidney | Cartilage sulfation, somatic cell growth |
| Angiotensinogen | | Liver, blood | Precursor of angiotensins, which affect blood pressure |

# Behavioral Endocrinology

# An Introduction to Behavioral Endocrinology

## Second Edition

### Randy J. Nelson
*The Johns Hopkins University*

Sinauer Associates, Inc. • *Publishers*
Sunderland, Massachusetts

## The cover

The underside of the throats of several male tree lizards (*Urosaurus ornatus*) collected from a single population in central Arizona; males extend these throat patches into a fan known as a dewlap, which is displayed to other males and to females. Males with blue dewlap coloration are aggressive and defend territories, whereas males without blue are much less aggressive and do not defend territories (see Chapters 3 and 8). The neuroendocrine mechanisms underlying the differentiation of these alternative male phenotypes parallel those involved in sexual differentiation in this species, which suggests that the morphological and behavioral differences between males arise in a manner similar to the development of differences between males and females (see Chapters 3 and 4). Photographs by Michael C. Moore and Christopher W. Thompson.

**An Introduction to Behavioral Endocrinology**, Second Edition

Copyright © 2000 by Sinauer Associates, Inc.
All rights reserved.
This book may not be reproduced in whole or in part for any purpose whatsoever without permission from the publisher. For information or to order, address: Sinauer Associates, Inc., P.O. Box 407, Sunderland, Massachusetts 01375-0407 U.S.A. FAX: 413-549-1118. Internet: publish@sinauer.com

**Library of Congress Cataloging-in-Publication Data**

Nelson, Randy Joe.
    An introduction to behavioral endocrinology / Randy J. Nelson.—2nd ed.
        p. ; cm.
    Includes bibliographical references and indexes.
    ISBN 0-87893-616-5
    1. Psychoneuroendocrinology. I. Title.
    [DNLM: 1. Behavior—physiology. 2. Hormones—physiology. 3. Physiology,
Comparative. 4. Psychophysiology. WK 102 N429i 1999]
    QP356.45 .N45 1999
    612.4'05—dc21

                                                                99-046279

Printed in U.S.A.

9 8 7 6 5 4 3 2

*For Morgan and Courtney*

# Contents

## Chapter 4   Sex Differences in Behavior: Animal Models and Humans   145

## Chapter 5   Male Reproductive Behavior   199

# Preface

When I wrote the first edition of this book, I had three main goals, and those goals remained important as I prepared this revision. First, I wanted to convey the excitement of a field that has continued to embrace the perspectives and contributions of diverse lines of research: understanding the interactions between hormones and behavior is a truly interdisciplinary effort that involves the study of phenomena ranging from the molecular and cellular to the social levels. Second, I wanted to give due credit to those scientists who laid the foundation of the field by presenting current hypotheses and theories within the context of their historical origins; I have expanded on that historical approach in this edition. Third, even though in some cases all or most of the relevant research in a given area has been conducted on rats or mice, and I have therefore necessarily restricted the discussion to these rodent species, I have attempted whenever possible to present behavioral endocrinology from a comparative perspective. In this edition, I have included new discussions of hormone–behavior interactions in fish, reptiles, amphibians, and even invertebrates. The advantage of this broadly comparative approach is that it illuminates the diverse endocrine and behavioral mechanisms that have evolved in animals to deal with common problems of survival and reproduction. Toward this end, the adaptive functions as well as the physiological mechanisms of hormone–behavior interactions are presented throughout the text. It is my hope that this integrative approach makes learning about behavioral endocrinology interesting, and provides a useful framework upon which you can arrange the details.

As was the case with the first edition, my motivation for revising this book was to have a teaching aid for my own course in behavioral endocrinology at The Johns Hopkins University. It sometimes seems that each week brings new and important research results that bear directly on issues the field, and, after five years in print, the book clearly required an update to maintain its usefulness. This is an exciting time for the field, and I was overwhelmed by all the fascinating and impressive new research now being conducted.

The most obvious change in this edition is the inclusion of a new chapter on hormones and stress. Stress—and how to cope with it—is a research area that impinges upon almost every aspect of behavioral endocrinology. Since the first edition appeared, many of the breakthroughs that have occurred are the result of novel molecular techniques, such as the deletion, overexpression, and insertion of specific genes into mice, and coverage of these methods is now an important part of this text. However, because approximately half of the undergraduate courses in behavioral endocrinology are taught in psychology departments, I have tried to employ a writing style and maintain a level of detail that will make the text accessible to students with a variety of scientific backgrounds. My assumption is that psychology students will have taken a course in biopsychology or neuroscience by the time they encounter this text, but I have tried to keep discussions of endocrine physiology and biochemistry to the minimum needed to understand the behavioral concepts under discussion, and, whenever possible, I have linked behavioral phenomena being described to common animals, such as dogs, to make the material more relevant to students' own experiences. Some topics covered in the text are controversial and will undoubtedly stimulate class discussion, so I have concluded each chapter with several potential starting points for such exchanges. Also, I have included a short list of additional readings that provide more detailed information on the material in each chapter. Needless to say, many new findings had to be omitted to keep the length of the book manageable, but if this edition captures even a small portion of the excitement and scope of current behavioral endocrinology research, I will be content.

### Acknowledgments

I benefited from the assistance of many people in the preparation of this book. I remain grateful to the reviewers of the first edition, including Elizabeth Adkins-Regan, Greg Ball, Jacques Balthazart, Dan Bernard, Eric Bittman, Elliott Blass, Jeff Blaustein, Sue Carter, Joe Casto, Greg Demas, Courtney DeVries, Don Dewsbury, Paul Gold, David Gubernick, Sabra Klein, Lance Kriegsfeld, Michael Leon, Margaret McCarthy, Martha McClintock, Jim McGaugh, Chris Moffatt, Celia Moore, David Olton, Emilie Rissman, Ed Roy, Ben Sachs, Barbara Sherwin, David Shide, Rae Silver, Cheryl Sisk, Chuck Snowdon (and his undergraduate students), George Wade, John Wingfield, Pauline Yahr, and Irving Zucker.

I was immeasurably helped in preparing this new edition by insightful, helpful, and remarkably kind comments by Elizabeth Adkins-Regan, Catherine Auger, Greg Ball, Jacques Balthazart, Tim Bartness, George Bentley, Staci Bilbo, Joan Blom, Robert Bridges, Silvana Chiavegatto, Tom Coombs-Hahn, James Dabbs, Greg Demas, Courtney DeVries, Debbie Drazen, Lori Flanagan-Cato, Alison Fleming, Nancy Forger, Stephen Gammie, Bruce Goldman, Elizabeth Gould, Elaine Hull, Sabra Klein, Lance Kriegsfeld, Vicky Luine, Chris Moffatt, Michael Moore, Kathie Olsen, Deb Olster, Mike Romero, Jay Rosenblatt, Ben Sachs, Randall Sakai, Jen Sartor, Jill Schneider, Rae Silver, Judith Stern, Anjali Trasy, John Wingfield, Amy Wisniewski, Ruth Wood, Kelly Young, and Irving Zucker. Most of these reviewers' suggestions for changes were incorporated into this new edition, but in some cases, laziness or stubbornness on my part prevented me from following the excellent advice I received from my friends and colleagues, and I remain responsible for any errors or other shortcomings that exist in the text.

I also thank Staci Bilbo, Donna Bilu, Courtney DeVries, Debbie Drazen, Joyce Hairston, Sabra Klein, Lance Kriegsfeld, Viollette Renard, Brian Spar, and Sue Yang for helping me track down various materials for this book. I am grateful to my many colleagues who kindly provided reprint copies of their papers, and I am especially indebted to many other colleagues, who are acknowledged individually in figure legends, for permission to use graphic or photographic material. I am particularly grateful to my colleague and wife, Courtney DeVries, for being critical when reading chapter manuscripts and uncritical at all other times.

I would also like to thank the team at Sinauer Associates, especially Peter Farley, the editor of this book. His careful attention to detail has greatly improved this edition. Others who deserve special mention are Kerry Falvey and Paula Noonan, production editors, Christopher Small, production manager, Wendy Beck and Janice Holabird, compositors, and Norma Roche, for her significant assistance with copyediting and suggestions for improvements in the style of presentation. This book is much better because of their hard work and uncompromising efforts.

Finally, I thank the hundreds of undergraduate students who have taken my course at Johns Hopkins over the past 13 years; they have provided many helpful suggestions on creating and improving the first edition.

# 1

# The Study of Behavioral Endocrinology

**D**oes anabolic steroid abuse cause violent behavior? Does an individual's sex drive wane with aging? Is the sex drive of women higher or lower than the sex drive of men? Can jet lag be cured with melatonin? Is mood affected by a woman's menstrual cycle? Do seasonal cycles of depression occur in people? Why are more men than women in prison for committing violent crimes? Does postpartum depression really exist? Is homosexuality caused by hormone concentrations that are too low or too high? Is the sexual behavior of women influenced by menopause? Can leptin curb our food intake? Many of us have pondered these questions during informal discussions with friends and family members. Researchers in the field of behavioral endocrinology, the study of the interaction between hormones and behavior, attempt to address these kinds of questions in a formal, scientific manner. In contrast to popular beliefs, hormones do not *cause* behavioral changes per se. Rather, hormones change the *probability* that a specific behavior will be emitted in the appropriate behavioral or social context.

The study of the interaction between hormones and behavior has been truly interdisciplinary: methods and techniques from one scientific discipline have been borrowed and refined by researchers in other fields. Psychologists, neuroscientists, entomologists, zoologists, anatomists, physiologists, endocrinologists, psychiatrists, and other behavioral biologists have all made contributions to the understanding of hormone–behavior interactions. This exciting commingling of scientific interests and approaches, with its ongoing synthesis of knowledge, has led to the emergence of behavioral endocrinology as a distinct field of study (Beach, 1975b).

## Historical Roots of Behavioral Endocrinology

Ebbinghaus (1908) stated that psychology has a short history but a long past, and the same can be said of behavioral endocrinology (Beach, 1974a). While the modern era of the discipline began only about 50 years ago, with the publication of the classic book *Hormones and Behavior* (Beach, 1948), some effects of hormones on behavior have been implicitly recognized for centuries.

The male sex organs, or testes, produce and secrete a hormone called testosterone, which affects sexual behavior, aggressiveness, territoriality, hibernation, and migration, as well as many other behaviors that differentiate males from females. The testes are usually located outside of the body cavity in mammals and can easily be damaged or removed. Thus, castration, the surgical removal of the testes, has historically been the most common manipulation of the endocrine system. For millennia, individuals of many species of domestic animals have been castrated to make them better to eat or easier to control, and the behavioral and physical effects of castration have been known since antiquity. Indeed, these effects were known to Aristotle, who described the effects of castration in roosters (and humans) with great detail and accuracy. For example, in *History of Animals*, written about 350 B.C., Aristotle reported that

> Birds have their testicles inside . . . Birds are castrated at the rump at the part where the two sexes unite in copulation. If you burn this area twice or thrice with hot irons, then, if the bird be full-grown, his crest grows sallow, he ceases to crow, and foregoes sexual passion; but if you cauterize the bird when young, none of these male attributes or propensities will come to him as he grows up. The case is the same for men: if you mutilate them in boyhood, the later-growing hair never comes, and the voice never changes but remains high-pitched; if they be mutilated in early manhood, the late-growths of hair quit them except the growth on the groin, and that diminishes but does not entirely depart.

For centuries, royalty employed men castrated before puberty, called eunuchs, to guard women from other men. For example, the Old Testament reports that these emasculated males were used to guard the women's quarters of Hebrew kings and princes (Esther 1:10). Castration in humans often has little or no effect on physical appearance or future sexual behavior when performed after the unfortunate individual attains sexual maturation; however, if human males are castrated before puberty, they will develop a characteristic physical appearance, marked by short stature and long arms (Figure 1.1), and sexual behaviors are unlikely to develop. The typical secondary male sex characters are also affected by prepubertal removal of the testes. For example, as noted by Aristotle, eunuchs never develop beards, and the pubertal change in voice does not occur. Normally during puberty, the vocal cords of males thicken in response to testosterone secreted by the testes. It is the thickened vocal cords that produce the deeper-pitched voice characteristic of males, just as the thick strings of a guitar produce deeper-pitched notes than the thin strings.

Castration was once a common practice in Europe and Asia—indeed, it continues to this day in some cultures (Box 1.1). Young boys with exceptional singing voices were castrated to prevent the pubertal changes in pitch. These singers became known as *castrati*. Although castrati were prized by church choirs for centuries, their popularity reached a peak in Europe during the 17th and 18th centuries with the development of opera, which made castrati the first superstars of the entertainment world (Heriot, 1974). The first castrato opera star, Baldassare Ferri, died in 1680 at the age of 70 with a fortune that was worth the equivalent of $3,000,000 today. In hopes of attaining this level of wealth and fame, young boys with musical aptitude were identified early, and poor families offered their sons outright to church leaders, singing teachers, and music academies. Thousands of boys lost their testes but never gained the celebrity or riches of the star castrati.

What did a castrato sound like? Essentially, the castrati had the range of a soprano, but the greater development of the male lungs gave their singing remarkable power. An early critic remarked, "Their timbre is as clear and piercing as that of choirboys and much more powerful; they appear to sing an octave

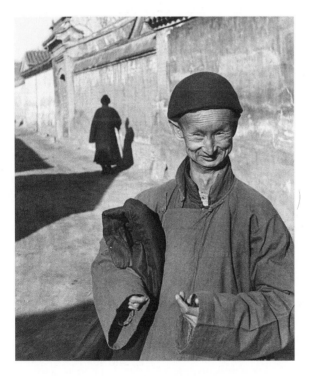

**1.1 Eunuch of the last imperial court,** photographed in China by Henri Cartier-Bresson in 1949. Note the lack of facial hair and unusually long arms.

Box 1.1

# The Hijras of India

Over a million eunuchs, called Hijras, are estimated to be currently living in India. Traditionally, the cultural function of Indian Hijras is to sing and dance at weddings and ceremonies associated with the birth of male children. The Hijras have become associated with fertility and form a sect within Hinduism; they worship Bahachara, a manifestation of the Hindu mother goddess. However, a significant minority of Hijras are Moslem. Although the Hijras claim the religious status of "sannyasis" (or celibates) because their genitalia (i.e., testes and penis) have been surgically removed, many work as prostitutes.

The Hijras are a heterogeneous population; most individuals have sexually ambiguous histories. Commonly, their genitalia were ambiguous at birth, or their sexual development was atypical during puberty (Nanda, 1990). Some Hijras engaged in homosexual sex during adolescence, and virtually all were reared as boys. The surgery is usually performed during an outdoor ritual that is accompanied by singing and dancing hijras. Both the penis and scrotum are removed in the rapid, but nonsterile, operation.

Although some Hijras work as prostitutes, the most common occupation of the Hijras is removing "bad luck." Because the Hijras consider themselves to have suffered the very worst luck that can befall a man (despite the "elective" nature of the surgery), they will accept a little more bad luck for a fee. Thus, it is customary for new homeowners to hire Hijras to dance through all the rooms to absorb any potential bad luck. Similarly, small groups of Hijras appear uninvited at weddings to dance away any potential bad fortune for the bride and groom. Despite a certain amount of traditional charm, the arrival of the garishly dressed Hijras at a wedding is seldom a welcome sight. If they are not given a substantial fee, then the Hijras will disrupt the wedding ceremony by cursing and exposing their disfigured genitalia. Not surprisingly, most families pay the fee to avoid the anatomy lesson, but these small extortions have made the Hijras rather unpopular in the cities of India. Also, rumors persist that young, homeless boys are taken in by the Hijras, who provide friendship and material goods, then transform them into eunuchs (e.g., Diamond, 1984). However, recent accounts of the Hijras failed to uncover any evidence of coerced or involuntary acceptance of the demasculinizing surgery (Nanda, 1990).

above the natural voice of women. Their voices . . . are brilliant, light, full of sparkle, very loud, and astound with a very wide range" (Heriot, 1974).

After 200 years, the tastes of the opera-loving public changed. The rise in popularity of the female soprano voice reduced the demand for the castrati, and they soon became an oddity. In 1849, the last great castrato, Giovanni Velluti, retired from opera to his villa in Venice.

### Berthold's Experiment

A useful starting point for understanding research in hormones and behavior is a classic 19th-century experiment that is now considered to be the first formal study of endocrinology. This remarkable experiment conclusively demonstrated that a substance produced by the testes could travel through the bloodstream and eventually affect behavior. Professor Arnold Adolph Berthold, a Swiss–German

**1.2  Arnold Adolph Berthold** of the University of Göttingen, who in 1849 conducted what is now recognized as the first formal experiment in endocrinology.

physician and professor of physiology at the University of Göttingen (Figure 1.2), demonstrated experimentally that a product of the testes was necessary for a cockerel (an immature male chicken) to develop into a normal adult rooster.

As you know, roosters display several characteristic behaviors that are not typically seen among hens or immature chicks of either sex. Roosters mate with hens, they fight with other roosters, and of course, roosters crow. Moreover, roosters are larger than hens and immature birds, and have distinctive plumage. On the other hand, capons, male chickens that have been castrated prior to adulthood in order to make them more tender to eat, do not show many behavioral and physical characteristics of roosters. They do not attempt to mate with hens and are not very aggressive toward other males. Indeed, they avoid aggressive encounters, and if conditions force them to fight, they do so in a "half-hearted" manner. Finally, capons do not crow like roosters.

The behavioral and physical differences among roosters, hens, capons, and immature chickens were undoubtedly familiar to Berthold when he planned his study, which began on the second day of August, 1848, and lasted for several months (Figure 1.3; Berthold, 1849). He placed six cockerels in three experimental groups, each consisting of two birds. He removed both testes from each of the two cockerels in the first group, and, as expected, these birds eventually developed as capons. They never fought with other males after castration, and they failed to crow; instead, Professor Berthold reported, they developed the "monotone voice of the capon." They avoided females and never exhibited mating behavior. Finally, these birds *looked* different than intact (uncastrated) adult males. Their bodies and heads were small, and their combs and wattles were atrophied and pale in color.

The second pair of cockerels was also castrated, but Berthold reimplanted one testis from each bird in its abdominal cavity after ensuring that all of the orig-

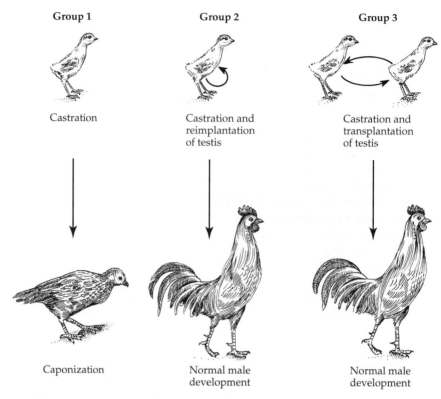

**1.3   Berthold's experiment.** The birds in Group 1 were castrated, and, when observed several months later, were smaller than normal roosters and failed to engage in rooster-typical behaviors. The birds in Group 2 were also castrated, but one of each bird's own testes was reimplanted in its abdominal cavity. These birds looked and behaved like normal roosters when adults. The two birds in Group 3 were castrated, and one testis from each bird was transplanted into the abdomen of the other. Several months later, these birds also looked and behaved liked normal roosters. Berthold found that the reimplanted and transplanted testes in Groups 2 and 3 developed vascular connections and generated sperm.

inal vascular and neural connections had been cut. Interestingly, both birds in this group developed normal rooster behavior. According to Berthold, they "crowed lustily, often engaged in battle with each other and with other cockerels, and showed the usual reactions to hens." Their physical appearance was indistinguishable from that of other young roosters; they grew normally and possessed highly developed combs and wattles that were bright red in color.

The remaining two birds were also castrated, but after the testes were removed, Berthold placed a single testis from each bird in the other's abdominal cavity. Like the cockerels in the second experimental group, these birds also developed the "voice, sexual urge, belligerence, and growth of combs and wattles" characteristic of intact males.

After observing all six birds for several months, Berthold dissected one of the cockerels from the second group and found that the implanted testis had attached itself to the intestines, developed a vascular supply, and nearly doubled in size.

Eventually, he examined all the implanted testes under a microscope and noted the presence of sperm.

Based on the results of this experiment, Berthold drew three major conclusions: (1) the testes are transplantable organs; (2) transplanted testes can function and create sperm (Berthold drew the analogy to a tree branch that produces its own fruit after having been grafted to another tree); and (3) because the testes functioned normally after all nerves were severed, there can be no specific nerves directing testicular function. To account for these findings, Berthold proposed that a secretory, blood-borne product of the transplanted testes (*productive Verhältniss der Hoden*) was responsible for the normal development of the birds in the second and third groups. It is worth noting that three of the four parameters Berthold used to formulate this hypothesis—mating, vocalization, aggression, and distinctive appearance—were behavioral.

In recent years, Berthold's experiment has been credited as the genesis of the field of endocrinology (and of behavioral endocrinology: Box 1.2), but his intriguing demonstration of non-neural control of behavior was apparently not embraced with great enthusiasm by his scientific contemporaries, as his paper does not seem to have been cited for nearly 50 years after its publication. Why, then, did Berthold conduct his study? His experiment was elegant in its simplicity, but unfortunately his report had no introduction, so we cannot know for certain what questions motivated him to conduct the work (Forbes, 1949). We do know that Berthold had previously authored a well-known physiology textbook and had actively conducted research.* A reading of his textbook makes it apparent that Berthold was a proponent of the pangenesis theory of inheritance. This theory, endorsed by many biologists prior to the discovery of how chromosomes and genes function, held that all body parts actively discharge bits and pieces of themselves into the blood system, where they are transported to the ovaries or testes and assembled into miniature offspring resembling the parents. As a consequence of this theoretical stance, Berthold had two concepts at hand when evaluating the results of his testicular transplantation study: (1) various parts of the body release specific agents into the blood; and (2) these agents travel through the bloodstream to particular target organs. Why Berthold did not go any further with his interesting finding is not known; he died 12 years later in 1861 without following up on his now-famous study.

## What Are Hormones?

Berthold took the first step in the study of behavioral endocrinology by demonstrating that the well-known effects of the testes were due to their production of a substance that circulated in the blood. Modern studies in behavioral endocrinology have documented effects of substances from many different glands affecting an even greater range of behaviors.

We now know Berthold's "secretory blood-borne product" as a hormone. **Hormones** are organic chemical messengers produced and released by special-

---

*For example, together with Robert Wilhelm Bunsen, for whom the ubiquitous piece of laboratory equipment was named, he discovered that hydrated oxides of iron can serve as an antidote for arsenic poisoning.

## Box 1.2
# Frank A. Beach and the Origins of the Modern Era of Behavioral Endocrinology

For some time before behavioral endocrinology emerged as a recognized field, its foundations were being laid by researchers in other fields. The anatomists, physiologists, and zoologists who were doing the majority of the work on "internal secretions" prior to 1930 often used behavioral end points in their studies. Soon thereafter, psychologists began making important contributions in the study of hormones and behavior. In the early decades of the 20th century, American psychology was undergoing a major change, both in ideology and methodology. Led by John B. Watson, students of the "science of the mind" were casting aside introspection as a method in favor of observation and experimentation. Watson argued that only overt behavior was observable, and psychologists began describing and quantifying all types of overt behavior.

Karl S. Lashley did his graduate work under Watson at Johns Hopkins University and eventually joined the faculty at the University of Chicago. Lashley investigated the effects of

Frank A. Beach (1911–1988)

ized glands called **endocrine glands**. Hormones are released from these glands into the bloodstream (or the tissue fluid system in invertebrates), where they may then act on target organs (or tissues) at some distance from their origin. Hormones coordinate the physiology and behavior of an animal by regulating, integrating, and controlling its bodily function. For example, the same hormones that cause gametic (egg or sperm) maturation also stimulate mating behavior in many species. This dual hormonal function ensures that mating behavior occurs when animals have mature gametes available for fertilization. Another example of endocrine regulation of physiological and behavioral function is provided by the metabolic system. Several metabolic hormones work together to elevate blood glucose levels prior to awakening in anticipation of increased activity and energy demand. This "programmed" elevation of fuel availability coordinates the animal's physiology with its behavior. Hormones are similar in function to neurotransmitters, the chemicals used by the nervous system in coordinating animals' activities. However, hormones can operate over a greater distance and over a much greater temporal range than neurotransmitters (Box 1.3).

removing parts of rats' brains to discover where in the brain various psychological processes were carried out; he was particularly interested in finding where memories were stored. Although he never published any reports on the interaction between hormones and behavior, Lashley was clearly interested in the subject (e.g., Lashley, 1938), and several of Lashley's students became important contributors to behavioral endocrinology, including Calvin P. Stone, Josephine Ball, and Frank A. Beach.

Beach, William C. Young (see Box 3.2), and Daniel Lehrman (see Box 7.2) were especially influential during the early studies of behavioral endocrinology. Beach's dissertation at Chicago, "The Neural Basis for Innate Behavior," examined the effects of cortical tissue destruction on the maternal behavior of first-time mother rats. In 1937, Beach began working as a curator in the Department of Experimental Biology at the American Museum of Natural History in New York, and began contributing to the museum's tradition of comparative behavioral experimentation. One study completed at the museum, which was a logical extension of Beach's dissertation work, is of special note: he began investigating the effects of cortical lesions on the mating behavior of male rats. Some brain-

damaged rats continued to mate, whereas others failed to do so. Beach was concerned that his lesions were interfering indirectly with the endocrine system, so he injected the nonmating brain-injured rats with testosterone, the primary hormone secreted from the testes. The treatment evoked mating behavior in some of the lesioned rats, and this modification of behavior by hormones prompted Beach to learn more about endocrinology.

Beach audited a course in endocrinology at New York University, but was distressed by the lack of information about the behavioral effects of hormones; the professor responded to Beach's complaint by allowing him to teach one session. While preparing for the lecture, Beach discovered that no comprehensive summary of hormone–behavior interactions existed, and he prepared such a review as a term paper for the endocrinology course. Several years later, Beach expanded his paper into an influential book, *Hormones and Behavior* (Beach, 1948). The publication of this book marked the beginning of the formal study of behavioral endocrinology. Beach is credited with the genesis of this scientific discipline, and he continued to provide intellectual leadership in shaping the field for the next 40 years.

Not all cells are influenced by each and every hormone. Rather, any given hormone can directly influence only cells that have specific **receptors** for that particular hormone. Cells that have these specific receptors are called **target cells** for the hormone. The interaction of a hormone with its receptor begins a series of cellular events that eventually lead to a genomic response wherein the hormone acts directly or indirectly to activate genes that regulate protein synthesis. The newly synthesized proteins may activate or deactivate other genes, causing yet another cascade of cellular events. Recently, some effects of hormones on behavior have been reported that are not caused by activation of the genetic machinery; these so-called nongenomic effects of hormones on behavior will be reviewed in later chapters. Importantly, sufficient numbers of appropriate hormone receptors must be available for a specific hormone to produce any effects. For example, if a capon had no receptors for testosterone, then implanting another testis (or giving testosterone hormone therapy) would not cause it to display testosterone-dependent traits. A common bias in behavioral endocrinology is the assumption that individual differences in the expression of a behavior reflect differences in hormone

## Box 1.3
# Neural Transmission versus Hormonal Communication

Although neural and hormonal communication both rely on chemical signals, several prominent differences exist. Communication in the nervous system is analogous to traveling on a train. You can use the train in your travel plans as long as tracks exist between your proposed origin and destination. Likewise, neural messages can travel only to destinations along existing nerve tracts. Hormonal communication, on the other hand, is like traveling in a car. You can drive to many more destinations than train travel allows because there are many more roads than railroad tracks. Likewise, hormonal messages can travel anywhere in the body via the circulatory system; any cell receiving blood is potentially able to receive a hormonal message.

Neural and hormonal communication differ in other ways as well. To illustrate them, consider the differences between digital and analog technologies. Neural messages are digital, all-or-none events that have rapid onset and offset: neural signals can take place in milliseconds. Accordingly, the nervous system mediates changes in the body that are relatively

**Neural transmission**

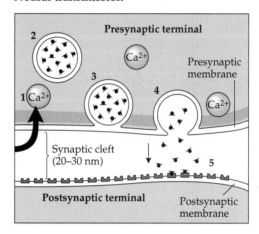

rapid. For example, the nervous system regulates immediate food intake and directs body movement. In contrast, hormonal messages are analog, graded events that may take seconds, minutes, or even hours to occur. Hormones can mediate long-term processes, such as growth, development, reproduction, and metabolism.

Hormonal and neural messages are both chemical in nature, and they are released and

concentrations in the blood. In other words, it is assumed that roosters that crow frequently have higher blood testosterone concentrations than roosters that rarely crow. To a certain extent this assumption is true. However, individual differences in hormone–behavior interactions usually reflect complex influences of hormone concentrations, patterns of hormone release, numbers and locations of hormone receptors, and the efficiency of those receptors in triggering signal transduction pathways that ultimately affect gene transcription.

Although hormones can influence target cells in many ways, they rarely change the *function* of a cell; rather, hormones commonly alter the *rate* of normal cellular function. Another way that hormones can affect cells is to change their morphology or size. For example, some athletes abuse anabolic steroids, which are synthetic hormones, because muscle cells grow larger after exposure to these substances. Hormones also may affect neuronal growth and development, as well as cell death (i.e., apoptosis) throughout the nervous system. While the examples we have discussed so far have all demonstrated how the presence or absence of a hormone may affect behavior, it is important to realize that the interactive relareceived by cells in a similar manner; however, there are important differences as well. As shown in the figure (opposite), in response to

**Hormonal communication**

the arrival of a neural impulse at a presynaptic terminal, there is an influx of calcium ions ($Ca^{2+}$) (1) that causes vesicles containing neural chemical messages called neurotransmitters to move toward the presynaptic membrane (2). The vesicles fuse with the membrane (3) and release the neurotransmitter into the synaptic cleft (4). The neurotransmitters travel a distance of only 20–30 nanometers ($30 \times 10^{-9}$ m) to the membrane of the postsynaptic neuron,

where they bind with receptors (5). As shown in the figure to the left, hormones manufactured in the Golgi apparatus of an endocrine cell (1) also move toward the cell membrane in vesicles (2) that fuse with the membrane, releasing the hormone (3). However, hormones then enter the circulatory system and may travel from 1 millimeter to 2 meters (4) before arriving at a cell of a target tissue, where they bind with specific receptors (5).

Another distinction between neural and hormonal communication is the degree of voluntary control that can be exerted over their functioning. In general, there is more voluntary control of neural than of hormonal signals. It is virtually impossible to will a change in your thyroid hormone levels, for example, whereas moving your limbs on command is easy.

While these are significant differences, the division between the nervous system and the endocrine system is becoming more blurred as we learn more about how the nervous system regulates hormonal communication. A better understanding of the interface between the endocrine system and the nervous system is likely to yield important advances in the future study of the interaction between hormones and behavior.

tionship between hormones and behavior is bidirectional: hormones obviously affect behavior, but, as we will see in later chapters, behavior can also influence hormone levels and effects.

## The Study of Behavior

Behavioral endocrinologists are interested in how the general physiological effects of hormones may eventually alter behavior, and how behavior may influence the effects of hormones. This book will describe, both phenomenologically and functionally, how hormones affect behavior. What is behavior? Generally, we think of behavior as "output," and because muscles are the most common output organs, or effectors, we tend to consider behavior to be coordinated movement. However, the flashing lights of fireflies, the production of electric shocks by eels, and the excretion of scents and chemicals by various species are also types of behavior. Sometimes the *lack* of movement is an important behavior, especially when used in stalking prey or avoiding predators.

## Problems of Behavioral Research

The goals of behavioral scientists are to determine what behaviors are relevant to the question being asked, to describe those behaviors, and to interpret their function. These goals are not as simple to achieve as they may sound, and there are several pitfalls that behavioral investigators must avoid. We will examine several of these problems in the context of a simple example: how might we begin to explain the singing of a robin (*Turdus migratorius*) that visits our backyard bird feeder each morning?

As soon as any observer begins to look at behavior, some degree of abstraction and bias is inevitable. When hens or roosters vocalize, we say that they "cluck" or "crow." However, the vocalizations of many birds are so melodious that we actually call them "singing." We may thus explain the bird's singing as a result of its being happy because we often sing when we are happy. This is obviously an anthropomorphic bias on our part. Behavioral scientists must take care not to attribute motives (hunger, fear, happiness) to animals based only on introspection, and must make an effort to observe behavior as objectively as possible.

Second, we must determine what other behaviors may be relevant to elucidating the behavior being examined. Even if an animal's behavior is videotaped continuously or observed directly for 24 hours a day, decisions must be made by the observer regarding which behaviors are meaningful and which are trivial in terms of answering the question at hand. In the case of the robin, for example, we must determine whether its presence at the bird feeder bears any relation to its singing.

Finally, to understand the causes (hormonal or otherwise) of any behavior, we must thoroughly describe the behavior (Tinbergen, 1951). When does the robin sing? What elicits its singing? Do all robins, or only some, engage in singing? As we saw in our discussion of Berthold's experiment, we must have a reasonably complete description of normal behavior before we can accurately assess the effects of any experimental manipulations on behavior.

## How Is Behavior Described?

We may classify descriptions of behavior within two categories: (1) descriptions of action and (2) descriptions of consequence (Dewsbury, 1979). In the former, the pattern of an animal's behavioral output is described with little or no reference to the effects of the behavior on the environment. Thus, descriptions of a lion's bared teeth, a firefly's flash of light, or a songbird's singing are descriptions of action. When classifying behavior by consequence, an observer notes the effect of the behavior on the environment; the observer may describe an animal's behavior as "gathering up nest material," "depressing a lever," or "inducing a female to visit." In practice, the two types of descriptive classifications can be combined to provide a rich description of animal behavior.

## The Simple System Approach

Even though we may ultimately be curious about the influence of hormones on human behavior, the unique and complex interactions of genes and environment make behavioral endocrinology studies of humans very difficult to interpret. For example, suppose that we observe that people in the upper twenty-fifth percentile of body mass tend to be more socially aggressive than individuals in the lower twenty-fifth percentile of body mass. The cause of the difference in behavior may reflect differences in body size, which may result from differences in concentrations of hormones that regulate growth and development. Alternatively, the differences in body mass may reflect differences in nutrition that affect brain development and thus the development of confidence in social situations. There is also the "chicken and egg" problem to resolve; that is, do hormones affect behavior directly by affecting the brain, indirectly by affecting body size, which in turn affects behavior, or does acting aggressive affect behavior, which in turn, affects body development? Furthermore, humans are reared in a wide variety of environments, which complicates the assignment of causation to individual variation in behavior. In order to untangle the contributions of various factors to hormone–behavior interactions, behavioral endocrinologists generally perform experiments on genetically identical animals in controlled environments. The development of behaviors and changes in hormone concentrations can be monitored throughout life under these conditions. Similar controlled experiments are virtually impossible to conduct on humans. Even though nonhuman animals represent "simple systems" relative to humans, it is important to appreciate that the behavioral repertoires of animals are extraordinarily varied.

Most research in behavioral endocrinology involves only a few types of simple behavior. This narrow focus on only a few behavioral measures is partially a response to the enormous variation inherent in observations of complex behaviors. There are advantages and disadvantages to this approach. The advantages of using simple behavioral indices include ease of replication and quantification. In this way, the simple system approach parallels the reductionist approach prevalent in physiological and biochemical analyses. On the other hand, the most apparent disadvantage to studying simple behaviors is the possibility that subtle but important interactions between hormones and behavior will be neglected and overlooked. Social and other environmental factors are often absent, or significantly reduced, in the laboratory, but may also be important in attaining a complete understanding of hormone–behavior interactions. There are certainly cases in which investigators have endeavored to observe the hormonal correlates of complex behavior. But commonly, the behavioral end point studied is as simple as the presence or absence of bird song, or the occurrence of mounting behavior among male rodents.

### Levels of Analysis

Once behaviors have been adequately described, we may proceed to ask about the causes of behavior (Alcock, 1997; Dewsbury, 1979; Tinbergen, 1951). For example, the zebra finch (*Taeniopygia guttata;* Figure 1.4), a native Australian songbird, is one of the most common species used to study bird song. The various notes zebra finches produce, the circumstances in which they sing, and even the specific muscles they use during singing have been extensively studied and described. Based on these descriptions, many researchers have begun to explore the causes of singing in male zebra finches (as in most songbird species, females and immature zebra finches do not sing in nature) by developing hypotheses and testing them by means of observation and experimentation.

The generic question an animal behaviorist asks at this point in the research may be simply expressed as "What causes animal *A* to emit behavior *X*?" (Sherman, 1988), so many researchers have asked, in effect, "What causes zebra finches to sing?" Surprisingly, there may be four types of correct answers to this basic question, based on four different **levels of analysis**: immediate causation, development, evolution, and adaptive function (Tinbergen, 1951).

**IMMEDIATE CAUSATION.** The level of immediate causation encompasses the underlying physiological, or proximate, mechanisms responsible for a given behavior. Typically these mechanisms are mediated by the nervous and endocrine systems, which influence behavior on a moment-to-moment basis during the life of an individual. Various internal and environmental stimuli as well as sensory and perceptual processes are involved in the short-term regulation of behavior. Accordingly, experiments designed to address questions of immediate causation often use physiological methods such as alterations of hormone concentrations or direct manipulations of the brain. In the case of zebra finches, these kinds of experiments have revealed that elevated blood concentrations of testosterone and increased rates of neural activity in certain areas of the brain are immediate causes of singing, so a correct answer to the question posed above might be that zebra finches sing because the level of testosterone in their blood is high. This class of

**1.4  Zebra finches.** These small birds have been used extensively in the study of the hormonal and neural bases of bird song. As with most songbird species, only the male zebra finch (right) sings in nature. Courtesy of Ellen Grass, Grass Instruments.

explanation is the one most frequently used by behavioral endocrinologists, and will be the primary focus of this book.

**DEVELOPMENT.**    The behavioral responses and repertoires of animals change throughout their lives as a result of the interaction between genes and environmental factors. Questions of development concern the full range of the organism's lifetime from conception to death. For example, the behavior of neonates is quite rudimentary in many species, but becomes more complex as they grow and interact with the environment. Hormonal events affecting the fetal and newly born animal can have pervasive influences later in life. While the majority of research at the developmental level of analysis has focused on how events early in ontogeny influence animals later in life, the decay of behavioral patterns during aging is also of interest to behavioral biologists pursuing developmental questions. Possible answers to our question from the developmental perspective might be that zebra finches sing because they have undergone puberty or because they learned their songs from their fathers.

**EVOLUTION.**    Evolutionary approaches involve many generations of animals and address the ways that specific behaviors change during the course of natural selection. Behavioral biologists study the evolutionary bases of behavior in order to learn why behavior varies between closely related species as well as to understand the specific behavioral changes that occur during the evolution of new species. Behaviors rarely leave interpretable traces in the fossil record, so the study of the evolution of behavior relies upon comparing existing species that vary in relatedness. An investigator working at the evolutionary level might say that zebra finches sing because they are finches, and that all finches sing because they have evolved from a common ancestral species that sang.

**ADAPTIVE FUNCTION.**    Questions of adaptive function are synonymous with questions of adaptive significance; they are concerned with the role that behavior plays in the adaptation of animals to their environment and with the selective forces that currently maintain behavior. At this level of analysis, it might be argued that male zebra finches sing because this behavior increases the likelihood that they will reproduce by attracting females to their territories and/or dissuading competing males from entering their territories.

Thus, there are four different possible types of causal explanations for a particular behavior, and there may be many correct answers to the question, "What causes male zebra finches to sing?" No one type of explanation is better or more complete than another, and, in practice, the levels of questions and explanations overlap and interact in many situations. Nevertheless, it is important that researchers specify clearly the level of analysis within which they are working when hypotheses are being generated for testing. Care must be taken to avoid comparing noncompeting hypotheses at the different levels of analysis (Sherman, 1988). For the sake of simplicity, these four levels of analysis can be grouped into sets of two, with questions of immediate causation and development grouped as "how questions" ("*How* does an animal engage in a behavior?"), and questions of evolution and function as "why questions" ("*Why* does an animal engage in a particular behavior?") (Alcock, 1997).* To construct an exhaustive explanation of the

---

*"How questions" have also been referred to as questions of *proximate causation,* and "why questions" as questions of *ultimate causation* (Wilson, 1975).

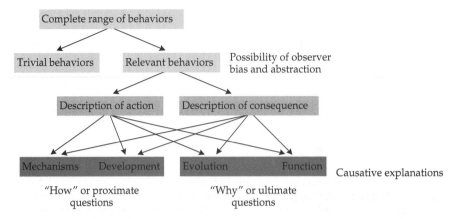

**1.5    Stages of behavioral research.** From the complete range of an organism's behavior, the behavioral scientist must first determine which behaviors are relevant to the question under consideration, a process that is inherently prone to undue abstraction or bias. Descriptions of relevant behaviors may focus on the actions themselves ("description of action") or on their environmental effects ("description of consequence"). Examination of the causes of behaviors may proceed at any of four levels of analysis that address either proximate ("how") or ultimate ("why") questions.

causes of bird song, then, we would want to study both *how* birds sing and *why* they sing (Figure 1.5). What developmental and physiological processes occur before and during singing? What is the evolutionary history of bird song? When, phylogenetically (during evolutionary history), did singing appear among birds? What adaptive advantages do singers enjoy relative to nonsingers?

Workers in different disciplines tend to favor particular types of questions and classes of explanations. For example, physiologists work almost exclusively at the level of immediate causation, whereas behavioral ecologists specialize in evolutionary and functional explanations of behavior. The types of explanations that individual scientists pursue in conducting their research reflect their tastes and their training, but their combined efforts allow us to gain the most comprehensive understanding of animal behavior.

## How Might Hormones Affect Behavior?

In terms of their behavior, one can think of animals as being made up of three interacting components: (1) input systems (sensory systems), (2) integrators (the central nervous system), and (3) output systems, or effectors (e.g., muscles) (Figure 1.6). Again, hormones do not *cause* behavioral changes. Rather, hormones influence these three systems so that specific stimuli are more likely to elicit certain responses in the appropriate behavioral or social context. In other words, hormones change the probability that a particular behavior will be emitted in the appropriate situation. This is a critical distinction that can affect how we think of hormone–behavior relationships. We can apply this three-component behavioral scheme by returning to our example of singing behavior in zebra finches.

As noted above, only the male zebra finch sings in nature. If the testes of adult male finches are removed, the birds stop singing, but castrated finches

**1.6   How hormones may affect behavior.** Behaving animals may be thought of as made up of three interacting components: input systems (sensory systems), central processing systems (the central nervous system), and output systems (effectors, such as muscles). Hormones may affect any or all of these three components when influencing behavior. Note that there is a bidirectional causal relationship between hormones and behavior in that an animal's behavior (or the behavior of conspecifics or predators) may affect its endocrine state.

resume singing if the testes are reimplanted, or if they are provided with the primary testicular hormone, testosterone. Singing behavior is most frequent when blood levels of testosterone are high. While it is clear from these observations that testosterone is somehow involved in singing, how might the three-component framework just introduced help us to formulate hypotheses to explore testosterone's role in this behavior? By examining input systems, we could determine whether testosterone alters the birds' sensory capabilities, making the environmental cues that normally elicit singing more salient. If this were the case, females or territorial intruders might be more easily seen or heard. Testosterone also could influence the central nervous system. Neuronal architecture or the speed of neural processing could change in the presence of testosterone. Higher neural processes (e.g., motivation, attention, or perception) also might be influenced. Finally, the effector organs, muscles in this case, could be affected by the presence of testosterone. Blood testosterone concentrations might somehow affect the muscles of a songbird's syrinx (the avian vocal organ). Testosterone, therefore, could affect bird song by influencing the sensory capabilities, central processing system, or effector organs of an individual bird. We do not understand completely how testosterone influences bird song, but in most cases, hormones can be considered to affect behavior by influencing one, two, or all three of these components, and our three-part framework can aid in the design of hypotheses and experiments to explore these issues. This conceptual scheme of how hormones and behavior interact will provide the major organization for this book.

## How Might Behavior Affect Hormones?

The bird song example demonstrates how hormones can affect behavior, but, as noted previously, the reciprocal relation also occurs; that is, behavior can affect hormone levels. For example, the sight of a territorial intruder may elevate blood testosterone levels in the resident male and thereby stimulate singing or fighting behavior (Wingfield, 1988). Similarly, male mice (Ginsberg and Allee, 1942) or rhesus monkeys (Rose et al., 1971) that lose a fight show reduced levels of testosterone for several days or even weeks afterward. Similar results have also been reported in humans. Testosterone concentrations are affected not only in humans involved in physical combat, but also in those involved in simulated battles. For example, testosterone concentrations were elevated in winners and reduced in losers of regional chess tournaments (Mazur et al., 1992).

People do not have to be involved in a contest directly to have their hormones affected by the outcome of the contest. For instance, male fans of both the Brazilian and Italian teams were recruited to provide samples to be assayed for testosterone before and after the final game of the World Cup soccer match in 1994. Brazil and Italy were tied going into the final game, but Brazil won on a penalty kick at the last possible moment. The Brazilian fans were elated and the Italian fans were crestfallen. When the samples were assayed, 11 of 12 Brazilian fans who were sampled had increased testosterone concentrations, and 9 of 9 Italian fans had decreased testosterone concentrations, compared with pre-game baseline values (J. M. Dabbs, personal communication, 1999).

Even anticipation of behavior may influence hormone levels. An anonymous contribution to the journal *Nature* (1970) provided an account by a gentleman whose work caused him to live in isolation for days at a time. Occasionally, he returned to his home and his fiancée. This man possessed a strong curiosity, and his isolated lifestyle presumably eliminated many of the usual distractions of modern life. In this peaceful milieu, he noted while shaving that his beard seemed thicker immediately prior to his visits to his fiancée. He began weighing the shavings, and noted that his beard thickened on days when he had sex with his fiancée. The rate of beard growth is correlated with blood concentrations of testosterone; high levels of testosterone increase the rate of beard growth, whereas low levels of testosterone are associated with slow beard growth. Our anonymous colleague suggested that his sexual behavior, as well as his *anticipation* of sexual behavior, caused an elevation in testosterone, which in turn increased beard growth.

You probably recognize that this is not a very robust demonstration of a hormone–behavior interaction because (1) only one experimental subject was used, (2) the experimental subject was aware of the experimental conditions, which, consciously or unconsciously, may have caused him to misread the scale on critical days, and (3) other conditions, such as the drying effects of the air during his travels home, could have accounted for some of the changes in beard growth. In other words, this letter described anecdotal evidence of a hormone–behavior interaction—evidence that is not compelling. More recently, testosterone concentrations were measured in four heterosexual couples over a total of 22 evenings (Dabbs and Mohammed, 1992). There were two different types of evenings. On 11 evenings, the samples were obtained before and after sexual intercourse; on the remaining 11 evenings, two samples were obtained during the evening, but there was no sexual intercourse. To avoid the logistic complications of drawing blood samples, testosterone was measured in the saliva of the participants. Engaging in sexual intercourse caused testosterone concentrations to increase in both men and women. The early evening saliva samples revealed no difference in testosterone concentrations between evenings when sexual intercourse took place and evenings when it did not. These results suggest that sexual behavior increases testosterone concentrations more than high testosterone concentrations cause sexual activity in humans (Dabbs and Mohammed, 1992). While this is certainly a reasonable conclusion, there are alternative explanations for the results of this study. For example, perhaps physical exercise alone increases testosterone concentrations. To rule out this possibility, additional studies are required in which the level of exercise is similar between experimental groups, but differs in sexual content.

## Classes of Evidence for Determining Hormone–Behavior Interactions

What sort of evidence *would* be sufficient to establish that a particular hormone affected a specific behavior or that a specific behavior changed hormone concentrations? Experiments to test hypotheses about the effects of hormones on behavior must be carefully designed, and, generally, three conditions must be satisfied by the experimental results to establish a causal link between hormones and behavior (Silver, 1978):

1. A hormonally dependent behavior should disappear when the source of the hormone is removed or the actions of the hormone are blocked.

2. After the behavior stops, restoration of the missing source or its hormone should reinstate the absent behavior.

3. Finally, hormone concentrations and the behavior in question should be covariant; that is, the behavior should be observed only when hormone concentrations are relatively high and never or rarely observed when hormone concentrations are low.

The third class of evidence has proved difficult to obtain because hormones may have a long latency of action, and because many hormones are released in a pulsatile manner. For example, if a pulse of hormone is released into the blood, and then no more is released for an hour or so, a single blood sample will not provide an accurate picture of the endocrine status of the animal under study. We might come to completely different conclusions about the effect of a hormone on behavior if we measure hormone concentrations when they are at their peak rather than when they are at their nadir. This problem can be overcome by obtaining measures in several animals and averaging across peaks and valleys, or by taking several sequential blood samples from the same animal. Another problem is that biologically effective amounts of hormones are tiny and difficult to measure accurately. Effective concentrations of hormones are usually measured in micrograms ($\mu$g, $10^{-6}$ g), nanograms (ng, $10^{-9}$ g), or picograms (pg, $10^{-12}$ g); they are sometimes expressed as a mass percentage relative to 100 ml of blood plasma or serum (10 $\mu$g% = 10 $\mu$g/100 ml = 0.1 $\mu$g/ml). The development of new techniques, such as the radioimmunoassay (see below), has increased the precision with which hormone concentrations can be measured, but because of the several difficulties associated with obtaining reliable covariant hormone–behavior measures, obtaining the first two classes of evidence usually has been considered sufficient to establish a causal link in hormone–behavior relations.

As we will see, the unique conditions of the laboratory environment may themselves cause changes in an animal's hormone concentrations and behavior that may confound the results of experiments; thus, it has become apparent that hormone–behavior relationships established in the laboratory should be verified in natural environments. The verification of hormone–behavior relationships in natural environments is not yet common, but it is a useful procedure for differentiating laboratory artifacts from true phenomena.

## Common Techniques in Behavioral Endocrinology

How do we gather the evidence needed to establish hormone–behavior relationships? Because we cannot directly observe the interactions between hormones and their receptors or their intracellular consequences, we must use various indirect tools to explore these phenomena. This section describes some of the primary methods and techniques used in behavioral endocrinology. Much of the recent progress in behavioral endocrinology has resulted from technical advances in the tools that allow us to detect, measure, and probe the functions of hormones. Therefore, familiarity with these techniques will help you to understand and assess the research to be discussed in subsequent chapters.

### Ablation and Replacement

The ablation (removal or extirpation) of the suspected source of a hormone to determine its function is a classic technique in endocrinology. Recall that this was the method Berthold used to establish the role of the testes in the development of rooster behavior. There are four steps to this time-honored procedure: (1) a gland that is suspected to be the source of a hormone affecting a behavior is surgically removed; (2) the effects of removal are observed; (3) the hormone is replaced, by reimplanting the removed gland, by injecting a homogenate or extract from the gland, or by injecting a purified hormone; and (4) a determination is made whether the observed consequences of ablation have been reversed by the replacement therapy. This technique is commonly used in endocrine research today. A complementary approach to the ablation–replacement technique is the observation of behavior in individuals with diseased or congenitally dysfunctional endocrine organs. When ablation occurs in the brain, it is often called a lesion.

The replacement component of this technique has been improved by technological advances, especially new recombinant DNA methods, that have made highly purified hormones readily available. Access to this virtually pure material has allowed researchers to rule out "contaminants" as a cause of the physiological or behavioral effects of a particular hormone. Also, recent studies have emphasized the importance of replacing hormones in patterns and doses similar to those found in nature rather than using a single pharmacological dose. This has been made possible by the availability of implantable timed-release hormone capsules and minipumps that provide precisely timed infusions of purified hormones.

### Bioassays

Once the existence of a hormone has been established, the next step is to identify the chemical processes involved in its actions. Classically, this has required a bioassay: a test of the effects of the hormone on a living animal. A living animal can serve as a reliable, quantifiable response system on which to test extracts and chemical fractions for biological activity.

A bioassay need not be conducted on the same species from which the hormone was obtained. For example, the crop sac of a pigeon (a structure that produces the "crop milk" fed to young pigeons; see Figure 7.5) can be used to measure levels of a hormone called prolactin in a rat. In incubating pigeons, prolactin stimulates growth of the epithelial cells of the crop sac to prepare it for the feeding of hatchlings; the height of the cells is correlated with the amount of prolactin in the pigeon's blood. To carry out a bioassay, researchers can inject different, known amounts of purified prolactin into pigeons, measure the resulting heights of the crop sac epithelial cells, and generate a dose–response curve (Figure 1.7). To measure the unknown prolactin levels of a rat, a tissue sample obtained

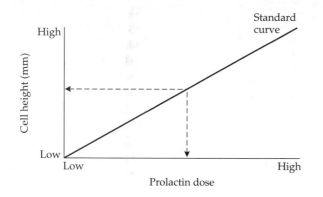

**1.7   A bioassay for prolactin.**
(Top) Photomicrograph of untreated pigeon crop sac. (Middle) Prolactin injection causes a marked increase in the height of crop sac epithelial cells; different known amounts of purified prolactin can be injected into pigeons to generate a dose–response curve (bottom). The levels of prolactin in pituitary extracts from some other animal (e.g., a rat) can then be measured by injecting a pigeon with an extract sample from the animal and comparing any resulting change in epithelial cell height with the dose–response curve (dashed line). Photomicrographs courtesy of C. S. Nicoll.

from the rat can be injected into a pigeon, and the resulting height of the epithelial cells measured and compared with the dose–response curve.

Probably the most famous endocrine bioassay was the "rabbit test" (or Friedman test) for pregnancy. The rabbit test was developed by Maurice Friedman in 1929 and was the most commonly used pregnancy test in North America until the late 1950s. This procedure tested for the presence of human chorionic gonadotropin (hCG; a hormone released from the implantation site of a blastocyst that prevents menstruation) in the urine of women. The urine was injected into a rabbit, and if hCG was present in the urine, the rabbit's ovaries would form corpora lutea (ovarian endocrine structures formed following ovulation; see Chapter 2) within 48 hours. The rabbit test had several advantages over the previously used Aschheim–Zondek mouse test (developed in 1928), which required six or more mice and at least 96 hours to complete. However, the rabbit test also had disadvantages. False positives could be obtained if the rabbit used was unduly stressed by the test procedure because stress can cause spontaneous corpora luteal formation in the *absence* of hCG.

Because biological systems are inherently subject to fluctuations induced by environmental conditions, it is essential that the conditions under which bioassays are conducted be rigidly defined. For example, in the Galli–Mainini or "frog test" for pregnancy, urine from a woman was injected into a male frog or toad. If the woman was pregnant and producing hCG, the animal would begin to produce sperm. The test provided results in 2–4 hours, and frogs were cheaper to maintain than mammals. However, there were variations in the sensitivity of the frogs: they had a greater tendency to yield "false negatives" during the summer.

Because the levels of hormones circulating in the bloodstream are generally very small, it is quite possible for contaminants to interfere with the results of a bioassay. Also, a bioassay is obviously only as good as the purified "standard" hormone used to calibrate the dose–response curve. For example, if the "purified" prolactin injected into a pigeon in the crop sac bioassay was contaminated by some other agent that suppressed cell growth, the resulting dose–response curve would not be accurate. Indeed, many early reports of endocrine effects on behavior and physiology were inaccurate because of contamination by hormones other than the so-called "pure" hormones. In recent years, with the advent of molecular biological tools to detect and measure biological products, the bioassay technique has been used less frequently.

**BEHAVIORAL BIOASSAYS.**    Several behavioral bioassays for hormones have been developed and used. The "water drive" of newts after injection of prolactin is one example. Prolactin causes newts to seek water; high levels of prolactin in a test sample cause a faster trip to water than low prolactin levels. A more common behavioral bioassay measured the behavioral effects of estrogens on the mating posture of female guinea pigs, and was used for many years as the most sensitive assay for measuring circulating levels of these hormones. Again, bioassays require rigorous standardization of test conditions for accuracy and reliability. Even minute amounts of estrogen-like plant compounds (phytoestrogens) in their food are sufficient to induce female guinea pigs to display a mating posture. Consequently, laboratory personnel who used guinea pigs for estrogen behavioral bioassays had to make certain that the animals' chow did not contain alfalfa or other phytoestrogen-rich ingredient(s).

### *Immunoassays*

Bioassays were useful because they measured a *biological* response to the hormone in question. In some cases, they allowed the determination of the presence or absence of a substance (as in the rabbit test), and in others they allowed quantitative measurement of specific hormones (as in the pigeon crop sac test for prolactin). However, bioassays usually required a great deal of time, labor, and the sacrifice of many animals for every assay conducted. The development of the **radioimmunoassay (RIA)** technique reduced these problems and increased the precision with which hormone concentrations could be measured.

The concept of RIA is based on the principle of competitive binding of an antibody to its antigen. An antibody produced in response to any antigen, in this case a hormone, has a binding site that is specific for that antigen. A given amount of antibody possesses a given number of binding sites for its antigen. Antigen molecules can be :labeled" with radioactivity, and an antibody cannot discriminate between an antigen that has been radiolabeled (or "hot") and a normal, non-radioactive ("cold") antigen.

The first step in a radioimmunoassay is to inject the hormone of interest into an animal to raise antibody; the antibody is then collected from the animal's blood and purified. To develop a standard curve, several reaction tubes are set up, each containing the same measured amount of antibody, the same measured amount of radiolabeled hormone, and different amounts of cold purified hormone of known concentration. The radiolabeled hormone and cold hormone compete for binding sites on the antibody, so the more cold hormone that is present in the tube, the less hot hormone will bind to the antibody. The quantity of hot hormone that was bound can be determined by precipitating the antibody and measuring its radioactivity. The concentration of hormone in a sample can then be determined by subjecting it to the same procedure and comparing the results with the standard curve (Figure 1.8).

As is the case with other techniques, there are limitations to this method. First of all, RIAs require a source of highly purified hormone in order to prepare an antibody against it. Thus, as with bioassays, the accuracy of RIAs is limited by the purity of the hormones used to calibrate the standard curve. Also, RIAs must be tested for specificity because of the possibility that the antibody recognizes other antigens in addition to the one of interest. For these reasons, when the results of an RIA do not agree with those of a bioassay, the bioassay may be considered more valid even if it is less precise.

The **enzymoimmunoassay (EIA)**, like the RIA, works on the principle of competitive binding of an antibody to its antigen. The major difference between the RIA and EIA techniques is that EIAs do not require radioactive tags. Instead, the antibody is tagged with a compound that changes optical density (color) in response to binding with antigen. The home pregnancy test is a familiar example of an EIA. These tests, like the rabbit test, are designed to give a yes-or-no answer. However, most EIAs are developed to provide quantitative information. A standard curve is generated, as for RIAs, so that different known amounts of the hormone in question provide a gradient of color that can be read on a spectrometer. The unknown sample is then added, and the amount of hormone is interpolated by the standard curves. A similar technique is called enzyme-linked immunosorbent assay (ELISA).

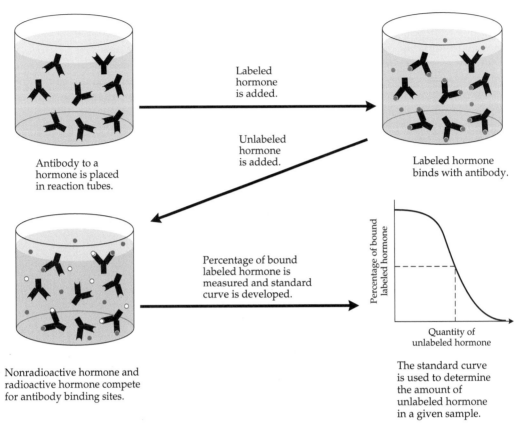

Antibody to a
hormone is placed
in reaction tubes.

Labeled
hormone
is added.

Unlabeled
hormone
is added.

Labeled hormone
binds with antibody.

Percentage of bound
labeled hormone is
measured and standard
curve is developed.

Nonradioactive hormone and
radioactive hormone compete
for antibody binding sites.

The standard curve
is used to determine
the amount of
unlabeled hormone
in a given sample.

**1.8  Radioimmunoassay.** Purified hormone injected into an animal acts as an antigen, and antibody is collected and purified. The hormone is radioactively labeled, and measured amounts of the labeled hormone are added to measured amounts of the collected antibody in several reaction tubes. The antibody binds with the radiolabeled hormone to form reversible hormone–antibody complexes. When different amounts of unlabeled hormone are added to the reaction tubes, this "cold" hormone competes for antibody binding sites and displaces "hot" hormone; increasing amounts of cold hormone will cause the radioactivity of the sample as a whole to decline. By measuring the radioactivity of each reaction tube, a standard curve can be developed that expresses the quantity of cold hormone as a decline in radioactivity. The hormone present in a blood sample can then be measured by using it as cold hormone in the same procedure and comparing its effect on measured radioactivity with the standard curve (dashed lines).

### *Immunocytochemistry*

Immunocytochemistry (ICC) techniques use antibodies to determine the location of a hormone in the body. Antibodies linked to marker molecules, such as those of a fluorescent dye (see Polak and Van Noorden, 1997), are usually introduced into dissected tissue from an animal, where they bind with the hormone or neurotransmitter of interest. For example, if a thin slice of brain tissue is immersed in a solution of antibodies to a protein hormone linked to a fluorescent dye, and the tissue is then examined under a fluorescent microscope, concentrated spots of fluorescence will appear, indicating where the protein hormone is located (Figure

**1.9   Immunocytochemistry.** Antibodies to a hormone can be linked to a dye and used to determine the location of a hormone in the body. If a slice of tissue is exposed to a solution of antibody linked to such a marker, the binding of the antibody will cause those parts of the tissue containing the hormone to selectively take up the dye, making them more visible under the microscope. A photomicrograph (×100) of a thin section of a rodent's brain, showing a tangle of neuronal dendrites; immunocytochemically marked cell bodies that contain gonadotropin-releasing hormone (GnRH) are prominent. Courtesy of Lance Kriegsfeld.

1.9). Fluorescent dyes used for ICC include fluorescein and rhodamine. Other commonly used markers are the enzyme horseradish peroxidase, for bright-field or electron microscopy; the enzyme alkaline phosphatase, for biochemical detection; and the iron-containing protein ferritin, for electron microscopy.

A common alternative ICC technique involves raising a second antibody against the primary antibody that recognizes the substance to be measured, then coupling the second antibody to a marker. Sometimes a primary antibody is linked to biotin, a water-soluble vitamin, which has a strong binding affinity to streptavidin, a bacterial protein. If streptavidin is coupled to a marker molecule, it can be used in place of a second antibody. A single biotin–antibody–antigen complex may link to multiple marker molecules, which essentially amplifies the signal indicating the presence of the antigen.

### Autoradiography

Many studies have demonstrated that hormone receptors are selectively concentrated in particular target tissues; estrogen receptors, for example, are concentrated in the uterus. Autoradiography is typically used to determine hormonal uptake and indicate receptor location. An animal can be injected with a radiolabeled hormone, or the study can be conducted entirely in vitro. Suspected target tissues are sliced into several very thin sections; adjacent sections are then subjected to different treatments. One section of the suspected target tissue is stained in the usual way to highlight various cellular structures. The next section is placed in contact with photographic film or emulsion for some period of time, and the emission of radiation from the radiolabeled hormone develops an image on the film. The areas of high radioactivity on the film can then be compared with the stained section to determine how the areas of highest hormone concentration cor-

**1.10 Autoradiography.** An animal is injected with a radiolabeled hormone and adjacent tissue slices are either treated with stains to reveal cellular structures or exposed to film. Those parts of the tissue that bind with the radiolabeled hormone darken the film, and when combined with the stained section, show which cell structures have taken up the hormone in the largest amounts. In this autoradiograph, cell nuclei in a monkey brain that have accumulated radiolabeled estrogen are seen as darker than the background neurons. Courtesy of Bruce McEwen.

relate with cellular structures (Figure 1.10). This technique has been very useful in determining the sites of hormone action in nervous tissue, and consequently has increased our understanding of hormone–behavior interactions.

### Blot Tests

Other techniques allow the determination of whether or not a particular protein or nucleic acid is present in a specific tissue. In the so-called blot tests, the tissue of interest is homogenized and lysed with detergent. The resulting homogenate is placed on a nitrocellulose filter. The filter is then incubated with a labeled substance that can act as a tracer for the protein or nucleic acid of interest: radiolabeled complementary deoxyribonucleic acid (cDNA) for a nucleic acid assay, or an antibody that has been radiolabeled or linked to an enzyme for a protein assay. If radiolabeling is used, the filter is then put over film to locate and measure radioactivity. In enzyme-linked protein assays, the filter is incubated with chromogenic chemicals, and standard curves reflecting different spectral densities are generated. The test used to assay DNA is called Southern blotting, after its inventor, E. M. Southern; the test used to assay RNA is called Northern blotting, and the test for proteins is called Western blotting.

### Autoradiography Using In Situ Hybridization

An important tool used at the cellular level to examine gene expression is called in situ hybridization. This technique is used to identify cells or tissues in which mRNA molecules for a specific protein—for example, a hormone or neurotransmitter—are being produced. The tissue is fixed, sliced very thinly, and mounted on slides, and either dipped into emulsion or placed over film and developed with photographic chemicals. Typically, the tissue is also counterstained to iden-

**1.11    In situ audioradiography.** The dark spots at the bottom of this slice of a rodent brain represent cells in the ventromedial hypothalamus (VMH) that contain mRNA for an oxytocin receptor. This tissue was treated with a specific cDNA that hybridized with the RNA that encodes for the oxytocin receptor. Courtesy of Thomas Insel and Larry Young.

tify specific cellular structures. A radiolabeled cDNA probe (hollow tube) is introduced into the tissue. If the mRNA of interest is present in the tissue, the cDNA will form a tight association (that is, hybridize) with it. The tightly bound cDNA, and hence the messenger RNA (mRNA), will appear as dark spots (Figure 1.11). The techniques previously described, such as blotting, can typically determine only whether or not a particular substance is *present* in a specific tissue, but in situ hybridization can be used to determine whether a particular substance is *produced* in a specific tissue, and recent advances in the technique allow for the quantification of the substance being produced. Also, blotting techniques cannot match the resolution or sensitivity of in situ hybridization.

### Stimulation and Recording

By using electrical stimulation to "turn on" specific neurons or brain centers, we can discover the effects of various endocrine treatments on the central nervous system. In this technique, a fine electrode is precisely positioned in the brain, and a weak electrical current is used to stimulate nerve cells. This technique has been used to study the releasing and inhibiting hormones of the hypothalamus (see Chapter 2).

The electrical activity of single neurons can be monitored through the use of single-unit recording, which involves the placement of very small electrodes in or near one nerve cell to record changes in its activity during and immediately after exposure to hormones. This technique can help to uncover the direct effects of various endocrine products on neural activity. Often, several neurons are recorded simultaneously and an average change in activity in multiple units is calculated.

### Pharmacological Techniques

The identification of hormones and neurotransmitters, and the development for medical purposes of synthetic **agonists** (mimics) and **antagonists** (blockers) of these chemicals, has told us a great deal about the functioning of the endocrine and neuroendocrine systems. Some specific chemical agents can act to stimulate or inhibit endocrine function by affecting hormonal release; these agents are called general agonists and antagonists, respectively. Other drugs act directly on receptors, either enhancing or negating the effects of the hormone under study; these drugs are referred to as receptor agonists and antagonists, respectively. For example, cyproterone acetate (CPA) is a powerful anti-androgen that has been used clinically as a treatment for male sex offenders (see Chapter 5). This antagonist binds to androgen receptors but does not activate them, thereby blocking the effects of androgen on behavior and physiology. Other examples of hormone agonists and antagonists will be presented throughout the book.

In the technique known as **cannulation**, hollow electrodes or fine tubes (cannulas) are inserted into specific areas of the brain and used to introduce substances into those sites. Davidson (1966a) used this technique to find out where in the brain testosterone acts to influence sexual behavior in rats. In Davidson's study, male rats were castrated, after which they were observed to cease mating. Testosterone was then introduced through cannulas into different areas of the brain in different rats; a control group of rats received cholesterol, the precursor of testosterone. Those animals that received testosterone in one specific location, the preoptic area of the hypothalamus, resumed sexual behavior; the rats that received cholesterol or received testosterone in other brain regions did not respond to the treatment.

Another type of cannulation involves inserting a small hollow tube into the jugular vein, carotid artery, or other blood vessel. In this way, specific hormones or pharmacological agents can later be injected directly into the animal without further disturbance, or blood samples can be obtained to correlate hormone levels with behavior. In a related technique, **anastomosis**, the blood systems of two animals are connected via cannulation tubing to see if the endocrine condition of one animal can cause a behavioral change in the other.

### Genetic Manipulations

With new advances in molecular biology, it is possible to perform specific genetic manipulations. In behavioral endocrinology research, common genetic manipulations include the insertion (transgenic) or removal (knockout) of the genetic instructions encoding a hormone or the receptor for a hormone. The genetic instructions for each individual are contained in its DNA, located in the nucleus of nearly every cell. These instructions are encoded in the form of four nucleotides, adenine (A), thymine (T), cytosine (C), and guanine (G). The specific order of these four nucleotides along the "rails" of the twisted double helix DNA molecule forms the genetic instructions for all organisms, from those as simple as slime molds to those as complex as mice and humans. Each gene represents the complex instructions for the production of a specific protein in the cell. Thus, nucleotide "syntax" is critical in conveying the instructions encoded in the genes. To inactivate, or knock out, a gene, molecular biologists scramble the order of the nucleotides that make up the gene (Aguzzi et al., 1994; Soriano, 1995). Among vertebrates, the identification of genes has been most successful among laboratory mice (*Mus musculus*). Consequently, mice are currently the most commonly used species in targeted gene deletion studies.

Knocking out a specific gene in a mouse is an arduous task that relies on several low-probability events. First, the gene of interest must be identified, targeted, and marked precisely. This has been accomplished for an astounding number of murine (mouse) genes during the past several years (Takahashi et al., 1994). Next, a mutated form of the gene is created (i.e., a piece of DNA that contains a marker gene or a genetically engineered, altered copy of the original gene; again, the altered order of the nucleotides renders the gene inactive). Mouse embryonic stem cells are harvested and cultured, and the mutated gene is introduced into the cultured cells by microinjection (Tonegawa, 1994). A very small number of the altered genes will be incorporated into the DNA of the stem cells through recombination (Bernstein and Breitman, 1989; Sedivy and Sharp, 1989). The mutated embryonic stem cells are inserted into otherwise normal mouse embryos (blastocysts), which are then implanted into surrogate mothers (Boggs, 1990; Le Mouellic et al., 1990; Steeghs et al., 1995). All of the cells descended from the mutated stem cells will have the altered gene; the descendants of the original blastocyst cells will have normal genes. Thus, the newborn mice will have some cells that possess a copy of the mutant gene and some cells that possess only the normal (wild-type) gene. This type of animal is called a **chimera**. If the mutated stem cells are incorporated into the germ lines (the cells destined to become the sperm and ova), then some of the mouse's gametes will contain a heritable copy of the mutant gene. If the chimera mice are bred with wild-type mice, then some of the offspring will be heterozygous for the mutation; that is, they will possess one copy of the mutant gene. If the heterozygous mice are interbred, then approximately one-fourth of their offspring will be homozygous for the mutation. These homozygous mice can then be interbred to produce pure lines of mice with the gene in question knocked out (Galli-Taliadoros et al., 1995). The product that the gene typically encodes will be missing from their progeny (Sedivy and Sharp, 1989). Behavioral performance can then be compared among wild-type (+/+), heterozygous (+/−), and homozygous (−/−) mice, in which the gene product is produced normally, produced at reduced levels, or completely missing, respectively. The comparison of +/+ and −/− littermates of an $F_2$ recombinant generation is probably the minimal acceptable control in determining behavioral effects in knockout mice (Morris and Nosten-Bertrand, 1996). The use of new inducible knockouts, in which the timing and tissue-specific placement of the targeted gene disruption can be controlled, will be an extremely important tool in future behavioral endocrinology research (Nelson, 1997). Similarly, the use of transgenic animals, in which there is overexpression of specific genes, will become an increasingly common technique in behavioral endocrinology investigations.

### *A Case Study: Effects of Leptin on Behavior*

Recently, a novel hormone was discovered that is released from adipose (fat) cells. This hormone was named leptin, a term derived from the Greek word *leptos,* which means "thin." Studies of the behavioral effects of leptin will be used to demonstrate how the various techniques described above are used to understand the biological functions of hormones.

For many years, specific mutations in mice have been recognized that cause extreme obesity in animals that are homozygous for the defective gene, known as *ob*. These animals may be considered natural knockouts for the *ob* gene. Two mutant strains that have been commonly used in studies of body mass regulation are the so-called *ob/ob* mice and *db/db* (diabetic) mice. The *ob/ob* mice have a pair of defective *ob* genes, and are hyperphagic (overeat), obese, and reproductively sterile (Figure 1.12). The *ob* gene normally codes for the hormone leptin; leptin is released by adipose cells into the bloodstream, where it travels to specific protein

**1.12  Behavioral effects of leptin.** Both of these mice have defective *ob* genes. This mutation typically results in a large increase in food intake and subsequent obesity. The mouse on
the right was treated daily with the protein encoded by the *ob* gene, called leptin. It weighs
about 35 grams; the untreated mouse weighs about 67 grams. A mouse with a normal *ob* gene
would weigh about 25 grams at this age. Photograph by John Sholtis.

receptors in the central nervous system and elsewhere to regulate feeding and
energy balance. Since its identification in 1994 (Zhang et al., 1994), many of the
techniques described in the previous sections have been used to understand the
behavioral functions of leptin.

For years, the effects of the *ob/ob* mutation on the ability to maintain normal
body mass in mice have been known. However, research into the mechanisms
underlying this mutation began in earnest only with the identification and
sequencing of the ob protein (i.e., leptin) (Zhang et al., 1994). Thus, researchers
had available a so-called experiment of nature in which leptin was depleted
(knocked out), and could determine the behavioral effects that resulted from a
lack of leptin. The leptin gene was cloned, and a copy of the gene was inserted
into a bacterial system; purified leptin was thus made available to researchers.
Using this purified leptin, a "replacement study" was conducted in which leptin
was provided to *ob/ob* mice to determine whether replacing their missing leptin
would ameliorate their hyperphagia, energy impairments, and obesity. It did.

The availability of purified leptin also allowed researchers to produce specific antibodies to this substance that could be used in developing assays to determine blood concentrations of leptin (e.g., Cohen et al., 1996). An RIA was
developed to determine the blood plasma leptin concentrations of obese and
diabetic humans to see whether leptin was implicated in human obesity or diabetes (McGregor et al., 1996); in this study, no connection was found. A leptin
ELISA was developed for rats and mice, which was used to determine that fasting or exposure to low temperatures caused circulating leptin concentrations to
fall (Hardie et al., 1996). Immunocytochemical localization techniques revealed

that leptin was present in both white and brown adipose tissue (Cinti et al., 1997) as well as other peripheral tissues.

Injections of leptin into the third or lateral ventricles of mice were found to reduce food intake (Campfield et al., 1995). To determine the site of action of leptin in the brain, purified leptin was labeled with a radioactive tag and injected into mice. Using autoradiography, dense, specific binding of the tagged leptin was found in the choroid plexus, a brain structure located in the dorsal part of the third ventricle, as well as the lateral ventricles (Lynn et al., 1996). This tissue was then used to clone a leptin receptor (Tartaglia et al., 1995). In situ hybridization showed that the mRNA for the leptin receptor was expressed in several brain regions, including the hypothalamus (Mercer et al., 1996; Zamorano et al., 1997).

In an effort to "cure" obesity, gene replacement therapy was attempted in mice and rats (Chen et al., 1996; Muzzin et al., 1996). The logic behind this effort was that mice deficient in the *ob* gene were obese because of a deficiency of leptin. If the leptin or the *ob* gene were replaced, then the individual should display normal food intake and body mass. When *ob/ob* mice were treated with a recombinant adenovirus expressing the mouse leptin cDNA, there was a dramatic reduction in both food intake and body mass (Muzzin et al., 1996). Similar findings were reported for rats (Chen et al., 1996). In addition to being obese, *ob/ob* mice are also sterile; treatment of *ob/ob* mice with recombinant leptin reverses the sterility (Chehab et al., 1996; Mounzih et al., 1997). These exciting findings suggested the possibility of treating obese humans with gene therapy. However, leptin appears to have weight-reducing properties only in rodents. Despite screening of thousands of obese humans, only two individuals have been found who displayed a mutation in the leptin gene (Montague et al., 1997), and the effects of leptin treatment on human obesity have been equivocal. Additional research is required to sort out the role of leptin in human and nonhuman energy balance.

Taken together, all of these techniques are useful in elucidating hormone–behavior relationships; later in the book, other specific techniques will be introduced as we examine the details of specific hormone–behavior interactions. In the next chapter, many of the fruits of these techniques will be presented in the context of a general introduction to endocrine anatomy, chemistry, and physiology.

## Summary

• Behavioral endocrinology is the study of the interaction between hormones and behavior. This interaction is bidirectional: hormones can affect behavior, and behavior can influence hormone concentrations.

• Hormones are chemical messengers released from endocrine glands. The endocrine system and the nervous system work together to regulate the physiology and behavior of individuals.

• Hormones induce changes in the rate of cellular function, and affect behavior by increasing the probability that a particular behavior will occur in the presence of a particular stimulus. Hormones can influence behavior by affecting an animal's sensory systems, integrators, and/or effectors. Peripheral structures can also be affected by hormones, and these effects can themselves influence behavior.

- Behavior is generally thought of as involving movement, but nearly any type of output can be considered behavior. A complete description of behavior is required before researchers can address questions of its causation. All behavioral biologists study a specific version of the general question, "What causes animal *A* to emit behavior *X*?"

- The four interacting levels of analysis that can be used for exploring and explaining the causes of behavior are immediate causation, development, evolution, and adaptive function.

- Three types of evidence are necessary to establish a causal link between hormones and behavior: (1) a behavior that depends on a particular hormone should diminish when the source of or actions of the hormone are removed, (2) the behavior should reappear when the hormone is reintroduced, and (3) hormone levels and the behavior in question should be covariant.

- Several techniques have been useful in advancing research in behavioral endocrinology: ablation–replacement; bioassays; modern assays that utilize the concept of competitive binding of antibodies; autoradiography; immunocytochemistry; electrical stimulation and single-unit recording; pharmacological methods; methods that make use of cannulation; and genetic manipulations.

## Questions for Discussion

1. What are some of the problems associated with attempting to determine causation in a hormone–behavior interaction? What are the best ways to address these problems?

2. An experimenter is interested in the effect of a particular hormone on migration behavior in butterflies. It is hypothesized that butterflies migrate because of high levels of this hormone. An alternative hypothesis is that the butterflies that migrate produce more offspring in subsequent generations. If the results of an experiment rule out the hypothesis that the hormone is required for migratory behavior, does that necessarily mean that the alternative hypothesis is true? Why or why not?

3. Hormones cause changes in the rates of cellular processes or in cellular morphology. Suggest some ways that these hormonally induced cellular changes might theoretically produce profound changes in behavior.

4. In recent years, investigations of hormone–behavior relationships have involved increasingly elaborate and precise methodology. Discuss the proposition that comparable increases in sophistication, quantification, and so forth are needed on the side of behavior. Give examples of desirable and undesirable approaches.

5. In lesion studies or studies of animals with specific genes deleted, the behavioral tests study the effects of the missing brain region or the missing gene, respectively. Discuss how these conceptual shortcomings can be overcome in evaluating the results of studies using these types of procedures.

## Suggested Readings

Beach, F. A. 1948. *Hormones and Behavior.* Paul Hoeber, New York.

Beach, F. A. 1975. Behavioral endocrinology: An emerging discipline. *American Scientist,* 63: 178–187.

Becker, J. B., Breedlove, S. M., and Crews, D. (eds.). 1992. *Behavioral Endocrinology.* MIT Press, Cambridge, MA.

Brown, R. E. 1994. *An Introduction to Neuroendocrinology.* Cambridge University Press, Cambridge.

Leshner, A. I. 1978. *An Introduction to Behavioral Endocrinology.* Oxford University Press, New York.

Tinbergen, N. 1951. *The Study of Instinct.* Oxford University Press, Oxford.

# 2

# The Endocrine System

In order to understand the interaction between hormones and behavior, a basic understanding of the endocrine system is essential. A comprehensive review of endocrinology is both beyond the scope of this book and unnecessary to understand hormone–behavior interactions conceptually. But a good basic knowledge of the general principles of endocrinology, the hormones found in animals, and the organs that produce hormones will help you in reading the discussions that follow. The goals of this chapter are to provide a solid general background in endocrinology for students who are unfamiliar with this topic; to provide a basic review for students who have previously studied endocrinology; and to serve all readers as a reference resource to aid in understanding the specific material in the following chapters. The major vertebrate endocrine organs involved in behavior and their various hormone products are described here, and this chapter is consequently rather densely packed with information. However, the individual hormones, their sources, and their physiological actions are also listed in tables on the endpapers of this book for easy reference and review.

When you have finished reading this chapter you should be able to answer the following general questions: Where do hormones come from? Where do hormones go? What do hormones do? The bulk of this chapter is devoted to providing specific answers to these three questions, but the general answers to these questions are straightforward: Hormones are produced by glands and secreted into the blood. They travel in the blood to target tissues containing specific receptors for the hormones. By interacting with their receptors, hormones initiate biochemical events that may directly or indirectly activate genes to induce certain biological responses. In some cases, hormone–receptor interactions result in nongenomic effects on cellular function. Because they are relatively fast, the nongenomic effects of hormones are being intensively studied in their role in mediating behavior.

In the first section of this chapter, the general principles of endocrine and neuroendocrine physiology are reviewed. Next, a description of the major endocrine and neuroendocrine glands and their location in humans is presented. In this context, the hormones associated with each gland will be briefly mentioned. Then hormone signal transduction, transcription, and translation is presented. Detailed descriptions of the hormones, as well as their physiological effects, are presented separately in the following section. The final section discusses the ways that hormones are regulated and the evolution of hormones.

## Chemical Communication

The endocrine system is only one example of chemical communication, which is a ubiquitous feature of life on earth. All levels of biological organization make use of some form of chemical messages, ranging from those used to mediate intracellular processes to the substances used in communication between organs, individuals, and even populations. In all these cases, information is communicated by the release of chemical agents and their detection by receptor activation.

This chemical mediation within and between cells, as well as between individuals and populations, is conducted by several interacting physiological systems. A key component of these interacting systems is the endocrine system; however, there are other systems of chemical mediation (Figure 2.1). For example, chemical mediation of intracellular events is called *intracrine* mediation. Some intracrine mediators may have changed their function over the course of evolution and now serve as hormones or pheromones (Bern, 1990). *Autocrine* cells secrete products that may feed back to affect processes in the cells that originally produced them. For example, steroid hormone-producing cells possess receptors for their own secreted products (O'Malley, 1995). Chemical mediators released by one cell that induce a biological response in an adjacent cell are called *paracrine* agents; nerve cells are well-known paracrine cells. Another example of paracrine processes is found during embryonic differentiation, when cells may release chemicals that induce or influence tissue development in neighboring cells. *Ectocrine* substances are released to the outside of an individual and induce a biological response in another animal; pheromones are examples of ectocrine agents.

Many of these chemical communication systems have been studied independently by separate groups of scientific specialists. For example, neuroscien-

**Intracrine mediation**

Intracrine substances regulate intracellular events.

**Autocrine mediation**

Autocrine substances "feed back" to influence the same cells that secreted them.

**Paracrine mediation**

Paracrine cells secrete chemicals that affect adjacent cells.

**Endocrine mediation**

Endocrine cells secrete chemicals into the bloodstream where they may travel to distant target cells.

**Ectocrine mediation**

Ectocrine substances, such as pheromones, are released into the environment by individuals to communicate with others.

**2.1   Systems of chemical mediation and communication.**  Chemical mediation occurs at all levels of biological organization, ranging from the intracrine mediation of intracellular processes to ectocrine communication, which takes place between individual animals or populations of animals.

tists have focused their studies on the chemical communication within the nervous system (i.e., neurotransmitters), endocrinologists have mainly studied the chemical communication processes within the endocrine system (i.e., hormones), and immunologists have focused their attention on the chemical communication within the immune system (i.e., cytokines). Although historically these three scientific disciplines have operated mostly independently of one another, it is becoming increasingly obvious that the chemical mediators from the nervous, endocrine, and immune systems interact significantly. For example, many immune cells have receptors for neurotransmitters, hormones, and cytokines. Similarly, many neurons have receptors for hormones and cytokines, as well as neurotransmitters. Furthermore, the structural features of receptors and the cellular and molecular mechanisms involved in signal transduction, signal amplification, and gene transcription among the nervous, endocrine, and immune systems are very similar. Thus, the hormone–behavior interactions that are the main focus of this book will also involve neuron–hormone–behavior interactions, as well as immune–hormone–behavior interactions. The separate categories of neurotransmitters, hormones, and cytokines reflect divisions within the field of biology, but may mask the integrative nature of the various chemical mediators. In a few cases, the anatomical locations of these chemical mediator interactions have been identified; however, in most cases, the site(s) or mechanism(s) of integration among the nervous, endocrine, and immune systems remain to be specified.

## General Features of the Endocrine System

The word *endocrine* is derived from the Greek root words *endon,* meaning "within," and *krinein,* meaning "to release," whereas the term *hormone* is based on the Greek word *hormon,* meaning "to excite" or "to set into motion."* **Endocrinology** is the scientific study of the endocrine glands and their associated hormones. As we will see, in some cases, a special type of hormone, called a **neurohormone**, is released into the blood by a neuron, rather than by a gland; **neuroendocrinology** is the scientific study of this transduction of a neural signal into a hormonal signal, and will be discussed later in this chapter.

The endocrine system has several general features:

1. Endocrine glands are ductless.

2. Endocrine glands have a rich blood supply.

3. Hormones, the products of endocrine glands, are secreted into the bloodstream.

4. Hormones can travel in the blood to virtually every cell in the body, and can thus potentially interact with any cell that has appropriate receptors.

5. Hormone receptors are rather specific binding sites, embedded in the cell membrane or located elsewhere in the cell, that interact with a particular hormone or class of hormones.

The products of **endocrine glands** are secreted directly into the blood (Figure 2.2a). Some glands in the body, known as **exocrine glands**, have ducts, or tubes into which their products are released. The salivary, sweat, and mammary glands are well-known examples of exocrine glands (Figure 2.2b). Some glands in the body have both endocrine and exocrine structures. The pancreas, for example,

*This derivation should not be taken too literally because, as we will see, hormones may have inhibitory effects as well as stimulatory ones.

(a) **Endocrine cells**

(b) **Exocrine cells**

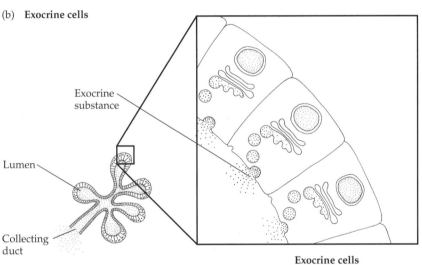

**2.2    A comparison of endocrine and exocrine cells.** (a) As noted in Chapter 1, hormones are secreted by endocrine cells into the bloodstream, where they may travel to distant target organs. (b) In contrast, exocrine cells, such as those found in the salivary, sweat, and mammary glands (and in parts of the pancreas), secrete their products into ducts that carry them to adjacent target organs or the external environment.

contains exocrine cells that secrete digestive juices into the intestines via ducts, while the endocrine compartment of the pancreas secretes hormones, such as insulin, directly into the blood system, where they travel throughout the body to regulate energy utilization and storage.

Some endocrine glands, such as the thyroid gland, are among the most highly vascularized organs in the body. As noted above, hormones are released into the bloodstream, and in many instances, the agents that regulate the endocrine glands themselves are transported to the glands via the blood system. The large supply of blood speeds the transport of hormones to their target sites. Although many endocrine glands are devoid of direct neural connections, in some cases neural control of vascular flow rates can indirectly influence endocrine activity.

Recall from Chapter 1 that hormones are organic chemical messengers produced and released by endocrine glands. Some hormones are water-soluble proteins or small peptides that are stored in the endocrine cell in secretory granules, or **vesicles**, each of which contains many hormone molecules suspended in a protein matrix. In response to a specific stimulus for secretion, the secretory vesicle fuses its membrane with the cellular membrane, an opening develops, and the hormones diffuse into the extracellular space. This process of extrusion is called **exocytosis**. The expelled hormones then enter the blood system from the extracellular space (see Figure 2.2a).

Other hormones, such as steroid hormones, are lipid-soluble (i.e., fat-soluble), and because they can move easily through the cell's phospholipid membrane, they are not stored in the endocrine cells. Instead, a signal to an endocrine gland to produce steroid hormones also serves as a signal to release them into the blood as soon as they are produced by the cellular machinery.

All cells in the body, except those in the lenses of the eyes, have a direct blood supply. Thus, the blood system provides direct access to virtually every cell, and hormones can potentially interact with any cell that has appropriate receptors. Protein and peptide hormones are soluble in blood, an aqueous (watery) solution. In contrast, steroids are not very water-soluble and must usually form a reversible bond with a carrier protein in order to travel through the blood.

Hormone receptors, which are either embedded in the cell membrane or located elsewhere within the cell, interact with a particular hormone or class of hormones. The receptor is analogous to a lock, and the hormone acts as a key to the lock. Receptor proteins bind to hormones with high affinity and generally high specificity. As a result of the high affinity of hormone receptors, hormones can be very potent in their effects, despite the fact that they are found in very dilute concentrations in the blood (some as low as one-millionth of a milligram [1 picogram] per milliliter of blood plasma). However, when the blood concentration of a hormone is high, binding with receptors that are specific for other, related hormones can occur in sufficient numbers to cause a biological response (i.e., cross-reaction).

When sufficient receptors are not available due to a clinical condition, or because previous high concentrations of a hormone have occupied all the receptors and new ones have yet to be made, a biological response may not be sustained (see below). Such a reduction in the numbers of receptors may lead to a so-called endocrine deficiency despite normal or even supernormal levels of circulating hormones. For example, a deficiency of testosterone receptors can prevent the development of male traits despite normal circulating testosterone concentrations. Conversely, elevated receptor numbers may produce clinical manifestations of endocrine excess despite a normal blood concentration of the hormone. Thus, in order to understand hormone–behavior interactions, it is sometimes necessary to characterize target tissue sensitivity (that is, the number and type of receptors a tissue has) in addition to measuring hormone concentrations.

## The Endocrine Glands

For our purposes, there are four classes of hormones: (1) peptides or proteins, (2) steroids, (3) monoamines, and (4) lipid-based hormones. In general, only one class of hormone is produced by a single endocrine gland, but there are some notable exceptions, as we will see below. The locations of the major endocrine organs in humans are depicted in Figure 2.3. Because the modern anatomical names for the endocrine glands typically originated from Greek or Latin terms that early anatomists used to describe the shape, location, or, occasionally, the function of a structure, the derivations for many of these names are provided as an aid to remembering and understanding the terms.

The **hypothalamus** is located directly beneath the thalamus (*hypo*, "below") at the base of the brain. The **pituitary** is located at the base of the skull in a bony depression called the sella tursica (*sella*, "saddle"; *tursica*, "Turkish"), and is connected to the base of the hypothalamus near the median eminence by a funnel-shaped stalk called the infundibulum ("funnel"), or pituitary stalk. The **thyroid gland** is an H-shaped organ located on the upper trachea. The **pancreas** resides within the curve of the duodenum (small intestine), behind the stomach and liver. The endocrine tissues of the **gastrointestinal tract** are somewhat primitively organized; small clumps of endocrine cells are scattered throughout the gut, rather than concentrated into a glandular organ. The **adrenal glands** are bilateral organs that are situated on top of the kidneys (*ad*, "toward"; *renes*, "kidneys"). The **pineal gland**, also called the epiphysis (*epi*, "over"; *physis*, "brain"), is located in the brain in mammals, between the telencephalon and diencephalon. The **gonads** are the

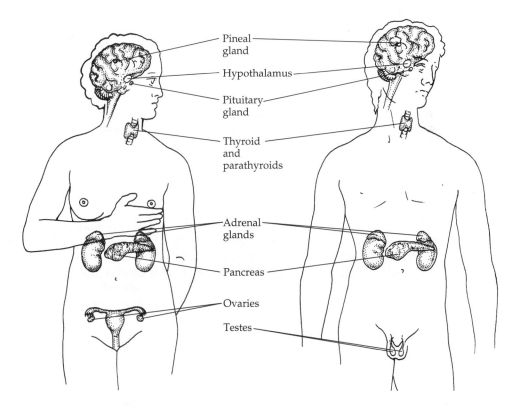

Pineal gland
Hypothalamus
Pituitary gland
Thyroid and parathyroids
Adrenal glands
Pancreas
Ovaries
Testes

**2.3   The major endocrine glands in humans.**

## Box 2.1
# Invertebrate Endocrinology

More than 90% of the animal species on this planet lack a backbone; these animals are called invertebrates. Although this book focuses on vertebrate animals, studies of hormone–behavior interactions among invertebrates have been extremely informative to those who wish to understand the basic principles of hormone–behavior interactions. Establishing the extent to which invertebrates and vertebrates have similar hormone–behavior interactions has provided insight into the evolution of these interactions.

Although the behavioral repertoires of invertebrates are remarkably complex and diverse, the organization of their nervous systems is relatively simple: the total number of neurons in the invertebrate brain may number in the hundreds compared with tens of billions in vertebrate brains. Many invertebrate species, such as the coelenterates (jellyfishes) or tunicates (sea squirts), have rudimentary nervous systems consisting of diffuse neural nets. Neuropeptides,

which are secreted from these nerve cells, can affect the firing rate of neighboring neurons or diffuse throughout the tissue fluid system to affect distant non-neural tissue. In more complex invertebrates, the neurons are often organized into discrete groupings called ganglia.

A circulatory system is present among complex invertebrates such as arthropods (insects and crustaceans) and mollusks (snails); these animals also possess distinct endocrine and neuroendocrine systems. Although all arthropods have a blood–brain barrier (BBB), many invertebrates lack a BBB, so that any neuropeptide secreted into the blood can affect any neuron (providing, of course, that the neuron in question possesses appropriate receptors).

The functions of invertebrate hormones are similar to those among vertebrate animals; that is, hormones modify bodily struct-

Neurosecretory cells produce **brain hormone**, which is released by the corpus cardiacum, and stimulates the prothoracic gland to secrete **ecdysone**.

Brain

The pupa does not produce juvenile hormone, so it metamorphoses into an adult.

As juvenile hormone wanes, the larva molts into a pupa.

The corpus allatum produces **juvenile hormone** in declining amounts, which inhibits pupation.

The release of ecdysone is episodic; each release stimulates a molt.

Adult

Metamorphosis

Pupa

Pupation

Fifth instar

Molt

Fourth instar

Third instar

Second instar larva

Molt

Molt

Molt

First instar larva

Molt

ures as well as physiological and behavioral functions. Invertebrate behaviors, including eclosion (hatching), courtship, mating, parental care, ecdysis (shedding the exoskeleton), oviposition (egg laying), migration, and aggression may be affected by hormones.

The main (neuro)endocrine glands in complex invertebrates (i.e., arthropods and mollusks) include the corpora cardiaca, corpora allata, protodeal nerve, and prothoracic gland. These glands secrete steroid, peptide, monoamine, and lipid-based hormones. In the silkworm moth (*Hyalophora cecropia*), one hormone, ecdysone, triggers molting, while juvenile hormone acts to keep insects in the larval stage. As the concentration of juvenile hormone decreases, larvae molt into pupae (see figure). Pupae do not produce juvenile hormone; thus, they molt into adults.

The behavioral effects of hormones tend to fall into one of four broad categories among invertebrates: (1) modifiers, (2) triggers, (3) primers, and (4) organizers (Truman, 1992). As in vertebrate animals, hormones function most commonly as modifiers of invertebrate behavior: in most cases, they do not "cause" behavior, but adjust the "gain" of the nervous system so that the threshold of stimuli that elicit a particular behavior is changed. For example, during cricket courtship, females become receptive upon hearing the calling of male conspecifics. One behavioral indication that a female is receptive is that she moves toward a male cricket (or an audio speaker) that is emitting calls; this behavior is called a positive phonotaxis. If the female is not mature, she ignores the calling or requires a much more intense stimulus before responding. Juvenile hormone, which is released from the corpora allata, causes maturation of this behavior. When the corpora allata are removed, immature female crickets never respond to males. Injection of juvenile hormone into adult female crickets that have had their corpora allata removed results in normal phonotaxis.

In some cases, hormones may directly trigger specific behaviors in invertebrate animals. One of the best-documented cases is the molting behavior of the hawkmoth (*Manduca sexta*)

(Ewer et al., 1997). Because arthropods outgrow their exoskeletons, they must shed them at the end of each molt. The shedding process requires a series of coordinated, stereotyped muscular movements during which the individual literally crawls out of its outer shell. This behavior is called *ecdysis,* and until recently it was thought to be triggered by a peptide called eclosion hormone (EH). *Eclosion* is the technical term for either the hatching of a larva from its egg or an adult arthropod leaving its pupal case. However, recent work suggests that EH is not the final activator of the ecdysis motor behavior, but rather is part of a neuropeptide cascade that triggers the behavior. The actual activator of ecdysis is a second peptide, known as crustacean cardioactive peptide; its release is controlled by EH via the up-regulation of the second messenger molecule cyclic GMP (Gammie and Truman, 1997).

As is the case with vertebrates, invertebrate hormones may also serve a priming function, preparing the nervous system to respond to subsequent hormonal signals. For example, EH can trigger the neuropeptide cascade that results in ecdysis only during a brief window of time late during each molt, but ecdysteroids, the steroid hormones that initiate molting, must first prime the system so that EH can exert its effects.

Among vertebrate animals, hormones have important effects on brain organization during development, particularly on sexual dimorphisms (see Chapter 3). Although many invertebrates do not use hormones to regulate sexual differentiation of the nervous system, hormones do cause brain differentiation of invertebrate species in which there are caste systems. That is, differential organization of the brains of worker bees and queen bees is mediated by hormones.

As the examples of the silkworm moth, cricket, and hawkmoth illustrate, hormones are important in mediating invertebrate behavior. The simplicity and diversity of invertebrate nervous systems and behaviors make this group of animals ideal for answering many questions about mechanisms underlying hormone–behavior interactions.

reproductive organs. In sexually reproducing animals, there are two types of gonads: as noted above, males have **testes**, often located in a sac outside the abdomen called the *scrotum;* females have **ovaries**, located in the abdomen. A temporary endocrine organ, the **placenta**, forms in the uterus of female mammals during pregnancy.

This section describes the structure of each of these glands in detail, and, in some cases, provides brief descriptions of their endocrine products (detailed descriptions of the hormones are presented in the following section). A brief description of invertebrate endocrinology is provided in Box 2.1.

### The Hypothalamus

The hypothalamus is made up of several collections of nerve cell bodies, or **nuclei**, at the base of the brain (Figure 2.4). The hypothalamus is a part of the brain,

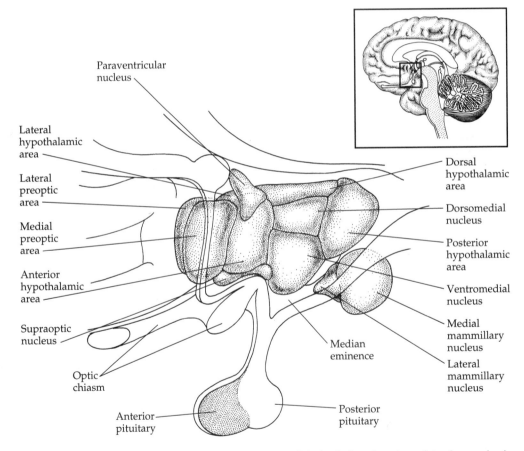

**2.4  The hypothalamus** is located at the base of the brain (inset), and consists of several collections of cell bodies called nuclei. The hypothalamic nuclei integrate neural information from higher brain sites and coordinate numerous physiological processes by means of specialized neurosecretory cells that produce and secrete neurohormones into the pituitary gland. This schematic rendering of the hypothalamus is a composite based on anatomical studies of rodents and humans.

and receives information via axons that form tracts, or projections, from various higher brain sites. This information is consolidated by several nuclei, which carry out many integrative processes, including the control of reproduction and metabolism (Griffin and Ojeda, 1988).

At the base of the hypothalamus, there are modified neurons specialized for the release of chemical messages. Although these **neurosecretory cells** function primarily as glands, they are morphologically similar to conventional neurons, having dendrites, axons, Golgi complexes, and neurotubules (for a review of basic features of the nervous system, see Rosenzweig et al, 1999). Their chemical messages, called neurohormones, are released from the nerve cell terminals in response to neuronal impulses in a manner analogous to neurotransmitters, but rather than being released into a synaptic space, they are released into blood vessels in the pituitary gland. This chemical communication system between the hypothalamus and the pituitary is one of the areas where the boundaries between the endocrine and nervous systems are blurred.

### The Pituitary Gland

The word *pituitary* is derived from the Latin word for "mucous"; early anatomists erroneously believed that this gland collected waste products from the brain and excreted them via the nose. The pituitary gland was once considered the "master gland" because it mediated so many physiological processes. While it is true that the pituitary orchestrates many processes, we now know that the pituitary itself is one of the most regulated glands in the endocrine system.

The mammalian pituitary, also called the *hypophysis* (from the Greek *hypo*, "below"; *physis*, "brain") is really two distinct glands fused into one (Kannan, 1987) (Figure 2.5). The two parts have very different embryological origins. The front

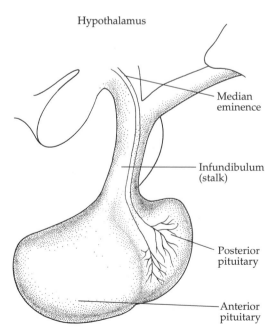

Hypothalamus

Median eminence

Infundibulum (stalk)

Posterior pituitary

Anterior pituitary

**2.5    The pituitary gland** has two distinct anatomical components in humans: the anterior pituitary and the posterior pituitary. The anterior and posterior pituitary have different embryological origins and different functional roles in the endocrine system.

part, the **anterior pituitary** (also called the *pars anterior* or *adenohypophysis;* from the Greek *aden,* "gland"), develops from an embryological structure called Rathke's pouch, which pinches off from the roof of the mouth and migrates to the final location of the gland. There the anterior pituitary joins the back part, or **posterior pituitary** (also called the *pars nervosa* or *neurohypophysis*), which is an outgrowth from the base of the brain. Thus, the anterior pituitary is derived from the soft tissues of the upper palate, and the posterior pituitary has a neural origin in the base of the brain. The area where the two parts of the pituitary join has a distinct anatomical organization in mammals, and is called the *pars intermedia*. Birds lack a distinct pars intermedia, and in some primitive vertebrates (for example, lampreys and hagfish), the two parts of the pituitary remain anatomically separate.

The hypothalamus communicates with the pituitary by two methods. Neurohormones from the hypothalamus reach the anterior pituitary via the **portal system**, a special closed blood circuit in which two beds of capillaries, one in the hypothalamus and one in the anterior pituitary, are connected by a vein (Figure 2.6a). The portal system ensures that blood flows primarily in one direction (although there can be some backflow), from the hypothalamus to the anterior pituitary, and also ensures that hormonal signals from the hypothalamus will be read by the pituitary rather than diluted in the general blood circulation. Evidence

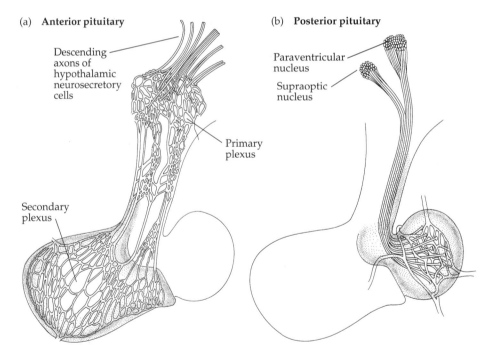

(a) **Anterior pituitary**

Descending axons of hypothalamic neurosecretory cells

Primary plexus

Secondary plexus

(b) **Posterior pituitary**

Paraventricular nucleus

Supraoptic nucleus

**2.6   Hypothalamic communication between the anterior and posterior pituitary.** (a) Hypothalamic neurosecretory cells synapse on the primary plexus of the portal system, a special closed blood system that bridges the hypothalamus and anterior pituitary. (b) Axons from hypothalamic neurosecretory cells that produce the neurohormones oxytocin and vasopressin extend down the infundibulum and synapse on blood vessels in the posterior pituitary.

for hypothalamic control of the pituitary via a portal system has been document-ed in all but the most primitive vertebrates.

A different set of hypothalamic neurosecretory cells directly innervates the posterior pituitary. Neurohormones are secreted directly into this structure, where they enter blood vessels and the general circulation (Figure 2.6b).

**THE ANTERIOR PITUITARY.**   The hypothalamic neurohormones secreted into the portal system are called by a variety of names, including *releasing factors, releasing hormones, inhibitory factors,* and *inhibitory hormones.* These small peptides act on the anterior pituitary to stimulate or inhibit the release of the anterior pituitary's own hormones. However, for the sake of simplicity, we will refer to these hormones as **releasing hormones**. When a stimulatory releasing hormone reaches the anterior pituitary via the portal system, the anterior pituitary releases appropriate hor-mones of its own. These pituitary hormones are also secreted into the portal sys-tem, but due to the "one-way" directional blood flow of the system, they join the general circulation, rather than traveling to the hypothalamus. The anterior pitu-itary hormones are called **tropic hormones** (from the Greek *trophe,* "nourishment") because they stimulate various physiological processes, either by acting directly on target tissues or by causing *other* endocrine glands to release hormones.

The anterior pituitary contains three distinct types of cells, each of which pro-duces a different group of tropic hormones (see below). Growth hormone, which acts on muscle and bone cells to increase their size, is an example of an anterior pituitary tropic hormone. As noted above, the anterior pituitary receives little neural input; however, the blood vessels in the anterior pituitary are innervated, and neural signals can increase or decrease the diameter of these vessels to alter blood flow rates and effectively alter hormone distribution.

**THE POSTERIOR PITUITARY.**   The posterior pituitary serves as a sort of reservoir for two neurohormones, oxytocin and vasopressin, which are actually manufac-tured in the cell bodies of the magnocellular neurons of the supraoptic and par-aventricular nuclei of the hypothalamus. Axons from these cells, which function both as typical neurons that conduct impulses and as endocrine cells, extend down the infundibulum and terminate in the posterior pituitary. Oxytocin and vasopressin made and packaged in the Golgi complexes of the neurosecretory cell bodies are transported down the axon and stored in vesicles at the nerve cell terminals in the posterior pituitary, from which they are released in response to a neural impulse. When the cell membrane is depolarized by a neural impulse, the hormones are released from the terminals by exocytosis and enter the blood-stream. Thus, a neuroendocrine reflex can occur in the posterior pituitary as fast as a neural impulse is conducted. The functional differences between the anteri-or and posterior pituitary are presented in Figure 2.7.

## The Thyroid Gland

The thyroid (Figure 2.8a) consists of many sphere-shaped, colloid-filled struc-tures called **follicles** ( *follicle,* "sac") (Figure 2.8b), which produce thyroid hor-mones in response to an anterior pituitary tropic hormone. The thyroid is unusual among vertebrate endocrine glands because it stores large quantities of these hormones; humans store sufficient thyroid hormone reserves for approxi-mately 90 days. A functional explanation for this storage ability is that thyroid

(a)

(b)

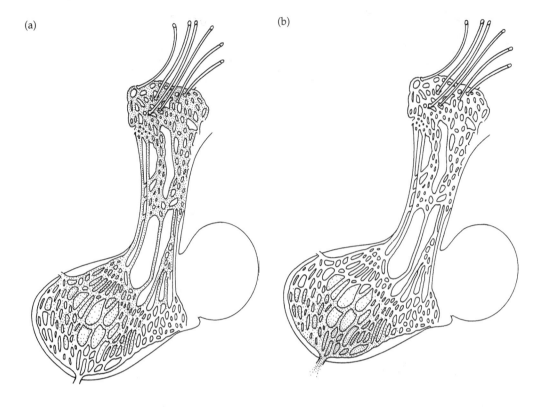

(c)

**2.7   A comparison of anterior and posterior pituitary function.** Hormone secretion from the anterior pituitary involves two stages. (a) Hypothalamic releasing hormones are secreted into the primary plexus of the portal system. They travel to the secondary plexus and diffuse into the anterior pituitary, where they reach target cells and act to stimulate or inhibit the release of the anterior pituitary's tropic hormones. (b) If a signal to release a tropic hormone has been received, the anterior pituitary releases the hormone into the secondary plexus. Because of the unidirectional blood flow in the portal system, the hormone leaves the pituitary and enters the general circulation. (c) Hormone secretion from the posterior pituitary, on the other hand, is a one-step process. When neurohormones are secreted from the terminals of the neurosecretory cells in the posterior pituitary, they immediately enter blood vessels that lead directly to the general circulation.

hormones are dependent upon dietary iodine, which is uncommon in many human diets.

Embedded in the thyroid are other endocrine cells called **C-cells,** which secrete a protein hormone called calcitonin that is involved in calcium metabolism. Also situated in the thyroid is the **parathyroid gland** (see Figure 2.8a, inset), which usually has several parts; in humans, two lobes are present in each upper layer of the thyroid. The parathyroid secretes a protein hormone, parathyroid hormone, that is also important in calcium regulation. However, the C-cells and parathyroid gland probably affect behavior only indirectly.

(a)

Parathyroids

Larynx

Thyroid gland

Trachea

**2.8    The thyroid gland** is a highly vascularized, H-shaped organ that partially surrounds the upper trachea in humans (a). Embedded in each upper layer of the thyroid are two lobes of the parathyroid gland (inset, rear view). (b) The spherical, colloid-filled follicles of the thyroid synthesize, store, and secrete thyroid hormones.

(b)

Secretory epithelium

Capillary

Interfollicular connective tissue

Colloid

### The Pancreas

As stated previously, the pancreas (Figure 2.9a) functions as both an endocrine and an exocrine gland. Most of the pancreas consists of exocrine cells that produce and secrete digestive juices into the intestines (Go et al., 1993), but nested throughout the exocrine tissue are islands of endocrine tissue called **islets of Langerhans** (Figure 2.9b). Within these endocrine islands are four cell types, α-cells, β-cells, δ-cells, and a few polypeptide-secreting cells, each of which secretes a different protein hormone (Figure 2.9c). For example, the β-cells secrete insulin, a hormone that is necessary for cells to utilize and store metabolic fuel.

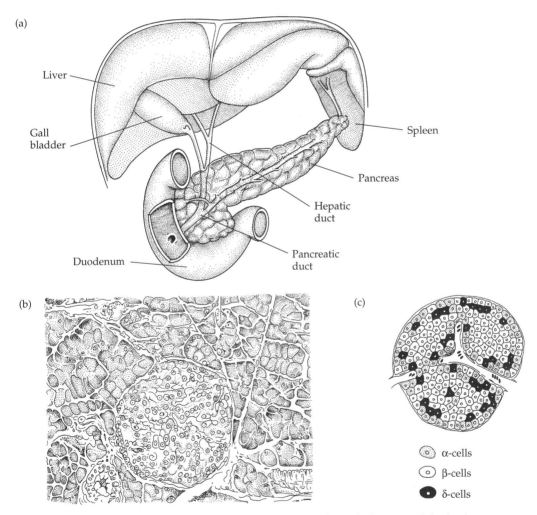

(a)

Liver

Gall bladder

Spleen

Pancreas

Hepatic duct

Duodenum

Pancreatic duct

(b)

(c)

α-cells

β-cells

δ-cells

**2.9   The pancreas** is located beneath the liver and rests in the curve of the duodenum, or small intestine (a). (b) While most of the pancreas consists of exocrine cells that secrete digestive fluids, islands of endocrine tissue called islets of Langerhans are also present. (c) The relative distribution of α-, β-, and δ-cells in a pancreatic islet; each cell type secretes a different protein hormone.

In many animals, the islets of Langerhans are innervated. In mammals, these cells are innervated by the vagus nerve, which stimulates insulin secretion when glucose concentrations in the blood increase, as they do after a meal. This mechanism allows an animal to anticipate the arrival of food in the intestine with a rapid secretion of insulin and thus promotes efficient movement of energy from the blood into the cells.

### The Gastrointestinal Tract

As mentioned above, the endocrine cells of the gastrointestinal tract are scattered throughout the gut, in what is considered to be a primitive organization. Also, the gastrointestinal hormones regulate the cells and organs in which they are produced. Such intracrine or autocrine chemical mediation is usually considered a more primitive mechanism than endocrine mediation (O'Malley, 1989).

There are three major gastrointestinal hormones—gastrin, secretin, and cholecystokinin—all of which are protein hormones that control various aspects of digestion. In addition to their gastrointestinal roles, many of these so-called gut hormones are also found in the brain and appear to have diverse and marked behavioral effects.

### The Adrenal Glands

The adrenal glands are located on the top of the kidneys (Figure 2.10a). Like the pituitary gland, each adrenal gland is actually two distinct organs in mammals (James, 1992). An outer gland, the **adrenal cortex** (*cortex*, "bark") surrounds an inner gland, the **adrenal medulla** (*medulla*, "marrow" or "innermost part") (Figure 2.10b). In many nonmammalian species, these two parts of the adrenal gland are separate.

THE ADRENAL MEDULLA.   The adrenal medulla is made up of **chromaffin cells**, so called because they have a high affinity for colored stains. During embryonic development these cells are derived from primitive neural tissue, specifically post-ganglionic sympathetic neurons, and after birth they function as part of the autonomic nervous system. In response to neural signals, the adrenal medulla releases three monoamine hormones—epinephrine, norepinephrine, and dopamine—into the general circulation. A class of protein hormones, the enkephalins, is also released from the adrenal medulla.

THE ADRENAL CORTEX.   The adrenal cortex is composed of three distinct zones in mammals (Figure 2.10b; Ganong, 1997). The outer region, the **zona glomerulosa** (*glomeruli*, "small balls"), represents 10–15% of the adrenal cortex, and is characterized by whorls of epithelial cells. The middle zone, the **zona fasciculata**, is the largest zone of the adrenal cortex and makes up 75–80% of this gland. The epithelial cells of the zona fasciculata are arranged as orderly bands (*fascicles*, "small bundles"). The **zona reticularis** is the innermost zone of the adrenal cortex. Here the epithelial cells are arranged in a somewhat disorderly fashion (*reticulum*, "net" or "network").

Human fetuses have very large adrenals that possess a fourth layer not found in adults. During fetal life, the zona glomerulosa, zona fasciculata, and zona reticularis account for only 20% of the adrenal cortex, while the other 80% of the cortex consists of the so-called *fetal zone*. The fetal zone undergoes rapid regression at birth, and its function remains unknown. There is no fetal zone per se in nonhu-

(a)  **Adrenal glands**

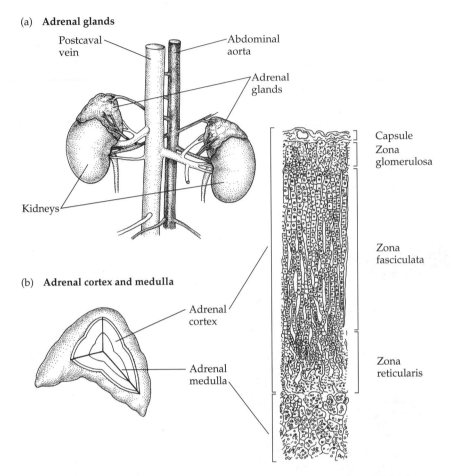

(b)  **Adrenal cortex and medulla**

**2.10    The adrenal glands** are located atop each kidney (a). (b) Each gland consists of two distinct regions, the cortex and the medulla. The adrenal cortex also has distinct cellular zones with different functional roles: the zona glomerulosa, marked by whorls of epithelial cells; the zona fasciculata, in which the epithelial cells are organized in orderly bands; and the zona reticularis, where epithelial cells have a disorderly appearance.

man animals, but an analogous layer of cortical cells appears perinatally in a number of laboratory mammals and has been named the *X zone*.

These anatomical divisions of the adrenal cortex represent functional divisions of hormone production. Although all three zones of the cortex produce steroid hormones, different types are produced in each zone. For example, aldosterone, a steroid hormone that regulates sodium levels in the blood, is produced only in the zona glomerulosa. Furthermore, each zone differs in the way its steroid production is controlled. For instance, the secretion of aldosterone from the zona glomerulosa is regulated by blood concentrations of sodium and via a blood plasma $\alpha_2$-globulin-derived hormone called angiotensin II (see Chapter 8), whereas the release of steroid hormones from the zona fasciculata and zona reticularis is regulated by tropic hormones from the anterior pituitary.

## The Pineal Gland

The pineal gland (Figure 2.11a) is unique among endocrine organs in the extent of its evolution, both structurally and functionally, among the vertebrates (Reiter, 1982). In all mammals examined, individual pineal cells (pinealocytes) function exclusively as secretory structures (Figure 2.11b; Hansen and Karasek, 1982). In nonavian and nonmammalian vertebrates, the pineal gland functions primarily as a photoreceptor organ and is often referred to as the "third eye" (Figure 2.11c; Eakin, 1973). The pineal also functions secondarily as a neurosecretory organ in these animals. In birds and some reptiles, the pineal cells possess rudimentary photoreceptive structures and also function as secretory cells. The avian pineal may also serve as an important biological clock.

**2.11  The pineal gland** is located within the brain, between the telencephalon and diencephalon (a). (b) The secretory cells of the mammalian pineal, known as pinealocytes, are nested in neural tissue, produce both serotonin and melatonin, and secrete melatonin. (c) In fishes, amphibians, reptiles, and birds, pineal cells act as photoreceptor cells or rudimentary photoreceptor cells. In mammals, the pineal consists of secretory pinealocytes.

The primary endocrine product of the pineal gland is melatonin. A number of small peptide hormones have also been found in the pineal, but thus far no functional role for these substances has been documented.

## The Gonads

The gonads have two functions, which are usually separately compartmentalized: (1) the production of gametes (sperm or ova) and (2) the production of hormones (Knobil and Neill, 1994). The hormones produced by the gonads, primarily steroid hormones, are required for gamete development and development of the secondary sex characteristics. These hormones also mediate the behaviors necessary to bring the sperm and ova together. The functions of the gonads are regulated by tropic hormones from the anterior pituitary.

**THE TESTES.** The testes are bilateral glands located in most mammals in an external sac called the scrotum, and in most other vertebrates in the abdomen. Several cell types exist in the testes. When looking through a microscope at a thin cross-section slice of a testis, you can identify the **seminiferous tubules**, long, convoluted tubes in which sperm cells undergo various stages of maturation, or spermatogenesis (Figure 2.12a). The heads of nearly mature sperm are embedded in specialized cells, called **Sertoli cells**, located along the basement membrane of the tubules; these cells provide nourishment to the developing sperm and also produce a peptide hormone, inhibin, that is important in regulating one of the tropic hormones from the anterior pituitary. The primary hormone-producing cells in the testis are interspersed among the tubules and are called the **Leydig cells** or interstitial cells (*inter + stit* = "standing between") (Figure 2.12b). The Leydig cells produce steroid hormones under the influence of tropic hormones from the anterior pituitary gland. The androgens are the primary type of steroid hormones secreted by the testes.

**THE OVARIES.** In mammals, the ovaries are paired glands located in the dorsal part of the abdominal cavity, normally below the kidneys (Figure 2.13a). Among many species of birds, only the left ovary is developed (Serra, 1983). Like the testes, the ovaries produce both gametes and hormones, and in the ovaries, as in the testes, the two functions are compartmentalized. However, active ovaries exhibit cyclic changes in both functions, whereas the testes are tonic, or constant, in their sperm-making and secretory activities during the breeding season.

The ovary has three functional subunits: **follicles**, which each contain a developing egg, or ovum; **corpora lutea**, structures that develop from follicles after the ovum is released; and supporting tissue, or **stroma** (Figure 2.13b). The functional potential of ovaries can be perceived microscopically early in their development. Within the fetal ovary are germinal epithelia that eventually develop into primordial follicles. The two ovaries of a human infant may contain half a million primary, or immature, follicles. No additional gametes are formed postnatally, and there is a continual degeneration of follicles throughout life through a process called atresia. Approximately 400 ova (eggs) are ovulated by a woman between puberty and menopause.

Each primary follicle consists of an oocyte (immature egg) surrounded by a monolayer of flattened epithelial cells called **granulosa cells**. The granulosa cells also appear to be the source of the peptide hormones, inhibin and activin, that are important in suppressing and enhancing, respectively, hormone secretion from

(a)  **Testis**

(b)  **Seminiferous tubules**

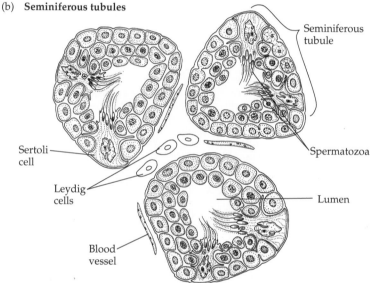

**2.12   The testes.** (a) A testis in cross-section, showing the seminiferous tubules and vas deferens. (b) Seminiferous tubules in cross-section, showing the heads of developing spermatozoa embedded in Sertoli cells and the steroid-secreting Leydig cells.

the hypothalamus and pituitary gland (see below). Under the influence of gonadotropic hormones secreted by the anterior pituitary, a certain number of oocytes mature during each ovarian cycle. As an oocyte matures, the follicle tends to move deeper into the stroma, and follicular cells increase in number via mitotic division. Surrounding the follicular cells, but separated from them by a basement membrane, are the **theca interna** and **theca externa** cells. The thecal cells secrete estrogens, the primary class of sex steroid hormones in females.

As the ovum continues to mature, its cell membrane becomes surrounded by an outer layer called the **zona pellucida**, and a multiple layer of epithelial cells surrounds the follicle. At this stage the maturing cell is called a secondary follicle. A space develops between the ovum and surrounding epithelial cells. This

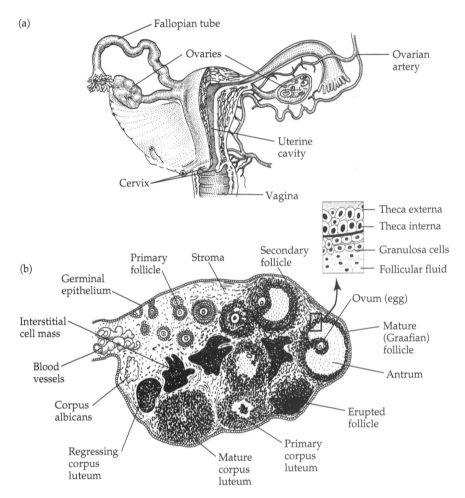

(a)

Fallopian tube

Ovaries

Ovarian artery

Uterine cavity

Cervix

Vagina

Theca externa

Theca interna

Granulosa cells

Follicular fluid

Secondary follicle

(b)

Primary follicle

Stroma

Germinal epithelium

Ovum (egg)

Interstitial cell mass

Mature (Graafian) follicle

Blood vessels

Antrum

Corpus albicans

Erupted follicle

Regressing corpus luteum

Primary corpus luteum

Mature corpus luteum

**2.13    The ovaries** are almond-shaped, bilateral glands about 4–6 cm long in humans, located in the abdomen of females (a). (b) A schematic diagram of one magnified mammalian ovary reveals several important anatomical features and the various stages of follicular and corpora luteal development. The inset shows different types of ovarian tissue as they are organized in the mature (Graafian) follicle, including the theca externa, theca interna, and granulosa cells. Prior to ovulation, the theca interna cells and the follicular cells collaborate to synthesize estrogens. After ovulation, the cells constituting the follicle enlarge and differentiate into luteal cells, and combine with the theca interna cells to form the corpus luteum, which secretes progestins.

space, called the antrum ("room"), fills with fluid prior to ovulation. As the antrum enlarges, the follicle is called a tertiary follicle. The antrum fluid is called the liquor folliculi (or follicle fluid), and is rich in steroid hormones. Just prior to ovulation, the follicle is at maximal size and is called a Graafian follicle. When the ovum is mature, it erupts from the Graafian follicle and travels to the mouth of the oviduct, through which it is transported to the uterus.

After the ovum is released, both the granulosa cells of the erupted follicle and the surrounding thecal cells undergo rapid mitosis, and capillaries generated from the theca vascularize the granulosa cells. In this way the follicle transforms into the corpus luteum ("yellow body"; so called because it appears orangish under a microscope). Although there is great species variation in the component tissues of the corpora lutea, in humans and many other mammals corpora lutea are derived from both granulosa cells and cells from the theca interna. The corpus luteum persists for some time on the surface of the ovary and produces another class of important sex steroid hormones, progestins. The corpus luteum eventually degenerates, leaving a scar called the corpus albicans ("white body"), which does not produce any hormones.

The stroma of the ovary consists of connective tissue and interstitial or granulosa cells. The interstitial cells of the ovary are probably analogous, if not homologous, to those of the testes. Sex steroid hormones are produced by these ovarian interstitial cells.

During the follicular phase (when the primary follicle is growing), the theca interna develops receptors for an anterior pituitary hormone called luteinizing hormone (LH), and produces androgens from cholesterol in response to LH stimulation of these receptors. The granulosa cells develop follicle-stimulating hormone (FSH) receptors, and in response to FSH from the anterior pituitary, convert androgens into estrogens. LH receptors are also expressed in the granulosa cells near the time of ovulation in response to FSH and estrogenic stimulation. Stimulation of these receptors by LH causes the granulosa cells to produce progesterone.

### The Placenta

The placenta is a temporary endocrine organ that develops in the uterus during pregnancy in mammals. It forms from tissues derived from both the blastocyst and the maternal uterus. The placenta is important in maintaining nutritional, respiratory, and excretory functions for the fetus(es). It is also the source of several steroid and peptide hormones that affect both the mother and the offspring. In fact, the most common pregnancy tests measure human chorionic gonadotropin (hCG), a hormone produced by the rudimentary placenta that forms immediately after blastocyst implantation. This hormone maintains corpora luteal function (and progesterone secretion) during pregnancy, and is part of the regulatory system that inhibits ovulation during pregnancy. The placenta is dislodged from the uterine wall during parturition (birth) and is expelled from the uterus at the end of pregnancy.

## Cellular and Molecular Mechanisms of Hormone Action

Now that you know something about the major endocrine glands and the hormones they produce and secrete, we will examine how hormones induce reactions at their target tissues. Hormonal messages, or signals, evoke intracellular responses via **signal transduction**: the chemical hormonal "message" is transformed into intracellular events that ultimately affect cell function. The sequence of events from the time a hormone binds to its receptor to the ultimate effects on a cell in a target tissue is called a **signal transduction pathway**. The initiation of these pathways in nerve cells is the most common mechanism by which hormones influence behavior.

### Hormone Receptor Types

Many different kinds of molecules constantly bombard the outer surfaces of cells throughout the body. However, few molecules have a greater effect on cellular function than hormones. The ability of a target cell to recognize and respond to a given hormone is mediated by the presence of specific receptor proteins, but only a small fraction of the total hormone-specific receptors needs to be activated to evoke the maximal cellular response. Steroid receptors differ in form and action from receptors for protein or peptide hormones, and we will now describe these differences in detail.

**STEROID RECEPTORS.**   Steroid or thyroid hormone receptors are located inside cells, either in the cytosol or in the nucleus. As mentioned earlier, steroids are lipid-soluble, and can penetrate the cell membrane to bind with these intracellular receptors. When the receptors bind to a specific steroid or thyroid hormone, they migrate to the nucleus (if they are not already there) to regulate gene transcription. These receptors are part of a superfamily that also includes receptors for vitamin D and retinoic acid receptors. We will discuss steroid receptors in more detail later in the chapter.

**PROTEIN OR PEPTIDE HORMONE RECEPTORS.**   Protein or peptide hormone receptors are found embedded in the plasma membrane and have at least three domains (a *domain* is a region of the receptor that has a specific recognized function), including (1) an extracellular domain that specifically binds to the hormone in question to form a hormone–receptor complex (in this context, the hormone can be called a *ligand*—the name for any molecule that binds to a receptor), (2) a transmembrane domain, and (3) a cytoplasmic domain (Figure 2.14). These cell membrane hormone receptors are dynamic, changing in form and position in the membrane, and they turn over with a rapid half-life. Though all protein hormone receptors share a basic structure, they can be divided into two functional classes: (1) those with  intrinsic enzymatic activity and (2) those which require an intracellular "second messenger" to exert their effects.

Receptors with intrinsic enzymatic activity have enzymes in the cytoplasmic domain that phosphorylate—activate—intracellular proteins. For instance, some of these receptors have a tyrosine kinase domain in the cytoplasm. Tyrosine kinase is an enzyme that catalyzes the transfer of a phosphate group from ATP to a protein kinase; in turn, the activated protein kinases phosphorylate various other enzymes that cause specific changes in cellular function or membrane permeability (Figure 2.15). In addition to tyrosine kinase receptors, this group includes guanylate cyclases that produce the second messenger cGMP from GTP inside the cell (e.g., natriuretic peptide receptors), tyrosine phosphatases that dephosphorylate proteins, and serine/threonine kinases that specifically phosphorylate serine and threonine residues (e.g., receptors for activin) (Hadley, 1996).

The second class of protein hormone receptor requires a **second messenger**—a molecular "middleman" such as an enzyme or another protein—to transduce the hormonal signal (Figure 2.16). These receptors are coupled to GTP binding and hydrolyzing proteins called **G proteins** that mediate intracellular effects; there are several different types of G proteins, all of which have 3 different sub-

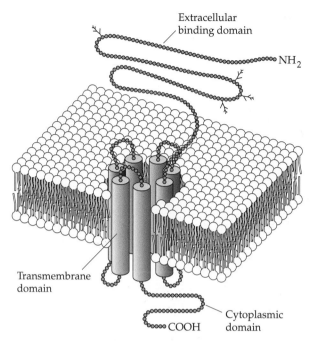

**2.14** **Protein hormone receptors** are embedded in the phospholipid bilayers of the cell membrane. These receptors consist of an extracellular binding domain to which the peptide or protein hormone binds, a complex transmembrane domain that may traverse the membrane several times, and a cytoplasmic domain within the cell membrane.

units, commonly labeled α, β, and γ. (Figure 2.17). When a hormone binds to a G protein receptor, the hormone–receptor complex most frequently activates an intracellular enzyme, adenylate cyclase, which in turn stimulates the formation of cyclic adenosine monophosphate (cAMP) inside the cell. This cyclic nucleotide then activate specific protein kinases in the cell. When formed in response to binding of a hormone or other ligand, cAMP is referred to as a second messenger(the hormone is the first messenger).* In some cases, G proteins open ion channels, causing an increased intracellular influx of calcium that eventually stimulates cAMP (or cGMP) production, which then activates specific kinases. Receptors linked to G proteins all have exactly seven transmembrane domains, and are sometimes called serpentine receptors (see Figure 2.14). The G protein receptor family includes glucagon, oxytocin, and vasopressin receptors.

Different cell types have different specific cellular responses to cAMP. For example, when epinephrine binds to its receptor, the ligand–receptor complex interacts with a stimulator G protein called $G_s$, which in turn interacts with adenylate cyclase. Through signal amplification, adenylate cyclase generates

*Because G proteins often mediate between the hormonal signal (first messenger) and the cAMP (or cGMP) second messengers, students often ask why G proteins are not called second messengers, and the cAMP (and cGMP) referred to as third messengers. Although this would be technically correct, the second messengers were discovered nearly two decades before the discovery of the G proteins, and the name has persisted.

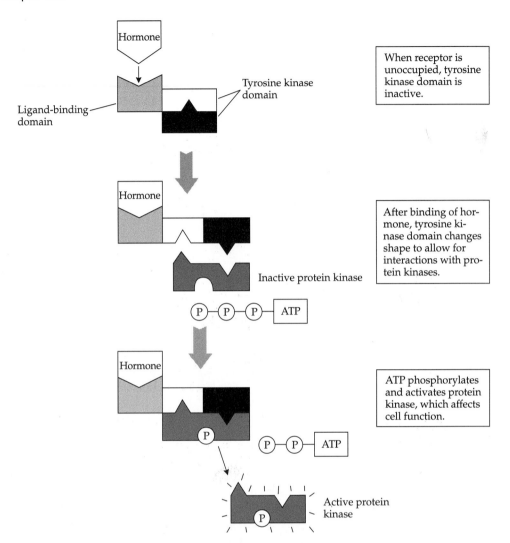

**2.15   Tyrosine kinase receptors are an important type of protein hormone–receptor.** When a peptide or protein hormone binds to its membrane-bound receptor, a conformational change (i.e., a change in the shape of the receptor molecule) typically occurs, which initiates a cascade of responses in the target cell. After binding to its hormone ligand, the receptor changes shape so as to permit interactions with a protein kinase and ATP. Phosphorylation activates the protein kinase, which can now activate other substrates within the cell. After some enzymatic degradation of the bound hormone, the receptor releases its ligand and returns to its unoccupied state and conformation.

many cAMP molecules (Figure 2.16; Norman and Litwack, 1987). (Cell membranes also may contain another G protein, called $G_i$ protein (i.e., inhibitory G protein); interaction with $G_i$ protein inhibits the cAMP mechanism.) We know that cAMP functions as the intracellular messenger for epinephrine because intracellular administration of cAMP duplicates all of the "hormonal" actions of epinephrine (Hadley, 1996). Once formed, cAMP can repeatedly combine with

**2.16    Signal amplification by second messengers.** When a receptor is occupied by its hormonal ligand, a cascade of changes occurs that greatly amplifies the original signal. An activated receptor induces an adjacent G protein molecule, consisting of α-, β-, and γ-subunits, to activate the enzyme adenylate cyclase (AC). AC, in turn, stimulates the production of many cAMP molecules, which activate many protein kinase molecules. At each step, there is a manyfold increase in the number of molecules activated, until finally, there is a significant change in the cell evoked by a single hormone binding to the membrane-bound receptor.

protein kinase A (PKA), an enzyme that phosphorylates (and thus activates) another enzyme called phosphorylase kinase in a variety of cells. Phosphorylase kinase then converts phosphorylase B into its active form, phosphorylase A, which breaks down glycogen into glucose to provide energy within the cell (Norris, 1996). In fat cells, cAMP activates a hormone-dependent lipase that causes hydrolysis of stored fats for energy. In heart or nerve cells, cAMP activates PKA, and may also bind to $Ca^{2+}$-gated ion channels, which can depolarize the cell membrane. In addition to these cytosolic mechanisms of cAMP signal transduction, cAMP may migrate to the cell nucleus and bind to a cAMP regulatory ele-

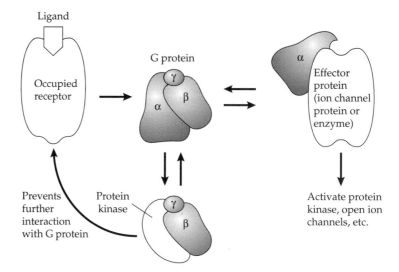

**2.17   G proteins** consist of three different subunits, which often dissociate after the protein receptor is occupied by its hormonal ligand. The α-subunit, which has GTP-binding and hydrolyzing ability, interacts with an effector protein (either an ion channel or enzyme) to open ion channels or activate various protein kinases. The β- and γ-subunits form a complex that binds to a protein kinase that may feed back to influence the hormone receptor.

ment binding protein (CREB). When bound to cAMP, CREB serves as a transcription factor that binds to DNA promoter regions in order to regulate gene transcription (see below).

There are signal transduction pathways that involve G proteins, but do not rely on cAMP or cGMP. One important example is the inositol triphosphate ($IP_3$)/diacylglycerol (DAG) pathway (Figure 2.18). As is the case with the G protein receptors we have discussed so far, the $IP_3$/DAG pathway begins with the binding of a hormone to an extracelluar receptor and the activation of its associated G proteins (see Figure 2.17) However, in this case, the dissociated α-subunit activates phospholipase C (PLC), resulting in the hydrolysis of phosphatidylinositol-4,5-biphosphate (PIP2), which leads to the formation of $IP_3$ and DAG. $IP_3$ mobilizes $Ca^{2+}$ from stores in the endoplasmic reticulum. These twin signals—that is, the rise in intracellular concentrations of both DAG and $Ca^{2+}$—evoke protein kinase C (PKC) binding to the cell membrane and activation of ion channels.

### Transcription, Translation, and Post-translational Events

The final common pathway through which hormones may affect behavior is by acting as **transcription factors**. The signal transduction pathways described above are diverse, and some, such as the cAMP pathway ultimately affect gene transcription, the process by which the sequence of nucleotides in a single strand of DNA is transcribed into a single strand of complementary RNA (Figure 2.19). Transcription factors bind to the beginning of the DNA sequence where the gene to be transcribed is located. In order to synthesize RNA, the two tightly twisted strands of DNA must be unraveled by agents called helicases. A gene consists of a

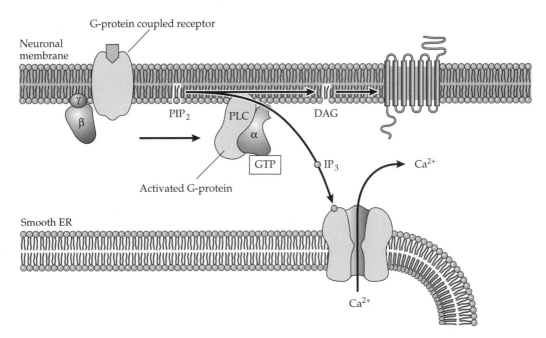

**2.18    Inositol triphosphate and diacylglycerol signal transduction** begins with the binding of
the hormone to its membrane receptor; the activated receptor is coupled to phospholipase C
(PLC) via a G protein. This evokes the hydrolysis $PIP_2$, and subsequent formation of $IP_3$ and
DAG. $IP_3$ mobilizes $Ca^{2+}$ from stores in the endoplasmic reticulum (and possibly moves $Ca^{2+}$
into the cell). The twin signals, the rise in intracellular DAG and $Ca^{2+}$ concentrations, evoke
PKC binding to the cell membrane and activation of $Ca^{2+}$ channels.

unique linear sequence of DNA. Among eukaryotic organisms, some of the
nucleotide sequences within the gene are noncoding sequences, called introns,
which alternate with coding sequences, called exons. There are special markers
denoting the start and end points of each gene. A distinct sequence of nucleotides,
called a promoter or facilitory region, marks the start of the gene. The binding of
a transcription factor to the promoter allows special enzymes, called RNA poly-
merases, to attach to the promoter and begin the process of RNA synthesis. The
sequence of RNA nucleotides, determined by the sequence of nucleotides along
the DNA, eventually determines the sequences of amino acids in the protein gene
product of the specific gene in question. After transcription, enzymes clip out the
intron sequences; then other enzymes splice together the remaining segments
(exons) to form messenger RNA (mRNA). The mRNA leaves the cell nucleus,
travels to the rough endoplasmic reticulum (RER), and serves as the template for
**translation** into a linear sequence of amino acids, which occurs on ribosomes.

When the protein being synthesized is itself a protein hormone, the first product of translation is called a **preprohormone** (Figure 2.20). At the amino terminal
end of the preprohormone is a certain amino acid sequence called the signal peptide. This peptide is separated from the preprohormone during further processing of the protein, yielding a **prohormone**, which is then packaged into vesicles
before being moved to the Golgi apparatus. Typically, additional post-transla-

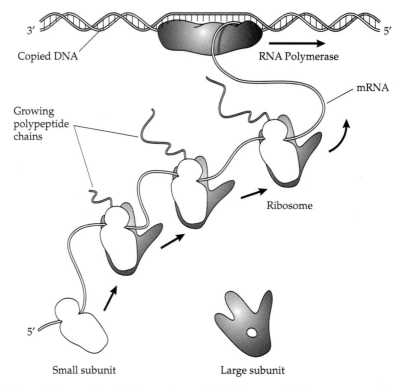

3′

Copied DNA

RNA Polymerase

mRNA

Growing
polypeptide
chains

Ribosome

5′

Small subunit

Large subunit

**2.19   Transcription and translation** can be nearly simultaneous. During gene transcription, the strands of the double-helix DNA molecule must be chemically "pried apart" by helicases. Then, transcription factors bind to the promoter region of a gene; this allows an RNA polymerase to transcribe the DNA and produce mRNA. As soon as the first part of the message has been transcribed, mRNA can leave the nucleus to be translated by the ribosomes. A complex of several ribosomes and mRNA is called a polysome.

tional processing of the prohormone by special enzymes occurs within the rough endoplasmic reticulum, the Golgi apparatus, and in the vesicles to yield the final version of the hormone (or hormones) for secretion. In some cases (e.g., thyrotropin-releasing hormone), the prohormone is cleaved into several molecules of the hormone; in other cases (e.g., proopiomelanocortin), several different hormones can be produced from a single prohormone (see below).

**2.20   The preprohormone** is the product of the mRNA at the ribosome. The signal peptide is required for transport of the prohormone into the endoplasmic reticulum. Later, the prohormone is cleaved to produce the hormone and the "inactive" fragment, which are both usually released from the cell.

Prepropeptide or preprohormone

Signal
peptide

Propeptide or prohormone

"Inactive"
fragment

# The Major Vertebrate Hormones

At this point, you should know where the major endocrine glands are located, as well as their primary physiological functions and how they are transduced. This section reviews in detail the four classes of hormones secreted by these glands: (1) **protein and peptide hormones**, (2) **steroid hormones**, (3) **monoamines**, and (4) **lipid-based hormones**. It is important and useful to discriminate among the four types of hormones because they differ in several important characteristics, including their mode of release, how they move through the blood, the location of their target tissue receptors, and the manner by which the interaction of the hormone with its receptor results in a biological response. Again, all of the hormones discussed here, as well as the glands from which they originate and their primary physiological function(s), are summarized in the tables on the endpapers of this book.

## Protein and Peptide Hormones

Most vertebrate hormones are proteins. **Protein hormones**, in common with other protein molecules, are made up of individual amino acid building blocks. Protein hormones only a few amino acids in length are called **peptide hormones**, whereas larger ones are called protein or polypeptide hormones. Protein and peptide hormones include insulin, the glucagons, the neurohormones of the hypothalamus, the tropic hormones of the anterior pituitary, inhibin, calcitonin, parathyroid hormone, the gastrointestinal hormones, leptin, and the posterior pituitary hormones. Protein and peptide hormones can be stored in endocrine cells and are released into the circulatory system by means of exocytosis (see Figure 2.2a). Protein and peptide hormones are soluble in blood, and therefore do not require a carrier protein to travel to their target cells, as do steroid hormones. However, protein and peptide hormones may bind with other plasma proteins, which slow their metabolism by peptidases (enzymes that break down peptides) in the blood. Hormones are removed from the blood via degradation or excretion. The metabolism of a hormone is reported in terms of its **biological half-life**, which is the amount of time required to remove half of the hormone (radioactively tagged) from the blood. Generally, larger protein hormones have longer half-lives than smaller peptide hormones (e.g., growth hormone has 200 amino acids and a biological half-life of 20–30 minutes; thyroid releasing hormone has 3 amino acids and a biological half-life of less than 5 minutes in humans) (Norris, 1996).

**HYPOTHALAMIC HORMONES.**    The peptidergic neurons of the hypothalamic median eminence secrete a number of releasing hormones and inhibiting hormones. These hypothalamic hormones are small peptides, ranging from 3 to 44 amino acid residues in length. The properties of releasing and inhibiting hormones are very similar to those of neurotransmitters. These hormones are best thought of as a special class of neurotransmitters that act on a variety of cells in the anterior pituitary. In fact, several of these hypothalamic hormones act as neurotransmitters elsewhere in the central nervous system.

Five releasing hormones—thyrotropin-releasing hormone (TRH), somatocrinin (or growth hormone–releasing hormone [GHRH]), gonadotropin-releasing hormone (GnRH), melanotropin-releasing hormone (MSH), and corticotropin–releasing hormone (CRH)—and one inhibiting hormone (growth hormone–inhibiting hormone, which is also called somatostatin) have been isolated and characterized (Figure 2.21). **Dopamine (DA),** a well-characterized neurotransmitter, and technically a monoamine, also serves as a neurohormone in the hypothalamus to inhibit the release of prolactin and melanotropin from the anterior pituitary; in these contexts, it is known, respectively, as prolactin inhibitory hormone (PIH) and melanotropin inhibitory hormone (MIH).

Although steroid hormones are structurally identical among all vertebrates, protein and peptide hormones can vary in their sequence of amino acids. Usually, the mammalian version of a hormone is isolated by researchers first. Because the sequence of amino acids ultimately affects the shape of the molecule, protein hormones from one group of animals may not activate the receptors in another group of animals. Injection of the mammalian version of GnRH into a frog, for example, would probably not affect its reproductive function. After conducting such an

**TRH**

pGLU*–HIS–PRO–NH$_2$**

*Denotes pyroglutamyl
**Denotes amide of C-terminal amino acid, thus prolinamide in TRH, glycinamide in GnRH, alanylamide in CRH, or leucinamide in GHRH.

**GnRH**

    1          3                              10
pGlu–His–Trp–Ser–Tyr–Gly–Leu–Arg–Pro–Gly–NH$_2$

**Somatostatin**

    1                                              14
Ala–Gly–Cys–Lys–Asn–Phe–Phe–Trp–Lys–Thr–Phe–Thr–Ser–Cys

**CRH**

    1
Ser–Gln–Glu–Pro–Pro–Ile–Ser–Leu–Asp–Leu–Thr–Phe–His–Leu–Leu–Arg–Glu–Val–Leu–
    20                                      30
Glu–Met–Thr–Lys–Ala–Asp–Gln–Leu–Ala–Gln–Gln–Ala–His–Ser–Asn–Arg–Lys–Leu–Leu–
        40  41
Asp–Ile–Ala–NH$_2$

**GHRH**

    1                              10                                  20
Tyr–Ala–Asp–Ala–Ile–Phe–Thr–Asn–Ser–Tyr–Arg–Lys–Val–Leu–Gly–Gln–Leu–Ser–Ala–Arg–
                                30
Lys–Leu–Leu–Gln–Asp–Ile–Met–Ser–Arg–Gln–Gln–Gly–Glu–Ser–Asn–Gln–Glu–Arg–Gly–
        40      44
Ala–Arg–Ala–Arg–Leu–NH$_2$

**2.21  Known amino acid sequences of releasing hormones.** The sequences of TRH, GnRH, somatostatin, CRH, and GHRH have been characterized. The sequence of melanotropin-releasing hormone has nearly been characterized in recent years. Melanotropin inhibitory hormone (MIH) and prolactin inhibitory hormone (PIH) appear to be dopamine.

experiment, it would not be prudent to conclude that GnRH is not involved in frog reproduction, although similar errors in logic have been made in endocrine investigations. Because species specificity is conveyed by the amino acid sequence of a hormone, it is important to identify the species-specific protein or peptide hormone before assigning functional roles to hormones in a new species under investigation. Some variants of GnRH are shown in Figure 2.22.

**ANTERIOR PITUITARY HORMONES.**    The hormones of the anterior pituitary are protein hormones that range from 39 to about 220 amino acid residues in length. If the anterior pituitary is removed from an animal, sliced very thin, mounted on a slide, colored with various stains to enhance visibility, and viewed through a microscope, a characteristic pattern of cells can be observed. One type of cell in the anterior pituitary stains readily with acidic stains, another type takes up basic stains, and a third type does not readily take up either acidic or basic stains. These types of cells are called acidophils, basophils, and chromatophobes, respectively. Through the use of recent techniques, particularly immunocytochemistry (ICC), we now know that specific types of hormones are made in these three cell types.

**Luteinizing hormone (LH)**, **follicle-stimulating hormone (FSH)**, and **thyroid-stimulating hormone (TSH)** are secreted by the basophils. They consist of 200–220 amino acids and have a molecular weight of approximately 25,000–35,000 daltons. Approximately 10–25% of the molecular structure of each of these three hormones is carbohydrate, and they are thus known collectively as glycoproteins. Each glycoprotein is composed of two subunits: $\alpha$ and $\beta$. These subunits have no biological activity separately; both subunits are necessary to produce a biological response. The $\alpha$-subunits of LH, FSH, and TSH are identical. The $\beta$-subunit imparts the function of the molecule, and also determines the species specificity. If the LH $\alpha$-subunit and the TSH $\beta$-subunit are combined, the result is a biologically active TSH molecule. LH and FSH are also known as **gonadotropins** because, in response to GnRH, they stimulate steroidogenesis in the gonads as well as the development and maturation of gametes. In response to TRH from the hypothalamus, TSH stimulates the thyroid gland to release thyroid hormones.

Growth hormone and prolactin are secreted by the acidophils and are similar in structure; both are simple proteins consisting of 190–220 amino acids.

|          | 1 | 2 | 3 | 4 | 5 | 6 | 7 | 8 | 9 | 10 |
|----------|---|---|---|---|---|---|---|---|---|----|
| Mammal | pGlu | His | Trp | Ser | Tyr | Gly | Leu | Arg | Pro | Gly–NH$_2$ |
| Chicken I | pGlu | His | Trp | Ser | Tyr | Gly | Leu | Gln | Pro | Gly–NH$_2$ |
| Catfish | pGlu | His | Trp | Ser | His | Gly | Leu | Asn | Pro | Gly–NH$_2$ |
| Chicken II | pGlu | His | Trp | Ser | His | Gly | Trp | Tyr | Pro | Gly–NH$_2$ |
| Dogfish | pGlu | His | Trp | Ser | His | Gly | Trp | Leu | Pro | Gly–NH$_2$ |
| Salmon | pGlu | His | Trp | Ser | Tyr | Gly | Trp | Leu | Pro | Gly–NH$_2$ |
| Lamprey | pGlu | His | Tyr | Ser | Leu | Glu | Trp | Lys | Pro | Gly–NH$_2$ |

**2.22    Primary structures of species-specific forms of GnRH.** Amino acid residues that are different from the mammalian form of GnRH are enclosed in boxes. Presumably, point mutations have occurred during evolution to yield the current forms of GnRH in different types of animals.

Growth hormone is released from the anterior pituitary in response to GHRH from the hypothalamus. Human growth hormone (hGH) has two disulfide bonds; growth hormone shows a fair amount of species specificity.*

**Growth hormone (GH)** stimulates somatic (body) growth. However, GH does not directly induce growth of the skeleton. Rather, it stimulates the production of growth-regulating substances called **somatomedins** by the liver, kidneys, and other tissues; the somatomedins cause bone to take up sulfates, leading to growth. GH and somatomedins also stimulate protein synthesis. GH promotes protein anabolism and acts as an anti-insulin. Other physiological effects of GH include fat mobilization, increased cell membrane permeability to increase the uptake of amino acids, changes in ion influxes, and increased blood sugar concentrations (hyperglycemia), as well as indirect effects on the thymus, an organ involved in immune function. Human GH also has inherent prolactin activity.

Human **prolactin (PRL)** has 198 amino acids and contains three disulfide bonds. The release of prolactin is stimulated by TRH from the hypothalamus. Prolactin is named for its well-known effect of promoting lactation in female mammals. However, the first function of prolactin discovered was the promotion of corpus luteum function in the ovaries of rats; thus, it was originally named *luteotropic hormone*. Several years passed before prolactin and luteotropic hormone were discovered to be structurally identical. The term *luteotropic hormone* has faded from current use; however, it reminds us that prolactin has many functions other than promoting lactation in mammals.

In fact, prolactin is a hormone that has been conserved throughout vertebrate evolution, and hundreds of different physiological functions of prolactin are known (see Table 2.1). These functions can be broken down into five basic classes of actions related to five different physiological processes: (1) reproduction, (2) growth and development, (3) water and electrolyte balance, (4) maintenance of integumentary structures, and (5) actions on steroid-dependent target tissues or synergisms with steroid hormones to affect target tissues. In terms of reproduction, prolactin stimulates the formation and maintenance of the corpora lutea in rats and mice, and may also be part of a luteotropic complex in other mammals. An example of the importance of prolactin to growth and development is seen in salamanders during their second metamorphosis from the terrestrial adult to the aquatic adult form; without prolactin, salamanders cannot undergo this metamorphosis. Prolactin has many osmoregulatory effects, especially in teleost (bony) fishes. Some species of minnows (such as *Fundulus heteroclitus*) are euryhaline; that is, they can migrate between seawater and fresh water. In the absence of prolactin, these minnows cannot adapt to fresh water (see Chapter 8). Pigeons and doves develop a specialized exocrine gland called a crop sac, which secretes a material called crop milk that is fed to the young (see Figure 1.7). Prolactin is important in the development of the crop sac, as well as the development of mammary glands in mammals. Finally, prolactin has synergistic actions on steroid-dependent target tissues. For example, prolactin is critical for maintaining LH receptors in the testes of some mammalian species.

*Lowercase letters are used with the hormone abbreviation to indicate the animal from which a particular hormone is derived. Growth hormone from rats, sheep (ovine), cattle (bovine), pigs (porcine), and mice (murine) would be abbreviated rGH, oGH, bGH, pGH, and mGH, respectively.

**Adrenocorticotropic hormone (ACTH)** is made in the chromatophores; it has 39 amino acids and weighs about 4500 daltons. Only the first 23 amino acids of the ACTH molecule are required to maintain its full physiological activity. ACTH is released in response to CRH from the hypothalamus, and stimulates the adrenal cortex to secrete corticoids (the mineralocorticoids and glucocorticoids).

ACTH comes from a much larger parent protein called pro-opiomelanocortin (POMC) (Figure 2.23). This giant precursor molecule can be cleaved into a variety of biologically active substances. In some cases, the precise signal that determines the cleavage pattern is not known, but in most cases, tissue-specific enzymes are responsible for the different fates of the large precursor molecule. Some of the other products of pro-opiomelanocortin include the lipotropins (which may mobilize fat), **melanoctye-stimulating hormone (MSH)**, a pigmentation regulator, and the endogenous opioids **β-endorphin** and met-enkephalin.

Because the MSH molecule is produced by cleavage of the ACTH molecule, all ACTH includes inherent MSH activity; therefore, all ACTHs are also MSHs. MSH has little or no effect on the adrenal cortex, but functions primarily to control

**2.23    Pro-opiomelanocortin (POMC)** is the precursor to a variety of biologically important substances, including ACTH, α-MSH, β-MSH, and the endogenous opioids β-endorphin and met-enkephalin. Cells in the anterior pituitary that secrete ACTH (corticotrophs) possess proteolytic enzymes (PC1/PC3), which cause primarily ACTH to be produced from POMC. Other hormones are produced from POMC in between the anterior and posterior pituitary, where other proteolytic enzymes are located.

pigmentation in nonmammalian and nonavian vertebrates. Melanocytes are pigment cells that contain melanin. MSH stimulates melanogenesis, the synthesis of melanin, therefore inducing a darker skin color. ACTH also results in melanocyte stimulation. Although the physiological function of MSH in mammals and birds is not well understood, this peptide does have some behavioral effects, which will be discussed in Chapter 10.

The opioids are endogenous (from within) "pain killers." They interact with opioid receptors throughout the central nervous system to ameliorate pain sensations. Exogenous opiates such as heroin and morphine also interact with these same receptors. ACTH and β-endorphin are secreted simultaneously in response to CRH. These two hormones come from different parts of the POMC precursor molecule (Nakanishi et al., 1979), and both are believed to be part of the stress adaptation response. ACTH stimulates glucocorticoid secretion, which helps an animal adjust to stressful conditions. Stressful challenges may also trigger the release of β-endorphin to reduce pain. The behavioral effects of β-endorphin will be discussed in subsequent chapters. The secretion of ACTH and β-endorphin increases after adrenalectomy, suggesting that the corticoids may feed back to control their release.

**POSTERIOR PITUITARY HORMONES.**    Two nonapeptides, oxytocin and vasopressin, are released from the posterior lobe of the pituitary in mammals. These nonapeptide hormones are often referred to as "octapeptides" despite their having nine amino acids. However, two cysteine molecules form a cysteine–cysteine dimer that has been counted as one amino acid "unit" in the peptide sequence.

The nonapeptides are produced from prohormones that also include a carrier protein, neurophysin. Thus, for each molecule of nonapeptide produced, one molecule of neurophysin is produced. There are two types of neurophysin: the prohormone prooxyphysin is hydrolyzed to oxytocin and neurophysin I, and the prohormone propressophysin is hydrolyzed to vasopressin and neurophysin II plus a short glycoprotein (Norris, 1996) (Figure 2.24). The relationship between the carrier protein and the nonapeptide is labile, and neurophysin increases the half-lives of vasopressin and oxytocin from 3 minutes to about 30 minutes in the blood when it is bound to them.

**Oxytocin** profoundly influences reproductive function in mammals. This hormone is important during birth, causing uterine contractions when the uterus is responsive to it. Oxytocin, or an artificial version of oxytocin, is often used medically to induce labor. Oxytocin cannot be used to induce abortions, however, because the uterus is responsive to it only when progesterone levels are low after high pregnancy-induced estrogen concentrations.

Oxytocin is also important in the suckling reflex. Oxytocin is released into the blood in response to sensory stimulation from the nipple, and travels through the general circulation to the mammary glands (Figure 2.25a). The myoepithelial cells surrounding the milk-collecting lumens of the mammary glands contract upon exposure to oxytocin, causing milk letdown (Figure 2.25b). This suckling reflex can become associated with environmental stimuli such that oxytocin is released in anticipation of the sensory stimulation arising from the nipples. Hence, the sight of the milkmaid or the sound of the milking machine may evoke milk letdown in cows, and women may respond to the cry of a hungry baby in the same way, because of prior associations between these sights and sounds and nipple stimulation.

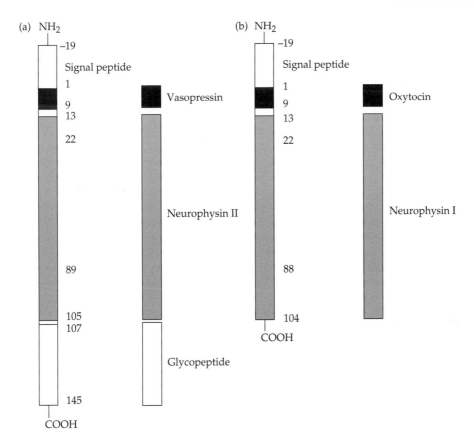

**2.24  Nonapeptide prohormones.** (a) Propressophysin (145 amino acids) is cleaved into vasopressin and neurophysin II plus an unnamed glycoprotein. (b) Prooxyphysin (104 amino acids) is cleaved into oxytocin and neurophysin I.

**Vasopressin,** also known as antidiuretic hormone (ADH) or arginine vasopressin (AVP), is another nonapeptide found in many mammals. ADH acts to retain water in tetrapod (four-footed) vertebrates. The afferent glomerular arterioles in the kidney contract in response to ADH, and the rate of filtration slows, resulting in water retention. Alcohol is a potent inhibitor of ADH secretion, thereby increasing the frequency of urination after imbibing. ADH also has pressor (hypertensive) effects during serious blood loss: it causes constriction of blood vessels in response to severe hemorrhage, which helps to slow blood flow and presumably enhances the probability of survival. One of the possible serious consequences of ADH-induced pressor effects is that the arterioles of the kidney may be completely constricted, and the kidney may become permanently damaged during hemorrhage-induced shock.

**THE THYROID HORMONES.**   The thyroid hormones are often considered to be monoamine hormones because they are derived from a single amino acid, tyrosine. However, the most common thyroid hormone, **thyroxine (T4)**, consists of two tyrosine residues and is thus considered a peptide hormone here. The thyroid gland releases its hormones in response to TSH stimulation from the anteri-

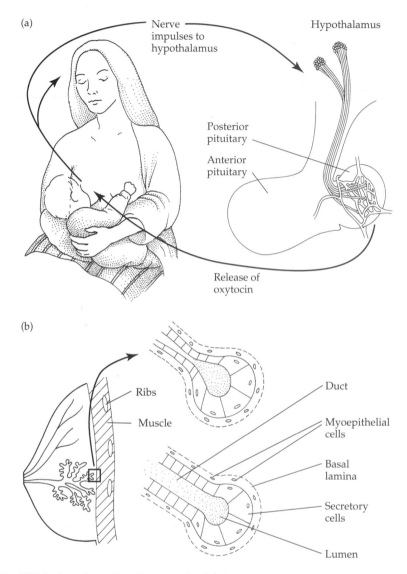

**2.25  Milk letdown is mediated by oxytocin.** (a) Upon stimulation of the nipple by a feeding baby, oxytocin is released, which causes the epithelial cells surrounding the lumens of the mammary gland ducts to contract (b). This response is subject to classical conditioning; a lactating mother may experience milk letdown after merely hearing a crying baby.

or pituitary. There are two biologically active thyroid hormones, both derived from a large, globular glycoprotein called thyroglobulin. The specific hormones are synthesized from iodinated tyrosine residues in the thyroglobulin molecule: essentially, inorganic dietary iodine reacts with water to form the "active" iodine that immediately binds to tyrosine residues in thyroglobulin. Binding of one active iodine atom to tyrosine at position 3 on the phenolic ring yields 3-mono-iodotyrosine (MIT). A second iodine attaches at position 5, resulting in 3,5-diiodotyrosine (DIT) (Figure 2.26); the 3 position is always more readily iodinated

(a)

**IODINATED
TYROSINES**

3-Monoiodotyrosine (MIT)

3,5-Diiodotyrosine (DIT)

(b)

MIT
+
DIT

DIT
+
DIT

**THYROID
HORMONES**

3,5,3′-Triiodothyronine ($T_3$)

Thyroxine ($T_4$)

**2.26   Thyroid hormone synthesis.** (a) The follicles of the thyroid produce a large glycoprotein molecule called thyroglobulin. Dietary iodine enters the bloodstream from the gut and is
transported to the thyroid gland, where tyrosyl components of the thyroglobulin molecule become iodinated and form monoiodotyrosine (MIT) and diiodotyrosine (DIT), the precursors of
the two main thyroid hormones. (b) Triiodothyronine ($T_3$) results from the combination of MIT
and DIT, and thyroxine ($T_4$) is formed by the combination of two DIT molecules.

than the 5 position. MIT and DIT are joined together through an ether linkage
(—O—) between the phenolic rings to form the thyronine structure called **triiodothyronine ($T_3$)**, one of the secreted thyroid hormones. $T_4$, also known as
tetraiodothyronine, is formed by the combination of two DIT molecules, and is
the most commonly secreted thyroid hormone.

Both $T_3$ and $T_4$ are fat-soluble. Like steroid hormones, they diffuse rapidly
across lipid-based cell membranes, but they need the help of a carrier protein to
travel through the blood. The thyroid hormones are easily removed from the
blood by the kidneys and liver if not bound to a carrier protein. About 99% of circulating thyroid hormones are reversibly bound to serum proteins. In humans,
about 75% of thyroid hormones are bound to $\alpha_2$-globulins, 20–30% are bound to
albumin or pre-albumin, and less than 1% are transported unattached in the blood.

The thyroid hormones act to increase oxidation rates in tissue. They have
three general effects in mammals. The thyroid is probably most commonly associated with its metabolic actions, especially its calorigenic, or heat-producing,
effects. Thyroid hormones can increase the rate of glucose oxidation and thus
increase the amount of metabolic heat produced in any given time. Also, it is
thought that thyroid hormones can uncouple oxidative phosphorylation, which
decreases the efficiency of adenine triphosphate (ATP) synthesis, allowing the
release of more heat. By analogy, if the motor of an electric fan heated up exces-
sively when turning the fins, this would indicate that the motor was inefficient in

converting electrical energy into movement. Because energy cannot be created or destroyed, it is released as heat. Likewise, a reduction in the efficiency of ATP synthesis increases the quantity of heat released per mole of glucose oxidized. There are some data suggesting that this function may be imprecise and that the uncoupling may not occur. An alternative hypothesis to explain the ability of thyroid hormones to increase oxidation rates suggests that they stimulate extramitochondrial processes that consume nutrients, but generate fewer moles of ATP.

Thyroid hormones are probably not as important in acute responses to cold as are the adrenal corticoids, but they do play an important role in adaptation to changing temperatures. Generally, thyroid activity in mammals is greater in winter than during the summer. In some nonhibernating mammals (for example, beavers and muskrats), however, thyroid activity is decreased during the winter. This is also true in hibernating species, but apparently the reduction in thyroid function does not directly cause hibernation.

The thyroid hormones also have specific effects related to carbohydrate, lipid, and protein metabolism, usually enhancing the effects of other hormones. For example, thyroid hormones can cause hyperglycemia (increased blood sugar levels), elevate lipid oxidation, and alter nitrogen balance.

Thyroid hormones are also important in growth and differentiation. Their growth-promoting actions are closely related to those of growth hormone and probably represent permissive actions (see below) on GH-sensitive target cells; that is, the effects of growth hormone probably cannot be expressed without prior or simultaneous exposure to thyroid hormones. We know that thyroid hormones mediate the secretion of growth hormones from the anterior pituitary. Thyroid hormones may also stimulate somatomedin production, thereby augmenting the actions of GH.

Thyroid hormones have both direct and indirect effects on behavior. Hypothyroidism, the insufficient production of thyroid hormone, can have a number of detrimental effects. The primary tissue affected by a lack of thyroid hormones is nervous system tissue. Hypothyroidism during development of the nervous system results in profound mental retardation, a syndrome called cretinism in humans; however, the addition of iodine to table salt has virtually eliminated this condition in industrialized countries.

Finally, the thyroid affects reproduction. Generally, sexual maturation is delayed in hypothyroid mammals. Spermatogenesis occurs in hypothyroid males, but blood levels of testosterone are reduced; as we have seen, a reduction in serum testosterone levels can greatly affect many reproductive behaviors. Ovarian cycles are irregular in hypothyroid female rats.

**THE PARATHYROID AND C-CELL HORMONES.**   The hormones produced by the parathyroid gland and by the C-cells of the thyroid are both protein hormones, and both are involved in calcium metabolism. **Parathyroid hormone (PTH)** is made up of 84 amino acids and has a molecular weight of about 9500 daltons. In terrestrial vertebrates, PTH elevates blood levels of calcium ($Ca^{2+}$) by increasing resorption of $Ca^{2+}$ from the bone and absorption of $Ca^{2+}$ from the gut via its effects on vitamin $D_3$. PTH also inhibits phosphate reabsorption from the kidney, which reduces $Ca^{2+}$ clearance.

**Calcitonin (CT)** is made up of 32 amino acids and has a molecular weight of approximately 3600 daltons. There is a disulfide bond between amino acids 1 and

7. CT is released from the C-cells of the thyroid in land vertebrates or from the ultimobranchial organ in fishes. CT acts in opposition to PTH to lower blood levels of calcium by inhibiting the release of $Ca^{2+}$ from bone. PTH and CT are both controlled directly by blood calcium levels; there are no pituitary tropic hormones involved in their regulation. The importance of CT in mammalian calcium regulation remains an open question.

**GASTROINTESTINAL HORMONES.**    Three major gastrointestinal hormones, secretin, gastrin, and cholecystokinin (CCK), are released into the circulation and act to supplement the actions of the autonomic nervous system during the process of digestion. Some of these so-called gut hormones have also been found in the brain, and several behavioral effects have been attributed to them (see Chapters 8 and 11).

Secretin is a small peptide consisting of 27 amino acids. It and other members of the secretin "family," including vasoactive intestinal peptide (VIP), share many amino acid sequences in common. The actions of secretin were first described by Starling and Bayliss in a series of papers that are generally considered to be the genesis of modern endocrinology (Box 2.2).The release of secretin by the duodenal mucosa is stimulated by the passage of food into the duodenum (small intestine). Secretin stimulates the acinar cells of the pancreas to produce water and bicarbonate ($CHO_3–$), which aid in digestion. Other actions of secretin include the stimulation of hepatic (liver) bile flow and pepsin secretion, as well as the inhibition of gastrointestinal (GI) tract movement and gastric acid secretion. Secretin also influences insulin release, fat cell lipolysis, and renal function.

There are several forms of the polypeptide **gastrin,** but the C-terminal tetrapeptide amide Trp-Met-Asp-Phe-NH$_2$ is common to all forms. Gastrin is produced by the gastrin (or G) cells in the antral glands of the stomach. Its release is promoted by acetylcholine or by vagus nerve stimulation. At low concentrations, gastrin stimulates the secretion of water and electrolytes by the stomach, pancreas, and liver, as well as enzyme secretion by the stomach and pancreas. Hydrochloric acid in the stomach inhibits gastrin secretion via negative feedback. Gastrin also inhibits water and electrolyte absorption by the ileum. At high concentrations, gastrin stimulates the growth of gastric mucosa, release of insulin, and smooth muscle contractions of the gut, gallbladder, and uterus. Gastrin also inhibits gastric secretion at high concentrations.

**Cholecystokinin (CCK),** also called pancreozymin, is another member of the gastrin family of hormones. CCK consists of 33 amino acids and causes the exocrine pancreas to secrete digestive enzymes. CCK also causes the gallbladder to contract and release bile. There are several additional gastrointestinal hormones, including bombesin, substance P, motilin, galanin, neurotensin, peptide YY, and neuropeptide Y. Many of these hormones have also been identified in the brain, where they appear to function as neurotransmitters or neuromodulators. **Bombesin,** for example, is a 14-amino acid peptide hormone that was originally isolated from frog skin (genus *Bombina*) and subsequently identified in the mammalian brain and GI tract. A gastrin-releasing peptide (GRP), consisting of 27 amino acids, isolated from the GI tract of hogs has virtually the same amino acid sequence as bombesin at one end of the peptide. Both GRP and bombesin stimulate gastrin release in isolated rat stomachs. Bombesin or a bombesin-like substance in the brain may be involved in feeding behavior in mammals. Other gut

## Box 2.2
# The Discovery of Secretin

Despite Berthold's early work in 1849, the "official" beginning of the scientific study of endocrinology dates to the first five years of the 20th century, when two British physiologists, W. M. Bayliss and Edward H. Starling, described the mode of action of the hormone secretin. Working in apparent ignorance of Berthold's earlier work, Bayliss and Starling convincingly demonstrated that chemical integration of physiological processes could occur independently from the nervous system, and that certain organs could release specific chemical agents that could travel through the blood and affect physiological processes at some distance from their source.

Normally, the pancreas secretes digestive juices when food enters the intestine. Building upon the earlier work of physiologists such as Claude Bernard and Ivan Pavlov, Bayliss and Starling denervated a loop of jejunum (intestine) in dogs. When they perfused the jejunum with weak acid, they observed the pancreatic secretory response. This finding demonstrated that the pancreatic response does not involve the nervous system, but must be stimulated by some substance that travels through the blood. However, when Bayliss and Starling injected the original stimulant, hydrochloric acid, directly into the blood, they did not observe a pancreatic secretory response. This result indicated the presence of a mediating factor. That mediating factor was found to be secretin, a hormone that is released from the cells of the duodenal mucosa in response to acidified food entering from the stomach. The hormone travels through the blood to the exocrine cells of the pancreas to stimulate the release of pancreatic digestive juices.

Bayliss and Starling published a series of elegant studies from 1902 through 1905. For example, they demonstrated the independence of secretin release and the pancreatic response from all neural influences by means of transplantation studies in which the intestinal loops containing the pancreas were moved to new locations without impairment of the secretin reaction. Their most convincing demonstration of the lack of neural involvement was obtained when the circulatory systems of two dogs were joined surgically. Introduction of acid into the duodenum of one dog stimulated secretion of pancreatic juices in both animals.

hormones that have been found in the brain and implicated in mammalian feeding behavior include substance P, neuropeptide Y, and galanin.

As noted in Chapter 1, **leptin** is a protein that appears to be secreted from adipose (fat) cells. At this point, little is known about its regulation, although there is a relationship between body fat mass and blood leptin concentrations. Leptin blood concentrations increase after a meal in concert with insulin release. If leptin is a "satiety" hormone, then it probably operates on the hypothalamus to reduce food intake, perhaps by affecting neuropeptide Y. Importantly, many of the gastrointestinal hormones operate on systems that are involved with energy balance (ingestive behaviors, activity, etc.), and also affect releasing hormones in the hypothalamus and tropic hormones from the anterior pituitary involved in reproductive regulation. The interaction between energy balance and reproduction will be considered in later chapters.

**THE PANCREATIC HORMONES.**    Three major peptide hormone products are secreted from the pancreas: insulin, glucagon, and somatostatin. **Insulin** is a protein hormone that has a molecular weight of about 6000 daltons. Insulin has three disulfide bonds in most vertebrates; it is made up of two short amino acid chains, called the A- and B-chains, linked together by two disulfide bonds. Proinsulin, the precursor of insulin, possesses a 33-amino acid C-chain in addition to the A- and B-chains (Figure 2.27). The insulin molecule has not changed in structure during the evolution of animals, and is evident in both vertebrates and invertebrates; in other words, insulin is a very conserved molecule. Many hormones act to increase blood glucose levels, but insulin is the only known hormone in the animal kingdom that can *lower* blood sugar. Consequently, anything that disrupts insulin action has a profound effect on blood glucose regulation.

The first place insulin acts after its secretion by the β-cells of the pancreas is the liver, where it promotes energy storage in the form of glycogen (sugar). Except for central nervous system tissue, all cells have receptors for insulin. When a cell's insulin receptors are activated, blood glucose is taken up into the cell, used, or stored in muscle (as glycogen) or adipose cells (as fat).

**Glucagon** is a simple peptide that is similar to those of the secretin family. Typically, glucagon has 29 amino acids and a molecular weight of approximately 3000 daltons. Once released from the α-cells of the pancreas, glucagon travels first to the liver, where it stimulates glycogenolysis, or the breakdown of stored glycogen. Glucagon thus acts in opposition to insulin and serves to increase blood levels of glucose.

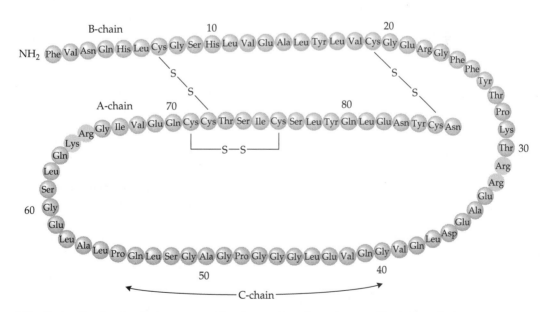

**2.27  Proinsulin,** the chemical precursor of insulin, consists of two short peptide chains called the A- and B-chains, which are bound by two disulfide bonds, and a 33-amino acid C-chain.

**Somatostatin** is an inhibitory hormone released from the δ-cells of the pancreas. Somatostatin consists of 14 amino acids and inhibits the release of insulin and glucagon, as well as the release of growth hormone from the anterior pituitary.

**THE ADRENAL MEDULLARY HORMONES.**    Enkephalins are released by the adrenal medulla in response to stress. A precursor protein consisting of 267 amino acids yields one leu- and six met-enkephalins. The individual enkephalins are released by the actions of trypsin-like enzymes on the proenkephalin precursor. As described above, enkephalins are also among the products derived from the POMC molecule and released by the anterior pituitary; however, the adrenal medullae are the major source of circulatory enkephalins. No definitive function has been assigned to adrenal medullary enkephalins. Because these hormones are released in response to stress, it is reasonable to suggest that they are involved in adaptation to stress.

**THE GONADAL HORMONES.**    Several peptide hormones are secreted by the gonads. Early in testicular development, a small peptide, **Müllerian inhibitory hormone (MIH)** inhibits development of the Müllerian duct system, the embryonic duct system that gives rise to the female accessory sex organs (see Chapter 3). The Sertoli cells in the testes and the granulosa cells in the ovaries also secrete different forms of **inhibin**, a hormone that feeds back to block the secretion of FSH from the anterior pituitary. Inhibin also actively inhibits aromatase, an enzyme involved in the formation of estrogens from androgens, in the granulosa cells of the ovary. A closely related peptide, **activin,** has been discovered in both the testes and the ovaries. Its physiological function has yet to be determined in the testes, but activin directly stimulates aromatase activity in the granulosa cells. The function of activin is not well understood, but this hormone is certainly a candidate to have regulatory effects on hormone–behavior interactions.

Another peptide hormone found in the ovaries of mammals is called **relaxin**. Relaxin, first identified in 1932, is an insulin-related peptide hormone that is produced in the corpora lutea during pregnancy. It functions to soften estrogen-primed pelvic ligaments to allow them to stretch sufficiently to permit passage of the relatively large head of a mammalian fetus through the pelvis during birth.

**THE PLACENTAL HORMONES.**    The placenta secretes a number of peptide hormones that can affect both the fetus and the mother. Some of these hormones are similar to hormones secreted elsewhere. For example, the placenta secretes prolactin and GnRH, which are chemically indistinguishable from those hormones released from the anterior pituitary gland. Other peptide hormones are unique to the placenta, but may augment the function of hormones from other sources. For example, chorionic gonadotropin(s) (CG), chorionic somatomammotropin (CS) (also called placental lactogen), chorionic corticotropin (CC), and chorionic thyrotropin (CT) act as "supplementary" tropic hormones to stimulate gonadal, mammary, adrenal, and thyroid functions. Recent evidence suggests that placental lactogen is important in initiating the onset of mammalian maternal behavior. Other hormones such as POMC, β-endorphin, and α-MSH are secreted by the placenta in vitro, and these hormones appear identical to the hypothalamic versions.

## The Steroid Hormones

The adrenal glands and the gonads are the most common sources of steroid hormones in vertebrates. Vertebrate steroid hormones have a characteristic chemical structure that includes three six-carbon rings plus one conjugated five-carbon ring. In the nomenclature of steroid biochemistry, substances are identified by the number of carbon atoms in their chemical structure (Figure 2.28). The precursor to all vertebrate steroid hormones is **cholesterol**. Although we mainly associate this waxy, artery-blocking substance with the bad cardiovascular consequences that can result from ingesting too much of it in our food, our bodies make substantial quantities of cholesterol from acetate in our livers. In addition to its role as a precursor to steroid hormones, cholesterol is important in many other biochemical reactions. The cholesterol molecule contains 27 carbon atoms. Thus, cholesterol is a $C_{27}$ substance, although cholesterol itself is not a true steroid.

As noted above, steroid hormones are fat-soluble and move easily through cell membranes. Consequently, steroid hormones are never stored, but leave the cells in which they were produced almost immediately. A signal to produce steroid hormones is also a signal to release them, albeit a rather slow one: the delay between stimulus and response in steroid production may be hours. On the other hand, steroid hormones are not very soluble in water, and, as you know, blood consists mainly of water. In the circulatory system, steroid hormones must generally bind to water-soluble carrier proteins that increase the solubility of the steroids and transport them through the blood to their target tissues. The target tissues have receptors for steroid hormones and accumulate steroids against a concentration gradient.

Upon arrival at the target tissues, steroid hormones dissociate from their carrier proteins and diffuse through the cell membrane into the cytoplasm of the target cell, where they bind to cytoplasmic receptors. The amino acid sequence of steroid hormone receptors is highly conserved among vertebrates. Each steroid hormone receptor comprises three major domains; the steroid hormone binds to the C-terminal domain, the central domain is involved in DNA binding, and the N-terminal domain interacts with other DNA-binding proteins to affect transcriptional activation (Hadley, 1996). The steroid–receptor complex is transported into the cell nucleus, where it binds to DNA sequences called hormone response elements and stimulates or inhibits the transcription of specific mRNA. The precise

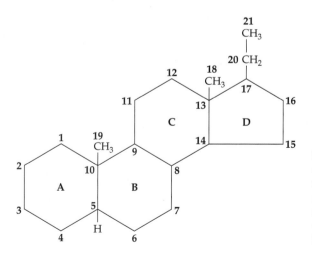

**2.28   Steroid chemical structure and nomenclature.** All steroids have a chemical structure characterized by three six-carbon rings plus one conjugated five-carbon ring. In the nomenclature of steroid biochemistry, each carbon atom is referred to by a number from 1 to 21.

mechanism by which the binding of a steroid–receptor complex to a specific hormone response element evokes activation or suppression of gene transcription remains unknown, but it appears certain that co-activator proteins are often necessary (Smith et al., 1997). The effects of environmental, social, or other extrinsic or intrinsic factors on the regulation of specific co-activators have not been studied, but represent yet another process by which individual variation in hormone–behavior interactions may be mediated (Smith et al., 1997). The transcribed mRNA migrates to the cytoplasmic rough endoplasmic reticulum, where it is translated into specific structural proteins or enzymes that produce the physiological response (Figure 2.29). Changes in the types of proteins a cell makes (i.e., the gene products) can often be observed within 30 minutes of hormone stimulation.

The actions of steroids on target tissues, therefore, are based on three factors: (1) the steroid hormone concentrations in the blood, (2) the number of available receptors in the target tissue, and (3) the availability of appropriate co-activators. Blood concentrations of steroid hormones are also dependent on three factors: (1) the rate of steroid biosynthesis; (2) the rate of steroid inactivation by catabolism, which occurs mainly in the liver; and (3) the "tenacity" (affinity) with which the steroid hormone is bound to its plasma carrier protein. The regulation of receptors and co-activators is currently a very active research area in molecular endocrinology.

**2.29  Steroid hormone receptors** are generally located in the cytosol (or nucleus) of a cell. The steroid hormone binds to its receptor to form a hormone–receptor complex (transcription factor), which binds to a hormone response element (HRE) on the DNA to begin transcription of mRNA. Some recent studies suggest that steroid hormone receptors also exist in the cell membranes, which have effects on cellular function that do not involve a genomic mechanism.

**THE C$_{21}$ STEROIDS: PROGESTINS AND CORTICOIDS.**    In response to various protein hormones from the anterior pituitary, cholesterol is converted into steroid hormones in the adrenals or gonads (Figure 2.30). The pituitary hormone induces an enzyme, called desmolase, that cleaves off the long chain of carbons from the top of the cholesterol molecule to yield pregnenolone, a C$_{21}$ steroid. There are two general types of C$_{21}$ hormones, **progestins** and **corticoids. Pregnenolone** is a progestin, and it is the obligatory precursor to all other steroid hormones. In other words, pregnenolone is a prohormone, a substance that can act as a hormone itself or can be converted into another hormone that has different endocrine properties. For example, pregnenolone can be converted to progesterone, another progestin. Progesterone is also a prohormone; it has several endocrine functions itself, and it is the major precursor for a variety of other C$_{21}$ steroids, including the corticoids and another progestin called 17$\alpha$-hydroxyprogesterone, which in turn is an important precursor of additional steroid hormone types.

Many progestins (e.g., pregnenolone and progesterone) are ubiquitous in vertebrates and are the obligatory precursors of all other steroid hormones (see Figure 2.30). Although named for their "progestational" or pregnancy-maintaining effects in rodents, progestins are found in vertebrates wherever steroidogenesis occurs. In mammals, progesterone is important in maintaining pregnancy and also in the initiation and cessation of mating behavior.

In response to hormone signals from the anterior pituitary, pregnenolone is converted in the adrenal glands to progesterone and then to the various corticoids. Like all steroid hormones, the corticoids appear to be released as they are produced. These steroids have behavioral effects associated with the maintenance of body functions, such as mediating salt appetite.

There are two types of corticoids: **glucocorticoids** and **mineralocorticoids.** Glucocorticoids are involved in carbohydrate metabolism and are often released in response to stressful stimuli; the two primary glucocorticoids are **corticosterone** (abbreviated B) and **cortisol** (F).* Most animals make either corticosterone or cortisol, but rarely are both glucocorticoids produced in large quantities. All reptiles and birds secrete corticosterone from their adrenals. Some mammals also secrete corticosterone; rats and mice excrete corticosterone exclusively. The primary glucocorticoid secreted by humans and other primates, however, is cortisol.[†]

Of the mineralocorticoids, **aldosterone** is the most important, as it is secreted by all terrestrial vertebrates and is important in ion exchange and water metabolism. Aldosterone is primarily responsible for retaining sodium ions (Na$^+$) and excreting potassium ions (K$^+$).

**THE C$_{19}$ STEROIDS: ANDROGENS.**    Just as a specific series of enzymes in the adrenals convert pregnenolone to the corticoids, specific enzymes found primarily in

---

*The adrenal steroids were initially fractionated or isolated before their biological functions were known. Each fraction was designated compound A, compound B, and so on. Later, when identified, they retained their original letter designations, but these abbreviations are now becoming obsolete and replaced by abbreviations such as CORT.

†It is important to be aware of this distinction between the two glucocorticoids. A physician–scientist recently argued that a procedure he was performing on mice was not stressful because "the levels of cortisol were very low." However, after he was persuaded to measure corticosterone, he discovered that his procedure indeed caused a substantial increase in this corticoid, which presumably reflected elevated stress.

**2.30  Biochemical pathways in steroid formation.**  The enzyme desmolase cleaves the chain of carbons from the top of the cholesterol molecule to form pregnenolone, a $C_{21}$ steroid that is the obligate precursor to all other steroids.

the gonads convert pregnenolone to several types of $C_{19}$ steroid hormones, called **androgens** because of their *andros* (male) *gen*erating effects (Figure 2.31).* These $C_{19}$ steroid hormones result from the enzymatic cleavage of the ethyl group from a progestin precursor at $C_{17}$. **Testosterone** and **androstenedione** are biologically important androgens, as is a biochemically reduced version of testosterone, **5α- and 5β-dihydrotestosterone (DHT)**.[†] These androgens are produced in the well-vascularized Leydig cells of the testes; the Sertoli cells are the source of androgen-binding proteins that carry androgens through the blood (see Figure 2.12b). Testosterone is typically reduced to DHT or converted to an estrogen in order to have a biological effect (see below). The zona reticularis of the adrenal cortex also produces a relatively weak androgen called **dihydroepiandrosterone (DHEA)**. For the most part, the physiological functions of DHEA remain unknown, but blood concentrations of this hormone decline as individuals age. Replacement of DHEA at appropriate small doses appears to ameliorate certain effects of aging, including decreased muscle strength and weakened immune function (Yen et al., 1995). Based on these preliminary studies, alternative medical care providers have advocated DHEA supplementation as a treatment to reverse some of the effects of aging. However, long-term studies on the effects of DHEA therapy on human health are lacking, and it is probably prudent to await the results of such studies before indulging in self-administration of an active steroid hormone.

Androgens have many physiological and behavioral functions. These steroid hormones are necessary for spermatogenesis and the maintenance of the genital tract (for example, the vas deferens). Androgens also maintain the accessory sex organs such as the prostate, seminal vesicles, and bulba urethra glands. The male secondary sex characters are also supported by androgens: well-known examples include the pattern and density of body hair in humans, comb size in roosters, and antler growth in deer. Some species show subtle morphological effects due to androgens; for example, in mice, the salivary gland and kidney structures are affected by androgens. The liver, heart, and kidneys are generally larger in male mammals than in females with similar body masses. Of course, androgens have many effects on behavior, including courtship and copulatory behaviors, aggressive behaviors, and other social behaviors.

Metabolism is greatly affected by androgens. These hormones stimulate respiratory metabolism and are well known for their protein anabolic effects. The increase in muscle mass that results from treatment with anabolic androgens motivates many people to abuse these compounds. However, because many organs have androgen receptors, long-term problems in the liver, heart, and kidneys can result from chronic exposure to high androgen levels as hypertrophy of these organs leads to a reduction in their functional efficiency. Reproductive problems are also common among people abusing anabolic androgens. Psychological problems have also been reported for long-term androgen users. In many cases, however, a subjective sense of "invincibility" allows steroid abusers to dismiss

---

*Androgens may also be synthesized in the adrenal cortex directly from corticoids if the appropriate enzymes are present. In certain congenital conditions in which excess converting enzymes are present, abnormally high levels of androgens may be produced by the adrenal glands, which can have masculinizing effects in females (see Chapter 3).

[†]The "5" in the name indicates that the reduction occurs with the addition of a hydrogen atom at carbon number 5; α and β refer to the orientation of the hydrogen molecule in space.

**2.31**  **Androgens,** such as testosterone and androstenedione, are formed by an enzymatic cleavage of the ethyl group from a progestin precursor at $C_{17}$.

warnings about the long-term health problems associated with androgen treatment (see Chapter 13).

**THE $C_{18}$ STEROIDS: ESTROGENS.**    Androgens are the obligatory precursors of all **estrogens** in the same way that progestins are the obligatory precursors of all androgens. Specific enzymes, primarily present in the ovaries, convert testosterone and androstenedione to estrogens by cleaving the carbon at position 19 from these androgen precursors (Figure 2.32). This process is called **aromatization** because the removal of the carbon leaves the estrogen with a phenolic A-ring, known as an aromatic compound. Biologically significant estrogens include 17β-estradiol, estrone, and estriol.

The interstitial tissues of the ovary (see Figure 2.13b) produce steroid hormones. The theca interna cells produce progestins, and enzymes in these cells act on those progestins to produce androgens. The blood flow in the ovary moves these androgens into the interstitial granulosa cells, where enzymes rapidly con-

**2.32   Estrogen,** such as 17β-estradiol, estrone, and estriol, are formed when the carbon at $C_{19}$ is cleaved from an androgen precursor in a process called aromatization.

vert them into estrogens. The follicles of the ovary also produce estrogens such as estradiol, estrone, and estriol as they mature. The corpora lutea produce progesterone in many vertebrate species, but also release estrogens, androgens, and perhaps oxytocin, a protein hormone.

Thus, ovaries produce substantial amounts of androgens, which are normally converted immediately to estrogens. However, in some cases, excess androgens are produced and enter the general circulation before they can be converted into estrogens, affecting female physiology and behavior. Also, if insufficient enzymes are present to convert androgens to estrogens in the ovaries, some androgens may be secreted into a female's blood circulation. On the other hand, if high levels of enzymes that convert androgens to estrogens are present in the testes, then estrogens will be secreted from the testes into the blood circulation of a male. Some androgens, such as dihydrotestosterone (DHT), cannot be aromatized and therefore cannot be converted to estrogens.

Estrogens have many functions. Estrogens initiate the formation of corpora lutea. They also affect the genital tract; for example, high levels of estrogens correlate with increased uterine mass. The secondary sex characters of female mammals are also influenced by estrogens. Estrogens also have several metabolic functions, including effects on water metabolism. For instance, estrogens favor the retention of water in humans. Estrogens are important in calcium metabolism. More bone is made in the presence of high estrogen concentrations. During human menopause, estrogen production diminishes, and bone erodes away in a degenerative process called osteoporosis. Finally, estrogens are very important in sexual behavior and may also play a part in maternal aggression (see Chapter 7).

The placenta also produces steroid hormones. Both estrogens and progestins can be produced in significant amounts by the placenta; it also produces some androgens and corticoids. The contribution of these hormones from the placenta to the development of behavior is not well understood at this time.

**A CAUTIONARY ASIDE.**   Although the androgens and estrogens are commonly referred to as *sex hormones*, it is important to emphasize that these hormones should not be considered "male" or "female." All male vertebrates produce some estrogens and progestins, and all female vertebrates produce androgens. The two sexes do differ in their relative concentrations of circulating androgens or estrogens, but this difference is due to the relative proportions of steroidogenic-specific enzymes in their gonads. Testes have more enzymes for making androgens and fewer aromatizing enzymes than do ovaries, but imbalances in the appropriate enzymes can lead to overt endocrine abnormalities. Androgens, with a few exceptions, are easily converted to estrogens. Importantly, testosterone can be considered a prohormone that is converted either to DHT or to an estrogen. Ovaries produce high concentrations of androgens, but high local concentrations of aromatizing enzymes rapidly convert those androgens to estrogens before they can enter the general circulation. Estrogens can theoretically be converted back to androgens, but this is an energetically expensive reaction and is rare in nature.

It is also important to emphasize that, while sex steroid hormones are *primarily* formed in the gonads, they can also be produced in the adrenals, along with glucocorticoids and mineralocorticoids. The production of these various types of steroid hormones is zone-specific: the presence or absence of various enzymes in each of the three layers of the adrenal cortex determines the type of steroid hormone produced there. An aberrant gene coding for an incorrect enzyme can lead to an ovary or adrenal gland producing great quantities of androgens. The behavioral effects of such genetic errors will be discussed in Chapter 3.

## The Monoamine Hormones

Monoamines are hormones that are derived from a single amino acid. There are two classes of monoamines that affect behavior: the **catecholamines** and the **indole amines**. Recall that the thyroid hormones are often classified as monoamines because they are derived from a single amino acid, tyrosine.

**ADRENAL MEDULLARY MONOAMINE HORMONES.**    The adrenal medulla is the main source of two catecholamines, **epinephrine** (adrenaline) and **norepinephrine** (noradrenaline); it also releases some dopamine (Figure 2.33). The catecholamines are derived from tyrosine, and are called catecholamines because each is a catechol (that is, a dihydroxyphenol) with an amine side group. In response to sympathetic neural signals, the adrenal medulla releases these hormones into the general circulation. Typical physiological stimuli that evoke catecholamine release include stress, exercise, low temperatures, anxiety, emotionality (fight or flight responses), and hemorrhage. In humans, norepinephrine and epinephrine are released at a ratio of 1:4 (James, 1992).

**2.33** **Epinephrine, norepinephrine, and dopamine** are catecholamines, so called because each is a catechol with an amine side group. Of the three catecholamines, only epinephrine (adrenaline) acts primarily as a hormone; norepinephrine and dopamine are released from the adrenal glands and act as hormones, but they serve mainly as neurotransmitters. Catecholamines are all derived from the amino acid tyrosine, which is hydroxylated to form 3,4-dihydroxyphenylalanine (DOPA). DOPA may be decarboxylated in the cytoplasm to form dopamine, which in turn may be hydroxylated to form norepinephrine. Norepinephrine can be changed to epinephrine by the addition of a methyl group to the amine.

The catecholamines influence both the circulatory and metabolic systems. They have five general effects: (1) increased heart rate and cardiac output; (2) vasoconstriction of the deep and superficial arteries and veins; (3) dilation of skeletal and liver blood vessels; (4) increased glycolysis; and (5) increased blood glucagon concentrations and decreased insulin secretion. All of these effects serve to prepare the body for action. Epinephrine and norepinephrine have similar physiological effects, but differ in several important respects. For instance, epinephrine elevates heart rate and affects metabolism more than norepinephrine. In contrast, norepinephrine is a more potent vasoconstrictor than epinephrine. The catecholamines affect their target cells via second messenger mechanisms.

**THE PINEAL GLAND HORMONES.**   Melatonin and serotonin are derived from the amino acid tryptophan. Melatonin is derived from serotonin in a two-step enzymatic reaction. These hormones are collectively called indole amines because the indole ring is common to both melatonin and serotonin (Figure 2.34)

**Serotonin** is the common name for 5-hydroxytryptamine (5-HT). Serotonin levels are high in the pineal gland during the light hours of the day, but diminish during the dark hours as serotonin is converted into melatonin. The enzyme N-acetyltransferase converts serotonin to N-acetylserotonin, which is transformed into melatonin (5-methoxy-N-acetyltryptamine) by the transfer of a methyl group from S-adenosylmethionine (SAM) to the 5-hydroxyl of N-acetylserotonin by the actions of hydroxyindole-O-methyltransferase (HIOMT). Serotonin and N-acetylserotonin are probably not released from the pineal gland in appreciable quantities. There is some evidence that the pineal gland secretes vasotocin, a nonapeptide, which may function as a regulator of reproductive activities (Reiter, 1982).

**Melatonin** is the major hormone secreted by the pineal gland. It is highly lipid-soluble and probably leaves the cell by diffusion in a manner similar to the steroids. The melatonin receptor has recently been characterized, but the specifics of its chemical nature remain elusive. The melatonin receptor gene codes for a 440-amino acid peptide that is found in the mammalian brain and amphibian skin (Weaver et al., 1989; Bittman and Weaver, 1990).

Melatonin is involved in regulation of puberty onset. Melatonin also inhibits secretion of LH and FSH in prepubertal rats (Reiter, 1973). The effects of melatonin on the seasonal organization of breeding will be described more fully in Chapter 9.

## The Lipid-Based Hormones

**Prostaglandins**, a family of lipid-based hormones, were discovered in the 1930s. Their first known function was an ectocrine one: these compounds are found in seminal fluid and cause uterine contraction or relaxation in the recipient. Since their initial discovery, there have been reports of a vast array of biological actions produced by the prostaglandins. However, prostaglandins probably affect behavior only indirectly in vertebrates. Conversely, among many invertebrate species, prostaglandins directly mediate behavior.

All prostaglandins possess a basic 20-carbon fatty acid skeleton, prostanoic acid, derived from essential fatty acids via cyclization and oxidation. The naturally occurring prostaglandins have been classified into four basic groups named E, F, A, and B. These groups are distinguished by differences in the cyclopentyl group of the fatty acid skeleton. Substitutions in the side chains and the extent of saturations provide a number of compounds within each group.

**2.34 Serotonin and melatonin** are formed from tryptophan. During the light hours of the day, tryptophan is converted in a two-step enzymatic reaction to serotonin. In darkness (shaded area), increased norepinephrine secretion causes an increase in *N*-acetyltransferase, the first of two enzymes that convert serotonin to melatonin. SAM = S-adenosylmethionine; HIOMT = hydroxyindole-O-methyltransferase.

Prostaglandins in the E and F series are involved in reproduction. High concentrations of prostaglandins coincide with degradation of the corpora lutea of the ovary. In other systems, prostaglandins mediate a large array of actions, often opposing ones; for example, prostaglandins both stimulate and relax smooth muscle. Prostaglandins also affect cardiac functioning. In some circumstances they act as a pressor agent, whereas in other situations they have an antipressor effect.

Prostaglandins have also been implicated in influencing cyclic nucleotide formation. Prostaglandins inhibit cAMP production in adipose cells, which can be stimulated by hormones such as epinephrine. In other cell types, prostaglandins can also stimulate cAMP formation, and often modulate the second messenger response that mediates the actions of many peptide hormones.

## How Hormones Are Regulated

There are two basic patterns of hormonal control: (1) hormones are regulated by the physiological by-products generated in response to their actions; and (2) hormones are regulated by the stimulatory or inhibitory effects of hormones. Within the second control system, there may be one, two, or three hormones in a regulatory chain, or there may be autoregulation via **negative feedback** directly from the circulating levels of the regulated hormone itself.

Parathyroid hormone provides an example of the first type of regulatory mechanism. When blood levels of calcium decrease, parathyroid hormone is released. When the action of the hormone has raised the concentration of blood calcium to some optimal level, parathyroid hormone secretion stops. Calcium levels in the blood are thus maintained in an optimal range (Figure 2.35a). This simple negative feedback system works much the way a thermostat controls the temperature in your home.

GnRH is an example of a hormone that is regulated by a multiple chain of negative feedback controls (Figure 2.35b). In response to environmental stimuli, some internal pacemaker, or some other intrinsic event, GnRH is released by the hypothalamus and stimulates the release of the gonadotropins from the anterior pituitary gland. The gonadotropins, in turn, stimulate steroid and gamete production in the gonads. The resulting steroid hormones feed back to turn off GnRH production in the hypothalamus, as well as shutting down gonadotropin secretion from the anterior pituitary. Peptide hormones from the gonads, such as activins and inhibins, may also be involved in the regulation of gonadotropins. The gonadotropins also feed back to shut down GnRH production, and GnRH also feeds back on the hypothalamus to regulate its own secretion (autoregulation). More detail regarding these multiple levels of control will be provided in Chapters 5 and 6.

In some cases, the feedback may drive hormone concentrations away from the preprogrammed setting. This sort of feedback loop is called **positive feedback**. Positive feedback is often involved when a relatively rapid endocrine response is necessary. Hormones associated with the stress response and with ovulation are regulated through a positive feedback system. Of course, positive feedback must be tightly controlled in short-term situations; otherwise, the equilibrium within the body will be seriously disrupted, with deleterious consequences for survival. Therefore, negative feedback is the most common type of regulatory mechanism in the endocrine system.

Hormones often affect their own receptor levels. For example, an increase in blood concentrations of prolactin stimulates the production of more prolactin receptors; this process is called receptor **up-regulation**. Similarly, high insulin concentrations reduce the number of insulin receptors in a process known as receptor **down-regulation**. Finally, hormones may regulate receptors for other hormones. Estrogens increase the number of uterine receptors for progestins. Such an effect, in which one hormone induces production of receptors for a second hormone, or otherwise brings about the conditions necessary for the second hormone to be effective, is called a **permissive effect**. Permissive effects are common in behavioral endocrinology.

Hormones are often released in spurts, a process called episodic or **pulsatile secretion**. For example, in male rhesus monkeys, GnRH is released in a pulsatile pattern. Every 45 minutes or so, a quantity of GnRH is released into the hypothalamic–hypophyseal portal system. Shortly thereafter, a pulse of LH is released into the general circulation. Several minutes later, a burst of testosterone is released from the testes, which suppresses further GnRH release for another 45–90 minutes. This pulsatile pattern of hormonal release has functional implications. If one chronically infuses high levels of GnRH into an animal, all of the GnRH receptors are soon occupied, and no further biological action is possible. A hormone-free recovery period during which receptors are replenished is necessary to allow

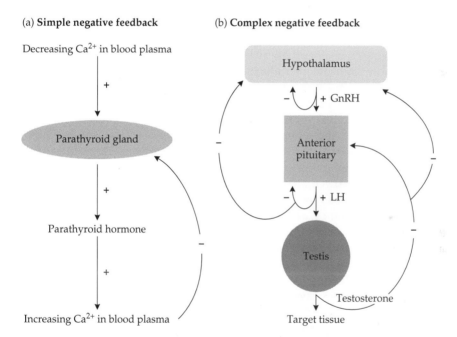

**2.35 Negative feedback.** (a) The parathyroid gland is regulated by a simple negative feedback mechanism. When levels of calcium in the blood decline, the parathyroid gland is stimulated to release parathyroid hormone, which causes blood calcium levels to increase. These increased calcium levels feed back to the parathyroid and inhibit the release of further parathyroid hormone until calcium levels decrease again. (b) A more complex negative feedback relationship exists among the hypothalamus, anterior pituitary, and testes. In response to certain external or endogenous stimuli, the hypothalamus releases GnRH, which stimulates the anterior pituitary to release gonadotropins such as LH. In turn, the secreted LH stimulates steroid synthesis and secretion in the testes. In addition to acting on target tissues, the steroid hormones feed back to inhibit activity in both the anterior pituitary and hypothalamus. In parallel, increasing levels of gonadotropin slow down its secretion from the anterior pituitary and GnRH secretion from the hypothalamus. Likewise, as GnRH is secreted, the hypothalamus responds to increasing levels of the hormone by slowing down its secretion.

a physiological response. The many factors that affect pulse frequency and amplitude will be discussed later in this book in terms of their effects on behavior.

## The Evolution of Hormones

Behavioral endocrinologists are often interested in the phylogenetic relationships among hormones, endocrine gland anatomy, and behavior. Examination of these relationships provides insight into the function and evolution of hormone–behavior interactions. For example, to understand the evolution of hormonal effects on bird vocalization, it might be useful to examine the distribution of steroid hormone receptors throughout the nervous systems of different types of birds that vocalize. Because we can estimate when various bird species diverged from common ancestors, the evolution of various brain centers and their interactions with hormones can be discerned through the use of the comparative method to study diverse bird species, such as roosters, starlings, and parrots. We can learn whether analogous or homologous neural structures are necessary for vocalization in birds, whether these structures serve similar functions in reptiles or amphibians, and whether these structures have retained this function in mammals. Do hormones affect vocalization in all types of birds? If not, which birds are affected by hormones? Is reptilian or amphibian vocalization affected by the same hormones or by different hormones? What about mammals? The comparative method potentially provides insight into many fascinating questions.

In most cases, the evolution of hormones has been an evolution in the *function* of hormones (Table 2.1). The chemical structures of steroid hormones are virtually identical among all vertebrate animals, but the functions of these hormones have changed many times across different species. Some protein hormones have also been conserved over evolutionary time and perform diverse functions. For instance, as noted above, insulin has been found virtually unchanged in species ranging from bacteria to humans (Norman and Litwick, 1987). Point mutations have occurred during the evolution of some other protein hormones, leading to species-specific versions of those hormones (e.g., GnRH; see Figure 2.22).

Peptide hormones have been identified within tissues of flies, worms, protozoans, and even bacteria, but these substances probably function as tissue growth factors; that is, these chemical messengers may have been released intracellularly to regulate cellular growth processes (Hadley, 1996; Norris, 1995). Cell-to-cell communication probably developed during the evolution of multicellular organisms so that processes could be synchronized among the various cells of an organism. Because receptors are necessary to mediate the effects of hormones on target tissues, there was probably simultaneous evolution of both hormones and receptors.

Studying the evolution of hormones, their receptor distributions, and behavior has provided behavioral endocrinologists with clues about how solutions to problems common to all species have evolved. During the process of natural selection, outcomes, not specific mechanisms, are selected. Consequently, vastly different mechanisms leading to similar outcomes have evolved among various species. In the following chapters, many hormone–behavior interactions that have led to increased survival and reproductive success will be described.

**Table 2.1**
## Selected functions of prolactin in nonmammalian animals

| Function | Group | | | |
|---|---|---|---|---|
| | **Fishes** | **Amphibians** | **Reptiles** | **Birds** |
| Reproduction | Growth and secretion of seminal vesicles<br><br>Parental behavior<br><br>Maintenance of brood pouch in male seahorse<br><br>Gonadotropic | Water drive (prior to breeding)<br><br>Secretion of oviductal jelly<br><br>Spermatogenic<br><br>Antispermatogenic<br><br>Ovulatory | Antigonadotropic | Production of "crop milk"<br><br>Formation of brood patch<br><br>Antigonadal<br><br>Parental behavior<br><br>Premigratory restlessness |
| Growth and development | Proliferation of melanocytes<br><br>Growth of seminal vesicles | Tail and gill growth<br><br>Limb regeneration<br><br>Brain growth in tadpoles<br><br>Proliferation of melanophores | Tail regeneration<br><br>Skin shedding | Feather growth<br><br>Epidermal hyperplasia in brood patch<br><br>Development of female reproductive tract |
| Water and electrolyte balance | Skin, buccal, and gill mucus secretion<br><br>Reduced gill $Na^+$ effux<br><br>Reduced gill permeability to water<br><br>Increased urinary water elimination and decreased salt excretion | Skin and electrolyte changes<br><br>Metamorphosis | — | Stimulation of nasal (orbital) salt gland secretion |
| Effects on integumentary structures | Inhibition of gill $Na^+/K^+$ –ATPase<br><br>Dispersal of yellow pigment | Skin yellowing in frogs<br><br>Proliferation of melanophores<br><br>Skin changes associated with water drive | Epidermal sloughing | Stimulation of feather growth<br><br>Stimulation of nasal gland secretion |
| Interactions with steroid-dependent targets or synergisms with steroids | Salt and water movement in gut<br><br>Synergism with androgens in seminal vesicles<br><br>Maintenance of brood pouch in male seahorses | Stimulation of oviductal jelly secretion<br><br>Spermatogenesis<br><br>Cloacal gland development | Antigonadal effects | Formation of brood patch<br><br>Parental behavior<br><br>Synergism with estrogens and progestins on female reproductive tract<br><br>Antigonadal effects |

*Source:* After Norris 1996.

## Summary

- Endocrinology is the study of the endocrine system. Endocrine glands are ductless glands that secrete their products, hormones, directly into the circulatory system. The anatomical locations of the major endocrine glands in humans are depicted in Figure 2.3. Tables listing the hormones and their primary physiological function are provided on the endpapers.

- The hypothalamus is located at the base of the brain. It integrates information from many higher brain sites into blood-borne signals, serving as one of the primary interfaces between the nervous system and the endocrine system. The hypothalamus secretes small peptide hormones that mediate anterior pituitary function. It communicates with the anterior pituitary through a portal blood vessel system, and with the posterior pituitary via nerve cell connections.

- The pituitary gland is really two distinct organs with different embryological origins that are fused together in most vertebrate species. The anterior pituitary produces and releases a number of tropic hormones, as well as protein hormones that regulate the production and release of other hormones and additional physiological processes. Two nonapeptide hormones are typically released from the posterior lobe of the pituitary. Oxytocin regulates smooth muscle contractions during milk letdown and birth; vasopressin monitors osmoregulatory functions.

- The thyroid gland is located in the upper thorax in most vertebrate species, and secretes two hormones in response to thyroid-stimulating hormone from the anterior pituitary. The thyroid hormones, triiodotyrosine and thyroxine, elevate oxidation rates in tissue. Situated in or near the thyroid gland are two additional endocrine structures, the parathyroid gland and the C-cells of the thyroid. These structures secrete protein hormones that regulate blood levels of calcium.

- The pancreas is both an exocrine and an endocrine organ. The endocrine compartment of the pancreas consists of islands of hormone-secreting cells nested throughout the exocrine tissue. These islets of Langerhans contain three cell types that release three different protein hormones: insulin, glucagon, and somatostatin. Insulin is the only hormone that can lower blood glucose levels. Glucagon works in opposition to insulin to elevate blood sugar levels. Somatostatin is an inhibitory hormone.

- The three major peptide gastrointestinal hormones—secretin, gastrin, and cholecystokinin—are secreted from specialized endocrine cells scattered throughout the gastrointestinal tract. These and other gut hormones have also been discovered elsewhere in the body, particularly in the brain, where they may have behavioral effects. In the gut, these hormones mediate the digestion process.

- The adrenal gland consists of two distinct organs. The outer part of the gland, the adrenal cortex, is arranged in three discrete bands of cell types, which secrete three distinct types of steroid hormones: mineralocorticoids, glucocorticoids, and sex steroid hormones. These steroids are primarily involved in mineral and carbohydrate metabolism. The adrenal medulla, or inner part of the gland, produces and releases two monoamine hormones, epinephrine and norepinephrine, which are important in the physiological response to stress.

- The pineal gland functions as a photoreceptor in nonavian and nonmammalian species. The indole amine melatonin is its primary endocrine product in most vertebrates thus far examined. Melatonin has many effects on reproduction, especially in terms of the timing of puberty or seasonal breeding patterns.

- The gonads are the reproductive organs, called testes in males and ovaries in females. The gonads have two major functions: production of gametes and production of sex steroid hormones. These two functions are compartmentalized in different cell types. In the testes, spermatogenesis occurs in the seminiferous tubules. The primary steroidal products of the testes are androgens. The ovaries produce ova (eggs), which develop in follicles in association with estrogen secretion. When the ova are shed from the ovaries during ovulation, the site of rupture develops into another steroid-producing structure called the corpus luteum. The primary steroidal products of corpora lutea are progestins.

- The placenta is a temporary endocrine gland that forms in the uterus of pregnant mammals. The placenta secretes protein and peptide hormones that can affect both the mother and fetus(es).

- There are four classes of hormones: (1) proteins and peptides, (2) steroids, (3) monoamines, and (4) lipid-based hormones. Peptide and protein hormones are made up of amino acid chains of various lengths. Protein hormone receptors are located on the cell surface and usually involve a second messenger to mediate the physiological response to the hormone. Steroid hormones are derived from cholesterol. These molecules are fat-soluble and thus travel through cell membranes easily; steroid receptors are typically found inside the cell.

- Monoamine hormones are derived from a single amino acid, whereas the lipid-based hormones are derived from lipids.

- Hormones are often regulated by negative feedback mechanisms, either by their own levels or those of other hormones or by regulatory physiological processes that involve the end products of the hormone.

## Questions for Discussion

1. Hormones control many aspects of physiology and behavior. Discuss the proposition that hormones themselves are exquisitely controlled substances.

2. One focus of behavioral endocrinology has been on correlating the blood concentrations of hormones with behavior. Recently, this focus has shifted to target tissue sensitivity to hormones. To what extent are hormone receptor numbers important in understanding hormone–behavior interactions?

3. How are comparative studies useful in understanding hormone–behavior interactions? Are there any negative consequences of comparative analyses?

4. Suggest a series of circumstances that might account for males having excess blood concentrations of estrogens. What endocrine errors might account for females having high circulating androgen concentrations?

## Suggested Readings

Brown, R. E. 1994. *An Introduction to Neuroendocrinology.* Cambridge University Press, Cambridge.

Ganong, W. F. 1997. *Review of Medical Physiology.* 18th edition. Lange, Los Altos, CA.

Gass, G. H. and Kaplan, H. M. 1996. *Handbook of Endocrinology.* CRC Press, Boca Raton, FL.

Griffin, J. E. and Ojeda, S. R. 1992. *Textbook of Endocrine Physiology.* Oxford University Press, New York.

Knobil, E. and Neill, J. D. 1994. *The Physiology of Reproduction.* Raven Press, New York.

Levy, A. and Lightman, S. L. 1997. *Endocrinology.* Oxford University Press, Oxford.

Norman, A. W. and Litwack, G. 1987. *Hormones.* Academic Press, New York.

Norris, D. O. 1996. *Vertebrate Endocrinology.* 3rd edition. Academic Press, New York.

# 3

# Sex Differences in Behavior

## Sex Determination and Differentiation

**B**oys and girls are different. Humans, like many animals, are sexually dimorphic (*di*, "two"; *morph*, "type") in the size and shape of their bodies, their physiology, and their behavior. The behavior of boys and girls differs in many ways. Girls generally excel in verbal abilities relative to boys; boys are nearly twice as likely as girls to suffer from dyslexia (reading difficulties) and stuttering. Boys are generally better than girls at tasks that require visuospatial abilities. Girls engage in nurturing behaviors more frequently than boys. Over 90% of all anorexia nervosa cases involve young women. Young men are twice as likely to suffer from schizophrenia as young women. Boys are much more aggressive and generally engage in more rough-and-tumble play than girls (Hines, 1982; Ruble and Martin, 1998). Many sex differences, such as the difference in aggressiveness, persist throughout adulthood. For example, there are many more men than women serving prison sentences for violent behavior. What accounts for these sex differences?

Behavioral endocrinologists, like most people, are interested in these and other behavioral sex differences. What are the proximate causes of behavioral sex differences? This question is one version of the enduring nature-versus-nurture question. As you probably already know, all behavior results from an interaction between environmental factors, including learning and cultural influences (nurture), and biological factors, including genes and physiological influences (nature). Students of behavioral endocrinology try to discern the extent to which the behavioral differences between males and females are mediated by environmental influences, including social interactions, and the extent to which they are mediated by physiological factors, especially hormones. Separating these influences can be difficult. Sex differences in some behaviors, such as snoring, are probably due exclusively to biological factors, whereas other behaviors, such as style of haircut, appear to reflect only cultural influences. But what about the pattern of play behavior? Is the difference in the frequency of rough-and-tumble play between boys and girls due to biological factors associated with being male or female, or due to cultural expectations and learning? If there is a combination of biological and cultural influences mediating the frequency of rough-and-tumble play, then what proportion of the variation between the sexes is due to biological factors and what proportion is due to social influences?

It is easy to speculate on these questions in a casual manner. Visit any preschool and watch three- or four-year-old children at play. Even when gender-neutral toys are provided, boys tend to play aggressive, rowdy games, whereas girls tend to engage in play activities in which cooperation is often valued. Again, are these differences mediated by biological influences or due to cultural influences? Perhaps children learn sexually dimorphic modes of behavior from TV or from their friends at nursery school—boys play with guns and trucks and girls play with dolls and tea sets. Of course, it is easy to produce examples of girls who enjoy rough-and-tumble play, and boys who enjoy playing nurturing roles. However, producing examples to support one's contentions is not the most effective way to determine the causes of a particular phenomenon. In order to ascertain the true causes underlying behavior, all biases must be eliminated from the data-gathering process. The most effective manner of obtaining information about an adequately described phenomenon is via the experimental method, primarily through the use of inductive reasoning (Platt, 1964).

Behavioral endocrinologists are particularly interested in the extent to which hormones mediate behavioral sex differences because it is known that steroid hormone concentrations differ between males and females from almost the first trimester of gestation. However, it is extremely difficult to ascertain the proximate factors underlying sex differences in human behavior experimentally. Although the critical experiments can be designed, they cannot ethically be performed on humans. Tracking hormone concentrations during sexual differentiation in utero could jeopardize the well-being of the fetus. To assess the role of hormones in rough-and-tumble play, children would have to be castrated and receive hormonal replacement therapy. Other children would have to be reared in social isolation to assess the contribution of social factors to aggressive play. Obviously, such studies are not possible. However, indirect evidence has been obtained from many converging sources that can help us to understand the behavioral differences between human males and females.

Three strategies that do not require experimentation on humans have been used to explore questions about the origin of human behavioral sex differences. First, animal models have been used to study **sexual differentiation**, the developmental process of becoming male or female, which occurs before or immediately after hatching or birth. The study of nonhuman mammals has established that hormone concentrations during sexual differentiation guide the development of many physiological, morphological, and behavioral characteristics that are displayed later in life. The second strategy has involved studies of people or nonhuman animals that have undergone anomalous sexual differentiation. For example, studying the behavior of girls who were exposed to a male-typical hormonal milieu in utero helps to separate the contribution of rearing conditions from the hormonal factors that may underlie behavioral sex differences. Finally, because child-rearing practices vary so greatly among different cultures, anthropologists, psychologists, and sociologists have looked for universal commonalities in the behavior of all children. Studies of sex differences in behavior that emerge consistently regardless of rearing conditions suggest that some such differences—in aggressive behavior, for example—are mediated by biological factors (Hines, 1982). Although this third approach will not be reviewed in great depth here, such behavioral surveys have indicated that several behaviors in humans may have significant biological bases that could override social effects. Of course, one could argue that human parents may universally treat their sons differently from their daughters and induce the sex differences in emitted behaviors. This argument is hard to refute because experimental controls are infrequent in long-term developmental studies of human behavior. Consequently, nonhuman animal studies have generally proved to be superior to human studies for understanding the sex differences underlying behavior because of the possibility for greater experimental control.

## Sex Determination and Differentiation

What is sex? What makes you male or female? There are several different ways to answer this very basic question (Figure 3.1). First, there is **chromosomal sex**, determined by the sex chromosomes the individual receives at fertilization. The homogametic sex in mammals is female (XX), whereas the heterogametic sex is male (XY). Chromosomal sex is fundamental during the process of sexual differentiation, and drives **gonadal sex**: the possession of either ovaries or testes. Females have ovaries, whereas males have testes. Gonadal sex is related to **gametic sex**. The ovaries of females produce large, immobile, resource-rich gametes called ova or eggs; the testes of males produce small, mobile, gametes called sperm. Females and males also differ on the basis of **hormonal sex**. Females of most vertebrate species tend to have high estrogen to androgen ratios of circulating steroid hormone concentrations; males have the opposite pattern. **Morphological sex** refers to the differences in body type between males and females. Male mammals are typically larger than females, and possess different external genitalia. In addition to size, males of many species differ from females in coloration, the presence of horns, antlers, and other ornamentation, and body shape. **Behavioral sex** can be

**3.1 Levels of sex determination.** Chromosomal sex, which is determined at conception, determines which gonads form in the embryonic individual. Gonadal sex determines the hormonal environment in which the fetus develops, and steers morphological development in a male or female direction. The resulting sex differences in the central nervous system and in some effector organs lead to the behavioral sex differences observed in later life.

discriminated on the basis of male-typical and female-typical behaviors. For example, females of many species often care for young, whereas males, especially male mammals, rarely provide parental care (see Chapter 7). Male and female birds of many species share equally in parental care, but they display other types of behavioral sex differences. For example, males of many avian species sing, but their female conspecifics do not.

Additional categories of sex classification exist among humans. For example, **gender identity** reflects the sex, or gender, that individuals feel themselves to be; gender identity usually corresponds to the expression of a **gender role**, a culturally based summary of behavioral sex differences. Finally, there is **legal sex**. You are recognized by governmental agencies as male or female because of an "M" or "F" on your driver's license, or some other official document. If individuals sporting "M" identification documents enter a women's rest room, they can be arrested in most parts of North America, even if they are exhibiting female-typical behavior (for example, wearing a silk evening dress). Sex differences occur at each of these organizational levels.

### Ultimate Causes of Sex Differences

Most of the animals with which you are familiar engage in sexual reproduction. In fact, most animal species currently on the planet engage in sexual reproduction. However, a survey of the entire animal kingdom reveals that many animals, especially insect species, breed asexually. There are several forms of asexual reproduction. The process of asexual reproduction among vertebrate animals is called **parthenogenesis**. In asexual vertebrate reproduction, there is only one sex: female. Parthenogenetic females produce genetically identical eggs that develop into female offspring that are all genetically identical to their mother. From the Darwinian perspective, reproductive success reflects the amount of genetic material an individual contributes to subsequent generations. Thus, asexual reproduction may seem like an extremely efficient system. This mode of breeding must have some distinct disadvantages, however, because so many animals breed sexually. One hypothesis about why asexual reproduction is rare among vertebrates is that asexual individuals, because they have such similar genotypes, provide lit-tle variation on which natural selection can act. Thus, if the conditions of its envi-ronment change, an asexual species could become extinct. Sexual reproduction, through the separation of chromosome pairs into haploid gametes and their recombination in each offspring, provides genetic variability and hence evolu-tionary flexibility (Howard and Lively, 1994). Those animals and plants that have the option of either sexual or asexual reproduction usually opt for sexual repro-duction when the environment becomes unstable. By analogy, would you rather have 100 lottery tickets with the same number or 50 tickets, each with a slightly different number? Another problem that can burden asexual species is the increased likelihood that pathogens may become specialized to exploit a single genotype (Ewald, 1994). Because pathogens reproduce faster than their hosts, they could rapidly evolve ways to override the immunological defenses of their hosts (Judson, 1997; Ladle et al., 1993). By shuffling the genetic material, host species reduce the odds that pathogens will be preadapted to exploit their offspring.

Sexually reproducing species have two sexes: male and female. Why do the two sexes differ in appearance and behavior? In other words, what are the *ulti-mate* causes of the behavioral differences between males and females? We cannot travel back in time to watch the slow evolution of sexual dimorphisms in a given species and note the ecological or social factors associated with the development of sex differences. But we can address these "why questions" by examining present-day species that show little or no sexual dimorphism and comparing them with species that are sexually dimorphic. When these comparisons are made, a striking relationship between sexual dimorphism and mating system becomes obvious. Species that are monogamous (have a single mating partner) display less sexual dimorphism than species that are polygamous (have multiple mating partners) (Trivers, 1972). In polygamous species, in which members of one sex compete to mate with the other sex, **sexual selection** may act to favor certain behavioral or morphological traits (Andersson, 1994).

Sexual selection is a subcategory of natural selection (Andersson, 1994; Trivers, 1972). Generally, the rule among animal species is that males compete and females choose. For instance, female deer choose to mate with bucks that con-trol the largest feeding areas (intersexual selection). Bucks obtain feeding areas prior to the breeding season by fighting among themselves and establishing a social hierarchy (intrasexual selection). The largest bucks usually have the largest antlers, and they typically win the most fights, move to the top of the hierarchy, and control the best feeding areas. Thus they are able to mate with the most females and pass on their genes to the most offspring (Lincoln et al., 1972). Consequently, females indirectly select for males with large body and antler size, as well as for aggressive behavior. Because males typically compete for females, they are usually bigger, more colorful, and more aggressive than females. In species in which the sex roles are reversed and females compete with one anoth-er for males (Box 3.1), the females are typically larger and more colorful than their male conspecifics (Trivers, 1972). Thus, sexual selection favors and probably amplifies sexual dimorphisms over time (Zahavi and Zahavi, 1997).

Although monogamy is asserted to be the most common mating system prac-ticed by humans (*Homo sapiens*) in Western societies, examination of many soci-eties suggests that humans are mildly to strongly polygynous; that is, each male

Box 3.1
# Behavioral Sex Role Reversals

In virtually every mammalian and avian species studied, males are more aggressive, weigh more, are more likely to establish and defend breeding territories, and (particularly among mammals) are less likely to provide parental care to the young than their female conspecifics. There are several notable exceptions to this dogma, however, and the study of these unusual cases is useful for shedding light on the more typical situation as well as for understanding how far the "generalities" of the interaction between hormones and behavior can be relied upon.

Female spotted hyenas (*Crocuta crocuta*) are socially dominant: in addition to eliciting submissive postures and vocalizations from males, they are also allowed first access to food (Frank, 1986; Kruuk, 1972). In addition to their masculinized behavior, females have masculinized external genitalia. Indeed, the species was once thought to be hermaphroditic because all individuals, even nursing mothers, possess scrota and penislike structures. The photographs show external genitalia of male (below, left) and female (right) hyenas. The vaginal labia in spotted hyenas are fused to form a fat-filled pseudoscrotum. The clitoris develops into a pseudopenis through which the urogenital tract passes. Females urinate, copulate, and deliver young through the urogenital tract. The pseudopenis possesses full erectile function, and both males and females routinely display erections as part of their social interac-

tions (Glickman et al., 1987). Erectile function in both sexes is observed from infancy. The extreme masculinization of female behavior and morphology appears to be organized by high maternal concentrations of ovarian androstenedione in pregnant females, which is converted to testosterone by the placenta (Glickman et al., 1987, 1992). Adult males exhibit higher androgen concentrations than adult females. Thus, adult concentrations of androgens do not appear to account for the difference in social dominance (see Chapter 10).

Spotted sandpipers (*Actitis macularia*) are birds that display atypical sex roles. Females establish and defend a feeding territory and engage in mate competition with other females for access to males (Fivizzani and Oring, 1986). Males incubate the eggs and brood the young with little or no assistance from the female. Prior to incubation, blood plasma concentrations of testosterone and dihydrotestosterone are substantially higher in males than in females. As incubation proceeds, testosterone levels in males plummet 25-fold. Mated females exhibit testosterone concentrations that are 7-fold higher than those of unmated females (Fivizzani and Oring, 1986). These hormone profiles are similar to those of other avian species in which males assist with care of the young. Thus, the reversal of sex roles in spotted sandpipers appears to be unrelated to adult hormone effects.

Photographs courtesy of Stephen Glickman.

may mate with more than one female (Alexander et al., 1979; Daly and Wilson, 1983; Martin and May, 1981; Murdock, 1967). Approximately 700 out of 850 human societies described in an extensive ethnographic catalog practiced polygyny (Murdock, 1967). Furthermore, as noted above, the sex differences observed among humans are atypical for monogamous animals, but are common in polygynous and promiscuous species. Human sexual dimorphisms include larger body size and strength (Alexander et al., 1979), later puberty (Bronson, 1988; Tanner, 1962), and higher mortality rates (Shapiro et al., 1968) in men than in women. Importantly, cross-cultural studies of humans have revealed *behavioral* sexual dimorphisms that are also consistent with those of other polygynous species, including increased courtship activity (Daly and Wilson, 1983), higher levels of aggression (Moyer, 1976), and reduced parental care (Clutton-Brock, 1991) in males as compared with females. Thus, the morphological, physiological, and behavioral differences between men and women may reflect the evolutionary history of the species' most common mating pattern, namely, polygyny.

Again, we cannot go back in time to test these ultimate hypotheses, but we can use them to make predictions about current behaviors, and we can conduct animal experiments designed to rule out our predictions. For example, males of polygynous species typically move around over larger areas than conspecific females or males of monogamous species, presumably because wandering around increases their chances of finding additional mates. One might predict that females and males of monogamous species will have poorer direction-finding skills or spatial aptitudes in general than males of these wide-ranging polygynous species. This prediction appears to be true when tested. Males of polygynous species, including rats, mice, meadow voles (a small field mouse; *Microtus pennsylvanicus*), and humans, are superior in spatial aptitudes to females of the same species (see below). Moreover, male meadow voles are superior in spatial abilities (navigating a maze) to male pine voles (*Microtus pinetorum*), a monogamous species of the same genus (Gaulin and FitzGerald, 1986).

The ultimate level of explanation is useful for guiding predictions about the proximate mechanisms that cause males and females to behave differently. The remainder of this chapter will review the proximate processes of sex determination and sexual differentiation. In other words, *how* do sexually dimorphic behaviors arise?

### Proximate Causes of Sex Differences

Because behavioral sex differences are so ubiquitous among animals, behavioral endocrinologists have focused significant effort on studying this phenomenon. One very important concept developed to guide this effort is the so-called **organizational/activational hypothesis**. This fundamental hypothesis of how hormones guide behavioral sex differences will be presented within its historical context. Basically, the organizational/activational hypothesis suggests that behavioral sex differences result from (1) differential exposure to hormones that act early in development to organize the neural machinery underlying the behaviors and (2) differential exposure to sex steroid hormones later in life that activate the neural circuitry previously organized. The workings of this process in several animal models commonly used to study behavioral sex differences will be described in detail below. Sex differences in brain structures, how these differences arise, and how these differences might mediate behavioral differences between males and females will also be reviewed in this chapter, as well as in Chapter 4.

A number of clinical syndromes exist among humans and nonhuman animals that cause anomalies in the process of sexual differentiation. Many of these syndromes are congenital; others are the result of endocrine treatment during gestation. The behavioral consequences resulting from these developmental irregularities in humans, as well as from animal studies in which these clinical syndromes are simulated, will be presented in this chapter. Issues of gender, sex role, and sexual orientation among humans, as well as cognitive sex differences, will be explored in Chapter 4.

There are real and substantial differences between males and females. Some of these sex differences may be apparent at birth; others appear later in development. Our goal is to understand how behavioral sex differences are mediated. But in order to do this, it is necessary to understand sexual differentiation in general. If we limit our discussion to mammals and birds, then basically, chromosomal sex determines gonadal sex, and all subsequent sexual differentiation is normally the result of differential exposure to gonadal steroid hormones. Thus, gonadal sex determines hormonal sex, which in turn influences morphological sex. Morphological differences in the central nervous system, as well as in some effector organs, lead to behavioral sex differences (see Figure 3.1). To understand the specifics of how sexually dimorphic behaviors arise, a discussion of embryology is necessary. This discussion will yield a rationale for the principles underlying behavioral sex differences.

## Mammalian Sexual Differentiation

The primary step in the process of mammalian sex differentiation occurs at fertilization. An ovum can be fertilized by a sperm bearing either an X or a Y chromosome. This event, called **sex determination**, has far-reaching consequences for the differentiation of the embryonic gonads, as well as subsequent behavioral differences. Each individual embryonic mammal, whether XX or XY, exhibits a thickened ridge of tissue on the ventromedial surface of each mesonephros (protokidney), known as the **germinal ridge** (Figure 3.2; Jost, 1979). At this stage, this embryonic gonad is said to be **indifferent** or **bipotential**. Whether the germinal ridge will develop into a testis or an ovary is determined by the cellular expression of the **testis determination factor**—a protein encoded by a gene known as *SRY* (sex-determining region on the Y chromosome) (Berta et al., 1990). The *SRY* gene is expressed in the indifferent gonads. It encodes the testis determination factor—a protein that binds to a specific hormone response element in the promoter region of other genes that it regulates (Harley and Goodfellow, 1995). When the protein products of these genes are produced, the middle (medulla) of the germinal ridge develops, and a testis forms (Berta et al., 1990). If the *SRY* gene is not expressed, then the outer part of the ridge (the cortex) develops, and an ovary is formed. It is possible for the *SRY* gene to be expressed in one gonad but not in the other, which leads to unilateral differentiation: in other words, a testis develops on one side while an ovary develops on the other side, suggesting that the testis determination factor functions only locally and is not a blood-borne agent. Partial expression of the *SRY* gene can lead to incomplete gonadal differ-

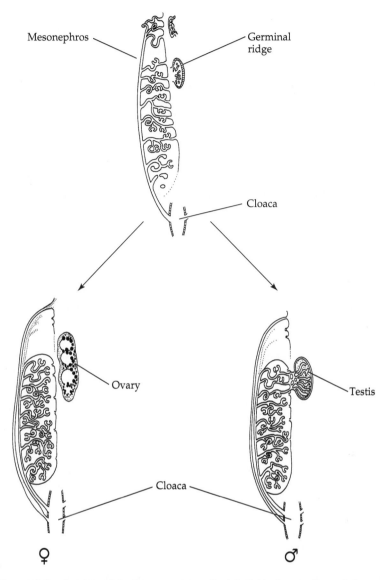

**3.2    Gonadal development of the human embryo.** Each individual, regardless of chromosomal sex, develops a thickening called the germinal ridge on the ventromedial surface of each mesonephros (protokidney). The germinal ridge is a bipotential gonad; it can become either an ovary or a testis. If the SRY gene is present and the testis determination factor (TDF) protein is expressed, the medulla of the protogonad develops, forming a testis. If no SRY gene is present, and TDF is not expressed, the cortex of the protogonad develops, and an ovary is formed.

entiation, yielding an ovotestis. Mice that are chromosomal XY males but do not have the *SRY* gene develop ovaries; similarly, XX transgenic mice into which an *SRY* gene has been inserted develop testes (Goodfellow and Lovell-Badge, 1993; McElreavey et al., 1995). In reptiles and birds, *SRY* is not a testis-determining gene.

Hormonal secretions from the developing gonads determine whether the individual develops in a male or female manner. The mammalian embryonic testes produce androgens, as well as peptide hormones, that steer the development of the body, central nervous system, and subsequent behavior in a male direction. The embryonic ovaries of mammals are virtually quiescent and do not secrete high concentrations of hormones (but see Arnold and Breedlove, 1985; Döhler et al., 1982). In the presence of ovaries, or *in the complete absence of any gonads*, morphological, neural, and, later, behavioral development follow a female pathway. (As we will see, however, low estrogen concentrations are probably required for *normal* female CNS and behavioral development.) Thus, the prevailing hypothesis about the initiation of sexual differentiation indicates that the gonads are differentiated by genetic influences (*SRY*), and that all other sexual differentiation reflects hormonal mediation. However, it is possible that some sex differences in brain and behavior might be mediated more directly by gene expression in nongonadal tissue (Arnold, 1996). For example, the *SRY* gene is transcribed in the hypothalamus and midbrain of adult male mice (Lahr et al., 1995). It is possible that these gene transcripts are translated, but there has yet to be a demonstration of such translation. Because only genetic males possess a Y chromosome, any gene located on the Y chromosome that may be involved in neural development is a candidate to mediate sex differences in brain and behavior directly, without invoking an endocrine mediator.

In contrast to the single, bipotential primordial gonad, dual anlagen (primordia) for the accessory sex organs are present early during ontogeny (Figure 3.3). The **Müllerian duct** system develops into the female accessory sex organs, which serve to connect the ovaries to the outside environment. The Müllerian duct system develops into the fallopian tubes, uterus, and cervix. The **Wolffian duct** system develops into the male accessory sex organs, which serve to connect the testes to the outside environment via the penis. Later-developing components of the Wolffian duct system include the seminal vesicles and vas deferens. During normal sexual differentiation, the Wolffian duct system develops in males, whereas the Müllerian duct system regresses. Conversely, in females, the Müllerian duct system develops, whereas the Wolffian duct system regresses. In humans, this process occurs during the first trimester of gestation.

In the presence of ovaries or in the complete absence of gonads, normal development of the Müllerian ducts is accompanied by complete regression of the Wolffian duct system. Again, no hormones are necessary to permit normal female development among mammals. Male development of the secondary sex organs requires two products from the embryonic testes: testosterone and a peptide hormone called **Müllerian inhibitory hormone (MIH)**. Testosterone is necessary to stimulate Wolffian duct development. Müllerian inhibitory hormone, as its name implies, causes the regression of the Müllerian duct system. If testosterone is absent early in development, then Wolffian duct development fails to occur. If MIH is not secreted at the proper time, then the Müllerian duct system develops. Because of the twin anlagen, it is possible for both systems to develop in a single individual.

In order for normal female morphological development of the accessory sex organs to occur, the embryo must become feminized (Müllerian duct development), as well as demasculinized (Wolffian duct regression). Normal male devel-

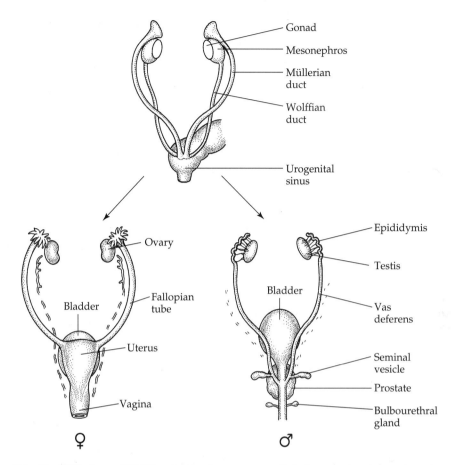

**3.3   The Müllerian and Wolffian duct systems** are normally both present early in embryonic development. In the absence of testicular hormones, the Müllerian duct system develops into the fallopian tubes, uterus, and upper vagina, and the Wolffian ducts regress. This is the normal course of events in female mammals. When testicular hormones are present, as is normally the case in male mammals, the Wolffian ducts eventually develop into the seminal vesicles and vas deferens, and the Müllerian ducts regress. Because anlagen for each of these duct systems are initially present in the embryo, it is possible in some circumstances for both systems to develop in a single individual.

opment requires both masculinization (Wolffian duct development) and defeminization (Müllerian duct regression). In other words, sexual differentiation of the accessory sex organs proceeds along two continua: (1) a masculinization–demasculinization scale and (2) a feminization–defeminization scale (Figure 3.4). **Masculinization** is the induction of male traits; **feminization** is the induction of female traits. **Demasculinization** is the removal of the potential for male traits, whereas **defeminization** is the removal of the potential for female traits. This nomenclature will be important for describing behavioral sex differences as well.

The difference in external genitalia is the most obvious difference between the sexes at birth and has been used for generations to assign the sex of humans. During embryological development, the urogenital sinus is surrounded on both

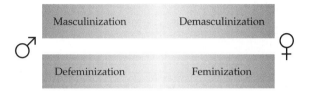

**3.4   Normal development of the accessory sex organs** occurs along two continua. Normal females must become feminized (Müllerian duct development) as well as demasculinized (Wolffian duct regression). Normal males must become masculinized (Wolffian duct development) as well as defeminized (Müllerian duct regression). Thus, sexual dimorphism in accessory sex organs, as well as in many behaviors, requires development along two separate continua, a masculinization–demasculinization continuum and a feminization–defeminization continuum.

sides by long thickened urogenital ridges that are flanked by two flaps of skin called the **genital folds** (Figure 3.5). In front of (anteroventral to) the urogenital opening, the two ridges meet to form a median outgrowth called the **genital tubercle**. The genital tubercle and folds are common to both sexes, and develop

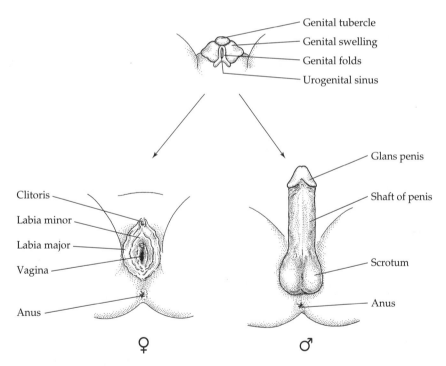

**3.5   Embryonic development of human external genitalia.**   During development, a single anlage for the external genitalia, called the genital tubercle, forms in front of the urogenital sinus. The urogenital ridges are flanked by two flaps of skin called the genital folds. In the absence of hormonal influence, a clitoris develops from the genital tubercle and the genital folds become the vaginal labia. In the presence of androgens, the urethral groove fuses, the genital tubercle develops into a penis, and the genital folds fuse into the scrotum.

**3.6   Normal development of the external genitalia** proceeds along a single masculine–feminine continuum. Because there is a single anlage for female and male external genitalia, the development of one type of genitalia precludes the development of the other.

into the external genitalia. Female humans, as well as many other species of mammals, possess a clitoris and vaginal labia, which develop from the genital tubercle and genital folds respectively. Males possess a penis, which develops from the genital tubercle, and a scrotal sac, which results from the fusing of the genital folds and eventually contains the testes. Consequently, development of one type of genitalia occurs at the expense of the other type. In other words, a single continuum of feminine to masculine external genitalia development exists (Figure 3.6).

Androgens are responsible for the differentiation of the external genitalia. In the absence of hormones, a clitoris develops from the genital tubercle and the vaginal labia develop from the genital folds. In the presence of androgens, the urethral groove fuses, the genital tubercle develops into a penis, and the genital folds fuse into the scrotum (Wilson et al., 1981). One of the androgenic metabolites of testosterone, 5α-dihydrotestosterone (DHT), is critical for this process of genital fusing. Testosterone is converted to DHT by an enzyme called **5α-reductase**, which is locally abundant in the embryonic genital skin of both females and males (Wilson et al., 1981). If unusually high concentrations of androgens are available to a female fetus, DHT conversion in the genital skin occurs, and the development of male-typical external genitalia proceeds. Males that congenitally lack the 5α-reductase enzyme undergo incomplete differentiation of the external genitalia and may be assigned the incorrect sex at birth (see Figure 3.11). Females that lack the 5α-reductase enzyme suffer no grave consequences, because normal female genital development occurs in the absence of sex steroid hormones.

### Anomalous Mammalian Sexual Differentiation

The process of mammalian sexual differentiation is summarized in Figure 3.7. This process is complex, and, as the case of 5α-reductase deficiency shows, the potential for error is present. People and nonhuman animals that have undergone such anomalous sexual differentiation are of interest to behavioral endocrinologists because they can serve as "experiments of nature," and, as such, they can provide important information about the workings of the normal process of sexual differentiation.

Errors in sexual differentiation have been recognized by humans since early in their history. One very old idea was that male babies came from the right testis and females came from the left. **Hermaphrodites**, individuals who possess both ovaries and testes, were thought to arise when both testes simultaneously contributed to the offspring. All human babies born with ambiguous genital development used to be called hermaphrodites (Ellis, 1945), but they are now considered

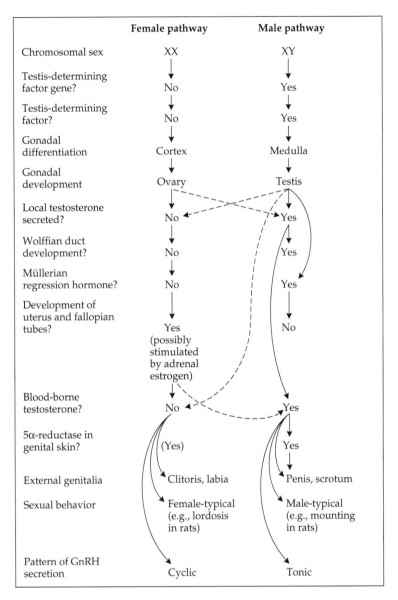

|  | Female pathway | Male pathway |
|---|---|---|
| Chromosomal sex | XX | XY |
| Testis-determining factor gene? | No | Yes |
| Testis-determining factor? | No | Yes |
| Gonadal differentiation | Cortex | Medulla |
| Gonadal development | Ovary | Testis |
| Local testosterone secreted? | No | Yes |
| Wolffian duct development? | No | Yes |
| Müllerian regression hormone? | No | Yes |
| Development of uterus and fallopian tubes? | Yes (possibly stimulated by adrenal estrogen) | No |
| Blood-borne testosterone? | No | Yes |
| 5α-reductase in genital skin? | (Yes) | Yes |
| External genitalia | Clitoris, labia | Penis, scrotum |
| Sexual behavior | Female-typical (e.g., lordosis in rats) | Male-typical (e.g., mounting in rats) |
| Pattern of GnRH secretion | Cyclic | Tonic |

**3.7  Sexual differentiation in humans** is complex, and there are several stages where errors can occur. Chromosomal sex determination takes place when an egg is fertilized by a Y- or X-bearing sperm. The normal developmental pathways for females and males are indicated by the solid lines; common developmental errors are indicated by the dotted lines, which show where individuals can be "shunted" onto the developmental pathway of the opposite chromosomal sex.

to be **pseudohermaphrodites**, because only one set of gonads is usually present. True hermaphrodites, with two sets of gonads, are extremely rare.

**ANOMALIES IN FEMALES.**    The female organization is basic among mammals. Because females are the so-called "neutral" or "default" sex, neither ovaries nor hormones are necessary for female development of the body prior to puberty. However, it is becoming increasingly clear that low concentrations of estrogens are critical for normal development of the female brain (Döhler and Hancke, 1978; Döhler et al., 1982; Toran-Allerand, 1984).

One out of every 3000 live births in humans exhibits **Turner syndrome**, characterized by a congenital lack of, or damage to, the second X (or a Y) chromosome (XO) (Figure 3.8; Zinn et al., 1993). Individuals with Turner syndrome are unambiguously sexed as girls at birth. The gonads rarely develop completely, but they are clearly recognizable as ovaries. The dysgenic ovaries fail to produce steroid hormones, however, so girls with Turner syndrome must be treated with sex steroid hormones in their mid-teens to induce puberty. The consequences of missing a second sex chromosome are widespread and are not limited to sexual differentiation. Additional endocrine problems associated with Turner syndrome are reflected in the slow growth rates of afflicted girls. Both neural and non-neural tissue are also affected; hearing loss and mental retardation, as well as kidney dysfunction and webbing of the neck, are observed in some individuals born with Turner syndrome. These individuals are of interest to behavioral endocrinologists because they are not exposed to steroid hormones prenatally or postnatally until the age of 16 or 17, when exogenous hormonal treatments begin.

Recently, an intriguing study was conducted that examined the role of gene imprinting on behavior in girls with Turner syndrome. Because females normally inherit one X chromosome from their mother and another X chromosome from their father, one of the X chromosomes in each cell is usually disabled so that normal transcription can occur. The process of inactivating either the maternal or paternal genes is called gene imprinting. Girls with Turner syndrome have only a

**3.8  Turner syndrome** results from a congenital absence of one of the X chromosomes. Without hormone therapy, these individuals do not undergo puberty. This 21-year-old XO woman is shown prior to estrogen therapy, and exhibits the short stature associated with the syndrome; however, she does not display other possible symptoms of Turner syndrome, such as webbed skin on the neck. Courtesy of John Money.

single X chromosome, which is either maternal ($X^m$) or paternal ($X^p$). $X^m$O girls tend to suffer from neurodevelopmental disorders of social cognition (e.g., autism) more than $X^p$O girls (Skuse et al., 1997). Because the X chromosome of all males necessarily comes from the mother, these results suggest that the vulnerability of males to cognition and social adjustment problems is not necessarily due to the presence of specific genes on the Y chromosome, but could rather be due to genes on the maternal X chromosome (which presumably act independently of sex steroid hormones). Alternatively, it is possible that pieces of the Y chromosome might be expressed in neural tissue to cause these behavioral difficulties because many individuals with Turner syndrome are so-called genetic mosaics (Henn and Zang, 1997), possessing cells with differing genetic contents. This issue will probably go unresolved for some time because it is virtually impossible to observe the chromosomal makeup of brain cells in living people (Skuse and Jacobs, 1997).

The most common reason for anomalous sexual differentiation in human females is prenatal exposure to androgens, either from exogenous or endogenous sources. Exogenous androgen exposure most commonly occurs during treatment of the pregnant mother with steroid hormones to maintain the pregnancy. Exposure to the artificial steroid hormones diethylstilbestrol (DES) and medroxy-progesterone acetate (MPA), for instance, often causes masculinization of reproductive function and subsequent behavior in the exposed children (see Chapter 4). Endogenous androgens are most likely to be secreted from one of two sources: the ovaries or the adrenal glands. For example, both males and females afflicted with congenital adrenal hyperplasia (CAH) possess fetal adrenal glands that produce high concentrations of androgens instead of cortisol. This does not cause sexual development problems in genetic males, but results in moderate to severe masculinization of the genitalia in afflicted females (Figure 3.9). The clitoris is enlarged into a penis-sized structure, and the labia may be fused into a scrotum-like organ. The anomalous genitalia can be corrected at birth by surgery, and the endocrine disorder can be treated by lifelong cortisol treatments.

**ANOMALIES IN MALES.**   There are more steps that require physiological intervention in male than in female sexual differentiation, and consequently more clinical problems in male sexual development can occur. For example, some XY individuals look and act like males throughout their lives, but during surgery for abdominal cramps, a uterus and small fallopian tubes are discovered. These individuals lack either Müllerian regression hormone or the receptors that respond to this hormone; all other components of their sexual differentiation are male-typical. This sort of error in sexual differentiation does not have important consequences for male behavior, but in other cases anomalous sexual differentiation produces dramatic behavioral effects.

Anomalous sexual differentiation occurs in XY individuals afflicted with androgen insensitivity syndrome, a condition also known as **testicular feminization mutation (TFM)**. The tissues of individuals with TFM do not possess functional androgen receptors. A genetic mutation on the X chromosome involving a single base pair substitution in the gene for the androgen receptor causes this insensitivity to androgens in rats (Yarbrough et al., 1990). Genetic XX females with this mutation have a second X chromosome that contains the normal gene for androgen receptors, so they suffer no ill effects from this condition. However, in genetic XY males, because a Y chromosome is present, the *SRY* gene is activated

**3.9    Partial masculinization** of the external genitalia in genetic females can be caused by prenatal exposure to progestins or by congenital adrenal hyperplasia (CAH). (Left) The mother of this individual was treated with progestins to prevent miscarriage after suffering symptoms of premature labor. Note the enlarged clitoris and fusing of the vaginal labia. (Right) Congenital adrenal hyperplasia, a condition in which the adrenal glands of genetic females secrete high levels of androgens, can cause varying degrees of masculinization of the external genitalia, including clitoral enlargement and fusing of the urethral groove. Courtesy of John Money.

and testicular development proceeds, accompanied by significant prenatal and postnatal androgen secretion. The testes also produce Müllerian regression hormone, which causes the regression of the Müllerian duct system. However, the Wolffian duct system is not stimulated to develop, even in the presence of androgens. In humans, there are several mutations that cause androgen insensitivity (Brinkmann et al., 1996). XY individuals born with TFM have perfectly normal-appearing female external genitalia and are sexed and reared as girls. The condition is usually discovered during adolescence when menstruation fails to occur. Upon examination, the vagina is discovered to be reduced in length. Because the Müllerian ducts failed to develop in these individuals, there are no uteri or fallopian tubes, and unfortunately, they are sterile. The testes are usually removed surgically and estrogen treatment is provided, although this treatment has been questioned by some individuals who have received it. Genetic male XY individuals with TFM display normal female body shapes and regard themselves unequivocally as female (Figure 3.10).

Behavioral endocrinologists are interested in TFM because this genetic defect has been discovered in several nonhuman species, including rats, mice, cattle, and

**3.10   Testicular feminization mutation (TFM)** is a condition caused by an absence of functional androgen receptors in genetic male (XY) individuals. Because individuals with TFM lack androgen receptors, the functional ratio of estrogens to androgens is high, and puberty, including development of secondary sexual characteristics, proceeds in a feminine direction. Although individuals with TFM exhibit a normal female body morphology, the gonads are testes, and the internal duct organs do not develop normally, resulting in sterility. Courtesy of John Money.

chimpanzees (Olsen, 1992), allowing experimental study of its physiological mechanisms. Also, individuals with TFM have normal receptors for, and normal concentrations of, the nonandrogenic hormones (such as estrogen) involved in sex differentiation, and thus provide researchers with the ability to separate the contributions of these hormones from those of androgens to typical behavioral sexual differentiation.

As noted above, another genetic dysfunction that leads to anomalous sexual differentiation is 5α-reductase deficiency. Genetic males (XY) with 5α-reductase deficiency are born with ambiguous genitalia and small, undescended testes. They are usually considered females at birth and reared as females. At puberty, testosterone masculinizes the body, which develops male-typical musculature and axillary hair growth, and the genitalia develop to resemble a male-typical penis and scrotum (Figure 3.11). The urethra usually opens at the base of the penis; this condition, called hypospadias, substantially reduces fertility. Because these individuals are exposed to male-typical hormones pre- and postnatally, but are reared as females until puberty, behavioral endocrinologists have studied them in order to understand the contribution of hormones versus rearing to human behavioral sexual differentiation.

**TRISOMIC ANOMALIES.**   Occasionally, babies are born with extra chromosomes. Approximately one infant in every 600 live births is born with **Klinefelter syndrome** (Figure 3.12a; Nielsen and Wohlert, 1990). These individuals possess an extra X chromosome (XXY). The presence of the Y chromosome is sufficient for the *SRY* gene to be activated and masculinization to occur, and these individuals are sexed as males at birth. Although the testes develop sufficiently to cause masculinization, these individuals are usually sterile because of reduced sperm pro-

**3.11   5α-reductase deficiency** results in incomplete genital masculinization. (Left) Note the incomplete fusing of the urogenital groove, the lack of penile development, and the presence of hypospadias, the opening of the urethra on the underside of the penis. Most individuals with 5α-reductase deficiency are sexed as girls at birth. (Right) The same individual at puberty. Although DHT is still not present, high blood concentrations of other androgens at puberty can activate DHT receptors and cause delayed and partial masculinization of the external genitalia. Despite pubertal penile development, hypospadias remains, which contributes to infertility. Because these androgen-induced changes in the external genitalia are accompanied by a change to a male-typical body type, some individuals with 5α-reductase deficiency who have been raised as females may take on a male gender identity and gender role at puberty. Courtesy of Julianne Imperato-McGinley.

duction. Mental retardation is also commonly observed among individuals with Klinefelter syndrome.

Approximately one infant in every 850 live births possesses an XYY genotype (Figure 3.12b; Nielsen and Wohlert, 1990). These individuals are considered male at birth, but in common with XXY individuals, XYY men may be sterile. The XYY genotype was once thought to result in increased aggressiveness because a survey of prison populations revealed that a disproportionately large number of these individuals were represented (Hook, 1973; Jacobs et al., 1965). It was proposed that the Y chromosome was responsible for aggressiveness in normal males; therefore, it was hypothesized that individuals with two Y chromosomes displayed increased aggression, which led to their imprisonment. Further analyses revealed that individuals with XYY genotypes were not necessarily more aggressive than XY males, but that they possessed two other traits that increased the likelihood of criminal prosecution: they were less intelligent than average and they were much taller than average. Thus, these individuals may not engage in more criminal activities than average, but apparently they tend to be apprehended more readily (Witkin et al., 1976).

In sum, possession of a single Y chromosome sets off a chain reaction that leads to the differentiation of the testes. Hormonal secretions from the testes lead

(a)

(b)

**3.12    Trisomic genetic anomalies.** (a) This 18-year-old XXY male shows the underdeveloped external genitalia, gynecomastia (breast development), and disproportionately long limbs characteristic of Klinefelter syndrome. (b) This young adult male with the XYY karyotype is well over 2 meters tall. As in Klinefelter syndrome, XYY individuals are sterile. XYY individuals were once thought to be unusually aggressive because of their disproportionate representation in prison populations, but recent studies have not found these individuals to be hyperaggressive, and have surmised that other characteristic traits of the syndrome, such as above-average tallness or below-average intelligence, may have caused disproportionate numbers of XYY individuals to be apprehended or prosecuted for criminal behavior. Courtesy of John Money.

to masculinization and defeminization. In the absence of these hormonal events, feminization and demasculinization occur. In the following sections, the similarities and differences in the process of sexual differentiation among mammals, birds, and other animals will be presented.

## Avian Sexual Differentiation

Studies of nonmammalian species offer intriguing insights into our own species by demonstrating alternative solutions to common problems of adaptation. The process of avian sexual differentiation is similar to that in mammals, but with several interesting differences. Among birds, females are the heterogametic sex (WZ), whereas males are the homogametic sex (ZZ). In the case of copulatory behavior, males are the default sex: in the absence of gonadal secretions, the male developmental track is followed, and the feminine pattern of development is attained by active hormonal secretion (Figure 3.13) (Balthazart and Ball, 1995). In other avian

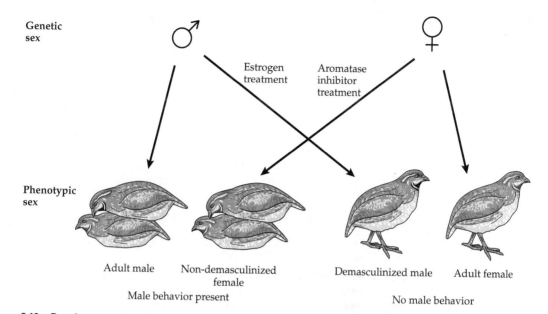

**3.13   Development of female copulatory behavior requires active hormonal secretion.**
The genetic sex of birds in the egg is either male or female. If only the presence or absence of male copulatory behavior is considered, then males generally show masculine patterns and females generally show feminine patterns of copulatory behavior. If estrogen is given to a genetic male bird in the egg, he is demasculinized. If a genetic female bird is given an aromatase inhibitor in the egg, preventing the formation of estrogens, she is not demasculinized, and shows male copulatory behavior as an adult. After Balthazart and Ball, 1995.

systems (i.e., the mechanisms underlying singing behavior), testicular hormones exert a masculinizing effect, whereas the absence of hormonal stimulation leads to the feminine pattern of no song (but, as noted below, it is still not clear what the mechanisms are for sexual differentiation of the neuronal system underlying bird song). For yet other aspects of differentiation, the default condition in birds is neither male nor female; rather, ovarian or testicular hormones must exert feminizing or masculinizing effects, respectively, during normal sexual differentiation (Adkins-Regan, 1987).

The presence of the W sex chromosome appears to cause the primordial gonad to secrete estrogens. The estrogens stimulate proliferation of the germinal epithelium in the left gonad, leading to ovarian cortical development. Only the left ovary of birds usually develops (Nalbandov, 1976). If chicken (*Gallus domesticus*) eggs containing ZZ chromosomal males are injected with estrogen, gonadal tissue develops into ovarian tissue. Similarly, when the embryonic gonads of one sex are grafted into an embryo of the other sex, or when embryonic gonads are grown together in culture dishes, ovaries are observed to feminize testicular development, but the presence of testes does not affect ovarian development (Haffen and Wolff, 1977).

Normal sexual differentiation of the avian Müllerian duct system provides an example in which neither the male nor the female pattern of development can be regarded as neutral. Like mammals, avian embryos of both sexes initially pos-

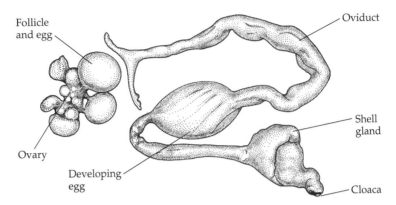

**3.14 Ovary and oviduct of a chicken.** Eggs (ova) are shown in the ovary at different stages of preovulatory development. Chickens ovulate virtually every day, and the egg travels down the oviduct to the shell gland, where a calcium-rich shell is laid down prior to oviposition (egg laying). Other birds have not been bred to be as prolific in their egg-laying behavior as chickens; typically most, but not all, songbirds and seabirds lay only 1–4 eggs per clutch and rear 1–2 clutches per year. After Nalbandov, 1976.

sess precursors to both Müllerian and Wolffian ducts. The Müllerian duct system develops in female chickens to form the oviduct and the shell gland (Figure 3.14), and regresses in male chickens during days 8–13 of incubation. Only the left duct develops in female chickens; the right duct regresses during days 9–18 of incubation. Thus, feminization of the accessory sex organs requires development of only the left components of the Müllerian duct system. If embryonic chickens or ducks are gonadectomized by focal X-irradiation prior to day 8 of incubation, then both duct systems persist; in other words, neither defeminization (regression of the Müllerian duct system) nor feminization (development of the left components of the Müllerian duct system) occurs in the absence of gonadal influences (Wolff and Wolff, 1951).

Sexually dimorphic avian behavior also reflects this variation in hormonal influences. In some cases, as in copulatory behavior, the masculine behavior pattern is the default condition, whereas the feminine pattern is produced by hormonal activation that causes demasculinization. In the case of other behaviors, testicular hormones exert a defeminizing or masculinizing effect, whereas the absence of hormonal stimulation leads to the feminine pattern.

## Alternative Reproductive Tactics and Male Polymorphism

There are other situations in which the default condition is neither male nor female, but rather, ovarian or testicular hormones must exert feminizing or masculinizing effects, respectively, during normal sexual differentiation of behavior. The previous sections have assumed that there are two distinct sexes–males and females. Within some species, however, there are multiple "types" (or morphs) of the same sex. Different types of males often look very distinct, and they often exhibit quite dissimilar behavioral patterns, as well as alternative mating tactics. In some cases, a subset of males within a population resemble females, whereas the alternative male types are different from females in appearance and behavior; in other cases, there are several different male morphs (polymorphism) within a population, all of which differ from females in appearance and behavior (Moore et al., 1998). Polymorphic males often pursue different tactics to achieve reproductive success. Some males are territorial and exclude other males from (and attempt to attract females to) their defended territories. Other males are "satellite" or "sneaker" males. Satellite males usually loiter near the edges of a territorial male's property and attempt to mate with females that are attracted to his territory. Sneaker males often resemble females; they "sneak" into a territorial male's property along with visiting females, then attempt clandestine matings with the females before the resident male discovers the deception.

Males that change phenotypes, either permanently or temporarily, during their lives are said to have plastic phenotypes (Moore, 1991). For example, male spring peepers (frogs of the genera *Pseudacris, Rana,* and *Hyla*) display one of two alternative mating tactics: they either vocalize to attract females, or remain silent near calling males and attempt to intercept females that are moving toward the callers. Calling is energetically expensive, and males can switch between these behavioral strategies on different nights (Lance and Wells, 1993).

Male morphs that permanently differentiate into a single phenotype for life are said to have fixed phenotypes (Moore, 1991). For example, male ruffs (*Philomachus pugnax;* a type of sandpiper) become either darkly colored and highly territorial or lightly colored with the behavioral characteristics of satellite males (Lank et al., 1995). Several species of fish, including sunfishes, swordtails, platyfishes, and midshipmen, display male polymorphism in appearance and mating tactics (Bass, 1996). One of the most interesting examples of alternative male phenotypes comes from the midshipman fishes.

There are two types of male plainfin midshipmen (*Porichthys notatus*) (Figure 3.15). Type I males build nests and attract females to their nests by generating an advertisement call, which sounds like a series of long-duration "hums." If you take a walk along a Pacific beach from Northern California to the Canadian border on a summer night, you are likely to hear the "songs" of the type I midshipman males calling females to their nests (Bass, 1996). A responding female inspects the nest, and if it meets her specifications, she deposits her eggs. After the female lays her eggs, the type I male fertilizes them, then maintains a vigilant defense of the clutch and the nest site against rivals. While guarding the eggs, he emits an aggressive call (or grunt) to warn away potential intruders (Bass, 1995). Type I males are nearly eight times larger than the type II males, which physically resemble females (Bass, 1995). Type II males never build nests, guard eggs, or vocalize to attract females; rather, they have evolved an alternative reproductive tactic as sneaker/satellite males. They swim into nest sites guarded by type I males and release sperm. Presumably, the type I males do not challenge them because they resemble females.

Type II midshipman males undergo sexual maturation nearly a year earlier than type I males, and this precocious puberty differentiates the two male phenotypes. However, it has not yet been established whether the difference in the timing of puberty is the primary determining factor in the developmental pathway leading to the different male morphs. Both types of males (and females) have detectable testosterone concentrations in their blood, with type II males dis-

**3.15    Different male phenotypes of the midshipman fish.** A nest containing a Type I male (center), a female (right), and Type II males (far right and lower left). Also shown on the left are newly hatched fry attached to a small rock by an adhesive disk at the base of the yolk sac. During the breeding season, male midshipman fish (*Porichthys notatus*) build nests under rocky shelters along the intertidal and subtidal zones of the western coast of the United States and Canada. Photograph by Margaret A. Marchaterre, courtesy of Andrew Bass.

playing the highest blood testosterone concentrations, followed by females, then type I males (Brantley et al., 1993). The primary teleost fish androgen, however, is 11-ketotestosterone. The 11-ketotestosterone concentrations in type I males are five times higher than their testosterone concentrations; neither type II males nor females have detectable 11-ketotestosterone levels (Bass, 1996). Only females have any detectable circulating estrogens. Presumably, these different patterns of steroid hormones activate receptors in various neural tissues involved in growth, reproductive behavior, and vocalization. Thus, one reasonable hypothesis is that 11-ketotestosterone mediates nest building and vocal courtship behavior in type I males.

In several lizard species, males also exhibit alternative behavioral mating strategies and body types. For example, male tree lizards (*Urosaurus ornatus*) display striking polymorphisms in the color of a body structure called a "dewlap" (Moore et al., 1998). The dewlap is a flap of skin attached to the throats of lizards that the males extend during courtship or aggressive encounters. Dewlaps of male tree lizards may be solid colors (typically orange, yellow, blue, or violet) or have a central spot surrounded by a contrasting background color (e.g., an orange spot surrounded by blue) (Hews et al., 1997). Nine different color morphs have been identified among tree lizards in Arizona, but most populations consist of two or three different male phenotypes. One well-studied population contains two types of males that are present in nearly equal proportions: (1) territorial males that have an orange dewlap sporting a blue spot, and (2) nonterritorial males with a solid orange dewlap (Thompson and Moore, 1992). The nonterritorial males display one of two dominant behavioral patterns: (1) sedentary satellite behavior or (2) nomadic behavior. The dewlap color and behavioral polymorphisms appear to be permanently organized early during post-hatching development (Moore et al., 1998). If immature males are exposed to high testosterone and progesterone concentrations, then territorial, orange–blue males result; if they are not exposed to high testosterone and progesterone concentrations, they develop into nonterritorial males with orange dewlaps (Figure 3.16). However, the nonterritorial tac-

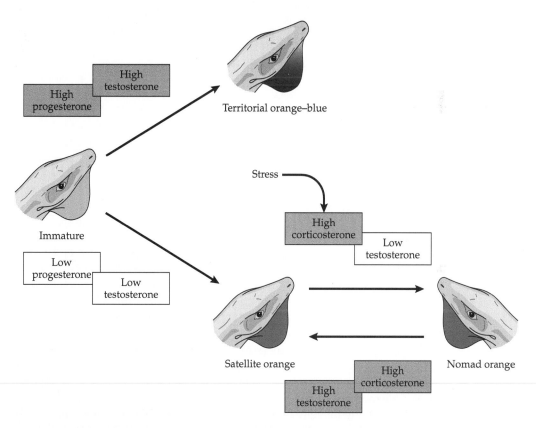

**3.16  Three types of male tree lizards** coexist in some Arizona populations: (1) territorial males, (2) sedentary nonterritorial males, and (3) nomadic nonterritorial males. The territorial males develop an orange dewlap with a blue spot; this morph results from early post-hatching exposure to high testosterone and progesterone concentrations. In the absence of high testosterone and progesterone concentrations, males develop a solid orange dewlap and become nonterritorial. In adulthood, if stressful environmental conditions result in high corticosterone concentrations, and thus lowered testosterone concentrations, nonterritorial males become nomadic; if low corticosterone concentrations, and thus higher testosterone concentrations, are present, nonterritorial males become sedentary. Territorial orange–blue males remain territorial regardless of environmental conditions and corticosterone concentrations. After Moore et al., 1998.

tics of the orange morphs appear to be affected by environmental conditions. Stressful ambient conditions (e.g., drought) cause sustained corticosterone secretion, which promotes nomadic, wandering behavior (Moore et al., 1998). Thus, the two male phenotypes are permanently fixed by early hormone conditions, whereas the flexibility of tactic switching (i.e., sedentary versus nomadic) among males with orange dewlaps is mediated by the temporary effects of corticosterone concentrations during adulthood.

## Environmental Sex Determination in Reptiles and Fishes

In mammals and birds, sex is determined by the genotype. If homologous sex chromosomes are present, then female mammals or male birds develop; if heterologous sex chromosomes are present, then male mammals or female birds develop. Sex determination is dependent *only* upon genotypic differences. Mammals and birds evolved from reptilian ancestral forms about 325 million and 150 million years ago, respectively. Some modern reptilian species, like mammals and birds, display genotypic sex determination. In some of these species males develop if homologous sex chromosomes are present, and in other species females develop if homologous sex chromosomes are present. However, in some lizards, most turtles, and probably all crocodilian species, environmental factors, not genotypic information, direct sex determination (Crews et al., 1988a; Korpelainen, 1990). Indeed, sex chromosomes are generally absent in these species (Crews and Bull, 1987).

The environmental factor most commonly involved in reptilian sex determination is temperature (Bull, 1980; Korpelainen, 1990), although water potential (concentration of salts) may also mediate sex determination in some species (for example, the painted turtle, *Chrysemys picta:* Gutzke and Paukstis, 1983). The embryos of a species with **temperature-dependent sex determination** are bipotential and can develop into a male or a female solely on the basis of the temperature at which the egg incubates. Relatively high temperatures (>30°C) produce males, and cool temperatures (<28°C) produce females in some lizard species, as well as in alligators (Crews et al., 1988a). The opposite pattern of temperature effects on sex determination is observed among many turtle species. Yet another pattern of temperature-dependent sex determination has been reported for snapping turtles and crocodiles: females are produced at the high and low extremes, whereas males are produced at intermediate temperatures (Figure 3.17; Bull, 1983). This mechanism could allow the mother to determine the sex of her offspring by varying the temperature of the nest in which her eggs are incubated. Although this is an extremely exciting possibility, there is no evidence thus far that sex ratio is manipulated by parental care (Clutton-Brock, 1991), nor is there any evidence that temperature exerts its effects by means of differential mortality in either sex (Crews et al., 1988a). Rather, incubation temperature determines whether the embryonic gonad develops into a testis or an ovary. The embryonic gonad in reptiles consists of distinct cortical and medullary tissue. If the cortical portion of the gonad develops, then an ovary develops; if the medullary portion of the gonad develops, then a testis develops. However, the physiological mechanisms by which temperature determines which portion of the gonad develops are unknown at this time (Crews et al., 1988a).

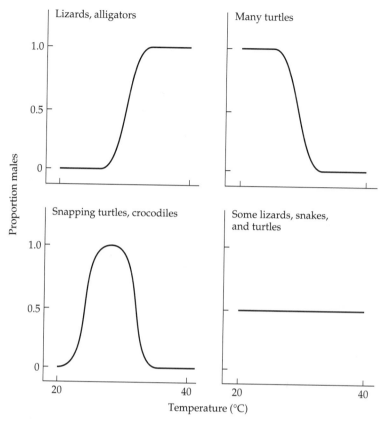

**3.17   Temperature-dependent sex determination in reptiles.** Exposure to relatively high ambient temperatures during incubation results in male-typical development among the offspring of some lizards and alligators, whereas in many turtle species, high temperatures during incubation result in female-typical offspring development. Relatively moderate temperatures result in male offspring in snapping turtles and crocodiles, while exposure of eggs to either high or low temperatures results in female offspring in these species. Sex determination in some reptilian species is unaffected by incubation temperatures. Because mammals and birds are kept at relatively constant temperatures during their embryonic development, the role of ambient temperature on the sex ratio of offspring in these species is unknown. Source: Crews et al., 1988a.

As in birds, steroid hormones influence gonadal differentiation, and steroid treatment can override temperature effects on gonadal development. That is, if eggs are incubated at male-producing temperatures but given estrogen, females develop; conversely, if eggs are incubated at female-producing temperatures but given androgen, males develop. The mechanism by which temperature affects steroidogenesis remains unknown. Presumably, the enzymatic conversions necessary for steroid metabolism are temperature-sensitive. It is possible that temperature controls the activity of aromatase (which converts testosterone to estradiol) or reductase (which converts testosterone to dihydrotestosterone) in reptilian gonads (Crews and Bergeron, 1994; Rhen and Lang, 1994). Thus, high temperatures might inactivate enzymes necessary for converting androgens to estrogens in some spe-

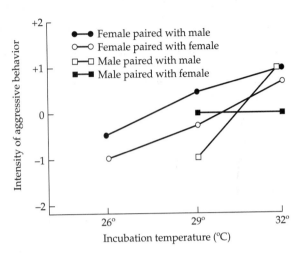

**3.18 Aggression in adult female geckos** can be influenced by incubation temperature. Relatively high temperatures (32°C) produce few female offspring, and relatively low temperatures (26°C) produce only female offspring in geckos. Females produced at low incubation temperatures display low levels of aggression as adults, compared with females incubated at high temperatures, which display male-like aggression as adults. −2 = fleeing; −1 = low posture; 0 = no response; +1 = high posture; +2 = attack. Source: Gutzke and Crews, 1988.

cies, whereas low temperatures could have the same effect in other species. The development of the reptilian gonads into testes or ovaries starts a cascade of events that results in subsequent male-typical or female-typical behaviors, respectively, in the adult reptile.

What happens if reptile eggs are maintained at intermediate temperatures? Based on the outcome of one study of leopard geckos (*Eublepharis macularius*), intermediate temperatures can have interesting consequences for adult sexual behavior (Gutzke and Crews, 1988). In this species, temperatures of 32°C produce mainly male geckos, but a few female offspring are also produced; temperatures of 26°C produce only females. When females hatched from these two incubation temperatures, as well as from a third, intermediate condition (29°C), were compared as adults in mating tests, female geckos from all three groups elicited equivalent amounts of courtship from males. Females from the low-temperature condition responded to male courtship with female-typical behavior. However, females from the high-temperature condition responded to courtship with male-typical behavior. Females incubated at intermediate temperatures displayed adult sexual behavior intermediate between the two extremes, showing some female-typical and some male-typical courtship behaviors. Interestingly, incubation at high temperatures increased adult levels of aggressive behavior in both sexes (Figure 3.18).

Like mammals and birds, animals with temperature-dependent sex determination remain the same sex throughout their lives (Crews et al., 1988a). However, some other animals, especially fishes, can switch sexes during their lifetimes! Several species of fish are hermaphrodites (Demski, 1987). **Simultaneous hermaphrodites** possess ovotestes that produce both eggs and sperm, and they alternate between two behavioral roles in providing eggs or sperm during spawning. There are also two types of **sequential hermaphrodites**: animals that begin life as one sex, then change to the other sex as adults in response to environmental or genotypic factors (Demski, 1987). Several species of sequential hermaphroditic reef fish have been identified, including wrasses, sea basses, gobies, anemonefishes, and parrotfishes (Bass, 1996). **Protogynous** types begin life as females, then

**3.19  Sequential hermaphroditism** in the striped parrotfish. (Left) Young females of this species have bold stripes, and defend territories along the edges of reefs. (Right) As females mature and grow in size, they change sex and adopt male-typical coloration and behavior, joining other males in defending large territories encompassing several "harems" of young females. Courtesy of Robert W. Warner.

change into males; **protandrous** types are first males, then change into females. Such sequential sex changes involve a change in gonadal type and function, a change in the dominant gonadal steroid secreted, a change in morphology (body type), and a change in behavior (Figure 3.19).

Stoplight parrotfish (*Sparisoma viride*) are coral reef fish that begin life as females and change into males (Cardwell and Liley, 1991a,b); in other words, these fish are protogynous. In many cases, the sex change is accompanied by a striking change in body coloration, from the female-typical "initial phase" coloration to the male-typical "terminal phase" coloration. Some individuals, however, undergo the sex change from female to male without the change in coloration. These female mimics compete with normal males by using a "sneaker" mating tactic. Normal terminal-phase males establish territories from which they exclude other males, and in which they court females. If a courted female releases her eggs, a female mimic may enter the territory undetected and fertilize some of the eggs. This alternative reproductive tactic is maintained in the population because of its occasional success in attaining fertilizations.

The sex change in parrotfish is accompanied by changes in the pattern of circulating steroid hormones. Females have undetectable concentrations of the primary fish androgen 11-ketotestosterone, moderate concentrations of testosterone, and high concentrations of 17β-estradiol. During the transition from initial to terminal coloration phases, concentrations of 11-ketotestosterone rise dramatically, and estrogen concentrations decline. Males have high concentrations of 11-ketotestosterone and testosterone, but low concentrations of estrogen. Injection of adult females with 11-ketotestosterone causes a precocious change in gonadal, gametic, and behavioral sex. Female mimics, which maintain the initial-phase coloration, do not display the increase in blood concentrations of 11-ketotestosterone.

Box 3.2
# William C. Young

William Caldwell Young was an important pioneer in behavioral endocrinology. Young received his undergraduate degree at Amherst College, where he worked with Professor Harold H. Plough. He published his senior thesis on the effects of high temperature on fertility in *Drosophila* (Young and Plough, 1926). Young attended the University of Chicago for his graduate training and worked in the laboratory of Carl R. Moore in the zoology department.

Carl Moore had earned his doctorate at the University of Chicago working in the laboratory of Frank Lillie. Moore had published a series of 11 papers with the generic title "On the Physiological Properties of the Gonads as Controllers of Somatic and Psychic Characteristics." He noted in his studies that, although castration of male guinea pigs resulted in rapid and nearly uniform degeneration of the epididymis and seminal vesicles, the timing of the cessation of sexual behavior varied enormously among individuals. Moore interpreted these results to suggest that reproductive behavior was "utterly capricious, unordered by hormonal events, and unrelated to variables of significance to reproductive biology" (Goy, 1967).

Young produced a classic study of epididymal sperm transport for his dissertation project and was awarded his doctorate in 1927. During the course of these studies Young became interested in the hormonal control of female mating behavior, but his mentor, Professor Moore, actively discouraged behavioral research because his own experience suggested that the variation inherent in behavioral studies was daunting.

Young joined the biology department at Brown University in 1928, and submitted a grant application to continue his work on the reproductive morphology and physiology of guinea pigs. While waiting for the funding agency's decision, he had "nothing better to do than investigate the inexpensive problem of the morphological changes associated with female sexual behavior in the guinea pig" (Goy, 1967). By the time he received the news that his application was not to be funded, Young and his research group had already started a productive line of research that used behavior as an indirect measure of ovarian activity (Dempsey, 1968). In 1939, Young moved to the Yerkes Laboratories of Primate Biology in Orange Park, Florida, where he interacted with R. M. Yerkes and other psychologists during his four-year tenure. His research began to include behavior as a primary object of study.

## The Effects of Hormones on Sexually Dimorphic Behaviors

As we have seen, the initial step in sex determination, the development of a testis or an ovary, triggers a cascade of events that results in sexually dimorphic behaviors (see Figure 3.7). In order to understand the interaction between hormones and behavior, behavioral endocrinologists have studied several animal models that show distinct behavioral sex differences. By studying the development, neural and hormonal bases, and molecular mechanisms of a simple behavior that is displayed by one sex but not by the other, researchers hope to elucidate general principles that can be expanded from these simple systems to explain more complex behavioral sex differences such as those displayed by humans.

Apparently, Young felt isolated in a nonacademic research setting (Goy, 1967), and left the Yerkes laboratory in 1943 to teach at Cedar Crest College. He then accepted an offer to set up an endocrinology laboratory in the anatomy department at the University of Kansas. This laboratory was very active, and studies of hormonal control of reproductive function, including mating behavior, were conducted there by a stellar team of graduate students and postdoctoral fellows, including M. Diamond, H. Feder, A. Gerall, R. Goy, J. Grunt, C. Phoenix, W. Riss, E. Valenstein, and others. The famous study of the organizational effects of prenatal androgen on guinea pig mating behavior was conducted in Young's Kansas laboratory (Phoenix et al., 1959). This study has been one of the cornerstones of modern behavioral endocrinology research. While at Kansas, Young also edited the third edition of *Sex and Internal Secretions,* published in 1961, which was the "bible" for reproductive biologists at that time, and continues to be an important sourcebook 30 years later.

In 1963, Young moved to the Oregon Regional Primate Center, where he became chairman of the reproductive physiology department. There, his organizational/activational hypothesis of behavioral sexual dimorphisms was examined in rhesus monkeys (Goy and Phoenix, 1972; Goy and Resko, 1972). William C. Young is one of the most important figures in behavioral

endocrinology because of his many significant research contributions, his theoretical contributions, which were profoundly important in framing research problems, and the graduate and postdoctoral students trained in his laboratories who continue to make important contributions to the field (Beach, 1981).

William C. Young (1899–1965)

## The Organizational/Activational Hypothesis

In 1959, W. C. Young (Box 3.2) and his colleagues published a classic study on the effects of prenatal and early postnatal androgen treatment on female reproductive behavior (Phoenix et al., 1959). This experiment rivals Berthold's study with roosters (see Chapter 1) in theoretical importance to behavioral endocrinology. Because of the profound effect of Young's study on shaping the field, this study will be described in detail.

Females and males of many species show sexually dimorphic mating postures. Female rodents stand immobile with arched backs and allow males to mount them. This mating posture is called **lordosis** (see Chapter 6). Males, on the other hand, mount females. Females rarely exhibit **mounting behavior**, the masculine behavior pattern, and males typically do not assume the lordosis posture, the feminine behavior pattern, when mounted by other males.*

Mating behavior in both sexes is under the control of gonadal steroid hormones. For example, castration of males stops mounting behavior, and testosterone replacement therapy restores mounting behavior to its original levels. Logically, we could conclude that testosterone causes mounting behavior. However, injection of adult females with testosterone does not increase their mounting behavior to male-typical levels. Females somehow lose the potential to exhibit male-typical behavior during development; in other words, the behavior of females is demasculinized. Similarly, castration of adult males and subsequent treatment with estrogens and progestins does not lead to the appearance of female-typical mating behavior. Males become defeminized during development; that is, they lose the potential to display female-typical behavior.

Professor Young and his research group sought to understand how these behavioral differences in hormonal response were mediated. They reasoned that hormonal events early in development must be responsible for the induction of feminine and masculine behavioral patterns in general, as well as for the shifting of the probabilities of masculine and feminine mating behaviors in females and males in the presence of the appropriate stimulus. In the experiments designed to address this hypothesis, testosterone propionate was administered to pregnant guinea pigs throughout most of their 69-day gestation period. Some pregnant females were given large doses of the hormone. At birth, some of the female offspring from these pregnancies possessed external genitalia that were indistinguishable from those of their brothers or of normal males. These females were labeled hermaphrodites by the researchers.[†] Another group of females was exposed to smaller doses of the androgen prenatally; these females had no visible abnormalities of the external genitalia and were referred to as unmodified females. The researchers waited for the guinea pigs to mature to examine their behavior in the second phase of the study.

In adulthood, both groups of androgen-exposed females, as well as androgen-exposed male and control male and female guinea pigs, were gonadectomized and then injected with estrogen and progesterone to stimulate female sexual behavior. Each of these animals was paired with a normal male guinea pig. Some time later, all of the animals were injected with androgens to stimulate male sexual behavior and paired with a normal conspecific female that was in mating condition. The results were impressive. Androgens given to guinea pigs early in life (1) decreased the ability of both experimental groups of females to display lordosis in adulthood, (2) enhanced the ability of both experimental groups of females to display mounting behavior in response to testosterone therapy, but (3) caused no deleterious effect on mounting behavior or other masculine behavioral patterns in males similarly treated.

---

*It should be noted here that this yes/no dichotomy is presented for clarity's sake; in reality, males of some strains of rats show lordosis regularly and females of some rat strains display frequent mounting behavior. A sex "difference" is often one of frequency, behavioral threshold, or the quality of the behavior.

[†]Actually, these females were pseudohermaphrodites because they all possessed two ovaries, but recall that it had become common in medicine to refer to individuals with ambiguous external genitalia as hermaphrodites (Ellis, 1945).

Not only were the data of considerable interest, but the conceptual framework in which the authors chose to cast them was rich and wide. Professor Young and his colleagues made the following speculations (Phoenix et al., 1959):

1. A clear distinction can be made between the prenatal actions of hormones in causing differentiation, or *organization*, of neural substrates for behavior and the actions of hormones in adulthood in causing *activation* of these substrates. This is a very important point, and provides the basis for the organizational/activational hypothesis of sexually dimorphic behaviors. During development, the sex steroid hormones organize or establish the components of the nervous system that will be needed for subsequent male- or female-typical behaviors. In the adult, these same hormones activate, modulate, or inhibit the function of these existing neural circuits.

2. Critical periods of perinatal development exist during which an animal is maximally susceptible to the organizing effects of steroids on neural tissue. (We now know that the timing of organizational effects of steroids may be broader in scope than originally formulated by Phoenix and his collaborators.)

3. Organization of the neural tissues mediating mating behavior is in some ways analogous to the differentiation of the genital tracts. That is, the nervous systems of males are normally masculinized and defeminized during development, whereas the nervous systems of females are normally feminized and demasculinized.

4. The organizing effects of steroid hormones on prenatal neural tissues are subtle and reflect alterations in function rather than structure, because even females whose external genitalia are not physically masculinized demonstrate behavioral masculinization and defeminization. (As you will soon learn, however, it has recently been established that changes in neural structures are associated with sexually dimorphic behaviors.)

5. The idea that prenatal hormones act to organize the neural substrates for behavior has possible implications for the study of behavior in primates, including humans.

This study profoundly affected the way behavioral endocrinologists conceptualized the interactions of hormones and sexually dimorphic behaviors. This groundbreaking study did not arise out of thin air, however, but was built upon three separate, but related, lines of research, involving (1) embryological studies showing that prenatal androgen exposure results in masculinized external genitalia, (2) studies of the effects of blood-borne substances in masculinizing the female twins of male cattle, and (3) endocrinological studies investigating the control of ovulation.

**PRENATAL ANDROGENS AND MASCULINIZED GENITALIA.**   Anatomists had studied the sexual differentiation of the body and had discovered what many of us have observed: the most striking sexual dimorphism in most species is that of the external genitalia. In one early study, pregnant rats were injected with androgens throughout their pregnancy (Hamilton and Gardner, 1937). Female rats whose mothers had received androgens during pregnancy were born with masculinized external genitalia: in other words, they developed penes. This study, as well as others, contributed to the development of the organizational/activational hypothesis by demonstrating that early endocrine treatments could masculinize or feminize anatomical and functional features.

**FREEMARTINS.**    The idea of hormonal regulation of the process of sexual differentiation was originally given impetus by studies of a phenomenon known as **freemartinism** (Lillie, 1917). A freemartin is a sterile female twin of a male found in cattle, sheep, goats, and pigs. Freemartins described in cattle have the following characteristics: (1) the freemartin calf is a sexually abnormal chromosomal female (XX) born as a twin to an apparently normal male; (2) about 90% of female cattle born as twins to males are freemartins; (3) the external genitalia of the freemartin are of the female type, and there is mammary gland development; (4) there is variable development of the internal genital tracts; and (5) the gonads are atrophic but resemble testes more than ovaries. To account for freemartinism, a hormonal theory was proposed suggesting that androgens produced by the male fetus are able to reach the female due to fusion of some of the placental blood vessels that supply the twins. Evidence to support this idea included the findings that such vascular connections (anastomoses) do occur in cattle, and that in the 10% or so of cases in which the female twin is fertile, the placental anastomoses are obliterated (Figure 3.20). That the male produced a blood-borne factor was deduced by the observation that the male twin seemed normal and the finding, based on histological techniques, that the prenatal testis was active prior to activation of the sibling's ovary.

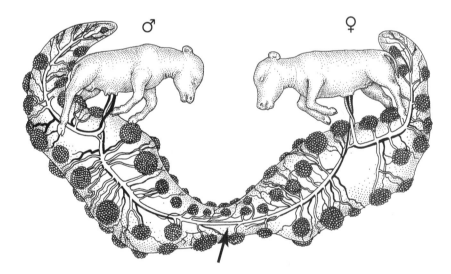

**3.20    Freemartins** are sterile female twins of a male found in cattle, sheep, goats, and pigs. It was hypothesized early in the 20th century that masculinizing factors travel from the male twin to the female through the vascular connections of the placenta because of a vascular fusion, or anastomosis (arrow), and affect the internal anatomy of the female. However, attempts to produce freemartins by administering androgens to pregnant cows have not been successful, and the mechanism underlying freemartinism remains unknown. After Lillie, 1917.

However, administration of androgens to pregnant cows never results in freemartins. Female fetuses of androgen-treated mothers have ovaries and internal genitalia of the female type (predominantly), but masculinized external genitalia. Thus one of the oldest questions about sexual differentiation is still unsolved. Apparently, the exchange of cells between twins during early pregnancy, or passage from the male to the female fetus of a nonsteroidal factor that favors testicular development, mediates the freemartin phenomenon.

**CONTROL OF OVULATION.** The third group of studies that laid the groundwork for the organizational/activational hypothesis examined the hormonal control of ovulation. Because studies of this process have continued to shed light on the mechanisms of sexual differentiation, they will be described in detail.

Female mammals display cyclic gonadal function, whereas males have more or less tonic reproductive function: that is, ovulation, the expulsion of a ripened egg from the ovary, occurs cyclically, whereas sperm production is constant throughout the breeding season. The reproductive behavior of the sexes follows these fundamentally different patterns of gamete production, with females displaying cycles of mating behavior and males displaying more or less continuous willingness to mate.

What causes these patterns? Gonadal function is driven by gonadotropins secreted from the anterior pituitary (see Chapter 2), but what drives the gonadotropins? Gonadotropin-releasing hormone (GnRH) secreted from the median eminence of the hypothalamus determines the pattern of release of luteinizing hormone (LH), a gonadotropin, from the anterior pituitary. In both male and female rats, this process begins when a series of LH pulses, 20–40 minutes apart (60 minutes in humans), are released into the circulation in response to pulses of GnRH from the hypothalamus; these pulses of LH often precede pulsatile releas-

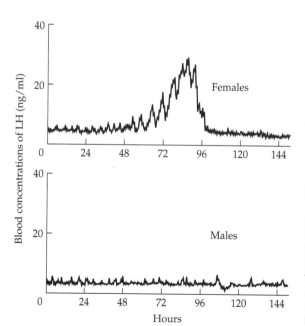

**3.21  LH profiles of female and male rats.** In both male and female rats, LH is released in a pulsatile fashion from the anterior pituitary in response to pulses of GnRH from the medial basal hypothalamus. In females, the pulse frequency and amplitude increase around the time of ovulation, as negative feedback mechanisms are temporarily overwhelmed by increasing blood estrogen concentrations and positive feedback mechanisms are engaged.

es of gonadal steroid hormones (Figure 3.21). Thus, the hypothalamus provides a pulsatile delivery of GnRH in both males and females, which subsequently drives the anterior pituitary, which eventually drives gonadal function. As circulating concentrations of LH and sex steroid hormones rise, they feed back to suppress further GnRH secretion (negative feedback). Similarly, the injection of steroid hormones suppresses GnRH and gonadotropin secretion in a dose-dependent manner.

In females, there is a steady increase in the amount of estrogen produced by the ovaries against the backdrop of continuous pulses of GnRH secretion and negative feedback endocrine regulation. Somehow, females escape from rigid negative feedback control. As estrogen accumulates in the blood, a surge of GnRH is released from a putative "surge center" in the hypothalamus. The surge of GnRH causes a surge of LH and follicle-stimulating hormone (FSH) secretion, which in turn stimulates ovulation via the positive feedback mechanism illustrated in Figure 3.22. This pattern can be demonstrated in the following manner. Injecting an ovariectomized rat with low doses of estrogen causes a reduction of GnRH and LH concentrations via negative feedback; injecting an ovariectomized rat with high doses of estrogen, however, causes an increase in GnRH and LH concentra-

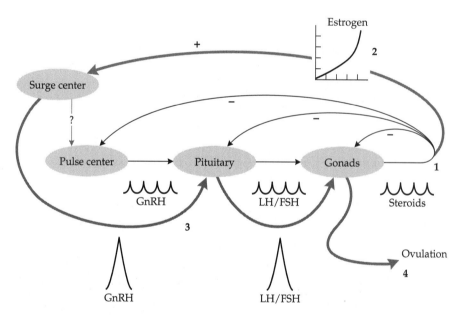

**3.22   Positive feedback and the control of ovulation.** Steroid secretion in both males and females is usually regulated by negative feedback (solid lines), whereby increasing gonadal steroid concentrations feed back to the gonads, anterior pituitary, and hypothalamus to slow secretion of GnRH, gonadotropins, and gonadal steroids. However, on a cyclical basis, females escape this rigid negative feedback control (1; shaded line), and blood concentrations of estrogen steadily increase (2). Through a positive feedback mechanism, the surge center responds to the rising estrogen concentrations by releasing a surge of GnRH, which stimulates the anterior pituitary to release corresponding surges of LH and FSH (3), which stimulate the gonads and cause ovulation (4). After ovulation, the negative feedback mechanisms are once again engaged, and LH and FSH secretion resume a pulsatile pattern.

tions by the process of positive feedback. Injecting a castrated male rat with low amounts of estrogen also causes reduction of GnRH and LH concentrations due to negative feedback. However, it has been shown that injections of even pharmacologically high doses of estrogens never result in a positive feedback response in male primates (Karsch et al., 1973). In monkeys, the preovulatory gonadotropin surge does not require elevated GnRH from the hypothalamus; the positive effect of estrogens on LH and FSH secretion in primates may reflect elevated numbers of GnRH receptors on LH- and FSH-producing cells (Karsch, 1987).

What is the basis of the sex difference in the regulation of endocrine function? Initially, it was proposed that the pituitary gland itself differs between the sexes. Females were thought to possess pituitaries that displayed cyclic function, whereas males were believed to possess pituitaries that displayed tonic function. According to this logic, a male does not normally ovulate because his pituitary does not display cyclic function—and more obviously, because he does not have an ovary. But if an ovary is transplanted into an adult male rat, he still does not ovulate. The notion that the pituitary gland was masculinized arose from pituitary gland transplant studies. In an extremely delicate operation, the pituitary gland can be surgically removed from a normal female rat and transplanted into a hypophysectomized female rat. If the transplanted pituitary gland is able to establish a blood supply, it can support ovulation in the recipient female. However, if the recipient of the transplanted female pituitary is a male with a transplanted ovary, ovulation is not observed. If female rats have testicular tissue implanted under the skin within a few days of birth, they also fail to sustain ovulation, either from their own ovaries or from transplanted ovaries. Similarly, the pituitary glands of male rats that are castrated within a few days of birth are able to support ovulation with an implanted ovary. On the basis of these results, it was reasonably concluded, first, that ovulation does not require neural input, because transplanted ovaries that establish vascular, but not neural, connections can ovulate, and second, that exposure to androgens early in life results in a masculine pattern of pituitary function that is incapable of sustaining ovulation, whereas lack of perinatal androgen exposure results in a feminine pattern of ovulation-supporting pituitary function (Pfeiffer, 1936). Conceptually, this argument was correct, but the facts were just slightly incorrect.

A series of papers reporting on the physiological control of ovulation in rabbits demonstrated that pituitary function is in fact controlled by the hypothalamus (Harris, 1937, 1948, 1955). These studies also demonstrated that the "male" pituitary can, in fact, sustain ovulation. If the pituitary is removed from a female rat and replaced by a pituitary from an adult male, then ovulation occurs, provided that vascular connections with the hypothalamus are established (Harris and Jacobsohn, 1952). Thus, the sexual dimorphism in the ability to support ovulation is not at the level of the pituitary, but rather, reflects changes induced by early androgen exposure upstream in the hypothalamus.

Many studies of the process of sexual differentiation have used rats rather than guinea pigs because investigators do not have to make endocrine manipulations via the mother, but can influence the sexual differentiation of each individual rat directly after birth. The masculinizing actions of the guinea pig fetal testis are completed approximately halfway through the 69-day gestation period, or about 35 days post-conception (Goy et al., 1964). Guinea pigs are *precocial* animals, which means that the young are born fully furred, able to walk about, and able to thermoregulate. In contrast, rats are *altricial* animals: their gestation period is only about 21 days, and they are born in a very immature state, blind and hairless, and unable to walk about or regulate their body temperature. Sexual differentiation in rats occurs during the first 10 days or so *after* birth, again about 35 days post-conception. This developmental pattern allows researchers to make endocrine manipulations in individual newborn rats. In rats, there is a critical period, or more properly, a period of maximal susceptibility to the effects of the hormones that induce behavioral sexual dimorphisms; if male rats are castrated at 1 day of age and implanted with an ovary as adults, ovarian cycles that are identical to female cycles are observed. However, if male rats are castrated at 20 days of age and implanted with an ovary as adults, no cycles in ovarian function are observed (Pfeiffer, 1935, 1936). Further studies have indicated that castration after 3 or 4 days of age also fails to preserve the potential for cyclic ovarian function in adult males. The secretion of testosterone by the male during the first several hours of life destroys forever the potential for the cycling that is seen in females.

The blood testosterone concentrations of male rat pups approach adult concentrations by about 6 hours after birth. This elevation in blood testosterone concentrations has been attributed to (1) release of the infant's testes from negative feedback suppression by placental gonadotropins and (2) retarded steroid clearance rates as steroid metabolism shifts from maternal systems to the infant's own liver function (Baum et al., 1988). This perinatal surge of testosterone appears to destroy the neuronal circuitry involved in the release of surges of GnRH from the hypothalamus, and thus permanently eliminates the potential for feminine positive feedback effects. In the absence of high concentrations of gonadal steroids, the neural circuitry involved in GnRH surge generation is spared. Male human babies also display this surge in blood testosterone concentrations at birth (Forest and Cathiard, 1975). However, they retain the ability to show positive feedback responses of gonadotropin release when injected with estrogens. In other words, the presence of positive feedback mechanisms associated with the hypothalamus–pituitary–gonadal axis is not a sexually dimorphic trait in humans, or in other primates examined (Hodges and Hearne, 1978; Karsch et al., 1973; Norman and Spies, 1986; see Chapter 4).

Where in the brain does the rodent sex difference in positive feedback occur? Recall that both males and females release LH in pulsatile bursts (see Figure 3.21). This pulsatile release of LH follows pulsatile bursts of GnRH in both sexes. In addition to these pulses of GnRH, females also show large, cyclic *surges* of GnRH that are not seen in males. The pulse generator in both males and females appears to be located in the arcuate nuclei and the ventromedial nuclei of the hypothalamus, which are often collectively considered to be part of the medial basal hypothalamus. However, most of the GnRH cells in females are located in the rostral aspects of the preoptic hypothalamus, that is, in front of the optic chiasm (Chappel, 1985). The surge generator is located in the region of the preoptic and suprachiasmatic nuclei (Figure 3.23; Pierce, 1988). As you will learn in Chapter 8, there are biological timekeepers located in these regions that control ovulation. A daily "minisurge" of GnRH is elicited by one of these clocks, and when this minisurge coincides with high estrogen concentrations, females' GnRH cells release large and rapid pulses of GnRH, resulting in a GnRH and LH surge. Destruction or sur-

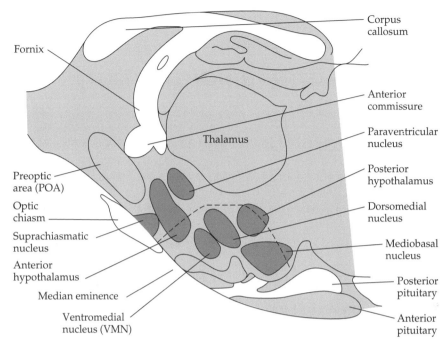

Fornix

Thalamus

Preoptic
area (POA)

Optic
chiasm

Suprachiasmatic
nucleus

Anterior
hypothalamus

Median eminence

Ventromedial
nucleus (VMN)

Corpus
callosum

Anterior
commissure

Paraventricular
nucleus

Posterior
hypothalamus

Dorsomedial
nucleus

Mediobasal
nucleus

Posterior
pituitary

Anterior
pituitary

**3.23    The surge and pulse centers of the hypothalamus.** Schematic sagittal view of rat brain showing the hypothalamic nuclei involved in the regulation of gonadotropin pulses and surges. Pulsatile gonadotropin secretion remains normal after isolation of the dorsomedial and medial basal hypothalamus in females (dotted line), but the periovulatory surges observed in normal females no longer occur, indicating that the female surge center is located in the hypothalamic nuclei adjacent to the preoptic area (POA).

gical isolation of these timekeeping cells prevents the surge of GnRH in response to estrogen treatment, but these procedures do not affect negative feedback; negative feedback in both males and females appears to be regulated in the medial basal hypothalamus.

Early exposure to androgens has been hypothesized to destroy the neural connections between the surge generators and the pulse generators. Another hypothesis states that androgenization may diminish pubertal estrogen binding to cytosol receptors so that surges are not observed (Gerall and Givon, 1992). Either hypothesis is consistent with the observation that no amount of estrogen treatment in adulthood can evoke a GnRH surge in males or in females treated with androgens perinatally: the underlying neural machinery is either not present or nonfunctional. As we will see, in some cases, early androgen treatment promotes death of neurons; in other cases, early androgen exposure spares neurons from death.

### Sexual Differentiation and Behavior

As Young and his colleagues demonstrated, the potential for feminine or masculine behavior, like other aspects of sexual differentiation, appears to be organized by early exposure to hormones. Subsequent studies of rats have confirmed this view (Figure 3.24). Female rats that are ovariectomized as adults and injected with

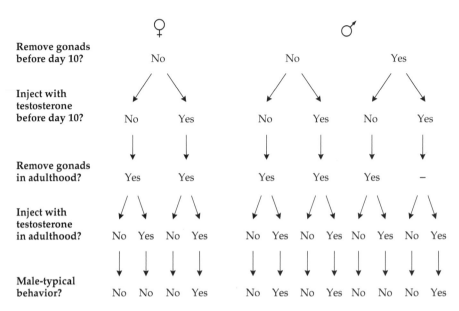

**3.24 Experimental protocol** for determining organizational versus activational effects of androgens on sexually dimorphic mating behavior in rodents.

androgens do not exhibit male-typical mounting behavior in the presence of other females that are sexually receptive. However, if female rats are injected with androgens prior to 10 days of age and injected again with androgens as adults, they do display male-typical mounting behavior in the presence of other females. Similarly, if male rats are castrated at 20 days of age and injected with estrogens and progestins as adults, they do not display feminine mating postures. But if male rats are castrated at 1 day of age and injected with estrogens and progestins as adults, female sexual behavior is observed; that is, these males exhibit lordosis when mounted by male conspecifics (Grady et al., 1965). Thus, exposure to androgens prior to day 20 of life permanently organizes the brain to permit the later expression of masculine behavior.

In addition to mating behavior, many adult behavioral sex differences in rats (for example, aggressive behavior, taste preferences, and parental behavior) are organized by steroid hormones perinatally and activated by steroid hormones in adulthood. The presence of such adult sexually dimorphic behaviors can be manipulated in a predictable way in infancy. Masculinization and defeminization of subsequent behavior occur when rats are exposed to androgens prior to 10 days of age; feminization and demasculinization of subsequent behavior occur when rats are not exposed to androgens prior to 10 days of age. Different sexually dimorphic behaviors do vary slightly in their organizational requirements. Small variations in the timing and dosage of androgen exposure do not influence all sexually dimorphic behaviors in rats equally; however, most behaviors are masculinized by androgen exposure on or before day 10 (Box 3.3) (Grady et al., 1965). Masculine behaviors are activated in adulthood by androgens; feminine behaviors are activated in adulthood by estrogens and progestins.

Box 3.3

# Early Effects of Androgen on Brain and Behavior Are Mediated by Activation of Estrogen Receptors

Recently, molecular biological techniques have been applied to the problem of sexual differentiation in rat brains. The results of these studies demonstrate the importance of neural estrogen receptors in masculinization and defeminization (McCarthy et al., 1993a). Recall that the DNA in the nucleus of each cell contains specific coding instructions for peptides. This "message" is carried by messenger ribonucleic acid (mRNA) from the nucleus to wherever protein production occurs in the cytosol. In the jargon of molecular biology, the mRNA sequence that codes for the protein that makes up the neural estrogen receptor is called the "sense" strand because it provides the message with the instructions for making the estrogen receptor. Once the mRNA sequence for a certain protein is known, a piece of DNA can be generated that consists of 10–30 complementary bases to the sense mRNA. This piece of DNA, technically called an oligodeoxynucleotide, is referred to as "antisense" because it consists of a sequence of bases that is the mirror image of the "sense" message. After entering a cell, the antisense binds to the mRNA and prevents the production of the protein that is normally coded by the mRNA.

In a study that demonstrated the role of estrogen receptors in sexual differentiation in the rat brain, 3-day-old female rats either received hypothalamic infusions of the oligodeoxynucleotide antisense for estrogen receptors, or were subjected to one of two control proce-

dures. Control rat pups were infused with either a scrambled series of 15 bases ("nonsense") dissolved in sesame oil, or the oil vehicle alone (McCarthy et al., 1993b). The females were then injected either with a low dose of testosterone propionate (50 mg), which usually produces slight masculinization in females, or with the oil vehicle.

When the females reached adulthood, they were ovariectomized and injected with estrogen and progesterone. One hundred percent of the females that were not subjected to early testosterone treatment showed lordosis behavior as adults (McCarthy et al., 1993b). Fewer than 20% of the females that received testosterone at 3 days of age and received oil infused into the hypothalamus exhibited lordosis as adults. Similarly, about 20% of the females that received testosterone at 3 days of age and received "nonsense" DNA infused into the hypothalamus exhibited lordosis as adults. In other words, these females were defeminized by the early testosterone treatment. However, infusion of the estrogen receptor antisense into the hypothalamus blocked many of the effects of early testosterone treatment; approximately 80% of these females showed lordosis behavior after estrogen and progesterone priming as adults. These results indicate that the organizational effects of early androgen exposure rely on the synthesis of estrogen receptors in the brain.

Recently, mice with targeted deletions (knockouts) of the α estrogen receptor were

---

Box 3.3 continued

produced (Korach, 1994). Because these mice develop with the estrogen receptor missing throughout life, one might predict that the males would not display normal male mating behavior. However, mating behavior was found to be fairly normal in male estrogen receptor knockout (ERKO) mice despite a lack of ejaculations (Ogawa et al., 1997). ERKO males were less aggressive than normal wild-type (WT) males. Because many so-called estrogen processes remained intact in the ERKO mice, the researchers re-evaluated their hypotheses about the role of estrogen receptors in the development of sexually dimorphic behaviors. It was discovered that an alternative form of the estrogen receptor (termed estrogen receptor β) persists in ERKO mice (see Chapter 5). It is now believed that the β isoform of the estrogen receptor might also modulate sex differences in brain and behavior. These results could also point to a role for androgens in inducing sex differences in the brain directly. Previous studies have indicated that androgens masculinize the amygdala without being converted to estrogens (Meaney and McEwen, 1986).

---

It is not androgen per se, however, that is responsible for the masculinization of neural organization. There is now overwhelming evidence that testosterone is aromatized to estrogen in the brain and that many of its masculinizing effects upon behavior are dependent on this cellular conversion (see Box 3.3; Gorski, 1993; Reddy et al., 1974). Indeed, an injection of estrogen before 10 days of age induces masculine organization of later sexual behavior among rats even *more* effectively than an injection of androgen (Booth, 1977; Feder and Whalen, 1965).

You may be wondering, if estrogens cause masculinization of the nervous system, then why are not all females masculinized? The ovaries of pregnant rats produce high concentrations of estrogen during gestation. Estrogen, like other fat-soluble steroids, could easily pass the blood–placental barrier, enter the fetal circulation, and theoretically cause masculinization in females. However, perinatal rats produce large quantities of a protein called α-fetoprotein, which actively sequesters circulating estrogens; the bound estrogens are removed through the placenta and metabolized by the maternal liver. Alpha-fetoprotein does not bind androgens effectively, however, so testosterone from the gonads of a male fetus reaches its brain, where it is aromatized to estrogen and masculinizes behavior. The α-fetoprotein protects female fetuses from estrogenic steroids, and because females normally have low circulating concentrations of androgens, masculinization does not occur. However, some artificial estrogens do not bind very well to α-fetoprotein (for example, DES), and these artificial estrogens, as we saw above, can have long-term ill effects on female health as well as masculinizing effects on female morphology and behavior.

### Environmental Influences on Mammalian Sexual Differentiation of the Nervous System

As noted above, the majority of behavioral sexual differentiation occurs postnatally in altricial rodents such as rats, mice, and hamsters. However, small and very subtle developmental events that occur *in utero* can also result in significant behavioral effects in adulthood. In addition to the effects of the intrauterine environment, differences in maternal care can also affect sexual differentiation. We discuss these effects in this section.

**EFFECTS OF THE INTRAUTERINE ENVIRONMENT.**    Although much of the process of sexual differentiation occurs postnatally, some sexual differentiation processes begin *in utero* for rats. For example, the position in the uterine horn where a female rat gestates can have important effects on subsequent adult physiology and behavior. Fetal rodents lie adjacent to one another in the uterine horns much like peas in a pod (Figure 3.25). Because the sexes are arranged randomly, a female fetus may be located between two sisters (a position designated 0-M for "no males"), between a sister and a brother (1-M), or between two brothers (2-M) (Clemens et al., 1978; vom Saal, 1979). This is a fine natural preparation for investigating whether there are postnatal effects on physiology and behavior of rodents from varying intrauterine differences. In these studies, rats are delivered by cesarean section and their intrauterine positions noted.

Only a summary comparing two positions, 0-M and 2-M female mice, will be presented here. Ultimately, there is no difference in reproductive capacity between 0-M and 2-M female mice in the laboratory; 0-M and 2-M females both become pregnant and produce equivalent numbers of offspring. However, interfemale aggression is higher in 2-M females than in 0-M females. Males spend more time with 0-M females than with 2-M females; that is, 0-M females are more attractive to males than 2-M females. The reproductive cycles of 0-M females are more easily inhibited by exposure to other adult females than those of 2-M females (see Chapter 6). Finally, 2-M females have longer ovarian cycles than 0-M females. Thus, intrauterine position can affect several physiological and behavioral characteristics of adult female rodents. In nature, enhanced aggressiveness or lengthened reproductive cycles could significantly affect fitness.

Maternal stress can also affect subsequent adult reproductive behavior. When pregnant rats are stressed by restraining them under bright lights several times per day, their male fetal offspring produce less androgen than control males (Ward and Weisz, 1980). In adulthood, the mating behavior of these male rats is adversely affected (Grisham et al., 1991; Ward and Reed, 1985), and certain parts of the nervous system are more female- than male-typical (see Chapters 4 and 11). In addition to these changes in copulatory behaviors, male rats that are prenatally stressed show reduced infanticidal behaviors, increased parental behaviors, and reduced aggressiveness (Ward, 1992). The amount of rough-and-tumble play of

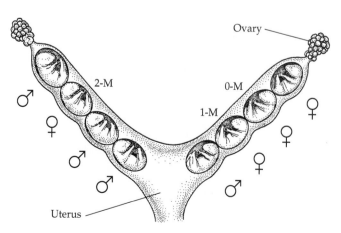

**3.25  Rat pups gestating in utero** are packed into the two uterine horns like peas in a pod. The sex of any given pup's neighbors in utero is entirely random. Thus, a female may gestate between two brothers (signified as 2-M), between a brother and a sister (1-M), or between two sisters (0-M). A female's uterine position in relation to male siblings can exert subtle influences on several behaviors later in life because it determines the degree of her exposure to androgens in utero.

prenatally stressed males is comparable to female levels (Figure 3.26) (Ward and Stehm, 1991).

**EFFECTS OF MATERNAL CARE.** Finally, sex steroid hormones can affect the way in which maternal care is delivered, which in turn can further affect sexual differentiation of behavior. Mother rats lick the anogenital regions of their newborn pups. The primary function of licking the pups is to stimulate the elimination of wastes, but newborn males require maternal licking if they are to develop normal adult mating behavior. Mother rats spend more time licking male pups than licking female pups (C. L. Moore, 1984, 1986; Moore and Morelli, 1979), apparently because mothers prefer the chemosensory cues associated with male pup urine. Testosterone contributes to this preference, because female rat pups injected with testosterone are licked as often as males. Mother rats that are made anosmic (unable to smell) do not lick their male offspring at higher rates, and these males display altered patterns of copulation in adulthood (see Box 4.2). Differential parental treatment of male and female infants has been reported for several primate species as well, including humans (Stewart, 1988). These differential behavioral interactions, as well as maternal stress, can have significant modifying effects on the neural tissues that may underlie sexually dimorphic behaviors (see Chapter 4).

## Conclusions

From these studies of rodents, three main principles of the sexual differentiation of behavior can be distilled: (1) gonadal steroid hormones have organizing effects upon behavior; (2) the organizing effects of steroid hormones are relatively constrained to a particular time during development; (3) an asymmetry exists in the effects of testes and of ovaries on the organization of behavior (but see Arnold and Matthews, 1988; Breedlove, 1992). The early effects of hormones are considered

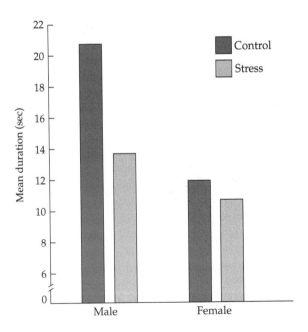

**3.26   Rough-and-tumble play is demasculinized in males by stress in utero.** When pregnant rats were stressed by exposure to bright lights during the last trimester of gestation, the average duration of rough-and-tumble play (at 31 days of age) in their male offspring was similar to that in females. After Ward and Stehm, 1991.

to cause permanent, irreversible behavioral characteristics (Arnold and Breedlove, 1985; Phoenix et al., 1959); for example, early androgen treatment causes relatively irreversible and permanent masculinization of rodent copulatory behavior.

These early hormonal effects can be contrasted with other reversible behavioral influences called activational effects (Phoenix et al., 1959). For example, androgens provided in adulthood activate male copulatory behavior by acting upon the structures organized earlier by these same hormones. The activational effects of hormones on adult behavior are temporary and usually wane soon after the hormone is metabolized. The organizational and activational effects of hormones may actually be quite similar when considered at the molecular level. The permanency of the effects of early exposure to androgens may reflect events unique to a limited period of development. For example, in rats less than 10 days of age, gonadal steroid hormones may prevent neuronal death or promote neuronal survival during a period of cell death (apoptosis) that is limited either temporally or developmentally (Gorski, 1993).

The notion of a critical period for organizational effects arises from the observation that these effects occur only during a specific temporal window of development. The mating behavior of rats, for example, can be masculinized by physiological concentrations of androgens only prior to about day 10. Masculinization can be induced between days 10 and 20 with pharmacological doses of androgen, but at some point (about day 25) no amount of androgen treatment can cause masculinization. This critical period reflects developmental processes that can be altered by steroid hormones only during particular stages of ontogeny; some of these developmental processes will be described in the next chapter. Increasing numbers of examples of organizational effects on adult behavior that occur later in life (for example, postpuberty) have been reported in recent years (Adkins-Regan et al., 1989; Bloch and Gorski, 1988; Cherry et al., 1990; Commins and Yahr, 1984; DeVries et al., 1985), suggesting again that the organizational and activational effects of hormones may be similar at the level of genetic mechanisms.

Finally, the asymmetry of gonadal effects on behavioral organization is striking. In the absence of gonads or steroid hormones, female-typical behavior patterns emerge; that is, behavior is feminized and demasculinized. Exposure to androgens causes the organization of male-typical behaviors; that is, behavior is masculinized and defeminized. This observation has led to the idea that females are the neutral or default sex in mammals, but recent studies indicate that hormones may be necessary for normal development of feminine behavior. Studies of avian sexual behavioral differentiation suggest that male birds are the default or neutral sex (see Box 4.1). To some extent, the asymmetry of testicular and ovarian effects on behavioral sexual differentiation in birds and mammals reflects the differential sensitivities (i.e., receptors) of the underlying neural tissue to estrogens and androgens. However, in both cases, estrogens ultimately act at the cellular level to masculinize and defeminize sexual behaviors.

## Summary

- Behavioral sex differences are common in humans and in nonhuman animals. Because males and females differ in the ratio of androgenic and estrogenic steroid hormone concentrations, behavioral endocrinologists have been particularly interested in the extent to which behavioral sex differences are mediated by hormones.

• Individuals of asexual vertebrate species produce only one sex: females. Production of offspring by asexual reproduction is very efficient, but such species risk extinction if environmental conditions change drastically because there is no genetic variation among the offspring. The recombination of genetic material during sexual reproduction produces genetic variation. Sexual species produce two sexes: females and males.

• The ultimate cause of sex differences appears to reflect sexual selection, a subcategory of natural selection. Animals with polygynous mating systems display more sexual dimorphism than monogamous animals. Humans, which are mildly to moderately polygynous, display several sexual dimorphisms, including larger body size, retarded puberty, increased courtship activity, higher levels of aggression, and reduced parental care in men as compared with women.

• The process of becoming female or male is called sexual differentiation. The primary step in sexual differentiation occurs at fertilization. In mammals, the ovum (which always contains an X chromosome) can be fertilized by a sperm bearing either a Y or an X chromosome; this process is called sex determination. The chromosomal sex of homogametic mammals (XX) is female; the chromosomal sex of heterogametic mammals (XY) is male. Chromosomal sex determines gonadal sex. All subsequent sexual differentiation is normally the result of differential exposure to gonadal steroid hormones. Thus, gonadal sex determines hormonal sex, which regulates morphological sex. Morphological differences in the central nervous system, as well as in some effector organs, lead to behavioral sex differences.

• The gonads and the external genitalia of both sexes result from a single primordial anlage; these organs differ between males and females along a continuum of masculinity and femininity. In contrast, there are dual anlagen for the accessory sex organs. Normal female development of these organs requires feminization (Müllerian duct development) as well as demasculinization (Wolffian duct regression). Normal male development requires masculinization (Wolffian duct development), as well as defeminization (Müllerian duct regression). Thus, sexual differentiation of the accessory sex organs proceeds along two continua: a masculinization–demasculinization scale and a feminization–defeminization scale. Masculinization is the induction of male traits. Feminization is the induction of female traits. Demasculinization is the removal of the potential for male traits, whereas defeminization is the removal of the potential for female traits. This nomenclature is also appropriate for describing behavioral sexual differentiation.

• The process of sexual differentiation is complex, and the potential for errors is present. Perinatal exposure to androgens is the most common cause of anomalous sexual differentiation among females. The source of androgen may be endogenous (as in congenital adrenal hyperplasia) or exogenous (exposure to DES or MPA). Turner syndrome results when the second X chromosome is missing or damaged; these individuals possess dysgenic ovaries and are not exposed to steroid hormones until puberty. Female mammals are the "neutral" sex; additional steps are required for male differentiation, and more steps bring more possibilities for errors in differentiation. Some examples of male anomalous sexual differentiation include 5α-reductase deficiency (XY individuals are born with ambiguous genitalia because of a lack of dihydrotestosterone and are reared as females, but masculinization occurs during puberty) and androgen insensitivity syndrome or TFM (XY individuals lack receptors for androgens and develop as females). By studying these individual "experiments of nature" in which the process of sexual differentiation is atypical, behavioral endocrinologists glean hints about the process of typical sexual differentiation.

• The process of sexual differentiation in birds is different from that in mammals; the homogametic sex is male (ZZ), whereas the heterogametic sex is female (WZ). Males appear to be the "neutral" sex among birds in most aspects of sexual differentiation. The embryonic ovary has the ability to feminize the embryonic testis.

• Some reptilian species are like birds in that the male is homogametic; other species resemble mammals in that the female is homogametic. In yet other reptilian species, sex chromosomes are absent and sex determination occurs in response to incubation temperature. Substantial variation in this process exists; high ambient temperatures evoke male development in some species, but female development in others. Some fish species possess the ability to undergo sex changes in adulthood in response to social or physiological cues.

• In some species, alternative mating strategies among males are associated with differences in body type and behavior, which are often regulated by changes in hormone secretion.

• Gonadal steroid hormones have organizing effects upon behavior. The organizing effects of steroid hormones are relatively constrained to the early stages of development. An asymmetry exists in the effects of testes and ovaries on the organization of behavior in mammals. Hormone exposure early in life has organizational effects on subsequent rodent mating behavior; early steroid hormone treatment causes relatively irreversible and permanent masculinization of rodent copulatory behavior. These early hormone effects can be contrasted with the reversible behavioral influences of steroid hormones provided in adulthood, which are called activational effects. The activational effects of hormones on adult behavior are temporary and may wane soon after the hormone is metabolized.

• Females undergo cycles of reproductive physiology and behavior that correspond to the cyclic release of eggs during the breeding season; males produce sperm at relatively constant rates throughout the breeding season and exhibit relatively constant reproductive behavior. The cyclic nature of female reproductive function is driven by the cyclic release of GnRH from surge generators located in the anterior hypothalamus. Both males and females display pulsatile release of GnRH from the medial basal hypothalamus. Exposure to androgens early in development abolishes forever the potential to generate GnRH surges, either by destroying the neural connections between the pulse and surge generators or by reducing estrogen receptor availability in the surge generator tissues.

## Questions for Discussion

1. What are some behavioral sex differences that you have noticed between boys and girls? Do you think that the sex differences you have noted arise from biological causes or are learned? How would you go about establishing your opinions as fact?

2. "Men are too aggressive to write and produce cartoon programs appropriate for children." Support and refute this statement based on sound scientific principles.

3. Why is it inappropriate to refer to androgens as "male" hormones and estrogens as "female" hormones?

4. Discuss the early hormone–anatomy correlates that were the conceptual forerunners of the organizational/activational hypothesis proposed by Young and colleagues.

5. Discuss the following proposition: The process of developing sexually dimorphic behaviors is conceptually similar to the development of sexually dimorphic accessory reproductive organs, and dissimilar from the development of sexually dimorphic external genitalia.

## Suggested Readings

Arnold, A. P. 1996. Genetically triggered sexual differentiation of brain and behavior. *Hormones and Behavior,* 30: 495–505.

Bass, A. H. 1996. Shaping brain sexuality. *American Scientist,* 84: 352–361.

Crews, D. 1996. Temperature-dependent sex determination: The interplay of steroid hormones and temperature. *Zoological Science,* 13: 1–13.

Gerall, A. A., Moltz, H., and Ward, I. L. 1992. *Handbook of Behavioral Neurobiology.* Vol. 11, *Sexual Differentiation.* Plenum, New York.

Gustafson, M. L., and Donahoe, P. K. 1994. Male sex determination: Current concepts of male sexual differentiation. *Annual Review of Medicine,* 45: 505–524.

Micevych, P. E., and Hammer, R. P. 1995. *Neurobiological Effects of Sex Steroid Hormones.* Cambridge University Press, Cambridge.

Phoenix, C. H., Goy, R. W., Gerall, A. A., and Young, W. C. 1959. Organizing action of prenatally administered testosterone propionate on the tissues mediating mating behavior in the female guinea pig. *Endocrinology,* 65: 369–382.

# 4

# Sex Differences in Behavior

## Animal Models and Humans

In North America, new parents are often sent congratulatory cards after the births of their babies. To gain some insights into the cultural attitudes about sex differences, a sample of these greeting cards was examined (Stern and Hildebrandt-Karraker, 1989). Not surprisingly, cards for boys were never pink and cards for girls were never blue; cards for boys also had fewer decorative elements such as lace, ribbons, hearts, and flowers than cards meant for girls. Pictures of toys and mobiles were more frequent on female cards; pictures of sports equipment and vehicles were more common on male cards. An analysis of the words printed on the cards revealed a sex difference in the verbal descriptions as well. For example, the word "sweet" was much more common on cards meant for girls than on cards meant for boys. These results suggest that people possess psychological schemas for the two sexes. One distillation of these observations is that boys are considered more "active," and girls are considered more "decorative" (Stern and Hildebrandt-Karraker, 1989). What are the bases for these schemas? Are the sex differences in activity, for example, the inevitable consequences of the differential endocrine environments of boys and girls, or are these differences imposed by cultural practices and beliefs? To untangle these issues, animal models are often used in behavioral endocrinology. Unlike the situation in humans, where sex differences are usually only a matter of degree (often slight), in some animals, only one sex exhibits a particular behavior. Studies of such behaviors are particularly valuable for understanding the interaction among behavior, hormones, and the nervous system. The goal of this chapter is to examine the factors that cause male and female brains to develop along distinct pathways underlying behavioral sexual dimorphisms.

When Young and his colleagues proposed the organizational/activational hypothesis of hormonal sexual differentiation (see Chapter 3), they drew an analogy between the effects of early testosterone exposure on the development of the accessory reproductive organs and its effects on the neural tissues underlying mating behavior. Because early exposure to hormones was found to change the probability of specific behaviors, and because all behavior is mediated by the nervous system, it was reasonable to suggest that hormones caused changes in the nervous system. However, the authors warned that, unlike the embryologists who

## Box 4.1
# The Organization of Avian Copulatory Behavior

Birds have been useful models for the study of neural sexual differentiation because they allow researchers to avoid one confounding factor that is present in the study of mammals. Because treatments that masculinize behavior usually masculinize the external genitalia of mammals as well, researchers found it inappropriate to assume that sex differences in behavior reflect changes in the nervous system. In other words, the sex differences in behavior might simply be due to the changes in external genital morphology (Beach, 1971). One way to resolve the controversy about the contributions of neural and non-neural changes to the development of sex differences in behavior is to discover structural changes in the nervous system that correspond to behavioral differences. Although sex differences in neural structure, neurotransmitter systems, and neuronal numbers have been reported in the mammalian nervous system (Breedlove, 1992), these morphological

differences have not been linked directly to the regulation of sexually dimorphic behaviors (Balthazart et al., 1996).

Another approach to this issue has involved studies of hormone–behavior interactions during the development of birds. Males and females of most avian species do not differ in external genital morphology: both sexes have a single cloacal opening. Thus, neural and genital morphological changes are not confounded in birds as they are in mammals (Adkins-Regan, 1987). Studies of avian sexual differentiation of behavior have provided the most convincing evidence that early hormone exposure changes the neural structures that control adult sexually dimorphic behaviors.

The Japanese quail (*Coturnix japonica*) is the avian species most commonly studied to understand the hormonal bases of mating behavior. Mating behavior is sexually dimorphic in quail. Males strut and crow before and after had found pronounced structural changes in the reproductive organs in response to perinatal androgen exposure, neurologists and psychologists interested in the effects of androgens on neural tissues were unlikely to find alterations so drastic. Instead, a more subtle change reflected in function rather than visible structure would be expected (Phoenix et al., 1959). So, most endocrinologists in the 1950s and 1960s believed that structural changes in the CNS mediated behavioral differences between the two sexes, but assumed that any underlying changes in brain tissue would be beyond the technical abilities of the day to observe. Despite the lack of any empirical data showing direct changes in neural tissue that mediated sexually dimorphic behaviors, hypothetical models of neural modulation in response to early hormone exposure flourished. Because the evidence of hormonally induced neural changes was indirect, other researchers resisted the temptation to speculate on mechanisms beyond their data. They explained changes in the adult copulatory ability of neonatally castrated rats, for example, by sensory deficiencies that resulted from inadequate penile development due to androgen deprivation (Beach, 1971). Thus, the effects of perinatal steroid hormone manipulations on subsequent adult behavior were explained as indirect effects on genital (non-neural) morphology (Box 4.1).

In the early 1970s, however, researchers discovered subtle, microscopic sex differences in the neural connections of the hypothalamus, and soon thereafter

---

copulatory mounting (Adkins, 1978). Castration of males reduces these male-typical behaviors, and testosterone therapy restores them (Adkins, 1975). Females never display copulatory mounting behaviors, and crowing and strutting occur less frequently than in males even when females are injected in adulthood with androgens (Adkins, 1975; Balthazart et al., 1983). Generally, estrogenic metabolites of androgens activate copulatory behavior in adult males, whereas androgenic metabolites of testosterone activate the strutting and crowing behaviors (Adkins, 1978; Adkins-Regan, 1996; Balthazart et al., 1985).

If eggs containing male quail embryos are injected with either testosterone or estradiol, the males exhibit fewer male-typical copulatory behaviors as adults than untreated males (Adkins-Regan, 1987). In other words, the males are demasculinized. These demasculinizing effects of testosterone or estradiol occur only prior to day 12 of the 17-day incubation period. If eggs containing female quail embryos are injected with androgens or estradiol, adult female behavior is relatively unaffected (Ad-

kins-Regan, 1987). In other words, the females are neither defeminized nor masculinized by the endocrine manipulations. Treatment of female quail in the egg prior to day 9 of incubation with an anti-estrogen (a substance that binds to estrogen receptors and prevents natural estrogens from binding) produced masculinization of adult copulatory behavior (Adkins, 1976). In other words, anti-estrogens prevented the demasculinization that is produced by the endogenous estrogens (Balthazart and Foidart, 1993).

Male and female quail do not differ in their concentrations of circulating androgens immediately post-hatching, but females do exhibit higher circulating estrogen concentrations during the last few days before hatching occurs (Balthazart and Foidart, 1993). Taken together, these results suggest that the estrogens secreted from the ovaries normally demasculinize the copulatory behavior of female quail. Male quail apparently do not secrete sufficient quantities of sex steroid hormones to demasculinize their own behavior.

macroscopic sex differences in brain organization were reported. It was shown that these sex differences in brain organization could be reversed by early hormonal manipulation. Even the most staunch critics of the organizational/activational hypothesis were eventually persuaded that early hormone treatment changed neural tissues underlying sexually dimorphic behaviors, and that these behaviors could be activated by the effects of gonadal steroid hormones on these same tissues in adulthood (e.g., Beach, 1975). Recent studies, however, have revealed that hormonal effects on the nervous system are not necessarily direct. Hormones may also act upon non-neural tissues, especially those that potentially change sensory input to affect neural development (Beyer and Feder, 1987; Fishman and Breedlove, 1987; Moore and Morelli, 1979; Moore et al., 1992).

## Neural Bases of Mammalian Sex Differences

The first clear-cut, but minuscule, sexual dimorphism in the brain was observed during electron microscopic examination of synapses in the **medial preoptic area (MPOA)**, an area just anterior to the hypothalamus in rats (Raisman and Field, 1973a). Because previous studies had shown that lesions or stimulation of the MPOA led to alterations in sexual behavior (see Chapter 5), the possibility of sex differences in the neural organization of this area was particularly intriguing. The researchers carefully counted and categorized the synapses in the MPOA that survived after neurons from another area of the brain, the stria terminalis, had been cut. They discovered that females had more synapses on dendritic spines and fewer synapses on dendritic shafts than males, whereas males had more synapses on dendritic shafts and fewer synapses on dendritic spines than females (Raisman and Field, 1973a). Dendritic spines are small outgrowths along the dendritic shafts that give dendrites possessing them a "rough" appearance. These spines have become the focus of much research, especially in learning and memory, because their number and function may vary in response to experience (Figure 4.1). In males castrated on day 1 of life, the female pattern of synapses was observed (Raisman and Field, 1973b). Similarly, in females injected with testosterone prior to 4 days of age, the male pattern of synaptic organization was observed. The functional meaning of these data remains unknown; in other words, how the observed sex differences in synaptic organization mediate behavior, or even *if* they mediate behavior, remains unresolved. However, this observation of sex differences in neural organization was extremely important because it began to fulfill the prediction made years before that a "more subtle change reflected in function rather than visible structure" was involved in mediating sex differences in behavior (Phoenix et al., 1959).

Since this early report, more obvious structural sex differences have been observed in mammalian brains. Because of its prominent role in the mediation of mating behavior in several species, the **preoptic area (POA)** of the hypothalamus has received special attention. For example, in rats, there is a collection of cell bodies (a nucleus) in the medial preoptic area that is five to seven times larger in males than in females (Gorski et al., 1978). The difference is so prominent that rat brains can be accurately classified as either male or female by examining with the naked eye thin slices dissected through the hypothalamus (Figure 4.2). This region of the preoptic area has been termed the **sexually dimorphic nucleus of the pre-**

Presynaptic neuron

Postsynaptic neuron

Dendritic spines

Shaft

**4.1   Synapses may form upon either dendritic spines or upon the shaft of a dendrite.** In the MPOA, male rats tend to have more synapses from non-amygdaloid neurons on dendritic shafts and fewer synapses on dendritic spines than females; females have more synapses on dendritic spines and fewer synapses on dendritic shafts than males. Hormone manipulations immediately postpartum can affect this pattern of neuronal connectivity.

optic area (**SDN-POA**) (Gorski et al., 1978). The SDN-POA of females treated early in life with androgens can approach the size of the masculine SDN-POA, whereas the size of the feminine SDN-POA can be attained in males by neonatal castration (Gorski, 1984). Presumably, the sex difference in the size of the SDN-POA could reflect differences in cell numbers or differences in cell size between males and females. The sex difference in the size of the SDN-POA is due to a decreased number of cells in females and castrated males; androgens or their estrogenic metabolites seem either to augment neurogenesis (Jacobson and Gorski, 1981) or reduce cell death in this region (Forger, 1998) (Box 4.2). Rats with testicular feminization mutation, which have deficient androgen receptors but normal estrogen receptors, display female-typical genitalia, but male-typical SDN-POA (Jacobson, 1980).

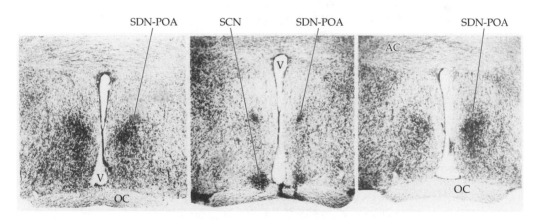

SDN-POA          SCN          SDN-POA                    SDN-POA

AC

V                V

V

OC               OC                                        OC

**4.2   The sexually dimorphic nuclei of the preoptic area (SDN-POA)** in rats are shown in cross-section in micrographs of a male (left), a female (center), and a female treated with testosterone as a newborn (right). Note that the SDN-POA of the male are substantially larger than those of the untreated female, but are equal in size to those of the testosterone-treated female. OC = optic chiasm; SCN = suprachiasmatic nucleus; V = third ventricle. Courtesy of Roger Gorski.

The functional significance of the sex difference in the size of the SDN-POA is not really known. Lesions to the entire POA disrupt normal mating behavior in a wide variety of species, including rodents and primates (Hart and Leedy, 1985). If only the SDN-POA is lesioned, females continue to display normal reproductive cycles (Arendash and Gorski, 1983). If only the SDN-POA is lesioned in males, they also continue to display normal mating behavior, or in some cases, exhibit temporary and mild copulatory dysfunction (Arendash and Gorski, 1983; DeJonge et al., 1989). Similar results have been documented with other species. For example, the sexually dimorphic region of the preoptic area/anterior hypothalamus is not necessary for male copulatory behavior in ferrets (Baum et al., 1990; Cherry and Baum, 1990).

Sex differences have been reported in several other brain structures of rodents. For example, the volume of the medial amygdala and the medial posterior area of the bed nucleus of the stria terminalis is about 20% larger in males than in females (del Abril et al., 1987; Mizukami et al., 1983). These two brain regions may be part of a sexually dimorphic neural circuit that includes the SDN-POA,

## Box 4.2
# The Spinal Nucleus of the Bulbocavernosus Muscle

One way to overcome the problems inherent in understanding the functional significance of neural sex differences is to study a sexually dimorphic system with a very simple function. One such mammalian system that has been studied extensively is located in the spinal cord. The spinal motoneurons that innervate the muscles attached to the base of the rat penis are located in a particular position in the spinal cord, and collectively are referred to as the spinal nucleus of the bulbocavernosus (SNB) (Breedlove, 1992). These neurons control the striated bulbocavernosus and levator ani muscles that are responsible for penile erection in rodents, as well as the external anal sphincter (see figure). The SNB is larger and has more cells in males than in females because the SNB in females, and the muscles that control erec-

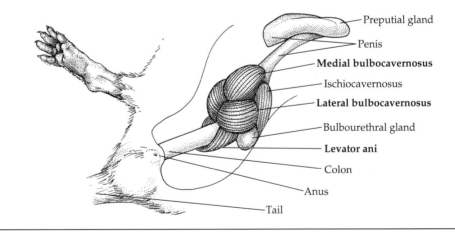

Preputial gland
Penis
**Medial bulbocavernosus**
Ischiocavernosus
**Lateral bulbocavernosus**
Bulbourethral gland
**Levator ani**
Colon
Anus
Tail

as well as the anteroventral periventricular nucleus (AVPv) (Simerly and Swanson, 1986). In contrast to the cell groups mentioned thus far, the AVPv is *larger* in females, or in males castrated before 10 days of age, than in intact males, and is the source of a sexually dimorphic projection to the arcuate nucleus (Simerly et al., 1996).

Several sexual dimorphisms in the nervous systems of humans have also been described (Table 4.1). In common with other mammals, a sexually dimorphic nucleus was discovered in the POA of humans (Swaab and Fliers, 1985). Because this nucleus resembles the SDN-POA of rats and is larger in males than in females, it was also named the SDN-POA. There has been some controversy, however, about the boundaries of the human SDN-POA and the consistency of the observed sex differences in its volume (see, for example, Allen et al., 1989). In other studies, the nuclei of the human POA have been subdivided into four smaller regions called the **interstitial nuclei of the anterior hypothalamus (INAH)**, abbreviated INAH-1, INAH-2, and so on (Allen et al., 1989). Under this neuroanatomical classification scheme, INAH-1 was considered to be equivalent to the SDN-POA, and,

---

tile function, are diminished in size or completely absent in adult female rats (Breedlove and Arnold, 1983a,b). Humans also have the bulbocavernosus muscle, but the sex difference is much less pronounced in humans than in rats (Forger and Breedlove, 1986). In men, the bulbocavernosus muscle has a similar function as in rats, contracting rhythmically during erection and ejaculation. Women retain a bulbocavernosus muscle, albeit smaller and modified in form. The motoneurons of Onuf's nucleus, the human homologue of the rat SNB, are more numerous in men than in women (Forger and Breedlove, 1986).

During fetal development, female rats have bulbocavernosus and levator ani muscles similar in size to those of males, and these muscles, which connect to the base of the clitoris in females, are innervated by the SNB (Rand and Breedlove, 1987). However, these muscles atrophy and the SNB motoneurons die in females around the time of birth. Androgen treatment spares the muscles and secondarily spares the SNB. Once the muscles have regressed, androgen treatment cannot restore the muscle cells, so the critical period of androgen effectiveness in sparing motoneurons in the SNB is defined

by the rate of muscular atrophy. The muscle cells, but not the motoneurons of the SNB, possess androgen receptors during the time of fetal sex differentiation (Fishman et al., 1990). Thus, androgen acts on the neural tissue of the SNB indirectly by preventing cell death (apoptosis) in the muscles directly. Androgens, but not estrogenic metabolites of androgens, prevent cell death. This assertion is based on the observation that genetic XY males with testicular feminization mutation, who lack functional androgen receptors but retain functional estrogen receptors as well as aromatase activity, exhibit feminine SNB and associated musculature (Breedlove and Arnold, 1981).

Environmental effects can also influence the size of the SNB. Mother rats spend more time licking and attending to the perianal regions of male than of female pups. Anosmic mothers reduced the time spent licking their male offspring, and these males exhibited a 10% reduction in the number of motoneurons in the SNB (Moore et al., 1992; Michel and Moore, 1995). This reduction in SNB size may contribute to adult deficits in male mating behavior. In utero stress and other factors can also feminize the SNB of male rats (Ward, 1992).

| Table 4.1 **Structural sex differences in the central nervous system of humans** | |
| --- | --- |
| **Brain region** | **Difference** |
| *Hypothalamus* | |
| SDN-POA | ♂ > ♀ |
| INAH-3 | ♂ > ♀ |
| Bed nucleus of the stria terminalis (BNST) | ♂ > ♀ |
| Suprachiasmatic nuclei (SCN) | ♀ > ♂[a] |
| *Spinal cord* | |
| Onuf's nucleus (no. of motoneurons) | ♂ > ♀ |
| *Structures associated with language* | |
| Planum temporale | ♀ > ♂[b] |
| Dorsolateral prefrontal cortex | ♀ > ♂ |
| Superior temporal gyrus | ♀ > ♂ |
| *Structures connecting the hemispheres* | |
| Corpus callosum (posterior portion) | ♀ > ♂[c] |
| Anterior commissure | ♀ > ♂ |
| Massa intermedia of thalamus | ♀ > ♂ |

*Source*: Forger, 1998.
[a]More elongated in ♀
[b]Left and right more symmetrical in size in ♀
[c]More bulbous in ♀

in contrast to the previous report, no sex differences were observed in this tiny brain region. The volumes of INAH-2 and INAH-3, however, were reported to be larger in men than in women (Figure 4.3; Allen et al., 1989). Even more recently, a sex difference in nuclear volume was reported in INAH-3, but not in INAH-2 (LeVay, 1991).

Because brain tissue from humans is obtained at different times after death and after great variation in fixation, it is not particularly surprising that contradictory results have been obtained. The report by LeVay (1991) has generated enormous debate because, in addition to the observation that INAH-3 was smaller in women than in men, INAH-3 was reported to be smaller in homosexual men than in heterosexual men (LeVay, 1991). Although sexual preferences have not traditionally been part of medical records, the sexual preference of the homosexual men in LeVay's sample was included in their health records because the vast majority of these men had died from complications resulting from AIDS. Their brains were compared with those of men whose sexual orientation was unknown, but assumed to be heterosexual, and who had died primarily from other causes. However, not all of the obvious potential confounding variables, namely, HIV infection, age, body size (people infected with HIV often have reduced body weight), brain size, and testosterone levels (males infected with HIV often show end-stage reductions in plasma testosterone levels), have been ruled out as causative factors underlying the differences in INAH-3 size between the hetero-

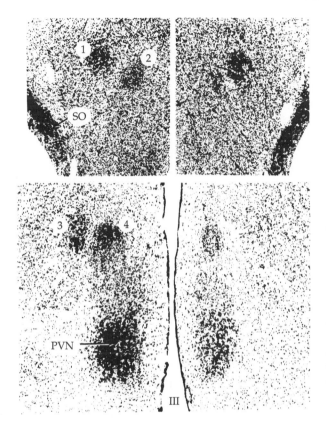

**4.3  The interstitial nuclei of the anterior hypothalamus (INAH).** Photomicrographs of the human anterior hypothalamus in cross-section, showing the four INAH in a male (left; 1–4) and the corresponding areas in a female (right). Precise quantitative procedures (Allen et al., 1989) have shown that the volumes of INAH-2 and INAH-3 are greater in men. The lower photomicrographs are taken from a region caudal to the area depicted in the upper photomicrograph. SO = supraoptic nucleus; PVN = paraventricular nucleus; III = third ventricle. Courtesy of Roger Gorski.

sexual and homosexual men (Byne and Parsons, 1993). These findings have fueled the debate on whether sexual orientation is mediated primarily by biological or by environmental factors, a debate that will be considered below.

Despite the importance of sexual dimorphisms in the size of brain structures as gross indicators of sex differences in brain function and behavior, structural differences in neural tissues have not been directly linked to behavior, especially in mammals. For example, the critical questions regarding what features in the brain are necessary and sufficient to account for sex differences in the ability of sex steroid hormones to activate adult sexual behavior remain, for the most part, unanswered (Balthazart et al., 1996). In addition to studies of nuclear volume, behavioral endocrinologists have examined sex differences in neurochemistry, neural connectivity, enzyme activation, hormone and neurotransmitter receptor distribution, and gene expression in the brains of males and females in an attempt to answer this question.

## Molecular Sex Differences in the Brain

One possible explanation for why adult hormone treatment elicits different sexual behaviors in males and females involves sex differences in neural estrogen or androgen receptors. In most early studies, no differences in steroid hormone binding sites were reported; however, recent studies using more sophisticated techniques have revealed some modest sex differences (Brown et al., 1992). For instance, sex differences in the distribution of corticosteroid receptors in rat brains have been reported. Mineralocorticoid binding in males was higher than in females throughout the hippocampus, although glucocorticoid binding in the brain was equivalent between the sexes, 3 days after both gonads and adrenal glands had been removed (MacLusky et al., 1996). These results may reflect sex differences in neural stress responses. Also, and more to the point, there are sex differences in the distribution of androgen and estrogen receptors throughout the nervous system (MacLusky et al., 1996).

Several studies that reveal sex differences in the distribution or regulation of neurotransmitters or their receptors have been reported. Only indirect links have been established between sex differences in neurotransmitter distribution and in the ability of steroid hormones to evoke adult sexual behavior, however. The innervation of several brain regions, including the lateral septum, by neurons that release vasopressin shows marked sex differences in rats (G. J. DeVries et al., 1983; van Leeuwen et al., 1985); however, the functional meaning of these sex differences remains obscure (G. J. DeVries, 1995).

In contrast to the unknown role of vasopressin in rats, a nanopeptide related to vasopressin, arginine vasotocin (AVT), has been shown to modulate several

**4.4　Sex differences in the bullfrog brain mediate calling behavior.** (Top) A male bullfrog calling. This behavior attracts potential mates and wards off competing males. (Bottom) Immunocytochemistry reveals greater numbers of cell bodies and fibers containing arginine vasotocin (AVT) in the preoptic area of a male bullfrog brain (right) than in the same region of a female brain (left). Top courtesy of Sunny K. Boyd; bottom from Boyd et al. 1992.

aspects of sexually dimorphic behavior in bullfrogs (*Rana catesbeiana*) (Boyd, 1997). Only male bullfrogs give the so-called "mate call," and only females respond to mate calls by moving toward the source of the call (phonotaxis). Males respond to other males' mate calls by emitting their own mate calls. Both sexes give "release calls" when mounted inappropriately. Injection of males, but not females, with AVT increases the rate of vocalizing. Injection of AVT causes females to be attracted to the source of a call (a male frog or a speaker). Six separate populations of AVT-releasing neurons have been found in bullfrog brains, and receptors for AVT are located in brain regions that are linked to important reproductive behaviors, including vocalization, phonotaxis, and locomotor activity. There are sex differences in the numbers of AVT receptors in the amygdala, hypothalamus, pretrigeminal nucleus, and dorsolateral nucleus (Figure 4.4). More importantly, steroid hormones affect AVT receptor availability. Estradiol modulates AVT receptor numbers in the amygdala of both sexes, and both estradiol and DHT affect AVT receptor numbers in the pretrigeminal nucleus of males. Thus, AVT seems to function as a neurotransmitter for reproductively relevant behaviors, and AVT activity is modulated by steroid hormones in bullfrogs.

Aggression in mammals is often mediated by the neurotransmitter serotonin. There are at least ten different types of serotonin receptors in mammals, and activation of one of three or four different receptors modulates aggressive behavior. In one study, using positron emission tomography (PET) and a selective radiotracer that binds only to the type 2 serotonin receptor, the distribution of this receptor was mapped in living, age-matched men and women (Biver et al., 1996). Significantly higher numbers of type 2 serotonin receptors were found in the brains of men (Biver et al., 1996). The mechanisms by which sex steroids influence serotonin or vasopressin receptor numbers and distribution have not been discovered.

As noted in Chapter 2, testosterone serves as a prohormone for the production of either estradiol or dihydrotestosterone (DHT) in many mammals and birds. One strategy for understanding the role of testosterone in evoking sex differences in neural tissue is to identify neurons containing testosterone receptors as well as enzymes that convert testosterone to other hormones (Hutchison and Beyer, 1994; Schlinger, 1997). Neurons that contain testosterone receptors and aromatase, 5α-, or 5β-reductase are likely candidates for part of a circuit mediating sexually dimorphic behavior(s) (Roselli et al., 1996, 1997). There are substantial sex differences in aromatase activity in several brain regions of rats, including the bed nucleus of the stria terminalis, the medial preoptic nucleus, and the ventromedial nucleus of the hypothalamus; aromatase activity was two to four times higher in males than in females in these areas (Roselli et al., 1997). Aromatase activity appears to be regulated by androgen receptors in the preoptic area and the hypothalamus; testosterone and DHT, but not estrogen, maintain aromatase activity in these regions in castrated rats. There is no sex difference in aromatase activity or aromatase mRNA in the amygdala, and neither aromatase levels nor aromatase mRNA expression were affected by steroid hormones in that area. These results suggest that adult sex differences in responsiveness to androgens may reflect differences in gene expression in neural circuits that are involved in regulating sexually dimorphic behaviors (Balthazart et al., 1996; Celotti et al., 1997; Roselli et al., 1997; Schlinger, 1997; and see below).

# Animal Models for Sexually Dimorphic Behaviors

## Bird Song

The best evidence that behavioral sex differences are the result of hormonally induced structural changes in the brain is found in birds (Nottebohm and Arnold, 1976). In contrast to mammals, in which structural differences in neural tissues have not been directly linked to behavior, structural differences in avian brains have been directly linked to a sexually dimorphic behavior: bird song. A subset of birds belonging to the order Passeriformes (the oscines, or songbirds) produce complex vocalizations that, for the most part, are learned during development. These complex, learned vocalizations are referred to as song. In most species of songbirds, song production is sexually dimorphic. Males usually sing more than females, although this sex difference is not constant across species. Male zebra finches (*Taeniopygia guttata*), like many male songbirds, sing in order to attract females and ward off competing males. Female zebra finches never sing, even after testosterone treatment in adulthood (Adkins-Regan and Ascenzi, 1987). In contrast, there appears to be no sex difference in the singing behavior of bay wrens (*Thryothorus nigricapillus*), a tropical duetting species in which males and females participate equally in producing two-bird song (Brenowitz and Arnold, 1985, 1986; Brenowitz et al., 1985; Brenowitz, 1997). Other species, such as canaries (*Serinus canaria*), fall somewhere between these two extremes; that is, females sing, but they sing less than males (Figure 4.5). These sex differences in behavior reflect sex differences in the neural centers of the brain that control singing (Arnold and Jordan, 1988).

**NEURAL BASES OF SEX DIFFERENCES IN BIRD SONG.**    In contrast to the early predictions of subtle, hormonally induced changes in brain structure (Phoenix et al., 1959), several brain regions in songbirds exhibit substantial sex differences in size. Two major brain circuit pathways, the efferent motor pathway and the auditory transmission pathway, have been implicated in the learning and production of

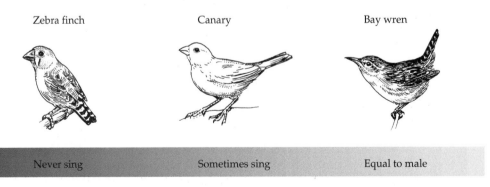

Zebra finch          Canary          Bay wren

| Never sing | Sometimes sing | Equal to male |

**4.5  Singing in female songbirds** falls along a broad continuum: females of some species, such as zebra finches, never sing in nature; females of other species, such as bay wrens, sing as frequently as male conspecifics. Most species are intermediate between these two extremes. For example, female canaries sing, but not as frequently as males, and their songs are generally less complex than those of males. After Brenowitz, 1997.

bird song (Arnold and Jordan, 1988). These pathways were first described in canaries and zebra finches (Nottebohm and Arnold, 1976; Nottebohm et al., 1982) and have been subsequently identified in several oscine species. Sexual dimorphisms in the sizes of nuclei in these pathways seem to parallel sex differences in singing behavior. For example, large dimorphisms exist in the size of several song control nuclei between male and female zebra finches (Bottjer et al., 1985; Nottebohm and Arnold, 1976), but these dimorphisms are less extreme in canaries, and are undetectable in bay wrens (Brenowitz, 1991; 1997; Brenowitz and Arnold, 1986; Brenowitz et al., 1985).

The efferent motor pathway is necessary for the production of song in adult birds. This pathway consists of the interconnected brain areas that control neural output to the syrinx (the avian vocal production organ). The locations of the nuclei in this motor pathway for a "generic" songbird brain are illustrated in Figure 4.6. The "high vocal center" (HVC) sends an efferent projection to the robust nucleus of the archistriatum (RA). A projection from RA travels to the tracheosyringeal division of the nucleus of the hypoglossal nerve (nXIIts), either directly or indirectly via the dorsomedial (DM) portion of the nucleus intercollicularis (ICo). From nXIIts, motor signals travel by way of the tracheosyringeal nerve to the syrinx. Lesions of the HVC and RA result in song production deficits in adulthood (Nottebohm et al., 1976; 1982).

Information from HVC can also reach RA through a more circuitous route (Bottjer et al., 1989; Okuhata and Saito, 1987). This second route, the auditory transmission pathway, has been called the "recursive loop" (Nottebohm et al., 1990). Information in the recursive loop travels from HVC to area X (a forebrain nucleus located in the parolfactory lobe), then to the medial nucleus of the dorsolateral thalamus (DLM), to the lateral portion of the magnocellular nucleus of

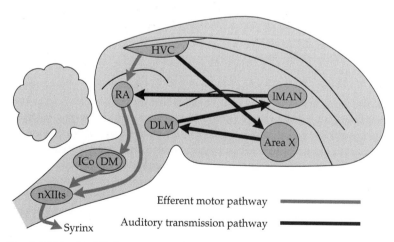

**4.6  The neural basis of bird song,** shown in a "generic" songbird brain. In species in which large sex differences in song frequency are observed, the nuclei involved in these brain circuits are larger in males than in females. Courtesy of Gregory Ball, Daniel Bernard, and Joseph Casto.

the anterior neostriatum (lMAN), and finally to RA. This recursive pathway has been implicated in the process of song learning.

The song learning process occurs in two stages. During the *sensory stage,* young birds hear and memorize the song(s) of adult birds. The sensory stage is followed by a *sensory–motor stage* in which birds try to reproduce the song that is stored in memory. Learning at this stage proceeds by trial and error. The sensory–motor stage ends when the bird can reproduce full adult song. At this point song is considered *crystallized* and is relatively impervious to change. Damage to the recursive loop in zebra finches, especially area X and lMAN, before species-typical song is crystallized results in song abnormalities (Bottjer et al., 1984; Scharff and Nottebohm, 1991; Sohrabji et al., 1990).

**HORMONAL INFLUENCES ON SONG CONTROL CENTERS.**    Because sexual dimorphisms in the size of their song control areas are so conspicuous, zebra finches have proved to be an excellent model species in which to study the effects of sex steroid hormones on the neural structures involved in song (Arnold et al., 1987). The HVC and RA of male zebra finches are three to six times larger than those of female conspecifics, and one song control region, area X, cannot even be discerned in females (Nottebohm, 1991; Nottebohm and Arnold, 1976). The larger size of these nuclei in males is due to the fact that the neurons in these nuclei are larger, more numerous, and farther apart (Arnold and Gorski, 1984; Arnold and Matthews, 1988). Although castration of adult zebra finches leads to a reduction in singing, it does not reduce the size of the brain nuclei controlling song production. Similarly, androgen treatment of adult female zebra finches does not induce changes either in singing or in the size of the song control regions. Thus, activational effects of steroid hormones do not account for the sex differences in singing behavior or brain nucleus size in zebra finches.

The sexual dimorphisms in brain nucleus size and subsequent singing behavior of zebra finches are organized early in development. Later, singing is activated by testosterone acting on the male-typical neural structure (Figure 4.7; Gurney and Konishi, 1980). Both male and female zebra finches have been studied, but only the results of endocrine manipulations of females will be presented here. Females treated with DHT soon after hatching and given no endocrine therapy as adults exhibited increased numbers of neurons in RA and HVC, but these nuclei were approximately the same size as those of untreated females. These females did not sing. If females were injected with DHT post-hatching, then treated with testosterone or DHT in adulthood, the RA and HVC were larger and had more neurons than those of typical females, but were smaller and had fewer neurons than those of typical males. These females also failed to sing as adults. Females that were injected with estradiol post-hatching but not treated with hormones as adults also did not sing. Their RA and HVC were larger in size and had more and larger neurons than those of untreated females, but these brain regions were still smaller and had fewer neurons than those of untreated males. If females were injected post-hatching with estradiol, then treated either with testosterone or DHT in adulthood, their RA and HVC approached the size of those of untreated males, and they sang! Thus, early exposure to estradiol increases sensitivity to androgens in adulthood. This pattern of hormonally mediated organizational effects is very different from those underlying other avian behaviors, such as quail copulatory behavior (see Box 4.1). The reasons underlying this difference remain

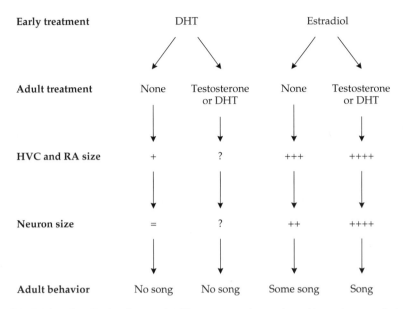

**4.7   Singing in zebra finches** is organized by estrogens but activated by androgens. Only females that are injected with estradiol after hatching and injected with either DHT or testosterone in adulthood show neural development comparable to that of males and display singing behavior. Thus, early exposure to estradiol is necessary for androgens to have the song-activating effects seen in adult male birds. The plus signs indicate the degree of increase in neuron number compared with normal females. After Gurney and Konishi, 1980.

unknown. Also, the source of the early estrogen in normal male development is uncertain. Presumably, the gonads produce androgens or estrogens that normally masculinize male zebra finches. However, castration fails to prevent masculinization of male zebra finches (Adkins-Regan and Ascenzi, 1990). Furthermore, the presence of functional testicular tissue does not masculinize the development of the song system in genetically female zebra finches (Wade and Arnold, 1996). Taken together, these results suggest that although hormones can masculinize the song control nuclei of female zebra finches, nonhormonal factors, perhaps specific activation of genes on the Y chromosome, normally induce masculinization of the zebra finch song system (Arnold, 1997).

**PHOTOPERIOD EFFECTS.**   Canaries also display sex differences in song production. Female canaries sing much less frequently than males, and their song is much less complex than that of males. However, the frequency of female singing can be increased to nearly male levels by injecting adults with androgen, which also causes a dramatic increase in the size of the adult female canary HVC and RA (Nottebohm, 1980a,b, 1989). Male canaries sing more frequently in spring than in winter, and they learn a new song each year. Their song production is mediated by day length—**photoperiod**—the number of hours of light per day. In the spring, the day length increases, the testes grow and secrete androgens, the frequency of singing increases, the song repertoire enlarges, and the HVC and the RA double in size. In autumn, when the day length decreases, the testes regress in size and androgen production virtually stops, the frequency of singing decreases, the song repertoire shrinks, and the HVC and RA regress in size as well (Nottebohm, 1989). Treatment with testosterone in autumn mimics spring hormonal conditions and supports song production.

The seasonal changes in brain nuclear volume are observed using a variety of cellular labels. There was some mild controversy about these seasonal changes in brain nuclear volume, related to the common use of Nissl stain to define the boundaries of the nuclei. Nissl stain is used to visualize the so-called Nissl bodies in a cell, which contain rough endoplasmic reticulum (ER), the sites of protein synthesis. The rough ER is found in the cytoplasm of cells and this is where the Nissl stains are concentrated, but variation in the degree to which Nissl stain is taken up by cells can lead to differences in measured sizes of cell nuclei that are more apparent than real. For example, Gahr (1990) reported that when brain sections were treated with other histological stains, they failed to display the seasonal changes in brain nuclear volume seen in Nissl-stained sections. However, many studies comparing Nissl stains with other histological techniques have failed to replicate Gahr's findings, and similar seasonal changes in nuclear volume have now been observed with several histological markers (see, e.g., Johnson and Bottjer, 1993; Smith et al., 1997; Soma et al., 1999). In one study, alternate slices of the brain were either stained with Nissl stain or treated for autoradiographic detection of neurotransmitter receptors. Autoradiography for $\alpha_2$-adrenergic receptors showed increases in the volume of the HVC in starlings with elevated testosterone concentrations as compared with the HVC of starlings with low testosterone concentrations, and these results corresponded exactly with the Nissl-stained material (Bernard and Ball, 1993). White-crowned sparrows (*Zonotrichia leucophrys*) display seasonal cycles of androgen secretion and song production, but one study of laboratory-reared birds did not display a seasonal cycle of changes in the song system nuclear volumes (Baker et al., 1984). Tramontin and Brenowitz (2000) hypothesized that laboratory-raised males may not have sufficiently high testosterone concentrations to induce changes in HVC volume; when they studied wild white-crowned sparrows, they found consistent volume changes in the HVC using both Nissl stains and immunocytochemistry (Brenowitz et al., 1998).

Estrogens are necessary to activate the neural machinery underlying the song system in birds. The testes of birds primarily produce androgens, which enter the circulation. The androgens enter neurons containing aromatase, which converts them to estrogens. Aromatase is generally localized in neurons lying near other neurons with estrogen receptors in the hypothalamus and preoptic area of songbird brains, as well as in limbic structures and in the structures constituting the neural circuit controlling bird song (Balthazart and Ball, 1995; Schlinger, 1997). Indeed, the brain is the primary source of estrogens, which activate masculine behaviors in many species (Schlinger and Arnold, 1992; Arnold and Schlinger 1993).

### Courtship Behavior of the Plainfin Midshipman Fish

As described in Chapter 3, there are two very different types of male plainfin midshipman fish. The so-called type I males are large, olive-gray colored, and attract females to their nests by calling with a persistent "humming" call, which has earned these fish the nickname of "canary bird fish." Type I males also engage in nest building and nest guarding behaviors. Furthermore, these males have high testosterone and 11-ketotestosterone concentrations. Importantly, their vocal mus-

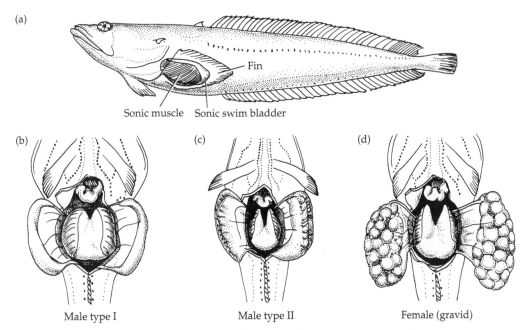

**4.8    The sonic muscle is used by type I male midshipman fish to attract females to their nests.** (a) The vocal organ is a pair of sonic structures attached to the swim bladder; contraction of the sonic organs vibrates the swim bladder like the skin of a drum. (b) The sonic organs of type I males are well developed compared with those of (c) type II males or (d) females. The ratio of sonic muscle mass to total body mass is six times greater in type I males than in type II males. In contrast, the gonad to body mass ratio is nine and twenty times higher in type II males and gravid females, respectively, than in type I males. After Bass, 1996.

cles and vocal motoneurons are large and exhibit a high discharge frequency matching the rhythm of the sonic muscle's pacemaker cells (about 20% higher than females or type II males) (Bass, 1996). In contrast, the type II males do not build nests, guard eggs, or vocalize to attract females. Rather, type II males are characterized as "sneaker" males. They follow females into type I males' nests and release sperm when the females release their eggs. Because type II males resemble females in size and color, the type I males do not exclude them from their nests effectively (Bass, 1996). The type II males do not vocalize, and their vocal system musculature and innervation is small and resembles that of females. The primary circulating steroid hormone in type II males is testosterone, and that in females is estradiol. Females are physically larger than type II males, but they also fail to engage in much vocal behavior.

The steroid hormone 11-ketotestosterone is produced only by type I males. This hormone is particularly effective in stimulating development of the sonic musculature and neural circuitry (Figure 4.8). The endocrine cascade leading to puberty occurs 3 to 4 months earlier in type II males and females than in type I males, precluding development of the sonic musculature and neural circuitry (Bass, 1996). The existence of two distinct male forms within a population exhibiting marked differences in behavior provides a great opportunity to study hormone–behavior interactions (see Figure 3.15).

### *Urinary Posture in Canines*

The difference in urinary posture between male and female dogs is a very well known sexually dimorphic behavior. The difference in body posture during urination is observed not only among domestic dogs, but also among wild canids (Martins and Valle, 1948). Although this might seem at first to be a silly topic for research, this sexually dimorphic behavior has provided endocrinologists with a useful measure in studies of sexual differentiation. If you were challenged to assign the sex of a dog 100 meters away, your task would be immediately simplified if you saw the dog raise one of its rear legs and urinate. If you have observed many dogs, then you are also in the position to state that the male dog has undergone puberty, because only male dogs that are sexually mature regularly display the raised-leg urinary posture. Females very rarely raise a leg when urinating, although adult males occasionally assume the squatting posture characteristic of female dogs. The important features of this behavior are that (1) it is sexually dimorphic; (2) the sexual dimorphism appears peripubertally; and (3) it is not a reproductive behavior per se. Behavioral endocrinologists have formalized these observations during controlled studies to elucidate the role of sex hormones in mediating this sex difference (Figure 4.9).

In a study that followed in the conceptual footsteps of the classic experiment conducted on guinea pigs by Phoenix and co-workers (1959), beagle puppies were subjected to several different early hormonal environments (Beach, 1974b). Beagles have a gestation period of about 58–63 days, and sexual differentiation begins late during gestation and continues for 10–15 days postnatally. To study hormonal effects on behavioral differentiation, some females were injected with testosterone 1–3 days after birth. The timing of the treatment for this experimental group was equivalent to that of the androgen treatment given to newborn rats to masculinize their mating behavior. Females of a second experimental group

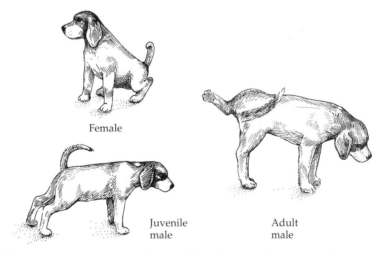

Female

Juvenile male

Adult male

**4.9  Urination postures of domestic dogs** exhibit a clear sex difference that has been exploited in studies of sex differentiation. Adult male dogs usually raise a rear leg and orient the stream of urine toward some target to mark it; adult females usually adopt a squatting posture. Puppies of both sexes usually assume a squatting position during urination, although male dogs begin to show a "lean-forward" urinary posture around the time of puberty. After Beach, 1974b.

were exposed to testosterone in utero by injecting their mothers with this steroid hormone late in pregnancy. This experimental treatment was reminiscent of the early endocrine treatment of guinea pigs, a species for which sexual differentiation occurs prenatally. A third experimental group simulated more closely what normally occurs for male dogs: female pups were exposed to testosterone in utero as well as immediately postpartum. Additional experimental groups included normal females that were ovariectomized in adulthood, males castrated at birth, and males castrated in adulthood.

With no additional hormone replacement therapy later in life, postpubertal female dogs that were exposed to testosterone both in utero and postpartum displayed the male urinary posture about 50% of the time. Many of their reproductive behaviors were also masculinized and defeminized. Their external genitalia, but not their internal sex organs, were masculinized; these females had a penis through which the urogenital opening passed (Figure 4.10). Females that were exposed to testosterone for shorter durations and control females rarely displayed the male-typical urinary posture. Males, even if castrated in infancy, began shifting from the juvenile squatting posture to the male-typical posture at about 4–6 months of age, the usual time of puberty (Beach, 1974b; Ranson and Beach, 1985). These experiments show that the sex difference in canine urinary posture is orga-

**4.10  Modified external genitalia of female dogs** resulting from androgen exposure. (Top left) Appearance of the external genitalia of a normal, untreated female. (Top right) A female treated with androgens in utero shows labial swelling and clitoral enlargement. (Bottom) A female treated with androgens in utero and immediately after birth shows a clitoris formed into a structure that is indistinguishable from a penis; this pseudopenis displays erectile function. Despite this masculinization of the external genitalia, these females have structurally normal ovaries and derivatives of the Müllerian duct system, and will show estrous bleeding through the pseudopenis if treated with estrogen in adulthood. From Beach et al., 1983.

nized by sex steroid hormones, but does not require their presence for activation of the behavior.

An interesting facet of the hormonal mediation of urinary posture of dogs is the way this behavior develops (Ranson and Beach, 1985). The developmental pattern of this behavior indicates that the male puppy's perception of his world changes as he moves through puberty. Initially, male and female puppies display similar squatting urinary postures. Peripubertal females do not exhibit place preference for urination, but as males mature, they begin to spend much time sniffing and exploring vertical objects in their environment. Objects with certain dimensions are preferred. As males become sexually mature, they lift a rear leg and direct the stream of urine onto these vertical objects (Ranson and Beach, 1985). These behaviors are the antecedents of the territorial marking behaviors that males will engage in throughout their adult lives. The process by which certain vertical objects become worthy of investigation and marking for males or perinatally androgenized females, but not typical females, requires further study. Studies of phenomena such as the development of marking in dogs and changes in tuning in weakly electric fishes (Box 4.3) could lead to important insights about how hormones change perception.

### Rough-and-Tumble Play in Primates

In rhesus monkeys and many other mammalian species, males engage in much more play behavior than their female peers throughout development (Hinde, 1966; Meaney, 1988; Pellis et al., 1997). A number of other play-associated social behaviors are also sexually dimorphic in rhesus monkeys. Males, using specific gestures, initiate play more often than females. Males also engage in more threat behaviors than females. A larger proportion of male play behavior involves simulated fighting or rough-and-tumble play as compared with the play behavior of females. Finally, males engage in pursuit play at higher rates than females (Goy and Phoenix, 1972). In order to understand these sex differences in play behavior, as well as other components of primate behavior, a series of studies was conducted on two populations of rhesus monkeys (Goy, 1978; Goy and Phoenix, 1972) and one population of marmosets (Abbott, 1984) treated with prenatal steroid hormones. The studies of rhesus monkeys (Goy, 1978) will be outlined here.

When pregnant rhesus monkeys were injected with androgen, the external genitalia of their female offspring were masculinized. When the behavior of these pseudohermaphroditic females was compared with that of females and males resulting from nonmanipulated pregnancies, it was found that males engaged in much more threat, play initiation, rough-and-tumble play, and pursuit play behavior than normal females (Figure 4.11). The pseudohermaphrodites engaged in these behaviors at frequencies that were between the observed rates for males and females (until the age of 4) (Goy and Phoenix, 1972). This sex difference is *not* dependent upon activational effects of hormones; in other words, the sex difference is organized prenatally. This sex difference is also not dependent on the presence of altered genitalia. By changing the timing of the androgen treatment, juvenile play could be affected independently of the external genitals (Goy et al., 1988). Castration or other postnatal endocrine manipulation did not affect the amount of threat, play initiation, rough-and-tumble play, or pursuit play. Interestingly, in order for these sexually dimorphic behaviors to be expressed at all,

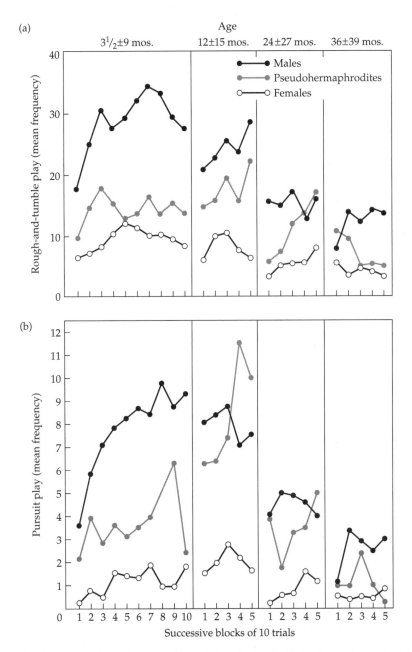

**4.11   The frequency of rough-and-tumble and pursuit play** is affected by early exposure to androgens. Rates of rough-and-tumble play (a) and pursuit play (b) at different ages are shown for normal males, normal females, and pseudohermaphroditic females treated in utero with androgens. Males engage in these play behaviors more frequently than normal females, but pseudohermaphrodites are intermediate between males and females, indicating that, in addition to the external genitalia, play behavior is masculinized by early androgen treatment. Source: Goy and Phoenix, 1972.

## Box 4.3
# Courtship Behavior of Electric Fishes

A sexual dimorphism of interest to behavioral endocrinologists exists in the electric discharge patterns of weakly electric fishes. Strongly electric fishes, such as the freshwater electric eel (*Electrophorus*) and saltwater electric rays (*Torpedo*), can generate hundreds of volts of electricity as an offensive weapon when hunting for prey, as well as a defensive weapon when threatened. In contrast, weakly electric fishes generate only a few volts, and use their low-voltage electrical signals for orientation, as well as during courtship. The two main groups of weakly electric fishes (the mormyriforms of Africa and the gymnotiforms of South America) both dwell among the vegetation along the murky bottoms of freshwater ponds and lakes. Because it is virtually impossible to study these creatures in the turbid water in which they live, the scenario that follows is derived from observations in laboratory tanks.

The electric organs of electric fishes are specialized effectors, called electrocytes, that have evolved from modified neurons, muscle cells, or muscle endplates. In weakly electric fishes, the electrocytes are arranged in an electric discharge organ located in the tail (see fig-

ure below). The fish "see" or orient in murky water by discharging electric signals and detecting any distortion in the pattern of their emitted signals (Carr, 1993). Animate objects are good conductors of electricity (filled circle) and elevate receptor activity; inanimate objects (open circle) depress receptor activity. This process is called electrolocation and is conceptually similar to the echolocation used by bats, moths, and other animals for orientation. The receptors for incoming electric signals are scattered along the body, but are concentrated along the midline of the fish. These receptors also detect electric signals emitted by conspecifics within short range (70–100 cm) (Hopkins, 1984), which is important for courtship behavior.

Courtship occurs in nature during the breeding season, which is closely linked to the seasonal rains. During the breeding season, if a mature male and female locate each other, courtship begins in earnest. In some species, males emit a rapid train of electrical "chirps" (Hagedorn, 1986). These "chirps" are actually silent electric discharges, but are named for the noise they make when the electric signal is transduced to sound via a loudspeaker. This

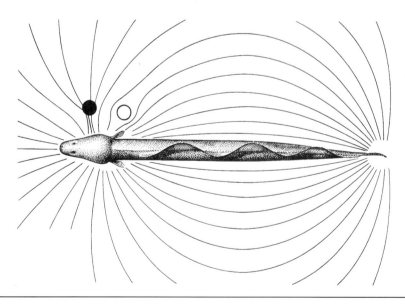

signal, or even a recording of this signal, is sufficiently potent to induce gravid (ready to spawn) females to release their eggs.

Although both sexes produce similar low-voltage signals during electrolocation, males usually produce much more electrical activity than females during courtship. Males, females, and sexually immature juveniles can be discriminated by the frequency pattern of their electric organ discharges (EOD; reviewed in Landsman et al., 1990). The EOD pattern in *Gnathonemus*, for instance, is sexually dimorphic. As shown in the figure below, Fourier transformations of a typical male and female EOD in *Gnathonemus petersii* show clear differences in the peak power spectral frequency (PPSF). Information about species, sex, and sexual maturation is transmitted to other fish by the electric signal. For example, individuals of the species *Sternopygus macrurus* display a species-characteristic wave pattern in their electric discharge. Sexually mature males discharge a wave pattern of 50 to 90 Hz (cycles per second), sexually mature females display patterns of 100 to 150 Hz, and sexually immature juveniles are intermediate between the adults (Hopkins, 1972). The sex difference in electric discharge patterns is often apparent only during the breeding season (Hopkins, 1988). The fish continuously discharge their electric signals as they navigate through their habitat, so information relevant to sexual reproduction is simultaneously broadcast.

Sex steroid hormones appear to be important in mediating electric signaling during courtship, as well as in influencing the frequency of the EOD. Treatment of females or juvenile fish of either sex with androgens, especially naturally occurring fish androgens (for example, testosterone and 11-ketotestosterone), produces electric discharge patterns similar to those of adult males in breeding condition, while castration of adult males shifts the pattern of electric discharge to one resembling that of conspecific females (Bass, 1986). The finding that hormone treatments can change adult female behavior shows that the sex difference in electric discharge pattern is due exclusively to activational effects of androgens. Sex steroid hormones also play activational roles in mediating the onset of electric signaling (Landsman and Moller, 1988).

Sex steroid hormones also appear to affect the sensory system mediating reception of electric signals (Bass and Hopkins, 1984). The electroreceptors of an individual fish are maximally sensitive, or "tuned," to its own unique pattern of electric organ discharges. This "tuning" obviously aids in electrolocation. Androgens, as well as shifting the EOD frequency, shift the receptor tuning to the new EOD. Androgens shift the tuning curve—that is, the sensitivity of the receptors—in a masculine direction in females (Bass and Hopkins, 1984). These results are especially intriguing because this model may yield evidence about how steroid hormones affect sensory receptors directly, and thus may provide a neural basis for understanding the sexual dimorphism in sensory abilities observed among many species (Hopkins, 1988).

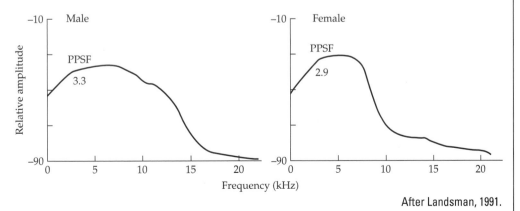

After Landsman, 1991.

appropriate social stimulation must be present during development. Rhesus monkeys that are reared in social isolation with access to only surrogate mothers do not develop the appropriate patterns of play. These results suggest that organization by hormones interacts with environmental factors to produce normal play behavior.

Human children also differ between the sexes in the amount of rough-and-tumble play they engage in, and there is some evidence suggesting that this difference, too, is organized prenatally by steroid hormones. In one series of studies, aggression was examined in children who were exposed prenatally to a synthetic progestin (MPA) that had been provided to their mothers to prevent premature labor (Reinisch, 1981). This progestin reportedly has androgenic effects, but does not usually cause masculinization of the external genitalia at low therapeutic doses; in some instances, prenatal exposure to MPA enhances feminine traits.

Seventeen female and eight male patients were compared with their unexposed, same-sex siblings in their responses to paper-and-pencil tests, as well as questionnaire data obtained from friends and family members (Ehrhardt et al., 1977). Girls exposed to prenatal progestins were considered to be ultrafeminine for some traits. They were very interested in clothes and playing child-rearing games, and were less often characterized as tomboys by themselves or by their peers than were unaffected girls. Despite this so-called *enhanced* feminization, girls exposed to MPA engaged in higher-energy play activities and excelled at athletic endeavors as compared with control females. In an earlier study, girls born with congenital adrenal hyperplasia, which results in exposure to high androgen concentrations early in development, also displayed elevated rates of energetic play, as well as initiation of fighting and rough-and-tumble play (Ehrhardt and Money, 1967; Ehrhardt et al., 1968a). In another study, both males and females exposed to MPA scored higher on aggression on paper-and-pencil tests than their unexposed siblings (Reinisch, 1981). However, although paper-and-pencil tests of aggressive behavior provide interesting data, direct observations of aggressive behavior provide more valid results (see Chapter 9). Taken together, the evidence suggests that gonadal steroid hormones may contribute to behavioral sex differences, especially in play behavior, among humans and other primates (Collaer and Hines, 1995).

## Sex Differences in Human Behavior

We have seen that many sex differences in behavior arise because (1) the neural substrates of the behaviors are organized by hormones early in development and (2) the behaviors are activated by hormones later in development (Baum et al., 1990). The mating behavior of male rodents, for example, is both organized and activated by steroid hormones. Other sex differences arise only from organizational effects of steroid hormones, such as rates of rough-and-tumble play in rhesus monkeys. Exposure to perinatal steroid hormones is sufficient to cause male-typical rates of rough-and-tumble play in the absence of postnatal hormonal effects. Behavioral sex differences may also be due only to activational effects, such as the electric discharge pattern of electric fishes (see Box 4.3). However, some sex differences in behavior may be unrelated to hormones, such as the learning of a sex role among humans. Behavioral endocrinologists aim to disentangle the contribution of hormones from the contribution of the environment to determine the cause of such behavioral sex differences.

As noted in Chapter 3, researchers cannot ethically manipulate hormone concentrations in humans to observe the subsequent effects on brain and behavior. Consequently, the potential effects of hormones on human brains and behavior must be inferred by observing the outcomes of so-called "experiments of nature," situations in which individuals have been exposed to atypical levels of hormones during some developmental period of their lives. Early exposure to MPA provides one example, and several other such conditions were covered in Chapter 3. The goal of studying the effects of unusual hormone exposures on human brains and behavior is to understand the effects of more typical endocrine events (Box 4.4).

Sexual differentiation in humans occurs early during gestation, near the end of the first trimester and throughout the first few weeks of the second trimester of pregnancy. Using the models developed in rodents, dogs, and rhesus monkeys, we can predict that exposure to high levels of sex steroid hormones during this time will masculinize and defeminize human brains and behavior, whereas low levels of steroid hormones early in development will tend to feminize and demasculinize brains and behavior. Two basic clinical populations have been examined in this regard: (1) individuals with congenital disorders that expose them to unusually high or low hormone levels during development, such as CAH, Turner syndrome, 5α-reductase deficiency, and TFM; and (2) individuals whose mothers were treated with steroid hormones during pregnancy for medical reasons (see Chapter 3). Exposure to prescribed hormones almost always occurs prenatally and may involve natural or artificial estrogens (such as DES), as well as progestins (such as MPA).

These clinical studies have many inherent flaws as compared with the animal studies previously described. In animal studies, individuals from inbred strains of genetically identical animals can all be treated with equal amounts of steroid hormones at the same time during development and examined under standard test conditions. The human clinical syndromes, on the other hand, are summaries of individual cases that may differ in the severity and timing of the disorder, or in the type, dose, and timing of the exposure to prescribed steroid hormones. Often the effects of prescribed hormones are confounded with the effects of the medical condition (for example, toxemia) that prompted treatment of the mother in the first place. Also, parental expectations may be affected, for instance, for children born with ambiguous genitalia (see Box 4.5).

It is important to keep in mind that there is more variation within each sex than between the sexes for virtually all human behaviors (Figure 4.12). That is, there is considerable overlap between males and females for most behaviors. With a sufficiently large sample size, relatively small differences in the performance or the frequency of a given behavior can be statistically significant, and these differences are reported in the scientific and popular press as "significant sex differences." Because there is often more variation *within* each sex than *between* the sexes, however, it is appropriate to talk about the "effect size," a measure of the variation between sexes corrected for the variation within each sex (Collaer and Hines, 1988; Forger, 1998). The effect size is "moderate" when the average difference between the sexes is about half the size of the standard deviation of the scores within each sex. For example, the sex difference in height between 16-year-old

Box 4.4
# Steroidogenic Effects of Chemical Pollutants

A number of commercial chemical agents, including many pesticides, some types of polychlorinated biphenyls (PCBs), and combustion products from plastics, can have pronounced estrogenic effects on animals (Raloff, 1994a,b). Although these substances are not steroids, they apparently mimic estrogens and bind to estrogen receptors. One of the first demonstrations that these chemical agents could affect reproduction was the link made in the 1950s between the now-banned pesticide DDT and the thinning of eggshells in many avian species. As you probably know, animals at the tops of food chains ingest all of the toxic chemicals that have accumulated in the bodies of the animals they consume. Birds that consume fish, reptiles, and insects are particularly at risk for contamination. Many bird species, including bald eagles, were put at risk of extinction by DDT, which caused abnormally thin-shelled eggs that parents were inadvertently crushing.

DDT also had other dramatic effects on reproduction in birds. One California gull population (*Larus californicus*) on Santa Barbara Island off the coast of California was heavily contaminated with DDT. When eggs did manage to hatch, the morphology of the offspring was markedly atypical. As you will recall, female birds normally develop only the left ovary and oviduct, but young females on Santa Barbara Island showed some development of the right reproductive tract as well. Young males also developed oviducts, and their right gonad often developed as an ovotestis (Fry and Toone, 1981). The behavior of adults was also atypical. Two parent gulls are required to obtain sufficient food to rear offspring successfully, but on Santa Barbara Island, most males were not engaging in reproductive behavior. Breeding males had become scarce in the population, which led to females predominating on the island; apparently many females mated with the scarce reproductively competent males, then shared nests in

female–female pairs. This rise in so-called "lesbian gulls" was thought to reflect the estrogenic effects of DDT on male mating behavior, because when eggs were experimentally treated with estradiol or DDT, males arising from those eggs demonstrated the same feminized structures and reduced sex drive as the males on Santa Barbara Island (Fry and Toone, 1981). Since the banning of DDT in 1972, the gull sex ratio on Santa Barbara Island has been slowly returning to normal levels, and the incidence of morphological and behavioral abnormalities is waning.

On the other side of the continent, biologists have been concerned with the dwindling numbers of the Florida panther (*Felis concolor coryi*). One reason for the decline in the number of panthers is human encroachment into their habitats, but these panthers also seem to exhibit increasingly high rates of cryptorchidism, a condition in which the testes remain in the abdominal cavity after birth (Raloff, 1994a). Normally, the testes develop near the kidneys and descend into the scrotum through the inguinal canals (small openings in the pelvis) around the time of birth. The scrotal sac has evolved a number of adaptations in mammals to maintain the testes at temperatures less than the core body temperature. Mammalian sperm are very sensitive to high temperatures and may be damaged by temperatures above 37°C. Failure of the testes to descend into the scrotum is associated with infertility because a high proportion of the sperm are damaged.

Only about 50 Florida panthers are estimated to remain in the wild, and the incidence of cryptorchidism was thought to be due to a genetic bottleneck, or reduction in genetic variation, in the dwindling population. Recent data do not rule out that possibility, but they also suggest that environmental estrogenic pesticides may be responsible for the increase in the incidence of cryptorchidism. When blood samples from Florida panthers were analyzed for steroid hormone levels, investigators discovered that several cryptorchid males had unusual hormone profiles showing higher circulating levels of estrogens than androgens, and that at least one female had higher circulating levels of androgens than estrogens. Investigators suspect that steroidogenic agents in the environment are responsible for the unusual steroid levels, and consequently, approximately 100 wildlife preserves in the southeastern United States that are managed by the U.S. Fish and Wildlife Service are now forbidden from using any known estrogenic chemicals, including pesticides and herbicides.

Are these steroidogenic agents affecting human reproduction? Probably. Thus far, disruptions in breeding attributed to environmental hormones have been reported for severely contaminated populations of amphibians, reptiles, birds, and mammals throughout the world. Humans, residing atop their food chain, may be ingesting far more of these steroidogenic agents than they might suspect. As with the Florida panthers, the rate of cryptorchidism in baby boys is apparently increasing (Carlsen et al., 1992); the incidence in the 1950s of about 1.6% of live births had nearly doubled by the 1970s to 2.9% in western Europe. The incidence of hypospadias, an abnormality in which the urethra opens on the underside of the penis, has also more than doubled in Great Britain between 1964 and 1983. Even more disturbing, testicular cancer, a cancer possibly associated with endocrine factors, is increasing sharply in several European and North American countries: the rate of testicular cancer has nearly tripled during the past half century, and the incidence appears to be increasing in industrialized countries (Giwercman and Skakkebaek, 1992).

Human fertility also seems to be waning in recent years. Although undescended testes can be moved to their correct location in the scrotum by surgical means, boys with this condition at birth often suffer fertility difficulties later in life. Across human populations, sperm counts appear to be declining. In 1940 the average density of human sperm was 113 million per millimeter of semen; in 1990 this figure had dropped to 66 million per millimeter in the United States and western Europe. Researchers also estimate that the volume of semen produced by men has dropped about 20% during the past 50 years, reducing sperm count per ejaculation even further (Carlsen et al., 1992). More recently, between 1981 and 1991, the ratio of normal spermatogenesis decreased significantly from 56.4% to 26.9%, with a parallel increase in the incidence of partial and complete spermatogenic arrest (Pajarinen et al., 1997). During this period, the size of seminiferous tubules decreased, the amount of fibrotic tissue in the testes increased, and testicular mass decreased significantly. These alterations in testicular characteristics over time could not be explained by changes in body mass index or in tobacco, alcohol, or other drug use. The authors of this study suggested that deteriorating spermatogenesis might be one important factor in the explanation of the declining sperm counts observed worldwide. Sperm count and fertility are affected by estrogens.

In addition to mimics of steroid hormones, several other so-called endocrine disruptors have been discovered in a wide variety of common chemical compounds. These include substances that interfere with thyroid hormones, growth factors, and prolactin. Although an important book, *Our Stolen Future* (Colborn et al., 1997), has motivated the U.S. federal granting agencies to begin funding systematic studies on the toxicology and developmental effects of endocrine disruptors, the effects of these chemicals on behavior remain, for the most part, unknown. Certainly, the extent to which human behavior has been affected by environmental steroidogenic agents remains unknown. Are aggressive, parental, or sexual behaviors in humans altered by the more than 500 measurable chemicals in our bodies that were not there prior to the 20th century? No one knows. It seems prudent to curtail the use of these substances until their effects on the reproduction and health of humans and nonhuman animals are understood.

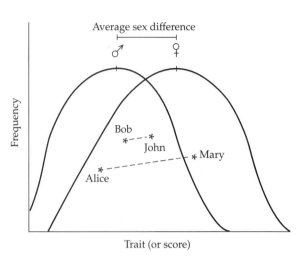

**4.12   Average sex differences in performance often reflect significant overlap between the sexes.** There are often greater differences in performance between individuals of the same sex (for example, between Alice and Mary in the figure) than between individuals of the opposite sex (for example, between John and Mary in the figure).

male and female humans has a moderate effect size (Table 4.2) (Kimura, 1992; Collaer and Hines, 1988).We will normally be discussing only slight behavioral sex differences as we discuss humans; this is very different from the research strategy using animal models in which only one sex displays a particular behavior. These caveats should be borne in mind as we discuss what these studies have revealed.

### Gender Role

The most prominent behavioral sex differences between men and women are observed in gender role, gender identity, and sexual orientation/sexual preference. Most, but certainly not all, women assume a feminine gender role, perceive themselves as female, and are sexually attracted to men. Similarly, most, but not all, men assume a masculine gender role, perceive themselves as male, and are sexually attracted to women. Estimates of the number of individuals who do not fall into these categories vary.

Every society has a set of expectations for the behavior of males and females. Children learn these expectations through their play activities and through shaping by their parents, caregivers, siblings, and peers. Young males may be scolded because "boys do not cry," or a young girl may be disciplined more harshly for fighting at school than her brother. The assumption of culturally based behavioral patterns that are specific to one's own sex is the adoption of a **gender role**. Gender roles are learned early in life, and it is difficult to reverse this early learning. For example, among the Nuer people of western Africa, the men tend cattle and the women cook meals (Evans-Pritchard, 1963). Men never cook in this society, and women never work with livestock. For these two tasks, the gender roles are distinct: cooking is considered a feminine gender role, whereas tending cattle is considered a masculine gender role. In North American society, gender roles are less distinguished by occupation than they were 30 years ago, but they still exist. Because gender roles differ substantially among human cultures and over time in the same culture, it has sometimes been assumed that gender roles are entirely mediated by environmental factors. Nonetheless, subtle influences of early endocrine conditions on subsequent gender roles can be demonstrated.

Table 4.2
**Effect size for behavioral sex differences in humans**

| Behavior | Approximate effect size[a] |
|---|---|
| Aggression | Moderate (♂ > ♀) |
| Rough-and-tumble play | Moderate–large (♂ > ♀) |
| Childhood activity levels | Moderate–large (♂ > ♀) |
| Overall verbal abilities | Negligible–small (♀ > ♂) |
| Speech production | Small (♀ > ♂) |
| Verbal fluency | Moderate (♀ > ♂) |
| Perceptual speed | Moderate (♀ > ♂) |
| 3-D visual rotation | Large (♂ > ♀) |
| 2-D visual rotation | Small (♂ > ♀) |
| Spatial perception | Small–moderate (♂ > ♀) |
| Overall quantitative abilities | Small–moderate (♂ > ♀) |
| Quantitative problem solving | Small–moderate (♂ > ♀) |

*Source:* Collaer and Hines, 1988; data from J. Cohen, 1977; Kimura, 1992; Forger, 1998.
[a]Effect sizes of ≥0.8 standard deviations are considered large, of ~0.5 standard deviations, moderate; of ~0.2, small; and of < 0.2, negligible.

For example, girls born with CAH display varying degrees of masculinization at birth. Typically, the endocrine dysfunction can be managed by exogenous hormone treatment and the masculinized genitalia can be surgically corrected. However, these girls display some degree of behavioral masculinization; as described by their siblings and parents, as well as in self-reports, they

1. Engage in increased physical activity with higher levels of rough-and-tumble play

2. Are characterized as "tomboys"

3. Prefer male playmates

4. Prefer male-typical as compared to female-typical toys

5. Engage in fewer games of simulated maternal behaviors

6. Display reduced interest in infant care

7. Manifest little or no interest in personal appearance or attractiveness

8. Are less likely to be interested in hairstyles, makeup, or jewelry

9. Engage in fewer fantasies about marriage and maternity, as compared with their unaffected sisters (Ehrhardt and Baker, 1974; Ehrhardt et al., 1968a,b).

Remember that none of these studies can be conducted in an "unbiased" way, because the parents, and often the child, know that there was a hormone dysfunction that required surgical modification of the genitalia. This knowledge may lead to subtle ambiguities in perception of the individual's gender and could result in exaggerated reports of masculine behavior. More recently, Berenbaum and Hines (1992) addressed the issue of parental biases by secretly observing play behavior among CAH girls and their unaffected sisters and first cousins during unsupervised play sessions. They found that the play behavior of CAH girls was significantly masculinized. In other words, the CAH girls played with toys typically preferred by boys. Given a choice of transportation and construction toys, books, board games, dolls, or kitchen supplies, CAH girls preferred to play with the toys generally preferred by boys and avoided by their unaffected female relatives. Of course, this preference for masculine toys could still reflect the biases of the parents or other environmental influences. However, one might expect that parents would be as likely to encourage feminine preferences in toys for their CAH daughters as for their unaffected daughters.

In the draw-a-person test (a psychological test during which a child is asked to draw a person; drawing a person of the same sex is considered to indicate satisfaction with gender role), both females and males with CAH drew the sex-appropriate picture (Hines, 1982). Incidentally, boys exposed to high prenatal androgen levels engaged in higher physical activity levels, more rough-and-tumble play, and were more likely to excel in aggressive sports than their unaffected brothers (Money and Ehrhardt, 1972). This was typically viewed as a good outcome by their parents. Although one may quibble about the relevance of the gender role identifiers used in this study 25 years ago to discriminate boys from girls (for example, preference for dolls as play objects), a subset of the results is strikingly similar to the behavioral data obtained with early androgen treatment of female rhesus monkeys (Goy and Phoenix, 1972).

Imperato-McGinley and her colleagues (Imperato-McGinley et al., 1974, 1979) have described a group of Central American males in whom an adolescent gender role change appears to be common. In the Santo Domingo region of the Dominican Republic live several families with a high incidence of 5α-reductase deficiency. The affected individuals are XY chromosomal males that lack 5α-reductase, the enzyme that converts testosterone to DHT (Savage et al., 1980). These individuals have ambiguous external genitalia and small, undescended testes at birth. They are generally reared as girls until puberty, when testosterone masculinizes their bodies and genitalia (see Figure 3.11). Most afflicted individuals successfully switch gender role from female to male at puberty. Of the twenty-one afflicted individuals studied in the original reports, only two retained the female gender role, and one of these was known to frequent a local female prostitute. Because these individuals were exposed to testosterone during development and puberty, the authors of the study argued that hormones are more powerful than rearing in determining gender role.

However, before this interpretation of the supremacy of hormonal factors over rearing conditions can be accepted, the process of change and the particular developmental and cultural backgrounds of these individuals must be carefully examined. These individuals have been given the colorful Spanish name *guevedoces*, which literally translates into "eggs at 12." In Papua New Guinea, the frequency of individuals with 5α-reductase deficiency is also relatively high, and this population has also been the subject of study (Herdt and Davidson, 1988). Individuals in the New Guinea study population with 5α-reductase deficiency also apparently undergo successful change in gender identity and develop a heterosexual male sexual orientation after puberty. The pidgin nickname for these individuals is "turnim-man" (Herdt and Davidson, 1988). The assignment of a special nickname for this syndrome in both cultures suggests that the nature of 5α-reductase deficiency is well known, and the possibility that rearing was unambiguously female for these individuals is suspect. Also, the afflicted individuals may have been motivated to switch gender roles because of the prestige and power afforded to males as compared with females in both societies.

As we have seen, early androgen exposure seems to result in male-like patterns of play. These findings occur cross-culturally and among different species (Goy and Phoenix, 1972; Meany, 1988; Hines, 1982; Pellis et al., 1997). However, virtually all other aspects of gender role agree with the sex of rearing. For example, boys (Meyer-Bahlburg et al., 1977) and girls (Ehrhardt et al., 1977) that were exposed in utero to MPA, an artificial progestin with androgenic effects, were completely satisfied with the male and female gender role, respectively.

### Gender Identity

The process by which individuals come to view themselves as either male or female reflects the development of **gender identity**. Gender identity is generally considered by clinicians to be irreversibly established by 4 years of age (Green, 1987; Money, 1988; Money and Ehrhardt, 1972; but see Diamond, 1996; Diamond and Sigmundson, 1997 for opposing views) (Box 4.5). To what extent is gender identity the result of parental influences and cultural expectations, and to what extent is it the result of perinatal hormonal influences?

Until recently it was generally accepted that the sex of rearing is the dominant feature mediating gender identity; that is, that the gender identity of children reflects the sex of rearing regardless of early endocrine environment. For example, girls born with CAH often display clitoral enlargement to the extent that visual assignment of sex at birth is difficult. However, if the problem is corrected surgically and there is no ambiguity about assignment of sex on the part of the parents, the girls generally develop normal female gender identity (Ehrhardt and Meyer-Bahlburg, 1981).

A potential problem for the notion that gender identity is primarily the result of parental influences is raised by the studies of *guevedoces* in the Dominican Republic (Imperato-McGinley et al., 1974, 1979). As described above, these genetic male individuals were reared as girls and had established a female gender identity, but changed their gender identity from female to male when their bodies became masculinized at puberty (Imperato-McGinley et al., 1974, 1979). Change of gender identity was observed even among a few individuals who had married men in their early teens, and then remarried women after puberty. These observations suggest that biological factors—namely, the presence or absence of androgens—mediate gender identity regardless of the sex of rearing. However, this conclusion must be tempered by the same two considerations that pertain to using these individuals to draw conclusions about gender role. First, as noted above, it is not at all clear that the sex of rearing was unambiguously female (Rubin et al., 1981). Because the 5α-reductase deficiency syndrome was so well known in this village, parents may have known that an unusual metamorphosis was possible at puberty, and they may have treated the affected individuals differently from genetic females, preparing them for a gender identity change. Also,

Box 4.5

# Ambiguous genitalia: Which course of treatment?

As was explained in Chapter 3, there are occasional developmental anomalies in sex differentiation that result in ambiguous external genitalia at birth. Prior to the 20th century, pseudohermaphrodites received no surgical treatment as newborns, and some earned their living displaying their bodies in sideshows. The figures show one such "bearded lady," Marie-Madeleine Lefort, in youth and old age. Lefort possessed traits of both men and women, and worked in carnivals throughout Europe in the 1800s (Dreger, 1998). It is now standard practice to surgically alter ambiguous genitalia shortly after birth, but the decisions involved in such procedures are far from simple.

Most experiments, including those described in this book, include large numbers of subjects in an effort to ensure that their findings will be generalizable to many individuals. In medical settings, physicians often base treatment decisions on guidelines that emerge from clinical trials that sometimes include thousands of patients. Sometimes this is impractical, however, because particular conditions occur only rarely. Physicians study rare cases in depth, and sometimes publish their findings as "case studies" or "case histories," which preserve patients' confidentiality and sometimes present hypotheses about the causes of a condition and the effectiveness of a given treatment.

Pseudohermaphroditism is fairly rare, and when a baby is born with ambiguous genitalia, physicians and parents must make treatment decisions based on a body of knowledge that has been gleaned from only a small number of cases. Although it is relatively easy to debate this issue from the comfort of the classroom, in the clinical setting a decision must be made quickly and in an emotionally charged atmosphere.

What are the options? One can determine the newborn's genetic sex and make surgical (and later endocrine) alterations so that the external genitalia match the genetic sex. This strategy assumes that genetic sex is supreme in determining psychosexual attributes such as gender identity or gender role. In contrast, one might assume that prenatal hormonal effects on the brain are reflected in genital development. According to this view, if the genitalia appear more female- than male-typical, then corrective surgery that enhances the female genital characteristics should be performed, and the individual should be raised as a female, and vice versa if the genitalia appear more male- than female-typical. The latter courses of action would be pursued regardless of chromosomal or gonadal sex, and based solely on genital appearance—an "anatomy is destiny" approach which assumes that environmental (i.e., rearing) factors are more important than early biological factors in determining psychosexual development.*

So imagine you are the physician in charge in the maternity ward, and a beautiful baby has been born with atypical genitalia. The parents are asking you what should they do. Until recently, virtually all physicians opted for the easiest surgical procedure and rearing the

*Both of these options suggest an acceptance that there are only two sexes and an assumption that making individuals fit into one of the two "normal" categories is a desirable goal of the medical profession. A third option is more daring, and has rarely been chosen in the past 40 years: that is, do nothing, in the belief that intersexuality is not an "error," but simply unusual. Recently, vocal spokespersons for intersexuals have expressed hostility toward surgical treatments. The imposition of "normality" by surgical means is often seen in hindsight as a judgmental assertion of abnormality, and intersexual individuals demand acceptance as born. This position was declared most elegantly by an anonymous author who noted, "I was born whole and beautiful, but different. The error was not in my body, nor in my sex organs, but in the determination of the culture, carried out by physicians with my parents' permission, to erase my intersexuality. "Sex error" is no less stigmatizing than "defect" or "deficiency." Our path to healing lies in embracing our intersexual selves, not in labeling our bodies as having committed some 'error.'"

child in a sex-specific manner that matched the altered genitalia, regardless of chromosomal sex, and these decisions were based on the classic and influential work of Dr. John Money and his colleagues at The Johns Hopkins University. Money's work on individuals born with ambiguous genitalia (reviewed in Money and Ehrhardt, 1972; follow-up studies are discussed in Money et al., 1986, and Money and Norman, 1987) had convinced him that babies are born neutral with respect to psychosexual development: if a child is raised unambiguously as one sex or the other, that child will develop a gender identity to match the sex assignment. Of course, for the sex of rearing to be unambiguous, the genitals must match the assigned sex. One classic case, now known as the "John/Joan" case, provided some of the strongest possible evidence for Money's position, and it has received a great deal of attention recently (including a feature in *Rolling Stone* magazine [Colapinto, 1997]) because the conclusions drawn in Money's original case study (Money and Ehrhardt, 1972) differ sharply from those of

a follow-up study reported nearly 25 years later (Diamond and Sigmundson, 1997).

The original case study described a little boy, given the pseudonym "John," who had his penis severely damaged during circumcision at 8 months of age; essentially, the penis was burned almost completely off. John was brought to Johns Hopkins Hospital several months later for a consultation, and it was decided that he should be reared as a girl (called "Joan" in the literature). A complete penilectomy was performed and a vagina was surgically constructed. (At the time, reconstructive penile surgery had not yet been perfected, whereas vaginal construction was a relatively straight-forward procedure.) The fact that John was genetically male, and had been born with normal male genitalia, made his case a particularly strong clinical test of the "sex-of-rearing" hypothesis. He also had a twin brother who could serve as a sort of "baseline control" when assessing the treatment's success. "John" became "Joan" at 17 months of age, which was, according to Dr. Money, within an acceptable

Courtesy of the Wangensteen Historical Library, University of Minnesota, Minneapolis, MN.

Box 4.5 *continued*

window of "early re-assignment." A series of follow-up reports indicated that Joan had successfully adopted a female gender identity, although she clearly displayed many "tomboyish" traits such as "abundant physical energy," a "high level of activity," and was "often the dominant one in a girls' group" (Money and Ehrhardt, 1972). Around the time of puberty, Joan and her family decided to end her participation in the study, and no more follow-up examinations were conducted by the Johns Hopkins research group.

Recently, Diamond and Sigmundson (1997) presented a startling report that Joan now lives as a man who had reconstructive surgery with a penile prosthesis, is married to a woman, and is a father to adopted children. In other words, his gender role and identity are now firmly male. Now known again in the literature as "John," he also reports that he experienced substantial mental anguish during childhood and adolescence, and a growing sense that he was not a girl. These feelings culminated in a decision at

age 14 to reverse his gender role and identity. The authors of this follow-up study claim that this outcome shows that biological factors are extremely powerful in psychosexual development. Essentially, Diamond and Sigmundson's report is the latest installment in a long series of doctrinal debates on this topic between Drs. Money and Diamond about the primacy of environmental versus biological factors in psychosexual development (Zucker, 1996).

Clearly, there is a strong interaction between biological and environmental factors in determining psychosexual development, and the truth is likely somewhere in between the two extreme positions. Unfortunately, this is not particularly helpful to physicians and parents agonizing over how to help babies born with ambiguous genitalia attain the best quality of life. Those of us who are used to conducting experimental studies never rely on a single incident or an "*N* of 1" (Favreau, 1993) to draw a firm conclusion. Additional studies on human psychosexual development are necessary in order to make sound clinical decisions in cases of anomalous sexual differentiation.

the society in this region of the world is strictly sexually segregated, and opportunities for work, education, and so forth are limited for women. Consequently, these individuals may have been motivated by social factors to change their gender identity from female to male. In other cases, changing gender identity is a long and difficult psychological process (Green, 1987). Thus, the extent to which gender identity is mediated by early hormone exposure or parental influences remains uncertain.

### Sexual Orientation/Sexual Preference

In most cases there is a marked sex difference in erotic attraction among humans: males are generally attracted to females and females are generally attracted to males. But this is not always true. The process of developing an erotic preference for same-sex partners is as complex as the process of developing an erotic preference for opposite-sex partners (Gorman, 1994). Very little is known about how heterosexuals form sexual attractions, and even less is understood about how homosexuals form sexual attractions. This section has a dual title because the terms used in discussions of this issue connote subtle beliefs about causality. The term **sexual orientation** suggests that homosexuality is the result of biological factors. The term **sexual preference** indicates to some that homosexuality is a lifestyle, a choice of same-sex erotic partners that is learned. The two terms will be used interchangeably here because, as with heterosexuality, both environmental and biological factors are likely to be involved in the development of homosexuality. This statement is based on the observation that monozygotic twins (with identical genes) do not always display the same sexual orientation (for example, Bailey and Pillard, 1991; Buhrich et al., 1991).

Because erotic attractions typically begin at puberty, sex steroid hormones have been assumed to be involved in their development (McClintock and Herdt, 1996). One common, but largely unsubstantiated, hypothesis about the cause of homosexuality is that the hormone levels of homosexuals are different from those of heterosexuals; that is, heterosexual men and homosexual women are attracted to women because of high androgen levels (or low estrogen levels) and heterosexual women and homosexual men are attracted to men because of low androgen levels (or high estrogen levels). However, many studies have failed to find any consistent evidence that adult homosexual men or women differ from their heterosexual counterparts in blood concentrations of androgens or estrogens. Some studies have reported lower blood androgen levels in homosexual than in heterosexual men, other studies have reported no differences, and a few studies have indicated that homosexual men have higher blood androgen levels than heterosexual men (reviewed in Bancroft, 1984; Meyer-Bahlburg, 1984). Similarly, there has been no consistent indication that hormonal imbalances underlie transsexuality, the feeling in an anatomically normal individual that he or she is actually a member of the other sex (Gooren, 1990a).

Some studies have suggested a difference in adult neuroendocrine regulatory mechanisms between heterosexual and homosexual men. For example, the positive feedback response to estrogen treatment was reported to be greater in homosexual than in heterosexual men (Gladue et al., 1984). Low doses of estrogens usually have a negative feedback effect on the secretion of gonadotropin in both sexes (Lacroix et al., 1979; Tsai and Yen, 1971; see above). However, treatment of women with high doses of estrogens evokes a surge of LH and FSH release after the initial suppression (a positive feedback response) (Tsai and Yen, 1971). These studies generated substantial interest because the results suggested that the brains, or at least the control mechanisms of gonadotropin secretion, of homosexual men were feminized relative to those of heterosexual men. These results seemed in accord with the previous studies of feminization and demasculinization of the neuroendocrine regulatory mechanisms associated with ovulation in rats (see Chapter 3). However, the sex difference in steroid effects on gonadotropin release is obvious in rats, but not in rhesus monkeys (for example, see Karsch et al., 1973). Male rats never show positive feedback effects of estrogen treatment unless they are castrated at birth and do not receive steroid hormone replacement treatment. Also, other studies of humans have noted a positive feedback effect in men under various experimental conditions (Barbarino et al., 1983; Kastin et al., 1972b; Kuhn and Reiter, 1976). Several subsequent experiments have failed to replicate the original finding that homosexual and heterosexual men differ in their neuroendocrine responses to estrogen treatment (for example, Gooren, 1986; Gooren et al., 1984; Hendricks et al., 1989). Thus, it appears that homosexual and heterosexual men cannot be reliably discriminated by their gonadotropin response to estrogen treatment.

If hormones are implicated in mediating human sexual preference, then exposure to hormones early in development may be involved. Again, it is not possible to manipulate early hormonal environments or even obtain blood samples from a human fetus without substantial risk to its well-being, and animal models are generally of limited use in understanding sexual orientation (Adkins-Regan, 1988) (Box 4.6). Consequently, experiments of nature must be examined to see whether changes in sexual orientation arise after unusual hormonal exposures. Studies of this type show that individual sexual preference does not necessarily reflect early endocrine events. For example, some XY individuals exhibit partial androgen insensitivity and are born with ambiguous genitalia. If they are surgically corrected and reared as girls, then these individuals are sexually attracted to men; if they are surgically corrected and reared as boys, then these individuals are sexually attracted to women

---

## Box 4.6
# Hormonal Influences on Mate Choice

Although there are enormous species differences in the type and extent of sexual dimorphism observed, nearly all animal species exhibit the following sex difference: females are generally attracted sexually to males and males are generally attracted sexually to females (Adkins-Regan, 1998). Despite the fact that this sex difference in attraction is a critically important component of individual fitness, little is known about the mechanistic processes that account for it. Studies at the ultimate level of analysis have investigated species preferences and individual partner preferences, but surprisingly few data have been collected that address the problem of sexual partner preferences (Adkins-Regan, 1998). In most cases, preferences have been experimentally determined using a two-choice test in which one individual (the "test" individual) can choose between mates A (e.g., a male conspecific) and B (e.g., a female conspecific); usually individuals A and B are tethered in some way so that the "test" animal can move freely between them. Recent evidence suggests that hormones can affect sexual preferences, but possibly via an indirect path.

The activational role of hormones on mate preference or mate choice remains ambiguous: when given a choice between a male and a female, gonadectomized "test" males usually

lose their preference to spend time with females. Similarly, gonadectomized "test" females usually lose their preference to spend time with males. Hormone replacement therapy typically restores the heterosexual preference. Importantly, however, no endocrine treatment in adulthood has been shown to reverse sex preferences. Thus, it seems that the activational effects of hormones function on sexual motivation, rather than on sexual preference.

However, some interesting studies on sheep have revealed that different hormone concentrations might account for differences in sexual preference (Perkins et al., 1995). Researchers at a USDA sheep breeding facility discovered that up to 16% of male sheep never mate with females during the breeding season. Approximately 6% of these males never show any sexual activity, but another 10% prefer males over females; that is, they are homosexual males. Homosexual ewes have not been identified. Homosexual rams display a level of estrogen binding in the amygdala (an almond-shaped structure in the brain that is often involved in aggression or reproductive behaviors) that is similar to that of females and much less than that of heterosexual rams (Perkins et al., 1995). The level of aromatase in the preoptic area of the brain is also lower in homosexual than in

(Money and Ogunro, 1974). Similarly, if XX individuals with CAH are surgically corrected and reared as boys, they develop a male-typical sexual orientation; females with CAH who are surgically corrected and reared as girls typically develop a sexual attraction to men (Money and Dalery, 1976; but see below).

At first glance, these studies provide powerful evidence that sexual preference is learned. But they do not rule out the potential effects of early hormone exposure. The decision for surgical correction in a male or female direction is not based on the whim of the surgeon; if there is substantial genital development, then a medical decision is made to modify in the male direction; if there is little genital development, then surgical modifications are made in the female direction. The extent of genital development probably covaries with the extent of androgen exposure, so again, the sex of rearing is confounded by early hormone exposure.

---

heterosexual rams (Perkins et al., 1995). Furthermore, homosexual rams have lower circulating testosterone concentrations than heterosexual rams (Perkins et al., 1995). Taken together, these results indicate that steroid hormone concentrations, receptors, and converting enzymes differ between male sheep that prefer females and those that prefer males. It is not know whether the difference in the brain is caused by behavior or vice versa. No studies have been conducted on humans to determine whether there is a similar difference in hormone binding between male heterosexual and homosexual individuals.

Recently, studies of the contribution of the organizational effects of hormones to partner preferences were conducted in monogamous zebra finches (*Taeniopygia guttata*) (Adkins-Regan et al., 1997; Adkins-Regan, 1998). Female zebra finches were exposed either to early treatment with estradiol (during the first 2 weeks post-hatching) or to no treatment, then housed for the next 100 days in an all-female or a mixed-sex aviary (Mansukhani et al., 1996). These females were then given testosterone in adulthood and tested for "social" partner and sexual partner preferences. Females reared in all-female groups were more likely to prefer other females in a two-choice test, regardless of their early hormone treatment; however, females that were both exposed to early estradiol treatment and reared in an all-female group not only preferred other females, but also formed pairs with females in the aviary. Perhaps females must interact with adult males to learn to choose them later in adulthood. In any case, these data suggest that, in contrast to adult hormone manipulations, steroid hormone manipulations early in life can reverse sexual partner preference.

Taken together, these results suggest that hormones interact with environmental conditions to elicit homosexual preferences. This may also be the case for humans, but again, it is difficult to conduct tightly controlled studies with humans.

A recent finding demonstrated the importance of the interaction between environment and genes in the sexual behavior of the fruit fly *Drosophila* (Zhang and Odenwald, 1995). These flies were genetically manipulated so that an ectopic tryptophan/guanine transmembrane transporter gene was activated. The activation of this single gene caused male recipients to vigorously court other males (Zhang and Odenwald, 1995). Mutations that removed this gene appeared to reverse this behavior. Notably, when wild-type flies lacking the mutation were courted by homosexual males, they altered their behavior and sexual preference and actively participated in the male–male courtship behaviors (Zhang and Odenwald, 1995). Thus, in *Drosophila*, both genetic and environmental factors can be shown to affect male sexual preference.

An example of hormones apparently reigning supreme in affecting sexual preference is observed among XY individuals with 5α-reductase deficiency. Despite being reared as girls, and in some cases married to men at an early age, most of these individuals switched gender roles and gender identities after puberty (Imperato-McGinley et al., 1974, 1979). Furthermore, the vast majority of individuals in this population displayed an erotic orientation toward women. Again, the sex of rearing may not have been unambiguously female (Rubin et al., 1981).

More recent studies have reported a slightly higher than typical rate of bisexual and homosexual *fantasy*, but again no significant differences in the incidence of bisexual or homosexual *behaviors*, among women with CAH whose genitalia were masculinized in utero by adrenal androgens (Money et al., 1984; Mulaikal et al., 1987; but see Migeon and Wisniewski, 1998). DES, a synthetic estrogen used to avoid miscarriages, has been reported to cause significant masculinizing and defeminizing effects in nonhuman animals (Hines, 1991), but the extent of behavioral effects of DES in humans remains somewhat controversial. For example, prenatal exposure to DES in humans may slightly increase the incidence of bisexual and homosexual activities to about 25% from 15–20% incidence in nonexposed women. Despite this finding, it is important to note that the majority (about 75%) of the women in this study who were exposed to an unusual prenatal endocrine milieu reported exclusively heterosexual preferences (Ehrhardt et al., 1985). Taken together, these studies indicate that prenatal sex steroid hormones may not play a primary role in sexual orientation.However, the incidence of homosexuality and bisexuality among the general population is not really known. The "increase in incidence" to about 25% is based on classic data that have recently been called into question (Kinsey et al., 1948). An alternative perspective would suggest that early hormonal environment is involved in sexual orientation, but the effects of elevated endogenous adrenal androgen or exogenous steroid treatment may not mimic the fetal conditions of high local concentrations or specific timing necessary for producing an effect.

The differences in neural organization recently discovered among heterosexual men, heterosexual women, and homosexual men are intriguing (see above). But the differences in brain morphology observed between homosexual men and heterosexual men could *result from*, rather than *cause*, homosexual behavior (LeVay, 1991; Breedlove, 1997). A recent study in which male rats were paired with individual ovariectomized females provides support for such a hypothesis (Breedlove, 1997). Some males were paired with ovariectomized females that were hormonally primed, and they engaged in frequent mating behavior. Other males were paired with females that did not receive hormone replacement therapy, and they never mated. The motoneurons in the spinal nucleus of the bulbocavernosus (SNB) mediate penile erection in rats (see Box 4.2). Microscopic sections of SNB tissue from these rats were stained with a Nissl stain, the same histological stain used in human postmortem studies to highlight cell bodies (LeVay, 1991). Adult male rats that had engaged in sexual behavior had smaller neuronal cell bodies and nuclei in the SNB as compared with noncopulators (Breedlove, 1997). These results indicate that adult sexual behavior can affect neural morphology. Taken together, sexual orientation or sexual preference is the result of a complex interaction between biology and environment, but there is no strong evidence that prenatal steriod hormone exposure directly orchestrates sexual orientation. The development of homosexual erotic atttraction remains as mysterious as the development of hetersexual erotic attraction (Gorman, 1994).

## Sex Differences in Cognitive Abilities

Sex differences in human brain size have been reported for years (Crichton-Browne, 1880; Swaab and Hofman, 1984), and, as discussed above, specific differences between male and female humans in the size or shape of certain brain regions have also been reported. These differences in brain structure are subtle, but can be readily discerned in most cases. Male and female humans certainly behave differently, and if human behavior reflects some manifestation of central nervous system activity or organization, then differences in brain activity or structure are to be expected. But because male and female humans overlap substantially in their behavioral repertoires (see Figure 4.12), any sex differences in the brain are expected to be subtle. Logically, as was the case for bird song, sex differences in brain morphology should be found in humans in regions where behaviors that are clearly sexually dimorphic are processed. Thus, an important strategy for studying human behavioral sex differences is to study behaviors that are sexually dimorphic and to map these behavioral differences onto sex differences in brain organization. The roles of these brain regions in mediating behavior can then be assessed by examining patients that sustain damage to the designated areas.

It should be emphasized here that there is no direct evidence that the sex differences in brain morphology thus far discovered mediate human behavioral sex differences. Similarly, there is no direct evidence that they do *not*. A further complication exists, as we saw above in the case of sexual orientation: if brain structural differences that correspond to behavioral differences do exist between males and females, it is still not certain whether they are the cause or the effect of the behavioral dimorphisms.

With these disclaimers in mind, there are several sex differences in cognitive abilities that are consistently observed cross-culturally and hence are good candidates to be mediated primarily by physiological factors; namely, sex steroid hormones. Corresponding sexual dimorphisms in the brain regions that are involved in these cognitive processes have also been found. This section presents a brief review of sex differences in perception and sensory abilities, lateralization of cognitive function, verbal skills, and visuospatial abilities among humans (reviewed in Velle, 1987).

### Perception and Sensory Abilities

Sensation and perception are possibly the most basic cognitive functions. Sensation is the initial processing of sensory information as it enters the nervous system through the sensory receptors. Perception is the transduction of this sensory information into biologically meaningful information. Sex differences have been widely reported in both sensation and perception. There are many subtle and a few marked differences between males and females in sensory and perceptual abilities.

There are three general areas of research into sensory and perceptual function: sensitivity, discrimination, and preference. To study sensitivity, experimental subjects are usually presented first with no stimuli, then gradually stimuli are presented and increased in small incremental steps until the subject reports a sensory experience. For example, a subject may be placed in a dark room and asked to stare at a wall and push a button whenever they perceive a pulse of light. The experimenter may initially flash only one or two photons of light, but continues to provide stronger stimuli until the subject reliably reports the presence of the light. To study discrimination, sensory stimuli that are closely related are presented to the subject and are made increasingly different by the experimenter until the subject reports the presence of more than one stimulus. For example, two equimolar sucrose solutions may be provided to the subject, who should not report any difference in taste. The experimenter then covertly increases the concentration of sucrose in one of the cups very slightly until the subject reports a difference between the two solutions. Preference can be determined in a straightforward manner. For instance, a subject might be water-deprived for 24 hours, then provided with cups of saline solution of varying concentrations and asked to sample all of the cups. The experimenter simply records the volume consumed from each cup to determine the preferred concentration.

**OLFACTION.**    The olfactory sensory system (the sense of smell) transduces information about airborne chemicals into central nervous system signals. There are important sex differences in olfactory sensitivity and odor identification ability. Women are approximately 1000 times more sensitive to musklike odors (for example, pentadecanolide and oxohexadecanolide) than men. The increased sensitivity of women to these odors begins at puberty and appears to be estrogen dependent (Koelega and Koster, 1974). However, for other odors, such as amyl acetate, a sex difference appears before puberty; girls are far superior to boys at detecting this odor at low concentrations. Periovulatory women, as well as women in early pregnancy, display enhanced olfactory sensitivity. Menstruating women and women tested late in pregnancy exhibit lowered olfactory sensitivities. Women are better than men at all ages at identifying odors, and this sex difference has been demonstrated in cross-cultural studies (Doty et al., 1984, 1985). These consistent and reliable sex differences in olfactory acuity, as well as variation in olfactory sensitivity observed across the menstrual cycle, during pregnancy, and in individuals with clinical endocrinological disorders, strongly suggest that sex steroid hormones influence olfactory sensitivity. For example, a study of women with irregular menstrual cycles showed that these women exhibit reduced olfactory sensitivity compared with women with regular menstrual cycles; fully 20% of the subjects were completely unresponsive to odors, but many of them did not recognize that they possessed a sensory impairment (Marshall and Henkin, 1971). The mechanism by which hormones affect olfactory sensitivity remains unspecified in most people.

An olfactory deficit in a clinical population of individuals indicates that olfaction and hormones may be only indirectly related in these people. Men with Kallmann syndrome possess small testes, are infertile, and are anosmic (cannot detect odors). Their olfactory deficit results from a congenital lack of olfactory bulb development during early ontogeny. Embryological studies have indicated that the hypothalamic neurons that secrete GnRH originate in the olfactory bulbs, then migrate to the hypothalamus (Figure 4.13; Schwanzel-Fukuda and Pfaff, 1989). In Kallmann syndrome, the lack of olfactory bulb development interferes with the migration of the GnRH neurons so that reproductive difficulties ensue

**4.13  Congenital absence of the olfactory bulbs in Kallmann syndrome** interferes with the migration of GnRH neurons to their proper destination in the hypothalamus. (Top left) Micro-projection drawing of a sagittal section through the brain and nasal region of a normal 19-week-old human fetus showing olfactory bulb development and a normal distribution of GnRH-immunoreactive cells in the nose and preoptic area (POA) of the brain (black dots). (Top right) Photomicrograph of the same section at higher magnification, showing a single GnRH-immunoreactive cell in the nose tissue, in a ganglion of the terminal nerve. (Bottom left) Microprojection drawing of another fetus, also 19 weeks old, with Kallmann syndrome. Note that the olfactory bulbs are absent and that no GnRH immunoreactivity is visible in the brain. GnRH-positive cells are seen as dots and heavy black lines in the nose, between the meninges, and on the dorsal surface of the cribriform plate (CP), the bony shelf upon which the olfactory bulbs are normally located. (Bottom right) Photomicrograph of this brain section, again at higher magnification, shows thick clumps and clusters of GnRH-immunoreactive cells in the nose. Courtesy of Marlene Schwanzel-Fukuda.

(Schwanzel-Fukuda et al., 1989). Thus, the sensory deficit is not affected directly by hormones in this case, but rather by a congenital condition that blocks normal olfactory bulb development as well as normal endocrine function.

**TASTE.**    The gustatory sense (taste) provides information to the nervous system about chemicals in solution. On tests of taste perception, women, on average, display more sensitivity than men. Typically, a drop of a representative solution is placed on the four areas of the tongue that have specific receptors for sweet, sour, salty, and bitter solutions. Solutions commonly used include sucrose, citric acid, sodium chloride, and quinine sulphate (Fikentscher et al., 1977). Women are superior to men in naming tastes and in discriminating tastes, especially bitter tastes (Doty, 1978). The physiological bases for these sex differences in the sensation and perception of taste in humans are unknown. Differential sex steroid hormone concentrations are suspected to be involved because the sex differences in taste perception arise after puberty, are exaggerated during pregnancy and the follicular phase of the menstrual cycle, and are diminished somewhat after menopause (Doty, 1978; Fleming, 1988; Fleming and Pliner, 1983).

Sex differences in taste preferences have also been reported in many species of laboratory animals. In the case of rats, the effects of hormones in mediating this sex difference are well known (Krecek, 1973; Valenstein et al., 1967; Wade, 1972; Zucker, 1969). Females display estrogen-dependent preferences for sweet tastes (for example, sugar or saccharin), organized by the lack of perinatal androgens and activated by estrogens in adulthood.

**AUDITION.**   Sound pressure changes are perceived by the auditory sensory system (hearing). There is ample evidence that women are more sensitive than men to sound. Women hear pure tones at lower thresholds than men; this is particularly true at higher frequencies and occurs at all ages (Corso, 1959). Similarly, tolerance for white noise (noise composed of all sound frequencies; an example of white noise is the hiss of an FM radio not tuned to a station) is significantly lower in females than in males. In children ranging in age from 5 to 12, the average noise tolerance level was about 82 decibels (dB) for boys and 73 dB for girls (Elliot, 1971); among college students ranging in age from 18 to 26, the average noise tolerance level was about 83 dB for men and 76 dB for women (McGuinness, 1972). (Remember that decibels are measured on a log scale, so a difference of 10 dB represents a doubling of loudness.)

In one interesting study of babies 12–14 weeks of age, the infants were trained by operant conditioning (rewarded for the appropriate behavior) to maintain visual fixation on a white circle (Watson, 1969). Both sexes could perform the task equally well under the right circumstances. In addition to demonstrating that human babies were capable of learning at a much earlier age than previously believed, this study also demonstrated a sex difference in reward contingencies. Girls could maintain visual orientation when a low-frequency tone was provided as the reward, but not when a visual stimulus was presented as the reinforcement. Baby boys performed the task better when the reward was visual. This study suggests that at a very young age, females react to auditory information preferentially, whereas males respond better to visual information. One might conclude from this study that physiological factors mediate these effects in such young children; however, this conclusion must be tempered by the observation that parents interact with baby girls differently from baby boys, and that this difference in interaction begins as soon as the sex of the child is known. Whatever the cause of the reinforcement preference, this auditory propensity in girls may be related to the increased verbal abilities displayed by girls relative to boys (see below).

In addition to hearing sounds, the ear also produces faint, echolike noises generated by the cochlea in the inner ear, called click-evoked otoacoustic emissions (EOAEs). These emissions are present from birth and remain relatively stable throughout life (in the absence of ear damage). They can be measured by inserting a very small speaker/microphone into the outer ear, sending a series of clicks into the ear, and recording the responses. Women generally have louder EOAEs than men, a sex difference that is present from birth, suggesting that this phenomenon is organized by early hormone exposure. In support of this notion, earlier studies reported that women with twin brothers have more male-like "quiet ears" (McFadden and Loehlin, 1995), presumably in response to exposure to prenatal androgens. A recent study reported that homosexual and bisexual women produce weaker EOAEs than heterosexual women (McFadden and Pasanen, 1998). There were no differences in EOAEs among male homosexual, heterosexual, and bisexual men. Importantly, there are few data suggesting that androgens from a male twin affect the brain and behavior of a female twin, or that there is an increase in the prevalence of homosexuality among females with twin brothers. Also, because there was significant overlap in the EOAEs between heterosexual and homosexual/bisexual women, it is not possible to predict homosexual behavior simply by measuring female otoacoustic EOAEs.

**VISION.**   The visual system transduces light energy into the electrochemical signals of the nervous system. As we have just seen, baby boys find visual information more rewarding than auditory information. With few exceptions, visual acuity is better in men than in women; that is, men see better than women. Sex differences also exist in tolerance of light intensity; on average, women tolerate higher levels of light intensity than men. Conversely, when subjects with good visual acuity are tested, women undergo dark adaptation more quickly than men (McGuinness, 1976). Visual perception, especially in regard to visuospatial abilities, is markedly better among males than females at all ages.

### *Lateralization of Cognitive Function*

The two cerebral hemispheres of the brain are somewhat specialized for processing distinct types of cognitive tasks (Wisniewski, 1998). In right-handed individuals, generally the right side of the brain specializes in spatial processing, whereas the left hemisphere is best at processing verbal information (Hines, 1982; Kimura and Harshman, 1984). This tendency for cognitive skills to be concentrated in one hemisphere is called cerebral specialization or **lateralization**. Males and females differ in the extent to which cognitive function exhibits cerebral lateralization: males tend to be more lateralized than females. That is, different cognitive functions tend to be more confined to separate hemispheres in males, whereas female cognitive function is generally more evenly distributed between both hemispheres.

Cerebral lateralization can be measured in several ways. Researchers take advantage of the fact that auditory information enters one ear and visual information enters one visual field, but then is processed by the contralateral hemisphere. For instance, auditory signals can be presented via headphones to one ear or the other. Commonly, a brief tone or a word is embedded in white noise, and the subject must indicate as quickly as possible when the signal is present. A variation of this technique involves presenting two signals (words) simultaneously to both ears; again, the subject must react as quickly as possible. The discrepancy in response speed or accuracy between the two ears reflects the degree of lateralization. A similar type of technique using a special apparatus called a tachistoscope to present visual stimuli to only one visual field has been employed to assess lateralization of visual processing.

People typically can detect sounds better with the right ear; that is, auditory processing is better in the left than in the right hemisphere. This facility has been referred to as the right-ear advantage. Perhaps not surprisingly, the processing of language and speech for most people occurs predominantly in the left hemisphere. However, men are much slower and make more mistakes in responding to auditory information arriving at the left ear than women, and women show less discrepancy than men in both response speed and response accuracy between the two ears and between the left and right visual fields. In other words, the brains of women are less lateralized than those of men for auditory and visual information. Additional support for this view comes from the clinical literature on verbal deficits caused by cerebral hemorrhages (strokes) (McGlone, 1980). In general, men who have suffered a stroke on the left side of the brain exhibit verbal deficits, but women with cerebral vascular damage on the left side may or may not exhibit a verbal deficit. If men suffer a stroke on the right side of the brain, their visuospatial abilities are affected. In many cases, women who suffer strokes on the right side do not exhibit any obvious decrement in cognitive or behavioral abilities. Thus, the masculine pattern of cognitive processing involves discrete lateralization of function, whereas the feminine pattern exhibits more equal distribution of cognitive function between the two hemispheres.

Prenatal steroid hormones can affect lateralization patterns. Women with Turner syndrome do not secrete steroid hormones prenatally and do not exhibit lateralization of auditory information (Gordon and Galatzer, 1980; Netley, 1977, 1983). These women may have other atypical features such as retarded mental development, however, which may affect these tasks independently of hormones. In contrast, women exposed to DES in utero displayed the male-typical pattern of increased lateralization of auditory and visual information as compared with their unexposed sisters (Hines, 1991).

Sex differences have also been reported in the lateralization of human brain morphology. The left hemisphere is slightly larger and weighs more than the right hemisphere of the human brain, but the weight difference between the two hemispheres is less pronounced in females than in males. The two hemispheres of the brain communicate with each other through several fiber pathways; one of these links is the corpus callosum. Sex differences in the size and shape of the corpus callosum, detected by magnetic resonance imaging and other techniques, suggest a neuroanatomical correlate that could account for the sex differences in lateralization of cognitive function (Figure 4.14), but there are many conflicting reports that fail to find a morphological sex difference in the corpus callosum (Allen et al., 1991; Crichton-Browne, 1880; deLacoste-Utamsing and Holloway, 1982; deLacoste et al., 1986; Wada, 1976).

### *Verbal Skills*

There is no sex difference in scores on modern standardized tests of intelligence (Hines, 1982). That is, boys and girls do not differ predictably in IQ. However, some subsets of the skills and abilities measured on intelligence tests show consistent, though small, sex differences in performance. On average, females excel at verbal tasks, perceptual skills, fine motor skills, and mathematical calculations, whereas males outperform females on targeted directed motor skills (e.g., guiding or interception of a projectile), quantitative tasks, and visuospatial abilities, including map reading, sense of direction, and mathematical reasoning (Bryant, 1982; Gladue et al., 1990; Hines, 1982; Kimura, 1992; Velle, 1987) (Figure 4.15).

Rostral                    Caudal              Rostral                    Caudal

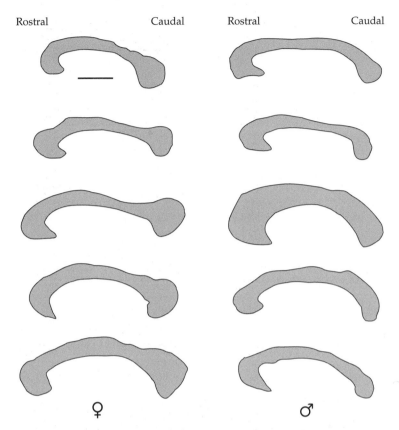

♀                                          ♂

**4.14  Possible sex difference in the human corpus callosum** is shown in these drawings based on midline cross-sections. In females, the caudal portion of the corpus callosum is more bulbous than in males. It has been suggested that some sex differences in the lateralization of cognitive function might be accounted for by differential numbers of axons in the caudal corpus callosum (splenium). Because this section of the corpus callosum connects the occipital lobes, which process visual information, sex differences in visual processing have also been attributed to sexual dimorphism in this structure. These suggestions are controversial. (Scale bar = 2 cm.) After deLacoste-Utamsing and Holloway, 1982.

Females generally display better language comprehension, faster language acquisition (both first and additional languages), and better spelling, verbal fluency, and grammar skills than males (Hines, 1991; Netley, 1983). Many of these sex differences in verbal performance arise after puberty, which makes them likely candidates to be mediated by hormonal effects (Maccoby and Jacklin, 1974); however, social and other environmental factors cannot be ruled out. No consistent effect of prenatal endocrine dysfunctions on subsequent verbal abilities has been demonstrated (reviewed in Hines, 1982).

Several studies have suggested a neuroanatomical basis for these sex differences in performance. In most people, the planum temporale, a flattened area of the temporal lobe, is larger in the left cerebral hemisphere than in the right. Based on earlier case studies of individuals with brain damage restricted to the planum

**4.15  Performance on certain tasks favor one sex over the other.** Specifically, women tend to outperform men on tests of perceptual speed, such as (a) finding the match to the house on the far left as quickly as possible. Women also do better than men in manual tasks that require fine motor coordination, such as (b) placing pegs on a board as quickly as possible. Women also excel over men on mathematical calculations (c). Men, on the other hand, are more accurate than women in target-directed motor skills such as catching a ball or (d) throwing a dart, regardless of previous sports experience. Men also do better than women in mathematical reasoning (e). Men excel over women at mentally rotating an object (f). After Kimura, 1992.

temporale, it has been concluded that this brain region is involved in speech. The asymmetry between the right and left planum temporale is less marked in women than in men (Wada et al., 1975). In other words, its size is less lateralized in females. In another study, the volume of the superior temporal cortex and the cortical volume fraction of Broca's area, which is also involved in speech, was about 20% larger in female than in male brains (Harasty et al., 1997), a finding that corresponds well with findings on sex differences in verbal function.

With the advent of new imaging tools such as functional magnetic resonance imaging (fMRI), it is now possible to view the living, awake brain and monitor

**4.16  Men and women use different parts of their brains to solve similar language tasks.** Among males, functional MRI (fMRI) reveals that brain activation during rhyming tasks is restricted to the left inferior frontal gyrus. In females, both the left and right inferior frontal gyri are activated, and the pattern of activation is more diffuse. From Shaywitz et al., 1995; courtesy of NMR Research/Yale Medical School.

specific brain region activity during the performance of a particular task. One recent study using fMRI revealed that men and women use different parts of their brains to solve similar phonological tasks. Nineteen males and nineteen females were asked to report whether or not two nonsense words rhymed. Among males, brain activation during this rhyming task was concentrated in the left inferior frontal gyrus region. In contrast, both the left and right inferior frontal gyri were activated in females performing the rhyming task, and the pattern of activation was more diffuse than for males (Shaywitz et al., 1995) (Figure 4.16). These striking data provide evidence that the brains of men and women operate differently when processing certain features of language.

### Mathematical Reasoning and Visuospatial Abilities

Sex differences in performance on mathematical reasoning tasks have been consistently observed within the general population for decades. In general, males outperform females on tests of mathematical reasoning ability, such as the mathematics section of the Scholastic Aptitude Test (SAT-M)(Benbow and Stanley, 1983; Gouchie and Kimura, 1991). The male-biased sex difference increases dramatically at the high end of performance: the sex ratio of seventh-grade boys to girls receiving SAT-M scores of 500 or above is 2.1:1; for scores of 600 or above, the ratio is 4.1:1; and for scores of 700 or above, the ratio is 12.9:1 (Benbow and Stanley, 1983). The activational effects of hormones are not likely to mediate this sex difference because this effect is observed prior to the onset of puberty (Wisniewski, 1998). There may be a complex relationship between rate of maturation, brain lateralization, handedness, and other social or biological factors that accounts for average sex differences in mathematical reasoning (A. B. Wisniewski, M. K. Galloway, and R. J. Nelson, unpublished manuscript).

On average, males perform visuospatial tasks better than females (McGee, 1979). Visuospatial tasks include mental rotation of objects, map reading, mental visualization of relationships among objects in space, solving maze problems, and shape recognition (see Figure 4.15) (Hines, 1991). The difference in visuospatial abilities between boys and girls is small or absent prior to puberty, but present after puberty, suggesting that hormonal influences could be involved.

Visualization of space, objects, or relationships among objects in space is a common test of visuospatial abilities. For example, an individual may be asked to go through the alphabet mentally as fast as possible and count the number of letters containing the sound "ee," including the letter *e* (Coltheart et al., 1975). This is a test of verbal abilities, and females are faster than males. In a visuospatial test, a person is asked to go through the alphabet mentally as quickly as possible and count all of the uppercase letters with a curve in their form (Coltheart et al., 1975). Males perform better than females at this task.

Similarly, males perform better at map reading and directional tasks. In one study, college students were placed in a windowless room and told to imagine that they were facing the front of a familiar building, the college administration building, for instance. With this imaginary orientation in space, they were requested to point to other familiar landmarks, such as the stadium or the clock tower. When the degrees of error in the students' estimated orientation reports were computed, it was found that men made fewer errors in estimation of direction than women (Bryant, 1982, 1991). Of course, college men may have more experience in navigating through space than college women. Boys may have been allowed to range farther from home than girls as they were growing up, or allowed to drive more frequently than girls. Because it is so difficult to account for differential experiential effects in humans, animal models, in which environmental experiences can be somewhat equalized, have been employed to understand these sex differences in spatial abilities.

**ANIMAL MODELS OF VISUOSPATIAL SKILLS.**   There is no perfect animal model for human visuospatial skills. However, animals can be taught to run mazes, a task that incorporates visuospatial (or perhaps olfactory–spatial) skills. A consistent sex difference in maze-running ability is observed among many rodent species (reviewed in Gaulin and FitzGerald, 1986; Haaren et al., 1990): males learn mazes faster and make fewer errors than females (see Chapter 11; McNemar and Stone, 1932). This sex difference in maze learning is thought to be mediated by hormonal effects on the hippocampus, a structure in the brain that is important for spatial learning (Williams and Meck, 1991). Recall from Chapter 3 that male meadow voles learn mazes better than female conspecifics, whereas there is no difference in maze-learning abilities between male and female pine voles (Gaulin and FitzGerald, 1986). The hippocampus of male meadow voles is approximately 10% larger than the hippocampus of females, but hippocampal size does not differ between male and female pine voles (Jacobs et al., 1990). Whether hippocampal size drives the difference in behavior or whether sex-related differences in experience in spatial habitats drive hippocampal size has recently been investigated; the results will be discussed in Chapter 10.

Sex differences in human cognitive behavior have been documented, but how do we gather evidence to determine the contribution of hormones to these differences in human behavior? Indirect evidence from people with atypical endocrine function suggests that early hormone exposure influences visuospatial abilities among humans. Individuals with Turner syndrome display a marked deficit in visuospatial abilities (Hines, 1982; Netley, 1983). Because these individuals possess dysgenic ovaries and produce no steroid hormones, these results are consistent with the idea that early exposure to androgen (or androgen metabolites) promotes subsequent visuospatial abilities. In some studies of females with CAH, who experience high levels of early androgen exposure, there have been reports of enhanced visuospatial abilities, but these reports have not consistently shown a clear trend (Hines, 1991). Similarly, exogenous prenatal hormone exposure does not consistently affect visuospatial abilities. Except for one brief report (Wada, 1976), there have not been reports of sex differences in brain regions that process visuospatial information corresponding to those that have been found in brain regions that process verbal information.

The organizational/activational hypothesis suggests that the human central nervous system is ordered in a male or female manner early in prenatal development by the presence or absence, respectively, of gonadal steroid hormones; behavioral sex differences arise when these prenatally organized neural circuits are activated by sex steroids secreted at puberty. Thus, sex differences in performance reflect differential prenatal exposure to steroid hormones. If the time frame of the organizational/activational hypothesis is expanded, an alternative view emerges. In a very interesting study, individuals that underwent puberty early were compared with individuals that underwent puberty late (Waber, 1976). Regardless of sex, early-maturing adolescents performed better than late-maturing adolescents on tests of verbal abilities. Late-maturing individuals outperformed early-maturing individuals on tests of spatial abilities. Because females typically undergo puberty at an earlier age than males, the differences in cognitive function between males and females could reflect differential brain organization mediated by *peripubertal* sex steroid hormones coincident with differential rates of brain maturation (Waber, 1976).

## Conclusions

A final note about sex differences in human performance: This area of research is highly politicized, both within and outside the scientific community. Some people see the discovery of sex differences in brain function, organization, or morphology as evidence of biological differences between the sexes in ability. Others view sex differences in the human brain as reflecting a social history of differential treatment of the two sexes, and thus as mutable. The data can be used either to maintain the status quo ("women are different biologically and therefore should not be expected to perform as well as men") or to effect change ("women and men are not fundamentally different and complete parity in opportunity should be a societal goal") (Harris, 1980). These issues are critical when, for example, the United States Employment Service indicates that successful candidates for technical–scientific occupations, jobs in diverse fields including architecture, engineering, chemistry, physics, and mathematics, require visuospatial aptitudes in the top tenth percentile (Harris, 1980). If career choices are made on the basis of these requirements, then people may sort themselves into career tracks because of their respective test scores. Thus, scientific data can be used to explain the enormous disparity between the sexes in these occupations.

It must be emphasized that the range of differences in brain morphology or function is greater *within* each sex than *between* the two sexes (Breedlove, 1994; Crichton-Browne, 1880; McGlone, 1980). Are studies of subtle differences in the human brain worthwhile? How are the data to be interpreted? These are difficult questions that require sensitive and carefully reasoned answers. A quote from Mrs. Fawcett, a leader of the women's movement in the late 19th century, nicely puts the debate into perspective:

> No one of those who care most for the women's movement cares one jot to prove or to maintain that men's brains and women's brains are exactly alike or exactly equal. All we ask is that the social and legal status of women should be such as to foster, not to suppress, any gift of art, literature, learning, or goodness with which women may be endowed (quoted in Romanes, 1887).

## Summary

• The organizational and activational actions of steroid hormones cause changes in neural tissue. Sexual dimorphisms in brain structure have been reported for a number of neural regions. Some of these dimorphisms are subtle, such as the differences in neural branching in the MPOA, but others are marked, such as the differences in the size of the rat SDN-POA. Other sex differences have been reported in brain structure and in neurotransmitter secretion, receptor numbers, and distribution patterns. In all mammalian cases, these neural sexual dimorphisms can be altered in a predictable fashion by early steroid hormone treatment. Sexual dimorphisms in the brain can be affected by circulating hormones in adults as well. However, the functional significance of sexually dimorphic brain structures in mammals is still under investigation.

• A strong relationship among hormones, brain structure, and sexually dimorphic behavior has been established in studies of bird song. The neural pathways underlying the production of bird song involve several interconnected nuclei, some of which show sexual dimorphism. The HVC and RA of male zebra finches, which sing, are three to six times larger than those of female conspecifics, which do not sing. The increased size of these areas in males is due to larger spacing among neurons, as well as more and larger neurons. Bird song is organized and activated by sex steroid hormones in some species, and only activated by hormones in other species. The sexual dimorphisms in brain nucleus size and subsequent singing behavior of zebra finches are organized early in development. In contrast, female canaries will sing if treated in adulthood with testosterone. Adult androgen treatment increases the size of the vocal control regions of the brain. Bird species in which both sexes sing exhibit no sex difference in the size of the neural structures making up the vocal control regions.

• Weakly electric fishes orient in the murky water of their habitat by discharging electric signals and detecting any distortion in the pattern of their emitted signals, a process called electrolocation. During courtship, the electric receptors detect signals emitted by conspecifics within a short range (70–100 cm). Sex steroid hormones play activational roles in mediating the onset, as well as the pattern, of electric signaling. Treatment of females or juvenile fish of either sex with androgens, especially naturally occurring fish androgens, produces electric discharge patterns similar to those of adult males in breeding condition. Castration of adult males shifts the pattern of electric discharge to resemble the pattern of conspecific females.

• The urinary posture of canines is sexually dimorphic. The male-typical urinary posture is organized by perinatal androgen exposure. Hormones during puberty are not necessary to activate the male-typical urinary posture.

• In rhesus monkeys and many other mammalian species, including humans, males engage in much more play behavior than their female peers throughout development. A larger proportion of male play behavior involves simulated fighting or rough-and-tumble play as compared with the play behavior of females. The sex difference in play behavior is organized prenatally, and castration or other postnatal endocrine manipulation does not affect the amount of threat, play initiation, rough-and-tumble play, or pursuit play among monkeys.

• Three common sex differences observed in humans are gender role, gender identity, and sexual orientation/preference. Gender role is the sum of culturally based behavior patterns that are specific to one sex or the other. Gender role appears to be primarily learned; however, there is currently great controversy about this topic. Individuals with early endocrine dysfunction may show adoption of an atypical gender role. Similarly, gender identity, whether individuals view themselves as male or as female, appears to be primarily learned. Studies of individuals with 5α-reductase deficiency who change gender role and gender identity at puberty suggest that hormones, rather than rearing, could determine gender role and/or gender identity.

• Very little is known about how heterosexuals develop erotic attractions, and even less is known about how homosexuals develop erotic attractions. Because erotic attractions typically begin at the time of puberty, sex steroid hormones have been assumed to be involved. A common hypothesis about the cause of homosexuality is that the hormone levels of homosexuals are different from those of heterosexuals. However, many studies have failed to find any evidence that adult homosexual men or women differ from their heterosexual counterparts in blood concentrations of androgens or estrogens. Evidence for effects of early exposure to steroids on sexual preference is also inconclusive.

• Sex differences in human brain size have been reported for years. More recently, sex differences in specific brain structures have been discovered. Sex differences in a number of cognitive functions have also been reported. Females are more sensitive to auditory information, whereas males are more sensitive to visual information. Females are also more sensitive than males to taste and olfactory input.

• Women display less lateralization of cognitive functions than men. On average, females generally excel in verbal, perceptual, and fine motor skills, whereas males outperform females on quantitative and visuospatial tasks, including map reading and direction finding. Although reliable sex differences can be documented, these differences in ability are slight; there is more variation within each sex than between the sexes in most cognitive abilities.

## Questions for Discussion

1. Imagine that you discovered that the brains of architects were different from those of nonarchitects; specifically, that the "drawstraightem nuclei" of the right occipital lobe were enlarged in architects as compared with nonarchitects. Would you argue that architects were destined to be architects because of their brain organization, or that experience as an architect changed their brains? How would you resolve this issue? Expand your arguments to include brain differences between homosexuals and heterosexuals.

2. What are the advantages and disadvantages of studying animal models to understand human behavioral sexual dimorphisms? Discuss the advantages and disadvantages of three different model systems. What characteristics of an animal model would provide an ideal experimental system for understanding human behavioral sexual dimorphisms?

3. Human reproductive organ pathologies have increased dramatically, and sperm counts have decreased substantially, over the past 50 years, possibly due to an increase in estrogenic substances in the environment. How would you go about establishing that human sexual behavior has also been affected?

4. Using organ discharge patterns in electric fishes and urinary behavior in dogs, discuss the proposition that hormones affect perception. Can you conceive of some possible ways how this might occur using a proximate level of explanation? Can you conceive of some possible reasons why this might occur using an ultimate level of explanation?

5. Are studies of individuals with endocrine dysfunction a reasonable way to understand typical sexual dimorphisms in human behavior? Why or why not?

6. Some individuals are born with genitalia that are not definitely male or neither female. Physicians and parents often must make choices about treatment and make a sex assignment at birth. Some adult individuals who were born with ambiguous genitalia claim that, in retrospect, they would have been happier "unaltered" than forced into one particular sexual category. Keeping these views in mind, what should physicians do or advise when individuals are born with atypical genitalia?

## Suggested Readings

Arnold, A. P. and Schlinger, B. A. 1993. Sexual differentiation of brain and behavior: The zebra finch is not just a flying rat. *Brain, Behavior & Evolution*, 42: 231–241.

Breedlove, S. M. 1994. Sexual differentiation of the human nervous system. *Annual Review of Neuroscience*, 45: 389–418.

Collaer, M. L. and Hines, M. 1995. Human behavioral sex differences: A role for gonadal hormones during early development? *Psychological Bulletin*, 118: 55–107.

LeVay, S. 1991. A difference in hypothalamic structure between heterosexual and homosexual men. *Science*, 253: 1034–1037.

LeVay, S. 1993. *The Sexual Brain.* MIT Press, Cambridge, MA.

Maccoby, E. E. and Jacklin, C. N. 1974. *The Psychology of Sex Differences.* Stanford University Press, Stanford, CA.

Migeon, C. J. and Wisiewski, A. B. 1998. Sexual differentiation: From genes to gender. *Hormone Research*, 50: 245–251.

# 5

# Male Reproductive Behavior

**M**ales of many species, including salmon, marsupial mice, and praying mantises, face certain death in order to mate. Stories abound in the natural history literature describing the heroic journeys of males of these and other species that overcome obstacles and dangers just to gain the opportunity to fight other males for the possibility of mating. Male elephant seals, for instance, migrate hundreds of kilometers to the northern California coast in order to set up breeding territories, and fight ferociously with their neighbors for the best real estate. Beachfront property is the best territory to control because females prefer locations close to the water and tend to mate with males occupying these prime spots. Females presumably prefer beachfront locations because their pups will be safer from terrestrial predators along the edge of the water. Once the territories are established, the high-ranking males are clustered around the water's edge, surrounded by lower-ranking males. As females come ashore, the lower-ranking males continually challenge the dominant males and try to mate with the females (Figure 5.1).

Why do male elephant seals expend so much energy fighting among themselves in order to secure a piece of the beach valued by females? Males occupying desirable waterfront territories mate with many more females than males located in peripheral areas because females prefer to mate with the males located in territories that provide the best place to deliver and nurse their pups (LeBoeuf, 1974). Although females directly choose the areas in which they want to rear their young, by doing so they also indirectly choose males possessing the constellation of genes that promotes the ability to fight and win against other males. The males' proximity to the water provides a reliable indication of these dominance traits. By mating with dominant, so-called "alpha" males, females increase the probability that their sons will possess the genes associated with reproductive success, and thus enhance their own fitness. Males are driven to fight for prime territories because if they fail to secure territories that are preferred by females, then they are unlikely to mate, but if they do secure prime territories, they have the chance to sire many offspring. Thus, the ultimate cause of males' strong motivation to mate is to increase their reproductive fitness.

Males and females differ in their potential rates of reproduction. Females produce relatively few, large, resource-rich gametes. The number of offspring a female

**5.1   A dispute over territory** between two male elephant seals. Waterfront areas are hotly contested among males of this species because females prefer to have their pups near the water—an easy escape route from terrestrial predators for themselves and their offspring—and thus prefer to mate with males that control these territories. Male elephant seals are highly aggressive: they have been known to accidentally crush their own offspring in an attempt to keep other males away from their territories. Courtesy of Burney LeBoeuf.

can produce in her lifetime is limited to the number of eggs she can produce or the number of young she can rear. Females generally invest much more than males in each offspring. A male, on the other hand, may produce billions of gametes in his lifetime, and invests relatively little energy in each one (see Chapter 7). A female elephant seal, for example, can produce and raise only one pup per year, but a male can potentially father many pups per year. Thus, the difference in potential reproductive success forms the basis of the different mating strategies of the two sexes (Box 5.1). Females improve their fitness by choosing the best male possible with whom to combine their genes; males can often best achieve reproductive success by seeking to mate with as many females as possible. In other words, females have generally evolved to be "choosy" and males have generally evolved to be "ardent." The proximate bases of sexual behavior reflect these ultimate, evolutionary factors.

---

## Box 5.1
# Battle of the "Sexes"

As noted in the previous two chapters, most animals are either male or female; that is, they possess either testes or ovaries. Males and females typically have conflicting interests as mating partners, and individuals have evolved behaviors to protect and promote their sex-specific self-interest. However, some animals, called hermaphrodites, possess both types of gonads and produce both eggs and sperm. Yet, even among hermaphrodites, conflicts of interest involving mating arise. For example, hermaphroditic animals often participate in elaborate courtship displays to determine which individual will donate sperm and which individual will donate ova during a particular encounter. In some circumstances, it is advantageous to donate sperm; in other cases, it is advantageous to provide ova.

One dramatic case in which it appears advantageous to donate sperm involves hermaphroditic flatworms (*Cotylea*) that typically mate in pairs. These flatworms rear up and literally fence with their penes (see figure). Each flatworm thrusts and parries, trying to stab an exposed area of its mating partner's body while trying to avoid getting stabbed (Michiels and Newman, 1998). An individual that successfully

After Michiels and Newman, 1998

pierces the body of its mating partner injects sperm that travel to the partner's ovaries to inseminate its ova. These "fencing" bouts are intense, and may last 20–60 minutes before one individual succeeds in inseminating the other. Apparently, the costs of producing eggs, and of mending the stab wounds, are sufficiently high to favor the selection of competition among these hermaphroditic flatworms to donate sperm.

These dueling flatworms exemplify the complexity of so-called "simple" organisms. In contrast to sexually reproducing animals, individual hermaphroditic flatworms may have identical, but incompatible, interests as mating partners; thus, as you might predict, cooperation between mating partners should be rare, and the mechanisms underlying aggression and reproductive motivation are probably linked.

# The Proximate Bases of Male Sexual Behavior

The physiological components of male sexual behavior are the topic of this chapter. More specifically, the interaction between the endocrine and nervous systems in mediating male mating behavior will be presented. Most of what we know about the physiological mechanisms underlying sexual behavior has been gained through studies of nonhuman animals, especially rodents; examples of these studies will be described below.

As described in Chapter 3, sex is a division of gamete types, and **sexual behavior** is behavior that has evolved to bring the two gamete types together. Male sexual behavior is defined as all the behaviors necessary and sufficient to deliver male gametes (sperm) to the ova. The hormones involved in gamete maturation—namely, the sex steroid hormones—have been "co-opted" over evolutionary time to regulate the web of behaviors necessary to bring the two sexes together for successful gametic union (Crews, 1984). **Sex drive**, the motivational force that propels individuals to seek sexual union, is a very powerful engine underlying the behavior of all animals, including humans. The sex drive tends to be strong in males, and the threshold for mating behavior tends to be low.

For purposes of description here, all male sexual behavior can be divided into two phases: (1) the appetitive phase and (2) the consummatory phase (Figure 5.2; Hinde, 1970). The **appetitive phase** is roughly equivalent to courtship and involves all of the behaviors the male uses to gain access to the female. Behaviors as diverse as searching for females, fighting for territory, advertising, or providing food for females may occur during courtship. Courtship functions as a communication opportunity during which information about species, readiness to mate, resources, and genetic endowments is shared. The appetitive phase lasts much longer than the second phase, called the **consummatory phase**, during which copulation occurs. Although separating mating behavior into these two phases is likely to divide a unified behavioral program artificially, this dichotomy remains valuable for

| | |
|---|---|
| Sex drive, libido | Performance, potency |
| Appetitive sexual behavior | Consummatory sexual behavior |
| Courtship behavior | Copulatory behavior |

Time

**5.2  Male sexual behavior** can be operationally divided into two components: seeking sexual encounters and engaging in copulation. The former component is variously referred to as sex drive, libido, appetitive sexual behavior, or courtship behavior; the latter is known as performance, potency, or consummatory sexual behavior. Males expend much more time and energy seeking copulation than actually copulating. This division of male sexual behavior into two phases is useful for heuristic purposes as well as in medical diagnoses because hormones can affect each component differently.

understanding the hormonal and neural bases of male reproductive behavior. Thus, the distinction between seeking sex (sex drive, motivation, or libido) and engaging successfully in a mating act (performance, potency) can be useful for heuristic purposes, as well as in medical diagnoses (Meisel and Sachs, 1994; but see Sachs, 1995b). Hormones affect both sex drive and sexual performance, but often to differing degrees.

Male sex drive is expressed overtly after puberty as the testes become active. The coincidence between the onset of sexual interest and puberty suggests that the testes influence sexual motivation. The observation that removal of the testes typically reduces the frequency of all male mating behaviors provides further evidence that the testes are important in the regulation of male sexual behavior (see Chapter 1). Post-castration treatment with androgens, the principal class of sex steroid hormones produced in the testes, restores reproductive behaviors to pre-castration levels. Thus, it is reasonable to conclude that androgens cause sexual behavior.

However, the statement that androgens *cause* sexual behavior requires some qualification. First, recall that hormones change the *probability* that a particular behavior will be exhibited *in a specific context*. Second, the effects of experience interact significantly with hormones to affect behavior. These two caveats are important to keep in mind when discussing the effects of hormones on behavior in general and on male sexual behavior specifically. One outdated model of hormone–behavior interactions arose from physiological models—the so-called hydraulic models—once proposed by ethologists to explain innate, reflexive fixed action patterns. According to these simplistic models, hormonal effects on behavior were analogous to a faucet: for example, if the "androgen spigot" was turned on, then male mating behavior or aggression ensued. But hormone–behavior interactions are far more complex than suggested by this model. About half the readers of this sentence have significant concentrations of androgens in their blood, yet they are reading, not copulating. How can we say, then, that androgens cause sexual behavior? It is more accurate to state that androgens, as well as other sex steroid hormones, appear to affect the likelihood of mating behavior by reducing the threshold for these behaviors in the presence of the appropriate stimuli in the appropriate social context. All other things being equal, a male with high blood androgen concentrations is more likely to copulate with a conspecific female than a male with low androgen concentrations. In other words, in terms of a stimulus–response paradigm of sexual behavior, hormones facilitate the male response, probably by affecting the perception and processing of the stimuli associated with the female. As we will see, androgens have many direct effects on the nervous system, such as regulating neurotransmitter levels as well as affecting the availability of neurotransmitter receptors and other proteins that affect neurotransmitter function (Hull et al., 1997).

Males vary in the frequency of their copulatory behavior, and vast species differences exist in the extent to which male reproductive behavior relies upon hormones. Similarly, enormous individual differences exist within any given species in both the frequency of sexual behavior and the extent to which sexual behavior is mediated by hormones. For example, the regulation of rodent sexual behavior is highly dependent upon hormones, but in primates, the control of sexual behavior is less dependent on hormones and more dependent upon socialization and learning. Compared with rats, then, primates are relatively less reliant on hormones to regulate sexual behavior. However, primates are not unique in this regard, and there is no evidence that species located "higher" on the phylogenetic scale have been emancipated from direct hormonal control of mating behavior as compared with so-called "lower" species. Examination of the regulation of mating behavior in nonmammalian animals also reveals varying degrees of hormonal dependence. An example of a reptile species (the red-sided garter snake) in which reproductive behavior is completely divorced from hormonal control will be presented to help counter the belief that humans are unique in this regard.

This chapter examines the endocrine mediation of sexual behavior among males, and will address many of these comparative issues. The chapter will also describe the ways in which hormones interact with the nervous system in males. Again, animal models, mainly rodents, have been helpful for understanding the physiological mechanisms underlying sexual behavior, both appetitive and consummatory, and research based on these models will be presented in detail below. But first, the history of research into the control of male sexual behavior will be briefly reviewed.

## Historical Origins of Research on Male Sexual Behavior

Castration virtually eliminates mating behavior among males of many species, a fact that has been known since the earliest recorded history (see Chapter 1). As noted in the 12th verse of the 19th chapter of the Gospel of Matthew in the New Testament, "There are eunuchs who are born so from their mother's womb; and there are eunuchs who are made so by men; and there are eunuchs who have made themselves so for the sake of the kingdom of heaven. Let him accept it who can." Some people have suggested that this passage indicates that Jesus believed that castration could clear the path to heaven. Members of the San Diego cult Heaven's Gate apparently believed this to be true. Eight of the 18 males, including the cult leader, who committed suicide together prior to their imaginary journey to a waiting "Mother Ship" reportedly had performed self-castration. There have been many religious sects throughout history that believed functional testes blocked rational and/or pious thought.

The English word *testicle* is derived from the Latin *testiculus*, a diminutive, but synonymous, form of the Latin term *testis,* which means "witness." The verb *testify* has a similar derivation. Witnesses in ancient Roman courts often covered their testes with their right hands and swore "on their virility" that they were about to state the truth (that is, provide *testimony*). This practice illustrates that a relationship among the testes, virility, and mating behavior has been well established for many centuries, but many misconceptions have arisen regarding the nature of the interaction between the testes and sexual behavior.

One common misconception about the regulation of male sex drive that persisted through the late 1800s was that distention, or swelling, of the seminal vesicles activates male sexual behavior (Carter, 1974). Neural stretch receptors were recent discoveries in the 1880s, and it was proposed by several researchers of the time that these receptors, activated by bulging seminal vesicles, induced copulation. Variations of the idea that male sex drive was the result of "pressure" sensations from the accessory organs that had to be relieved lasted well into the 20th century (for example, Ball, 1934a; Nissen, 1929). Anecdotally, many men report "pressure" in their testes or seminal vesicles when they are sexually aroused. A major piece of scientific evidence supporting the "distended seminal vesicle" theory came from work on frogs in mating condition (Tarchanoff, 1887, cited in Steinach, 1894). Male frogs were reported to continue copulating despite removal of major portions of their anatomy, including their testes; after physical separation from their partners, castrated frogs would immediately re-mount the female. However, draining the seminal vesicles led to the rapid separation of the pairs and loss of subsequent sexual activity for the male. Thus, neural impulses from the full seminal vesicles were thought to generate sexual behavior, or more commonly, sex drive. Apparently unaware of Steinach's research or Berthold's work (see Chapter 1), Cunningham (1900) also suggested that male sex drive was a manifestation of neural impulses from the testes.

Steinach, apparently influenced by the writing of Freud, postulated the existence of an incipient sexuality that existed prior to puberty and was triggered by nervous impulses from the swelling reproductive glands. He believed that once the process was initiated, psychic influences or sensory input could send the mechanisms underlying reproductive behavior into action. He attempted to reduce mating behavior in rats by removing their seminal vesicles; however, this procedure had little effect upon their mating behavior (Steinach, 1894). As will be described later, some of Steinach's views on the regulation of sexual behavior, especially the importance of sensory information, remain part of current hypotheses.

Rather than confirming the pressure hypothesis, subsequent research supported the idea that hormones from the testes generate male mating behavior. But even the presence or absence of gonads is not the only mediating factor in male sexual behavior. As mentioned above, sexual experience also affects post-castration responses. Virtually all sexually inexperienced male rats exhibit mating behavior when given the opportunity to interact with estrous females soon after castration, but their interest in females wanes in about 2 weeks. Males with prior sexual experience, on the other hand, vary in how long they maintain reproductive behavior after castration; some males lose interest in females rapidly, while others continue to mate for weeks.

Steinach and his early 20th-century contemporaries were aware of the effect of sexual experience in determining the rate at which post-castrational reductions in male sexual behavior would occur in domesticated animals. For instance, tom-cats with sexual experience prior to neutering may continue to engage in copulatory behavior for months after the testes are removed, usually to the chagrin of pet owners (Dunbar, 1975). Even Aristotle noted in his *Historia Animalium* that castrated bulls occasionally continued to copulate with cows. It was also well known during the 19th century that men who lost their testes through disease or accident maintained sexual behavior for some time, often indefinitely, after the injury. According to Pfüger (1877, cited in Steinach, 1894), one way in which the difference between human sexual behavior and that of other animals could be explained was on the basis of humans' unique mental faculties, that is, their "psychic qualities, the vigor of men's fantasies, and their powerful memories."

Certainly, "psychic" qualities must be called forth as an explanation for the claims made by Charles Edouard Brown-Séquard, at the Société de Biologie de Paris in 1899 (Brown-Séquard, 1899). Ten years earlier, Brown-Séquard, a prominent researcher, had published findings in the *Archives de Physiologie Normale et*

*Pathologique*, claiming that injections of endocrine extracts had astounding rejuvenating effects on several physical parameters, including sexual vigor. At the Société in 1899, Brown-Séquard sought to demonstrate his findings: he injected himself with an aqueous solution of homogenized dog and guinea pig testes. He claimed that the injections had amazing restorative effects; his claims prompted sales of endocrine extract "treatments" (Figure 5.3). However, androgens were later discovered to be lipid-soluble steroid hormones; therefore, water-based injections are unlikely to have produced the behavioral effects reported by Brown-Séquard, because they would have been unlikely to contain many androgen molecules. The improvements in stamina that he noted were probably the result of a "placebo effect" produced by his belief in the treatment. Although his final studies on himself overshadowed a career of bona fide accomplishments in endocrine research, the furor created by Brown-Séquard's demonstration initiated medical interest in the sex steroid hormones, for which he must be given credit.

As noted in Chapter 3, a masculine or feminine behavior pattern is not determined simply by the presence or absence of a particular behavior, but is often a matter of the frequency of, or the threshold for, a certain behavior. Quantitative measures of male sexual behavior are therefore an important means of describing it. One of the earliest attempts at quantification of mammalian sexual behavior was made by Calvin P. Stone, a psychologist, who determined the age at which male rats first exhibited copulatory ability (Stone, 1922). He tested males for mating behavior every day from 21 to 60 days of age, and discovered that the aver-

**PROFESSOR**

# BROWN SEQUARD'S
METHOD.

## EXTRACTS OF ANIMAL ORGANS.
Testicle Extract,
Grey Matter Extract,
Tyroid Gland Extract, &c., &c.

*Concentrated Solutions at 30%.*

These preparations, completely aseptic, are mailed to any distance on receipt of a money order.  Directions sent with the fluids.

Price for 25 Injections, $2.50.
Syringe Specially Gauged, (3 cubic c.,) $2.50.

*Used in the Hospitals of Paris, New York, Boston, etc.*
Circular Sent on Application.

## New York Biological and Vaccinal Institute,
Laboratory of Bovine Vaccine and of Biological Products.
*GEO. G. RAMBAUD, Chemist and Bacteriologist, Superintendent.*
PASTEUR INSTITUTE BUILDING, NEW YORK CITY.

**5.3  A 19th-century advertisement for extracts based on Brown-Séquard's fallacious claims.** Hoping to capitalize on Brown-Séquard's findings, charlatans sold "rejuvenating" preparations.

age age at which first copulation was observed was about 50 days (Stone, 1924). Stone also determined that developing male rats maintained copulatory ability for about 14 days after castration (Stone, 1927), and reported that substantial variability exists in the maintenance of intermale aggressiveness and mating behavior after castration.

In addition to measuring sexual performance, psychologists developed ways of measuring the strength of the sex drive (for example, Tsai, 1925; Warner, 1927). Given a choice, they asked, will a rat prefer to satiate its hunger, thirst, or sexual drive? What levels of deprivation are necessary for one biological need to override another? And how much pain will an individual bear to reduce its sex drive? The sex drives of individuals of many species were quantified by a battery of motivational tests (for example, Nissen, 1929; Stone et al., 1935; and see below). Remember that "motivation" is a psychological hypothetical construct; like "learning" or "attention," motivation cannot be measured directly. Only performance on a test designed to indirectly assess such a hypothetical construct can be measured.

Early in the 20th century, the ablation–replacement technique (see Chapter 1) was used to determine the behavioral effects of sex steroid hormones. For instance, a series of studies suggested that ovarian grafts in castrated young male rats or guinea pigs modified their subsequent behavior and physiology so that they "became" females (Steinach, 1910, 1913). In guinea pigs, growth of the mammary glands and milk secretion were reported, but these findings were never replicated completely. On the other hand, grafts of testicular tissue in young females influenced their development so that they became masculinized as they matured. These latter findings have been replicated many times in several species. A secretion from the interstitial cells of the transplanted gonad was proposed as the controlling factor in these transsexual changes, because the secondary sex characters of the opposite sex were not manifested unless the implanted gonad developed vascular connections (Steinach, 1940). We now know that the organizing properties of the steroid hormones from the testes cause the appearance of male-like characters in early-treated females (see Chapter 3).

An obvious refinement in experiments addressing endocrine effects on male sexual behavior was the discovery of the active agents in the testes that were responsible for observed behavioral effects. After the estrus-inducing hormone from the ovarian follicle was discovered to be lipid-soluble, the search for the *andros*-generating hormone began. Injections of an extract of bull testes dissolved in oil were found to produce a rapid regeneration of capons' combs (McGee et al., 1928). Pure crystalline hormone from testicular tissue was soon isolated and named *testosterone* (David et al., 1935). A year later, preparation of synthetic testosterone from cholesterol became feasible, and large amounts of the hormone rapidly became available for clinical and experimental studies. Several investigators demonstrated the restoration of sexual behavior in castrated male rats after injections of testosterone propionate, a stable, injectable form of testosterone (Moore and Price, 1938; Shapiro, 1937; Stone, 1938a,b, 1939). For example, a dose–response experiment revealed that 50–75 µg of testosterone propionate per day was necessary to maintain adult male mating behavior after castration (Figure 5.4; Beach and Holz-Tucker, 1949).

Many early researchers who attempted to link hormones and behavior came to approach their work, both theoretically and methodologically, with a "one hor-

**5.4   Testosterone treatment maintains sexual behavior after castration.**  Mating behavior declines after castration in male rats, but can be maintained by testosterone treatment. The maintenance of sexual behavior by testosterone is dose-dependent: in this study, only rats receiving testosterone doses of 100 μg/day or greater displayed sexual behavior at pre-castration levels. Source: Beach and Holz-Tucker, 1949.

mone equals one behavior" philosophy (reviewed in Beach, 1948). Differences in behavior were thought to represent differences in the underlying hormone that controlled the behavior in question. However, we now know that hormonal effects on behavior rarely reflect this type of unitary relationship. For example, male copulatory behavior can be restored in castrated males by injections of *either* estrogens or androgens (Ball, 1937; Beach, 1942c). Massive doses of testosterone propionate also can cause *either* feminine or masculine mating behaviors in castrated males. These results indicate that the action of any particular sex steroid hormone cannot be behavior-specific; every individual probably possesses the behavioral repertoire of both sexes, but one set of responses appears to have a lower threshold for expression in the presence of a particular hormone(s) (Beach, 1948). It has been shown that aromatization of androgens into estrogens occurs in the nervous system, which accounts for many of these puzzling results in nonprimates. Nonetheless, the empirical observations that both estrogens and androgens can support mating behavior in castrated males led eventually to an appreciation and understanding of the neural bases of reproductive behaviors and to the formulation of modern theories of hormone–behavior interactions. Current views about the hormonal regulation of behavior focus on the substrate or target tissues of the hormones, and research is now aimed at elucidating how differences in behavior reflect differences in target tissue sensitivity.

## Male Sexual Behavior in Rodents

As with other areas of behavioral endocrinology research, most work on the effects of hormones on male reproductive behavior has been performed on laboratory rats (*Rattus norvegicus*), and many current theoretical considerations have arisen from these studies. Consequently, many of the concepts we discuss will be illustrated with examples from studies of rat mating behavior. In order to understand what these studies have revealed about the hormonal and neural bases underlying male reproductive behavior, a thorough description of rat mating behavior is necessary.

## Male Mating Behavior: A Description

In rats and many other rodent species, there are three easily distinguishable behavioral components of the consummatory phase of male mating behavior: (1) mounting, (2) intromission, and (3) ejaculation. In most standard mating tests, one male and one female are introduced into a glass enclosure (usually an empty aquarium). Prior to mounting, several precopulatory male behaviors are observed; these behaviors are relatively easy to quantify and provide a useful measure of male sexual motivation. **Mount latency**, for instance, is the period of time from the introduction of the male and female until the first mount. Sexual motivation is considered high if mount latencies are low, and vice versa. The mount latency can be altered by placing some sort of obstacle between the male and the female and observing how long it takes the male to overcome the obstacle. This common test of sexual motivation is called an "obstruction" test; the so-called Columbia University obstruction test, using a physical barrier or an electrified floor, was often used in research of this sort (for example, Stone et al., 1935; Warner, 1927) (Figure 5.5). In other tests, the male must run on a treadmill that is moving away from the female, climb a ladder, or press a bar. Presumably, high motivation for sex can be inferred if the male passes the obstruction at a high speed or endures great pain. Males unmotivated for sex will not work or suffer to obtain access to a female.

Soon after introduction of the pair, the male begins to investigate the female, sniffing her mouth and anogenital region (Stone, 1922). Moments later, he attempts to mount her. If she is in estrus, or mating condition, the female exhibits the lordosis posture, which facilitates an intromission (Figure 5.6a). **Mounting** is operationally defined as the male assuming a copulatory position, but failing to insert his penis into the female's vagina. In some cases, males may mount the side or head of the female, and occasionally males may mount other males. In other cases, males may not mount at all. During time-limited tests, 1 hour, for example,

**5.5    The Columbia University obstruction device** was used to measure sexual motivation. In this version, a rat is placed in the entrance compartment (A), and the time it takes to cross the electrified floor (B) to gain access to another animal in the holding compartment (D) is operationally defined as a measure of sexual motivation. When males require little time to cross the grid, they are considered highly motivated. The door to the holding compartment (C) opens when the rat reaches the release plate (E) on the floor. After Warden et al., 1935.

(a)

(b)

**5.6   Sexual behavior in rats.** A male rat first investigates the anogenital region of a female, and if she
is in estrus, he will mount her with his forepaws
clasped against her hindquarters. This tactile stimulation causes her to display the lordosis posture,
arching her back and deflecting her tail (a). Lordosis
facilitates intromission, or insertion of the male rat's
penis into the vagina, accompanied by thrusting of
his hindquarters (b). After several seconds, the male
dismounts, grooms himself, and soon remounts. After several intromissions, the male ejaculates,
forcefully expelling semen into the female rat's
vagina (c). Courtesy of Ronald Barfield.

(c)

some males consistently fail to initiate sexual behavior by mounting. Males may
fail to mount a female because of low sex drive, decreased penile sensitivity, or
reduced erectile potential. One measure used to describe sexual behavior is the
**intermount interval (IMI),** or the average time between successive mounts.

   **Intromission** can be defined as the penis entering the vagina during a mount.
In rats and mice, intromission is associated with thrusting motions of the
hindquarters (Figure 5.6b), but in many species, thrusting is not observed. For
example, male guinea pigs and rabbits ejaculate during the first intromission and
complete copulation within a few seconds without thrusting. Counting the number of intromissions prior to each ejaculation provides a useful measure of reproductive behavior for males that exhibit multiple intromissions; however, the
utility of this measure is limited because interindividual differences are common.
Another common measure of male sexual behavior is the **inter-intromission
interval (III),** the average time between successive intromissions.

   **Ejaculation** is the forceful expulsion of semen from the male's body via the
urethra. Ejaculation is behaviorally defined in rats as the culmination of vigorous
intravaginal thrusting accompanied by the arching of the male's spine and often
the lifting of his forepaws off the female prior to withdrawal (Figure 5.6c). During
ejaculation, a sperm plug is often deposited in the vagina. In some rodent species,
this plug effectively blocks intromission by other males until the sperm have had
the opportunity to fertilize the estrous female. In laboratory tests, the number of
intromissions to ejaculation, as well as the ejaculatory latency, the time from the
first intromission to ejaculation, is also typically recorded. The mating potential
of any given male is determined by the number of ejaculations during a time-limited test or by the number of ejaculations prior to his attaining sexual satiety

(Sachs and Meisel, 1988). Most male laboratory rats can ejaculate 5–8 times during an unlimited-time mating test (Ågmo, 1997).

Male rats normally "sing" after an ejaculation; a special ultrasonic detector is required to hear these vocalizations, which are in the 20–22 kHz range. Observers can detect singing by noting the rapid shallow respirations that correspond with the ultrasonic vocalizations. After ejaculation, male rats usually become sexually inactive and rather lethargic. The male may groom his genitals, then lie down and sleep. He virtually ignores the female. This postejaculatory sequence of behaviors is not due to ejaculation per se, because artificial electro-ejaculation does not induce these behaviors.

The time between an ejaculation and the onset of the next copulatory series is called the **postejaculatory interval (PEI)**. The PEI is less than 30 seconds in golden hamsters (*Mesocricetus auratus*) (Bunnell et al., 1976), about 5–15 minutes in laboratory rats, and may last for hours or days in some other species (Dewsbury, 1972; Money, 1961). The PEI is generally considered to be composed of two separate periods, an absolute refractory phase and a relative refractory phase (Beach and Holz-Tucker, 1949). Males are completely nonresponsive to sexual, mildly painful, and other stimuli during the absolute refractory phase. A new or very potent sexual stimulus may elicit responsiveness in a male rat during the relative refractory phase (see below). A male rat with a PEI greater than 90 minutes is usually considered sexually "exhausted" or satiated (Ågmo, 1997).

**DIVERSITY OF MALE MATING PATTERNS.**   Male sexual behavior in mammals can be classified into several categories based on the presence of the following features (Dewsbury, 1972) (Figure 5.7; Table 5.1): (1) copulatory lock, (2) intravaginal

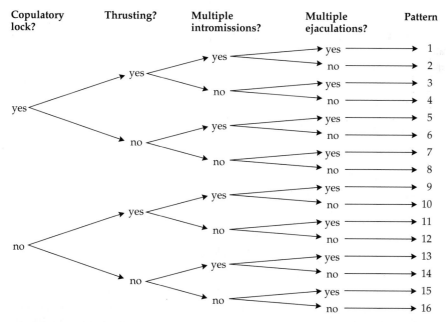

**5.7  Male copulatory patterns in mammals** can be classified by the presence or absence of four basic behaviors that occur during a mating bout: copulatory lock, thrusting, multiple intromissions, and multiple ejaculations. Species can be grouped according to the sixteen different mating patterns that emerge from this classification scheme. Source: Dewsbury, 1972.

## Table 5.1
## Examples of copulatory patterns in mammals

| Common name | Taxonomic name | Lock? | Thrust? | Multiple intromissions? | Multiple ejaculations? | Pattern[a] |
|---|---|---|---|---|---|---|
| Dog | *Canis familiaris* | Yes | Yes | No | Yes | 3 |
| Wolf | *Canis lupus* | Yes | Yes | No | Yes | 3 |
| Golden mouse | *Ochrotomys nuttalli* | Yes | No | No | Yes | 7 |
| House mouse | *Mus musculus* | No | Yes | Yes | Yes | 9 |
| Montane vole | *Microtus montanus* | No | Yes | Yes | Yes | 9 |
| Rhesus monkey | *Macaca mulatta* | No | Yes | No | Yes | 11 |
| Bonnet macaque | *Macaca rudiata* | No | Yes | No | Yes | 11 |
| Meadow vole | *Microtus pennsylvanicus* | No | Yes | No | Yes | 11 |
| Norway rat | *Rattus norvegicus* | No | No | Yes | Yes | 13 |
| Mongolian gerbil | *Meriones unguiculatus* | No | No | Yes | Yes | 13 |
| Bison | *Bison bison* | No | No | No | Yes | 15 |
| Black-tailed deer | *Odocoileus hemionus* | No | No | No | No | 16 |

[a]See Figure 5.7.
*Source:* Dewsbury, 1972.

thrusting, (3) multiple intromissions, and (4) multiple ejaculations. Animals that show genital lock, such as dogs, have a penis that swells after ejaculation, which facilitates sperm transport to the female; this process may take several minutes, during which time it is virtually impossible for the pair to disengage (Figure 5.8). Males of some species, such as guinea pigs, do not show pelvic thrusting and ejaculate with a single intromission. Male rats, on the other hand, engage in about 20 mounts and 10 to 15 intromissions prior to the first ejaculation, but these values vary among rat strains; additional intromissions are usually required for each subsequent ejaculation (Beach and Jordan, 1956).

The various patterns of male copulatory behavior have been related to the ecology of particular species, and several broad generalizations can be made (Dewsbury, 1972). For example, predator species are more likely to lock than prey species; prey species cannot risk being immobilized for long periods of time, and there are few prey species that require lengthy sperm transport periods (see Table 5.1). Animals that mate at night are more likely to engage in genital locking than diurnal creatures, presumably because of a similar lack of predation pressures. Virtually all rodent species that lock (for example, golden mice, *Ochrotomys nuttalli*, and southern grasshopper mice, *Onychomys torridus*) are nocturnal.

### Hormonal Correlates of Male Mating Behavior

As we have seen, testosterone is necessary for the maintenance of mating behavior in rats. Castration leads to a reduction in sexual responsiveness; both motivation and performance wane. For most rodent species, sexual behavior is markedly reduced immediately after castration. Sex drive also declines rapidly after the testes are removed. Castrated males will not investigate females, nor will they work or suffer pain to reach them. If castrated animals are examined during daily

**5.8  Sexual behavior in the dog.**  A male dog first investigates the anogenital region of a female (top). If she is in estrus (mating condition), she will allow the male to mount her (middle left). The hindquarters of the male thrust with increasing intensity until ejaculation occurs some seconds later. After ejaculation, the penis remains "locked" in the vagina, and the male steps over the female as he dismounts (middle right). They remain in this copulatory lock for several minutes to facilitate sperm transport (bottom). After Beach and LeBoeuf, 1967.

mating tests, the timing of the disappearance of components of sexual behavior follows a characteristic pattern. The effects of castration are observed within days. Males first begin to take longer to initiate mounting and intromissions (Meisel and Sachs, 1994). Another early effect of castration is that fewer intromissions occur prior to ejaculation. This may seem paradoxical: fewer intromissions before ejaculation may appear to reflect *increased* reproductive performance. However, a male that normally has eight intromissions prior to ejaculation is not necessarily a more efficient or effective copulator than one that typically has fifteen intromissions before ejaculation. Fewer intromissions may be less likely to provide the female with sufficient stimulation to induce a progestational state (see Chapter 6), resulting in a failure of blastocyst implantation (Wilson et al., 1965). By a week

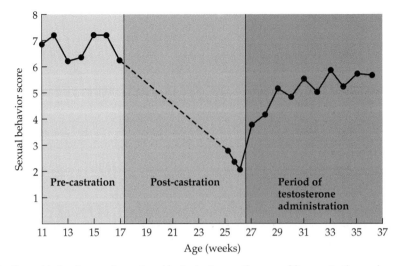

**5.9    Sexual behavior can be restored by testosterone therapy.** After castration, guinea pigs displayed marked declines in sexual behavior, but testosterone replacement therapy gradually restored sexual behavior to pre-castration concentrations. Source: Valenstein and Young, 1955.

or two post-castration, rats cannot mate to ejaculation. The inability to ejaculate is soon followed by a decline in the number of mounts with intromissions, and finally the male no longer mounts females.

The effects of castration on male rodent reproductive behavior can be reversed by testosterone treatment (Figure 5.9). The restoration of copulatory behaviors after sustained androgen therapy mirrors the disappearance of these behaviors: first mounting recurs, followed by intromissions, then ejaculations. Of course, neither intromissions nor ejaculations can occur in the absence of mounting, and ejaculations will not be observed in the absence of intromissions, yet it is theoretically possible that all the behaviors could be restored simultaneously. However, they generally reappear sequentially over the course of several days (Larsson, 1979). This rigid sequential ordering of behavior suggests, although it does not prove, that mounting, intromission, and ejaculation behaviors have different sensitivities to testicular hormones.

If androgen replacement therapy is initiated immediately after castration (maintenance treatment), then lower amounts of hormone are required to maintain reproductive behavior than are necessary to restore sexual behavior some time later, after it has stopped (restoration treatment) (Figure 5.10; Davidson, 1966b). Continuous exposure of brain and sensory neural tissue to androgens apparently preserves their responsiveness to these hormones. Similarly, male hamsters arousing from hibernation may require a large pulse of androgens to activate their reproductive systems (Berndtson and Desjardins, 1974).

Two androgens, testosterone and androstenedione, a weakly androgenic precursor of testosterone, can maintain mating behavior in castrated rodents (Sachs and Meisel, 1988). Dihydrotestosterone (DHT), another product of testosterone, does not prevent the post-castration decline in reproductive behavior, regardless of whether it is provided at the time of castration or post-castration (Feder, 1971).

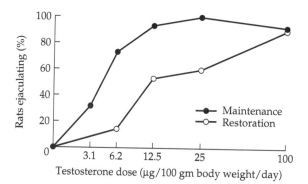

**5.10 Maintenance versus restoration of sexual behavior by testosterone therapy.** The amount of testosterone necessary to restore full sexual behavior is greater if the treatment begins after all sexual behavior stops (restoration regimen) than if it begins immediately after castration (maintenance regimen). Presumably, the restoration regimen requires higher doses because androgen receptors decrease in number if not maintained by circulating androgens. Source: Davidson, 1966a.

In contrast to DHT, estradiol, an estrogen, is very effective in activating mating behavior in castrated male rodents (Davidson, 1969; Södersten, 1973). As you know, both testosterone and androstenedione can be aromatized to estradiol and other estrogens, but DHT cannot be converted to an estrogen (see Chapter 2). Taken together, these findings suggest that testosterone and androstenedione produce their behavioral effects after being first converted to estrogens. Further support for this hypothesis arises from the observation that injecting castrated rats with specific estrogen receptor blocking agents renders subsequent androgen therapy ineffective in sustaining copulatory behavior (Beyer et al., 1976). DHT is not completely without effect; estradiol plus DHT treatment restores the mating behavior of castrated rats to the level of gonadally intact individuals (Feder et al., 1974). DHT appears to be important for maintaining penile tactile sensitivity (see below). In general, estradiol appears to affect the central nervous system to promote mating behavior, and DHT affects neurons in the periphery to maintain tactile sensory feedback. Thus, testosterone from the testes appears to function primarily as a prohormone providing estrogens to the CNS and DHT to the periphery to regulate sexual behavior.

Penile responses can be tested by placing a rat or mouse on its back and retracting the penile sheath to the base of the glans penis (Sachs, 1995a). The pressure of the sheath causes the erection reflex of the glans, which is due to the engorgement of the corpus spongiosum (Box 5.2) with venous blood. An erection of the corpus cavernosum is depicted in Figure 5.11. If the pressure on the penis continues, penile reflexes called "flips" are noted. Flips are due to the action of the corpus cavernosum and the striated penile muscles. Intense glans erections, called cups, are observed after prolonged penile stimulation. These three penile responses are similar in form to those observed both during normal sexual behavior (*in copula*) and during artificial stimulation (*ex copula*) (Meisel et al., 1984; Sachs, 1995b). Developmental studies of male rats show a remarkable coincidence between the average age of onset of erections and mounts (40.0 versus 40.8 days, respectively), flips and intromissions (44.0 versus 43.8 days, respectively), and cups and ejaculations (about 47.5 days in both cases) (Sachs and Meisel, 1979). This coincidence in development between penile reflexes and copulatory behaviors suggests a functional relationship, as well as separate underlying mechanisms and possibly different sensitivities to hormonal regulation for each of the three components of mating behavior.

## Box 5.2
# Anatomy of the Penis

There are two important structural components of the penis, the paired corpora cavernosa and the corpus spongiosum. Both components are critical erectile tissues comprising smooth muscle and blood vessels and are usually associated with a set of striated muscles. The corpora cavernosa and the corpus spongiosum usually function together during tumescence and detumescence, but they may become functionally dissociated.

In humans, the corpora cavernosa are twin "tunnels" of highly vascular tissue that occupy most of the penile body. A muscle called the ischiocavernosus is connected to the base (crura) of each corpus cavernosum. The glans and the central tissue of the penis make up the corpus spongiosum. Some species have a bone, called the os penis, located within the corpus spongiosum. In rats, the bone is present only in the glans; in other species, such as dogs, the os penis is found in the penile body. The base of the corpus spongiosum is connected to the bulbospongiosus striated muscle in primates, which is called the bulbocavernosus muscle in other species, including rodents.

There is great diversity in penile morphology across species. Some species possess such distinctive penes that they can be classified taxonomically by this organ. This species-specific penile morphology has evolved to maximize fertilization of conspecific females. Enormously diverse mechanisms of penile erection have also evolved among mammals, involving different combinations of smooth muscle, vascular tissue, and striated muscles. In rats, penile erections are mainly the result of neural signals that contract striated muscles, causing erection of the glans penis (see figure). In humans, penile erections are the result mainly of vascular changes that cause the corpora cavernosa to fill with blood, resulting in tumescence of the penile body (Tanagho et al., 1988).

Recently, the innervation of the penis and the details of how penile erection in humans is mediated have been established, but the details are incomplete (McConnell et al., 1982; Tanagho

If animals fail to mate after castration, ascertaining whether sexual performance, sex drive, or both functions have been affected by the surgery is difficult. One way to differentiate between the effects of hormones on sex drive and on mating performance is to isolate the brain—presumably the source of sex drive—from the spinal cord. We know that the entire erectile repertoire is programmed in the spinal cord, because appropriate stimulation causes a rat with a spinal cord severed from the brain to show erections, as well as the penile reflexes underlying intromission, thrusting, and ejaculation (Meisel and Sachs, 1994). The term "sex drive" implies that the brain is "driving" behavior through *excitatory* messages to the periphery via the spinal cord. Although the brain does send some excitatory signals (see Box 5.2), it acts primarily to *inhibit* the spinal mechanisms of erection (Beach, 1967; Sachs and Bitran, 1990). In spinally transected rodents, the stimuli required to induce an erection are much less than the stimuli necessary for inducing erections in intact males. As we shall see, clinical data suggest an inhibitory influence of the human brain on erectile function as well.

et al., 1988). It has been known for over a century that it is possible to induce penile erections with electrical stimulation of certain pelvic nerves in rats and dogs (Eckhardt, 1863). Direct electrical stimulation of the rat cavernosus nerve results in tumescence of the penile shaft—because of corpus cavernosum blood engorgement—but not tumescence of the glans (Burgers et al., 1991; Quinlan et al., 1989). The latter may be the result of a somatic response produced by the erect corpora cavernosa; contraction of the bulbocavernosus muscle may compress the erect shaft against the os penis in the glans, resulting in straightening of the glans.

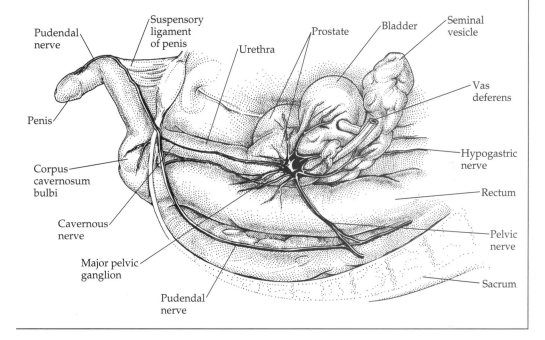

If spinally transected rats are also castrated, their penile reflexes begin to wane after 24 hours, and disappear after 12 days (Hart et al., 1983). The loss of penile responses after castration follows an ordered pattern similar to the degradation of post-castration mating behavior: cups, then flips, and finally erections disappear (Davidson et al., 1978). (As discussed previously, however, the order of decline and restoration of copulatory behaviors is somewhat constrained by the nature of the chaining of these processes.) These results suggest that androgens are necessary, but not sufficient, for erections. Appropriate penile stimulation is necessary for penile erection, and androgens reduce the amount of stimuli required for a penile response to be observed.

Normal penile reflexes are maintained or restored by testosterone. In one study, castrated rats were implanted with Silastic capsules of testosterone that varied in length (from 2 to 18 mm). The hormone seeps out of the capsules at a constant rate; therefore, longer capsules result in more hormone being released into the body tissue fluid per unit of time. Animals bearing capsules longer than

**Stimulation on**

5 seconds          7 seconds          12 seconds          15 seconds

**Stimulation off**

22 seconds          25 seconds          27 seconds

**5.11   Erection in rats** can be induced by bilateral electrical stimulation of the cavernosus nerve, as seen in these sequential video images of a 22-second stimulation period. Tumescence begins between 5 and 7 seconds after the initiation of stimulation; detumescence is brisk and occurs within 5 seconds of cessation of the electrical current. Courtesy of David Quinlan.

6 mm exhibited penile reflexes comparable to those of noncastrated males. A 6 mm capsule produced average blood plasma testosterone concentrations of 0.79 ng/ml, well below the average blood testosterone concentrations of gonadally intact males (1.95 ng/ml) (Table 5.2; Davidson et al., 1978). Thus, blood plasma testosterone concentrations are typically well above the minimum necessary to maintain copulatory behaviors or penile reflexes, so a slight decrease, even 30%, from normal blood androgen concentrations should not be expected to influence mating behavior. Even an average reduction of blood testosterone concentrations of 50% would probably not affect behavior.

Testosterone per se also does not seem to directly regulate penile responses. Rather, testosterone serves as a precursor to DHT, which directly regulates penile responses. DHT has been found to maintain or restore penile reflexes to pre-castration levels in both spinally transected and spinally intact rats; estradiol, another testosterone metabolite, does not seem to affect penile reflexes (Gray et al., 1980; Hart, 1979; Meisel et al., 1984). Castrated rats implanted with Silastic capsules of estradiol maintained mating *behavior* at a level comparable to gonadally intact animals; however, the rate at which penile reflexes decreased in estrogen-treated males was similar to that in untreated castrated individuals (Meisel et al., 1984). Thus, it appears that testosterone, after being aromatized to estradiol in neural tissue, mediates copulatory behavior, whereas testosterone, after conversion to

Table 5.2

**Frequency of sexual reflexes, latency to first reflex, and plasma testosterone concentrations in intact, castrated, and testosterone-treated male rats**

| Treatment | Sexual reflex | | | Latency (min) | Plasma testosterone (ng/ml) |
|---|---|---|---|---|---|
| | Erection | Flip | Cup | | |
| Intact | 22.2 | 4.2 | 1.3 | 5.5 | 1.95 |
| Castrated | 12.3 | 0.5 | 0.04 | 9.9 | <0.2 |
| Testosterone implant | | | | | |
| 2 mm | 18.4 | 2.4 | 0.04 | 6.5 | 0.40 |
| 6 mm | 22.5 | 6.0 | 0.6 | 5.4 | 0.79 |
| 18 mm | 20.8 | 3.5 | 1.0 | 6.5 | 1.09 |

*Source:* Davidson et al., 1978.

DHT, mediates penile reflexes and sensitivity to tactile feedback (Meisel and Sachs, 1994). Again, testosterone appears to act as a prohormone from which steroids affecting central nervous system processing and peripheral sensory receptor sensitivities are produced to ensure successful copulation.

### Brain Mechanisms of Male Mating Behavior

Behavior is mediated by the central nervous system. The results of the experiments discussed above suggest that hormones produce their effects on male reproductive behavior by acting on the central nervous system tissues controlling reproductive behaviors. But what are the neural systems underlying reproductive behavior? In order to answer this question, a number of neural manipulations have been employed. Historically, brain lesioning techniques have been used to find out where in the brain sexual behavior is regulated. The logic behind lesioning techniques is that removal of a critical component of the neural mechanism underlying sexual behavior should result in disruptions of sexual behavior. Initially, rather large lesions were performed to study sexual behavior. Perhaps not surprisingly, removing the entire neocortex of rats diminished their sexual behavior; removal of the frontal cortex also effectively disrupted rat copulation (Larsson, 1962; Lashley, 1938). More recently, researchers have tried to limit the scope of brain lesions to locate more precisely the brain areas that regulate sexual behavior.

THE PREOPTIC AREA.   The region of the brain anterior to the hypothalamus, especially the preoptic area (POA) (Figure 5.12), appears to be critical for integrating environmental, physiological, and psychological information prior to and during successful copulation (Crews and Silver, 1985; Sachs and Meisel, 1988). The POA contains several nuclei from which axons project to other brain regions. The region of the POA along both sides of the midline of the brain is called the medial preoptic area (MPOA), and some studies have focused on this specific area of the POA. In virtually all species studied to date, lesions of the POA in adult males eliminate sexual performance, although sexual motivation appears unaffected: male rats with POA lesions fail to mount females even when tested 8 months after surgery, although they will press bars or run mazes to gain access

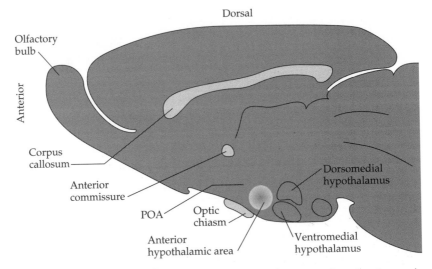

**5.12** **Regions that are essential to the control of sexual performance in male rats** seen in a schematic sagittal section of the brain. The preoptic area (POA) appears to be especially important for the integration of environmental, physiological, and psychological information prior to and during successful copulation; POA lesions reduce or eliminate male sexual behavior in virtually every vertebrate species examined. The POA apparently regulates endocrine function by interacting with hypothalamic nuclei and mediates parasympathetic functions associated with male copulation. After Pfaff, 1980.

to females (Ginton and Merari, 1977; Heimer and Larsson, 1966). Neither testosterone treatment nor access to multiple females compensates for POA lesions.

What does a POA lesion accomplish? It destroys cell bodies that send out axons to many other parts of the brain. Many of these neurons use dopamine as their neurotransmitter, so postsynaptic dopaminergic neurons that receive messages from these POA neurons are deprived of input (Hull et al., 1997). Treating POA-lesioned male rats with lisuride, a chemical that mimics dopamine, transiently activates copulation in these animals, with many of them copulating to ejaculation (Hansen et al., 1982). Presumably, the dopaminergic neurons destroyed by a POA lesion are part of a neural circuit that integrates and regulates copulatory behavior. In the absence of dopamine–receptor interactions "downstream" from the POA, copulatory behavior is not observed. By replacing the dopamine with an agonist that can interact with and excite neurons "downstream" from the POA, copulatory behavior is restored. If this hypothesis is true, then drugs that increase dopamine synthesis or stimulate postsynaptic dopamine receptor sites should also facilitate copulatory behavior among intact male rats, and this has been observed to be true (Ahlenius and Larsson, 1984; Napoloi-Farris et al., 1984; Paglietti et al., 1978; Sachs, 1995b). Similarly, one might predict that drugs that suppress dopaminergic activities would reduce male rat sexual behaviors, and this has also been observed to occur (for example, Ahlenius and Larsson, 1984; Napoli-Farris et al., 1984). The claim that dopaminergic axons are mainly responsible for mediating male copulatory behavior in rats is strengthened by the observation that no other pharmacological treatment, including GnRH or naloxone, reinstates copulatory behavior in POA-lesioned rats. Taken together, these results indicate that dopaminergic neurons destroyed by POA lesions are necessary for normal copulatory behaviors in male rats (Mas, 1995) (see below).

Social history can dramatically affect the outcome of POA lesions in young rats. Juvenile male rats with POA lesions reared in social isolation never copulate as adults (Twiggs et al., 1978), but, in sharp contrast to the profound copulatory deficits observed in adult rats after POA lesions, similar lesions in juvenile rats have virtually *no* effect on adult copulatory behavior if the lesioned rats are reared in heterosexual groups (Twiggs et al., 1978). Exactly what component of group living ameliorates the effects of POA lesions remains unspecified. A reasonable hypothesis is that social interactions somehow elevate dopamine levels. This result is intriguing because it shows the importance of social conditions in mediating rodent brain plasticity and reproductive function after a substantial neural insult, and because social conditions also play a major role in the development of normal sexual behavior among primates (Money, 1988).

Remote cues from females result in so-called non-contact erections in rats (Sachs et al., 1994). These non-contact erections are analogous to psychogenic erections in humans that occur in response to visual, auditory, chemosensory, or imaginative stimuli (Meisel and Sachs, 1994). Thus, studies of non-contact erections should help us to trace the neural circuits involved in sexual arousal or motivation prior to copulation. Lesions of the medial amygdala (see below) inhibit non-contact erections; however, lesions of the bed nucleus of the stria terminalis (BNST) or paraventricular nucleus of the hypothalamus (PVH) cause only mild impairments, and lesions of the medial preoptic area have no obvious effect (Liu et al., 1997b).

**THE CHEMOSENSORY SYSTEM.**    Olfaction is critical for successful expression of male reproductive behavior among many rodent species. Chemosensory cues are also critical in mediating many other social interactions. Experimental blocking of the sense of smell usually results in social and reproductive behavioral deficits.

The **olfactory bulbs** are located at the front of the brain (see Figure 5.12) and are actually made up of two anatomically distinct regions, the main olfactory bulbs and the accessory olfactory bulbs (Figure 5.13). The olfactory neurons are bipolar cells located in the olfactory neuroepithelia at the rear of the nasal cavity. Their axons form the first cranial nerve and terminate in the main olfactory bulbs (Scalia and Winans, 1976). In many mammalian species, a portion of the olfactory neuroepithelium is discretely organized into a **vomeronasal organ** (also called Jacobson's organ), an encapsulated structure on each side of the nasal septum located near the floor of the nasal cavity (see Figure 5.13; Moulton, 1967). Rodents have highly developed vomeronasal organs, but this structure is regressed or absent in some primate species (for example, great apes and humans) and aquatic mammals. The neurons of the vomeronasal organ connect to the accessory olfactory bulb via the vomeronasal nerves (Alberts, 1974; Moulton, 1967; Wysocki, 1979).

Historically, several methods have been used to impair the chemosensory system in order to ascertain its behavioral and physiological role (reviewed in Alberts, 1974; Murphy, 1976). The most common such technique is olfactory bulbectomy (surgical removal of the olfactory bulbs), but this method has some drawbacks. Removal of the olfactory bulbs destroys approximately 4% of the entire central nervous system in rodents (Cain, 1974). Consequently, substantial neural damage

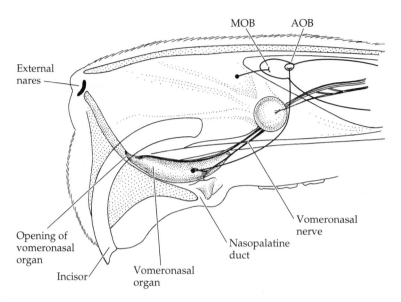

MOB   AOB

External
nares

Opening of
vomeronasal
organ

Incisor

Vomeronasal
organ

Nasopalatine
duct

Vomeronasal
nerve

**5.13   The vomeronasal organ (VNO)** and other major components of the rodent chemosensory system, seen in a lateral view of the guinea pig snout. This structure may be absent in most primate species, but is essential to normal rodent reproductive behavior. When male rodents engage in anogenital investigation of females prior to mounting, vaginal chemosignals are maneuvered to the roof of the mouth, then "pumped" through the nasopalatine duct into the opening of the VNO. Other signals may enter via the external nares (nostrils) and may be pulled down to the VNO from the floor of the nares. Neural information moves from the VNO to the accessory olfactory bulbs via the vomeronasal nerve bundle; thus, information originally obtained from activation of VNO receptors is processed by the accessory olfactory bulbs. Information from the olfactory receptors is processed separately in the main olfactory bulbs. MOB = main olfactory bulb; AOB = accessory olfactory bulb. After Wysocki, 1979.

can occur, and separation of the effects of such damage from the effects of sensory loss after bulbectomy is not always possible. Also, the olfactory bulbs integrate nonsensory functions as well as sensory functions (Alberts, 1974), and the proportion of damage to sensory versus nonsensory functions caused by olfactory bulbectomy may vary among species. Finally, the procedure is irreversible.

Several acute, somewhat reversible, methods of impairing olfaction have been used to reduce the neural damage associated with olfactory bulbectomy. One frequently used technique is intranasal infusion of zinc sulfate ($ZnSO_4$) (Alberts, 1974; Alberts and Galef, 1971), which temporarily destroys the olfactory neuroepithelia, rendering the animal anosmic (unable to smell). The chemosensory receptors in the nasal cavity regenerate after several weeks. Two problems with using $ZnSO_4$ are uncertainty about its side effects and about the extent of the olfactory impairment (Murphy, 1976). Anesthesia of the nasal epithelia is another method used to produce acute olfactory impairment (for example, Doty and Anisko, 1973).

The results of olfactory bulbectomy have varied among studies and among species. Surgical ablation of the olfactory bulbs of sexually naive rats had no discernible effect on subsequent mating behavior in one early study (Stone, 1922). In contrast, a later study revealed that many bulbectomized rats were sexually impaired; some stopped mating completely after the surgery (Beach, 1942a). Sexually naive rats exhibited profound behavioral deficits after bulbectomy in other studies (Beach, 1942a; Bermant and Taylor, 1969). Further analyses of the impairments in mating behavior following olfactory bulbectomy revealed that male rats failed to achieve ejaculation after a series of intromissions or simply did not initiate copulation at all, suggesting that both sexual performance and motivation were impaired by olfactory bulbectomy (Larsson, 1969). Olfactory bulbectomy completely eliminated sexual behavior in male house mice (*Mus musculus*) (Rowe and Smith, 1972; Whitten, 1956a), but removal of the olfactory bulbs had variable effects on the copulatory behaviors of male guinea pigs (*Cavia porcellus*) (Beauchamp et al., 1977). Local anesthesia of the nasal mucosa (Doty and Anisko, 1973) and olfactory bulbectomy both virtually eliminated sexual behavior in male golden hamsters (*Mesocricetus auratus*) (Murphy and Schneider, 1970; Winans and Powers, 1974).

Copulation can be activated in olfactory-bulbectomized rats by techniques that increase the general level of arousal in the animals. Thus, a mildly painful tail pinch or an electric shock to the flank will stimulate bulbectomized rats to copulate to ejaculation. Such arousal "therapy" is only temporarily restorative; additional arousing stimuli must be administered prior to subsequent mating sessions conducted a few days later (Meisel et al., 1980). These findings suggest that olfactory bulb tissue or neurons that are connected to the bulbs are part of a neural circuit involved in male sexual motivation among rodents.

Inputs from both the main olfactory neurons and the vomeronasal organ are apparently necessary for rodent mating behavior (Guillamón and Segovia, 1997). Olfactory bulbectomy tends to destroy both the main olfactory bulbs and the accessory bulbs, so differentiation of the contributions of the olfactory and vomeronasal inputs requires manipulations of the respective sensory receptors. While treatment with $ZnSO_4$ alone had no effect, destruction of the vomeronasal nerve alone stopped mating behavior in about one-third of the male hamsters tested (Powers and Winans, 1975). Thus, the vomeronasal organ has an important, but not critical, role in normal reproductive behavioral function in these animals. In contrast, ablation of the vomeronasal organ of male house mice and pine voles (*Microtus pinetorum*) eliminated the surges of LH associated with the presence of females and stopped mating behavior (see below) (Lepri et al., 1985; Lepri and Wysocki, 1987; Wysocki et al., 1983). Because the deficits of vole and mouse mating behavior are similar following either olfactory bulbectomy or vomeronasal organ ablation, the vomeronasal organ/accessory olfactory bulb system appears equally or more important in mediating mating behavior than the olfactory neuroepithelia/main olfactory bulb system.

**THE ROLE OF THE AMYGDALA.**    Projections from the accessory and main olfactory bulbs travel to the **amygdala** (from the Greek for "almond"), an almond-shaped structure located in each temporal lobe of the brain that is critical for the integration of sensory information important in sexual behavior. Two regions of the amygdala have been studied in rodents: the basal and lateral collections of nerve cell bodies (the basolateral nuclei) and the cortical and medial nuclei (corticomedial nuclei) (Figure 5.14). Removal of the basolateral nuclei of the amygdala generally does not affect the reproductive behavior of male rodents, but does reduce sexual motivation (Everitt, 1990). Lesions of the corticomedial nuclei, on the other hand, increase the ejaculation latencies of rats (Giantonio et al., 1970),

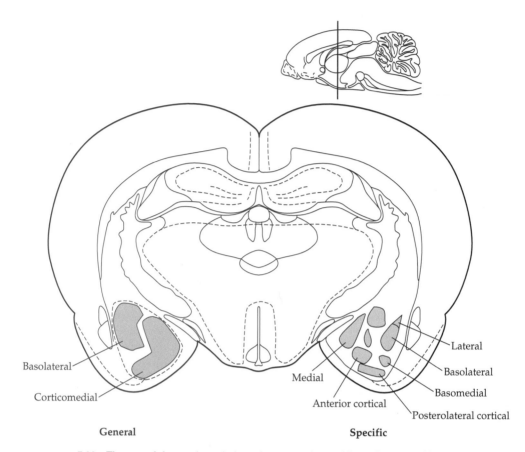

**5.14   The amygdala,** an almond-shaped structure located in each temporal lobe, seen in a schematic drawing of a coronal section of the rat brain. Two general amygdaloid regions, the basolateral and corticomedial nuclei (left), have been studied extensively because they receive neural input from the main olfactory bulbs. Destruction of the corticomedial nuclei, but not the basolateral nuclei, severely affects male copulatory behavior in rodents. The specific nuclei of the basolateral and corticomedial amygdala that receive olfactory input are depicted (right).

and completely abolish copulation in male hamsters (Lehman and Winans, 1982). Information from the amygdala is relayed to the MPOA via the stria terminalis and the ventral amygdalofugal pathway. Predictably, lesions of these relay structures produce reproductive deficits similar in nature to corticomedial amygdala lesions (Figure 5.15; Giantonio et al., 1970).

Exposure to the chemosignals in the vaginal secretions of female hamsters produces sex-specific behaviors in the recipient animal: females mark over the scent, whereas males initiate copulatory behavior aimed at the source of the scent (Swann and Fiber, 1997). Although these behaviors are markedly different, the responses of both sexes to the chemosignals of female hamsters involve the main olfactory system. In females, the neural circuitry involved includes the medial nucleus of the amygdala and the posterior medial subdivision of the bed nucleus of the stria terminalis. In addition to these two neural components, the magnocellular subdivision of the medial preoptic area is activated in males exposed

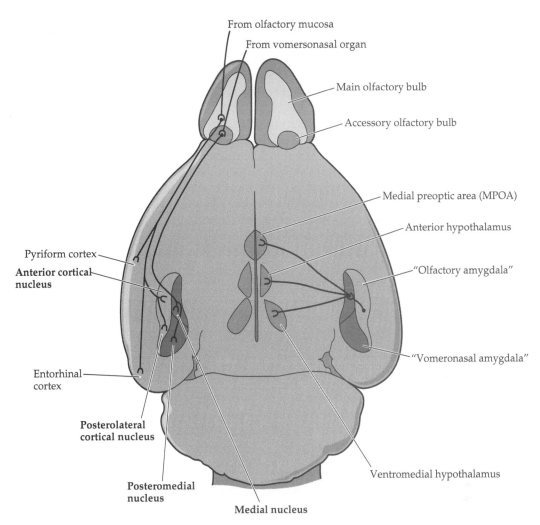

From olfactory mucosa

From vomersonasal organ

Main olfactory bulb

Accessory olfactory bulb

Medial preoptic area (MPOA)

Anterior hypothalamus

Pyriform cortex

Anterior cortical nucleus

"Olfactory amygdala"

Entorhinal cortex

"Vomeronasal amygdala"

Posterolateral cortical nucleus

Ventromedial hypothalamus

Posteromedial nucleus

Medial nucleus

**5.15    Neural pathways in the rat olfactory system** shown in a schematic horizontal section. (Left) Axons from the olfactory mucosa synapse in the main olfactory bulb, where sensory information is sent to pyriform and entorhinal cortex and the anterior and posterolateral nuclei of the amygdala; axons from the vomeronasal organ (VNO) synapse in the accessory olfactory bulb, which sends axons to the medial and posteromedial nuclei. (Right) Because of these projections, the cortical portion of the amygdala can be considered the "olfactory amygdala," and the medial portion the "vomeronasal amygdala." The olfactory amygdala innvervates the vomeronasal portion, where signals are sent to central structures including the medial preoptic area (MPOA), the anterior hypothalamus, and the ventromedial hypothalamus. Courtesy of Ruth Wood.

to female vaginal secretions (Swann and Fiber, 1997). The bed nucleus of the stria terminalis of males can be activated by vaginal secretions only if plasma testosterone concentrations are sufficient (i.e., only in gonadally intact males) (Swann and Fiber, 1997).

**ELECTRICAL STIMULATION AND RECORDING STUDIES.**    In addition to lesion studies, researchers have employed electrical stimulation and recording studies to locate the neural circuitry underlying male reproductive behavior. Generally, electrical stimulation of a brain site produces a behavioral response that is opposite from the effect of destroying the area. Recording of the electrical activity in the brain in response to specific stimuli can also reveal what parts of the brain are involved in a behavioral response.

Recall that POA lesions, especially MPOA lesions, disrupt copulatory behaviors. Electrical stimulation of the MPOA accelerates ejaculation in male rats (Malsbury, 1971; Van Dis and Larsson, 1971). The MPOA appears to be crucial for integrating important external and internal information. Prior to making a successful mating response, a male rat must orchestrate and organize a multitude of stimuli. The environmental context, including the time of day, and stimuli associated with the estrous female, as well as the endocrine state of the male and his memories of previous sexual encounters, if any, must be processed and integrated in the MPOA. Lesions of the MPOA not only disrupt sexual behavior, but also interrupt several other motivated behaviors, including maternal behavior (see Chapter 7), locomotory behavior (King, 1979), drinking (Mogenson et al., 1980; Rolls and Rolls, 1982), and thermoregulatory behaviors (Satinoff and Prosser, 1988; Szymusiak and Satinoff, 1982).

Male rats must integrate auditory, olfactory, and tactile sensory cues in order to mate successfully. The MPOA appears to be critical for processing this sensory information (Hull et al., 1997; Melis and Argiolas, 1995). Early studies found that adult male rats with no previous sexual experience required at least two of these three sensory inputs, and it was thought that it did not matter which two sensory channels were available. Rats with previous sexual experience were thought to require only one source of sensory information to engage in successful copulation (Beach, 1942b; Stone, 1923). Current views suggest that olfaction and somatosensation (tactile cues) are critical for the expression of appropriate copulatory behaviors, although the specific somatosensory requirements for male copulatory behaviors remain unknown (Stern, 1990).

As the male's brain processes incoming olfactory sensory information, a sufficiently powerful stimulus evokes a neural response from the MPOA, which results in the appropriate motor output, as well as a burst of GnRH release from the hypothalamus, which begins an endocrine cascade resulting in elevated testosterone secretion (Purvis and Haynes, 1974). Chemosensory stimuli from an estrous female induce electrical activity in the MPOA as well as in the olfactory bulbs of a male rat. Castration of the male does not affect the electrical activity in the olfactory bulbs; in other words, the chemosensory cues associated with the female continue to be processed at this early level of sensory input into the brain. However, the electrical activity of the MPOA, several synapses downstream from the olfactory bulbs, is no longer evoked by estrous female odors. The neurally coded sensory signal from the bulbs no longer influences the output of the MPOA of castrated males (Pfaff and Pfaffmann, 1969). Testosterone replacement therapy appears to amplify the chemosensory signal so that the MPOA again responds with neural activity (Figure 5.16).

**IMPLANT STUDIES.** As we unravel the basic neural circuitry underlying sexual behavior, we should presumably discover where exactly hormones interact with the central nervous system to mediate mating behavior. Brain implant studies have provided some clarification of these questions. Implants of crystalline testos-

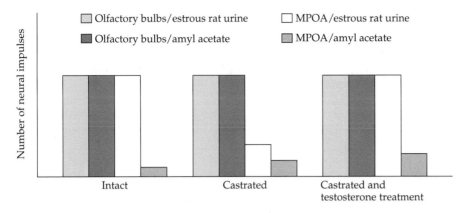

**5.16 Castration reduces neural responsiveness in the MPOA.** Electrical recording in the olfactory bulbs and MPOA of intact male rats reveals that the odor of estrous females causes increased neural activity in both regions. After castration, estrous odors continue to increase neural activity in the olfactory bulbs, but not in the MPOA. Testosterone replacement therapy restores MPOA responsiveness to estrous odors to the levels seen in intact rats. Source: Pfaff and Pfaffmann, 1969.

terone into the MPOA of castrated male rats facilitated copulation in 100% of the animals; conversely, no castrated rats with crystalline cholesterol (a hormonally inert precursor of testosterone) implants in the MPOA mated (Davidson, 1966a). Implantation of testosterone into the MPOA of castrated male rats and simultaneous treatment with an androgen aromatization inhibitor resulted in mating frequencies much lower than those observed in castrated males with MPOA implants of estrogen (Christensen and Clemens, 1975). These results again suggest that testosterone exerts its effects on mating behaviors via aromatization to estrogen. Recall that systemic injections of low doses of DHT did not affect the reproductive behavior of castrated male rats. However, DHT injections paired with implants of estradiol into the MPOA elicited full copulatory behavior in castrated males (Davis and Barfield, 1979), providing additional evidence that estradiol mediates central mechanisms of mating behavior, whereas DHT is important in maintaining peripheral sensitivity in castrated males (Davis and Barfield, 1979). Nevertheless, androgens must be able to interact with central androgen receptors to initiate male sexual behavior. Male sexual behavior was inhibited in males that received intracranial implants of hydroxyflutamide, an androgen receptor blocker, into the preoptic area or hypothalamus, but not the amygdala or the septal region, which are parts of the limbic system involved in motivation (McGinnis et al., 1996).

**AUTORADIOGRAPHIC AND IMMUNOCYTOCHEMICAL STUDIES.** To gain additional information about where sex steroid hormones might exert their influence upon behavior, autoradiographic studies have been performed to map the distribution of sex steroid receptors in the central nervous system. After an injection of radiolabeled testosterone, evidence of receptor binding is found in several specific regions of the rat brain involved in sexual behavior: (1) the MPOA, (2) the bed nucleus of the stria terminalis, and (3) the corticomedial nuclei of the amygdala (Figure 5.17; Sar and Stumpf, 1977). Other brain regions, such as the ventromedi-

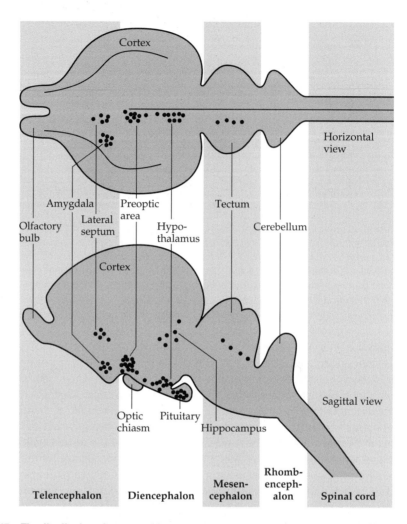

**5.17    The distribution of sex steroid receptors** depicted in a hypothetical generalized vertebrate brain. Note that most steroid receptors are clustered in the POA, the lateral septum, the
amygdala, the hypothalamus, the hippocampus, and the pituitary. After Morrell and Pfaff, 1978.

al nuclei of the hypothalamus (VMN) and arcuate nucleus (AN), were also heavily labeled, but lesion studies suggest that these nuclei are not directly involved
in the control of male mammalian mating behaviors. That is, males perform normally in mating tests after lesions of the VMN and AN.

Because testosterone can be converted to other androgens or to estrogens inside of neurons, binding studies that specifically examined estradiol and DHT receptors have also been conducted to ascertain the separate roles of these steroid
hormones in specific neural target tissues. The distribution of cells that concentrate labeled DHT in the rat brain is essentially identical to the pattern of testos-
terone-concentrating cells (Sar and Stumpf, 1977). The distribution of estrogen-
concentrating cells is more extensive than that of androgen-concentrating neurons
(Commins and Yahr, 1985; Sheridan, 1978), extending from the MPOA into the
forebrain. Both androgen and estrogen receptors mediate male sexual behavior.

Recall from Chapter 2 that an enzyme called aromatase converts testosterone to estradiol. In rodents, aromatization of testosterone into estradiol in the brain is required for the expression of normal male mating behavior (Christensen and Clemens, 1975; Clancy et al., 1995). A radiolabeled antisense RNA probe for rat aromatase mRNA can be used to show where in the brain aromatase mRNA is present (Roselli et al., 1997). Aromatase mRNA has been detected in many areas of the rat brain; the MPOA, VNH, and the medial and cortical nuclei of the amygdala are especially rich in aromatase activity (Roselli et al., 1997). Castrating male rats caused aromatase mRNA concentrations in the MPOA and hypothalamus to drop after 7 days; androgen replacement therapy (either testosterone or dihydrotestosterone), but not estrogen treatment, restored aromatase activity and aromatase mRNA concentrations in those brain regions (Roselli et al., 1997). Neither aromatase activity nor mRNA levels in the amygdala were affected by castration. Thus, testosterone serves as a prohormone in mediating male sexual behavior. DHT can regulate aromatase mRNA transcription and/or stability in specific rat brain regions, whereas estradiol can activate neural circuits regulating male sexual behavior.

Much of the neural circuitry involved in mediating male mating behavior has been confirmed and extended by tracking the activation of so-called **immediate early genes (IEGs)** (Pfaus and Heeb, 1997). In neurons, these genes are activated early during the signal transduction process whereby extracellular signals result in the expression of specific genes. The nature and function of the "activation" of IEGs remain controversial (Pfaus and Heeb, 1997); nevertheless, the presence of their protein products is thought to indicate the initial activation of the genetic machinery of neurons. The protein products of IEGs, such as the fos, jun, and egr-1 families, can be detected by immunocytochemical methods. Analysis of IEG protein products in neurons has confirmed that copulatory stimuli activate neurons in several steroid-concentrating brain regions, including the MPOA, lateral septum, BNST, PVH, VMN, medial amygdala, ventral premammillary nuclei, central tegmental field, mesencephalic central gray region, and perpendicular nuclei (Pfaus and Heeb, 1997) (Figure 5.18; also see Box 10.3). Although devoid of intracellular sex steroid hormone receptors, the ventral and dorsal striatum and the cortex also display significant activation after sexual behavior. Note that the MPOA, BNST, and corticomedial amygdala are regions of the brain that other methods have shown to be critical for regulating male sexual behavior. Although many nonspecific stimuli can "activate" neurons and increase IEG expression, it is a reasonable strategy to use IEG expression as one of several tools to identify neural circuits involved in sexual behavior.

**MICRODIALYSIS STUDIES.**   Presumably, neurotransmitter function must be affected if hormones are to influence behavior. In the case of male sexual behavior, dopamine seems to play a central role (Melis and Argiolas, 1995; see above). Although many other neurotransmitters are involved, a discussion of the effects of hormones on every neurotransmitter system is beyond the scope of this book. We will look at dopamine as an example of how hormones and their receptors function to affect neurotransmission.

Some neurotransmitters act to stimulate sexual behavior, whereas other neurotransmitters act to inhibit it (Table 5.3). Dopamine appears to facilitate male sexual behavior by removing tonic inhibition (Chevalier and Deniau, 1990) of brain regions that mediate sensorimotor abilities (Hull et al., 1997). Three major inte-

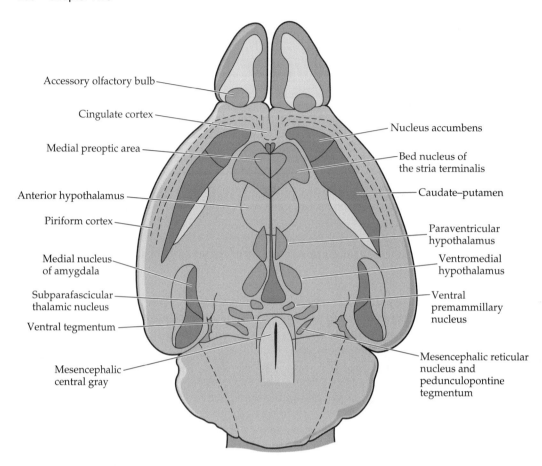

Accessory olfactory bulb

Cingulate cortex

Medial preoptic area

Anterior hypothalamus

Piriform cortex

Medial nucleus of amygdala

Subparafascicular thalamic nucleus

Ventral tegmentum

Mesencephalic central gray

Nucleus accumbens

Bed nucleus of the stria terminalis

Caudate–putamen

Paraventricular hypothalamus

Ventromedial hypothalamus

Ventral premammillary nucleus

Mesencephalic reticular nucleus and pedunculopontine tegmentum

**5.18   Brain regions in rodents that show fos induction after sexual stimulation.** This schematic illustration of a horizontal section of rat brain depicts the various regions that are activated during male sexual behavior. After Pfaus and Heeb, 1997.

grative dopaminergic systems regulate sexual motivation, genital responses, and bodily postures during copulation in male rats (Hull et al., 1997): the nigrostriatal tract, the mesolimbic tract, and the medial preoptic area. Sensory input from an estrous female before or during copulation evokes the release of dopamine in each of these three tracts (Mas, 1995; Hull et al., 1995). The nigrostriatal tract is the largest dopaminergic system and mediates the initiation of movement. The nigrostriatal tract is damaged in humans with Parkinson's disease, which is characterized by tremors, slow movements, and impairments in the initiation of movement. In rats, the nigrostriatal tract appears to be involved in the muscular movements associated with mounting females (Robbins and Everitt, 1992). The mesolimbic tract is important in reward and appetitive behaviors such as brain self-stimulation, drug addiction, and food, alcohol, and water intake, as well as sexual behavior (Hull et al., 1997). The mesolimbic tract terminates in the nucleus accumbens, and blocking or stimulating dopamine receptors in this region decreases or restores, respectively, behaviors associated with sexual motivation (Pfaus and

**Table 5.3**
**Effects of various neurotransmitters on male sexual behavior**

| Neurotransmitter | Effect on copulation | Effect on penile erection |
|---|---|---|
| Norepinephrine | $\alpha_1$ receptor activity $\uparrow$ copulation | $\alpha_1$ receptor activity $\downarrow$ reflexive erection |
| | $\alpha_2$ receptor activity $\downarrow$ copulation | $\alpha_2$ receptor activity $\uparrow$ reflexive erection |
| | $\beta_1$ receptor activity has no effect | $\beta$ activity inhibits reflexive erection |
| | $\beta_2$ receptor activity $\uparrow$ copulation | ($\beta$ receptor subtype not specified) |
| Dopamine | Presynaptic activity $\downarrow$ copulation | Postsynaptic activity $\uparrow$ reflexive erection, but $\downarrow$ spontaneous erection |
| Serotonin (5-HT) | $5\text{-HT}_{1A}$ activity $\uparrow$ copulation | $5\text{-HT}_{1A}$ activity $\downarrow$ erection |
| | $5\text{-HT}_{1B/1C}$ activity $\downarrow$ copulation | $5\text{-HT}_{1C}$ activity $\uparrow$ spontaneous erection |
| | $5\text{-HT}_2$ activity $\downarrow$ copulation | $5\text{-HT}_2$ activity $\downarrow$ spontaneous erection |
| $\gamma$-Aminobutyric acid (GABA) | $\text{GABA}_{A/B}$ activity $\downarrow$ copulation | $\text{GABA}_{A/B}$ activity $\uparrow$ spontaneous erection |
| Acetylcholine | Inconclusive | Inconclusive |
| Endorphins | Activity $\downarrow$ copulation | Activity $\downarrow$ erection |
| Neuropeptide Y | Activity $\downarrow$ copulation | No effect |
| Oxytocin | Activity $\uparrow$ copulation | Activity $\uparrow$ spontaneous erection |

$\uparrow$ = facilitates; $\downarrow$ = decreases.
*Source:* Meisel and Sachs, 1994.

Phillips, 1991; Everitt, 1990); however, activation of the nucleus accumbens may only enhance generalized appetitive behavior.

As noted above, lesions of the MPOA impair sexual performance, but spare sexual motivation, in male rats (Everitt, 1990). However, more recent ideas indicate that the MPOA contributes to sexual motivation (Hull et al., 1995, 1997). The MPOA is critical for male sexual behavior in all vertebrate animals thus far studied (Meisel and Sachs, 1994). This structure receives input from and sends output to virtually every sensory modality (Hull et al., 1997). This reciprocity in connections provides a means for the MPOA to modulate sensory processes, and for sensory information to affect the integration of sexual motivation. Many neurons within or connected to the MPOA possess receptors for sex steroid hormones (Simerly and Swanson, 1986). Similarly, steroid hormone receptors are embedded within the membranes of many neurons constituting nondopaminergic neurotransmitter systems.

In microdialysis, a very small (200–300 µm diameter) probe (hollow tube) is inserted into the brain. The probe is usually filled with cerebrospinal fluid, and neurotransmitters, hormones, and their metabolites diffuse into the tube from the surrounding extracellular fluid. Microdialysis samples are usually obtained continuously while animals are awake and active. The samples can be analyzed using high power liquid chromatography (HPLC). Microdialysis has revealed a consistent pattern of increased dopamine concentrations in the MPOA of males in the presence of an estrous female rat housed behind a perforated barrier (Hull et al.,

1997). A variety of other stimuli, including access to highly palatable food or a male conspecific, did not affect MPOA dopamine secretion. Castration attenuated the female-induced elevation of dopamine in the MPOA (Du et al., 1998). Dopamine appears to integrate sensorimotor information in the MPOA, resulting in facilitation of male sexual behavior (Figure 5.19) (Hull et al., 1997).

Dopamine also seems to facilitate sexual behavior in primates (Hull et al., 1997; Melis and Argiolas, 1995). Treatment of male rhesus monkeys with a dopamine agonist, apomorphine, resulted in dose-dependent enhancements of sexual responses toward females that males could see, hear, and smell, but not touch. For instance, low doses (25–100 μg/kg) of apomorphine caused yawning, whereas moderate doses (50–200 μg/kg) caused penile erections and masturbation, occasionally to ejaculation (Pomerantz, 1990). Interestingly, the males required the presence of a female in order to show these sexual behaviors. These results are reminiscent of the effects of testosterone in facilitating male sexual behaviors in the presence of the appropriate stimuli, and they also suggest that hormones mediate male primate behavior by acting via dopaminergic pathways. Apomorphine also induces penile erections in normal and impotent men (Lal et al., 1984, 1987).

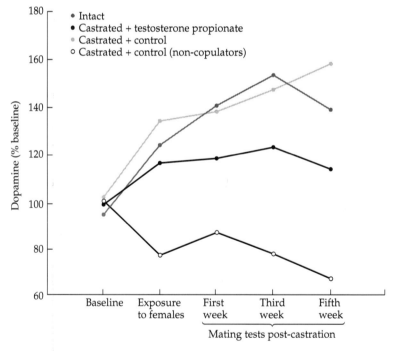

**5.19    Extracellular dopamine in the MPOA is elevated by cues from the female.** Dopamine concentrations in the MPOA of male rats were measured by microdialysis in the presence of an estrous female rat housed behind a perforated barrier. In the absence of the precopulatory rise in dopamine, males failed to copulate when the barrier was removed. In contrast, males that showed an increase of approximately 50% in extracellular dopamine in the MPOA copulated with females, regardless of testosterone concentrations. After Hull et al., 1995.

**GENE KNOCKOUT STUDIES.**    As described in Chapter 1, new advances in molecular biology make it possible to perform specific genetic manipulations. An increasingly common genetic technique used in behavioral endocrinology studies is the removal (knockout) of the genetic code for a specific hormone or its receptor. Virtually all of the knockout studies of hormone–behavior interactions to date have been performed on mice (*Mus musculus*) (Nelson, 1997). Thus far, male sexual behavior in mice has been examined in a few knockout varieties. For example, mice that have had the gene encoding the μ-opioid receptor deleted displayed reduced their mating activity (Tian et al., 1997). The μ-opioid receptor mediates the pain-attenuating features of endogenous and exogenous opioids such as morphine and heroin. The "pleasurable" aspects of copulation may require the μ-opioid receptor (van Furth et al., 1995).

Nitric oxide (NO) is well established as a neurotransmitter (Nelson et al., 1997) (Box 5.3). NO is formed from nitric oxide synthase (NOS) and arginine. There are three isoforms of NOS. Male mice that lack the gene that codes for the neuronal isoform of NOS (nNOS –/–) displayed persistent mounting behavior, even toward anestrous females that refused to cooperate with their mating attempts (Nelson et al., 1995). Testosterone concentrations were not elevated in these nNOS –/– mice.

Recently, another gas, carbon monoxide (CO), has also been implicated as a neurotransmitter (Dawson and Snyder, 1994). Mice with targeted deletions of the gene encoding heme oxygenase-2 (HO2–/–), an enzyme that produces endogenous carbon monoxide in neurons, displayed altered mating behavior. HO2–/– mice showed markedly diminished ejaculatory behavior (Burnett et al., 1998). When ejaculations were elicited by neural stimulation ex copula, HO2–/– mice were dramatically impaired (Burnett et al., 1998). In many cases, the effects of a particular missing gene on sexual behavior are pursued only when a breeding colony of knockout mice either fails to produce offspring or increases at a reduced rate. In these cases, the investigators did not anticipate the impairments of male sexual behavior (Burnett et al., 1998; Nelson et al., 1995; Tian et al., 1997).

In contrast to the serendipitous, unexpected, and somewhat subtle results of the targeted deletion of the genes encoding the μ-opioid receptor, nNOS, and HO2, the deletion of genes encoding androgen or estrogen receptors would be expected to result in predictable, severe defects in male mating behavior. However, male estrogen receptor knockout (ERKO) mice show only subtle deficits in male sexual behavior, mainly reduced ejaculations (Eddy et al., 1996; Ogawa et al., 1995); otherwise, they show mounting and intromission behaviors comparable to those of normal, wild-type (WT) mice (Ogawa et al., 1995). If male ERKO mice are castrated and implanted with Silastic capsules filled with testosterone (which leaks out at a constant rate), so that their blood concentrations of testosterone are all similar, a deficit in the rate and onset of intromissions is observed as compared to WT mice (Rissman et al., 1997b).

Recall from Chapter 3 that, based on the results of early injections of estrogen receptor antisense RNA, estrogen receptors appear to be necessary for the organization of masculinization and defeminization of behavior (McCarthy et al., 1993a). How do we reconcile the results of these studies with the results of the ERKO studies, in which male ERKO mouse mating behavior was essentially unaffected (Ogawa et al., 1995)? One hypothesis is that there might be other forms of

## Box 5.3
# Erectile Dysfunction, Nitric Oxide, and Viagra

Approximately 50% of men over the age of 40 have some degree of erectile dysfunction. Because penile erections are mainly vascular events, medical problems such as diabetes, high blood pressure, high cholesterol, and heart disease, all of which affect blood flow, are frequently underlying causes. Therefore, it is important for individuals experiencing erectile dysfunction to be screened for these conditions. Furthermore, if these conditions are not treated, there could be a progression of erectile dysfunction.

Androgens are essential for the expression of normal sex drive (libido) in men, but their role in the maintenance of the erectile response in humans is controversial. Castration in rats causes both a loss of penile reflexes and a marked reduction in the erectile response to electric field stimulation (EFS) of the cavernosal nerve. Both of these effects can be reversed by testosterone or DHT, but not estradiol, replacement (Lugg et al., 1995).

However, nitric oxide (NO) has emerged as a key mediator of erection. The physiological mechanism of penile erection involves a release of NO in the corpora cavernosa (the paired chambers in the penis where blood is trapped) during sexual stimulation (Burnett, 1995). Nitrates such as nitroglycerin are broken down to NO, a very transient and reactive free radical that not only acts as a vasodilator, but is vital in the regulation of mitochondrial respiration in both skeletal muscle and other organ systems. NO is produced in normal amounts by the vascular endothelial tissues to facilitate blood flow, stimulate cellular respiration, and help prevent plaque formation on interior vessel walls. NO also appears to function as a neurotransmitter. However, NO is a very toxic free radical that can cause substantial tissue damage in high concentrations, especially in the brain. In stroke, for example, large amounts of NO are released from nerve cells to cause damage to surrounding tissues.

In the penis, NO is released from both neuronal and endothelial sources (Nelson et al., 1997). NO combines with the enzyme guanylate cyclase, which converts GTP to cyclic guanosine monophosphate (cGMP). The resulting ele-

Viagra (sildenafil citrate)

the estrogen receptor gene that persist in ERKO mice. Recently, in vivo autoradiography studies indicated that neurons in ERKO mouse brains were concentrating radiolabeled estrogens (Shughrue et al., 1996)! A second isoform of the estrogen receptor, which binds estradiol-17β with high affinity, was isolated in rat prostate and ovarian tissue (Kuiper et al., 1996); this second estrogen receptor has been termed ERβ, whereas the originally described receptor is now called ERα (Shughrue, 1998). It is possible that male mice with targeted deletions of the gene encoding the β form of the estrogen receptor might display impaired male sexual behavior. It is also plausible that other genes encode alternative estrogen receptor molecules, and that one of these alternative estrogen receptors is critical in mediating sexual behavior in male mice.

vation of cGMP concentrations in the penis produces smooth muscle relaxation in the corpora cavernosa, allowing the inflow of blood.

Recall that the loss of penile reflexes in rats following castration can be reversed by testosterone or DHT replacement. Production of the synthetic enzyme (nitric oxide synthase) that produces NO and a byproduct, citrulline, from arginine is also dependent upon DHT (Lugg et al., 1995; see also Box 8.1). DHT production wanes in men after the age of 40, so the increased prevalence of erectile dysfunction at this age might reflect the interaction between DHT and NO.

In March 1998, the Pfizer Pharmaceutical Company released the drug Viagra (the generic name is sildenafil citrate; see figure at left) for the treatment of erectile dysfunction. Sildenafil acts by potentiating the effects of NO on the mechanism of penile erection; it enhances the effect of NO on cGMP by inhibiting the enzyme phosphodiesterase type 5 (PDE5), which breaks down cGMP in the corpora cavernosa. Individuals can take sildenafil 30–60 minutes prior to sexual activity. When sexual activity stimulates NO release, inhibition of PDE5 by sildenafil causes increased levels of cGMP in the corpora cavernosa, resulting in the desired smooth muscle relaxation and inflow of blood to the corpora cavernosa. Thus, sildenafil does not cause an erection

per se, but enhances or potentiates an erection. Current evidence suggests that sildenafil does not affect sexual motivation.

Sildenafil at recommended doses (50–100 mg) has no effect on penile erection in the absence of sexual stimulation. At appropriate doses and in the presence of sexual stimulation, however, sildenafil is remarkably effective. One study showed a covariant relationship in sildenafil dosage and the number of patients reporting improvement in erectile function: with a 25 mg dose of sildenafil, 63% of patients reported improvement, while 82% reported improvement with a 100 mg dose (see figure below). Although anecdotal information suggests that sildenafil also enhances female sexual performance, no controlled studies have been conducted at this time.

Shortly after its release, Viagra became the fastest-selling drug in history. At $10 per pill, typical estimates call for annual Viagra sales to reach $5 billion by the year 2002.

## Conclusions

How do steroid hormones affect male mating behavior? Taken together, the studies on rodents that have been described suggest that steroid hormones activate certain genes in neurons. Recall that neurons, like other cells, have a cell nucleus, and within the nucleus are genes located along the chromosomes. DNA transcription turns on the cellular mechanisms within neurons to produce proteins (see Chapter 2). Generally, steroid hormones activate certain genes that increase DNA transcription and protein production by other genes. The result of this genomic expression may be an increase or a decrease in the number of hormone receptors, or a change in the presence or amounts of enzymes that affect neurotransmitter or neurohormone production, neurotransmitter receptor production, or even recycling of neurotransmitters. For example, dopamine may not be recycled quickly in some circumstances; increased dopamine concentrations in the MPOA stimulate male sexual behavior (Bitran et al., 1988; Hull et al., 1995, 1997). Thus, a genomic signal initiated by steroid hormones that reduced dopamine recycling rates, thereby increasing dopamine concentrations, could stimulate male copulatory behavior in the appropriate social context. New protein synthesis in response to steroidal influences on neuronal genes may allow new neuronal connections to be made, facilitating sensory input associated with estrous females or even memories of prior sexual encounters (for example, Pfaff and Pfaffmann, 1969; Stern, 1990). For instance, implants of testosterone into the MPOA of rats stimulate dendritic branching and other structural changes there (Meisel and Sachs, 1994). These effects are presumably due to testosterone effects on genes that code for specific structural proteins.

Mating behaviors are very complex, and many endocrine, neural, and environmental stimuli interact to produce successful copulation. Further discoveries of the physiological mechanisms by which hormones affect male mating behavior await our understanding of precisely how a change in protein synthesis in a brain region becomes amplified into a behavioral response.

### Social Influences on Male Mating Behavior

The endocrine and neural mechanisms underlying mating behavior in male rodents have been discussed up to this point. As we know, hormones affect behavior by changing the thresholds at which specific behaviors are displayed in response to particular stimuli. But many environmental factors, including social cues, can modulate hormone–behavior interactions. One environmental stimulus that greatly affects males is the presence of females. Females affect both sexual motivation (appetitive behavior) and performance (consummatory behavior) among males.

If a male rat is placed in a box with an estrous female, he will mate to satiation; that is, he may ejaculate seven or eight times over the course of several hours. He is operationally defined as sated when no mating behavior is observed for 45 minutes or longer. However, if a new female is introduced into the mating arena, the so-called sated male often immediately resumes copulation. This phenomenon has been termed the "Coolidge effect," in honor of an anecdote involving the former President and First Lady of the United States (Bermant et al., 1968).*

The Coolidge effect, the enhanced mating performance of males with novel females, is a striking phenomenon in some species, including rats and cattle, but in general it is not a very robust effect among mammals. Among humans, there are many anecdotal reports of enormous individual differences in the stimulatory effects of novel females on males' copulatory performances, but not very many

---

*According to the story, President Coolidge and his wife were visiting a farm in the Midwest and were given separate tours by the owners. Both President and Mrs. Coolidge noted during their tours that only one rooster was associated with the large flock of hens. Mrs. Coolidge asked the farmer how many times per day the rooster engaged in romance. "Several times a day," the farmer replied. "Please relay that information to the President," responded the First Lady, apparently impressed by the rooster's performance. Later, during his tour, President Coolidge was given this same information about the copulatory prowess of the rooster. The President pressed further, "Same hen each time?" "Oh no," replied the farmer, "A different hen each time." "Please relay that information to Mrs. Coolidge."

convincing data. There is a complete absence of this phenomenon in some other species. For example, males of some monogamous rodent species do not show the Coolidge effect; for a male prairie vole (*Microtus ochrogaster*), the opportunity to mate with a novel female results instead in resumption of copulation with his mate (Getz et al., 1987; Gray and Dewsbury, 1973). The endocrine bases, if any, of the Coolidge effect remain unspecified. However, its neurobiological bases may involve an augmentation of dopamine release in the nucleus accumbens (mesolimbic tract) during copulation (Fiorino et al., 1997).

In order to study the effects of hormones on reproductive behavior in the laboratory, the physical space in which the animals interact is often simplified. Typically, the mating behavior of rats is assessed in a small, empty aquarium. The rich complexity of the natural habitat, including space, odors, and escape paths, is eliminated to control as many variables as possible during the experiment. This simplification of the physical space in which behavior is examined may make experiments easier to analyze, but it also removes much of the rich environmental texture that may play important roles in the regulation of behavior.

Natural sexual behavior may be unintentionally constrained by these simplified testing environments. The stimuli associated with copulation normally induce luteal function and subsequent progesterone production in female rats (see Chapter 6). The timing of the vaginal stimulation caused by copulation may be important for inducing luteal function; thus the interval between, and the pacing of, intromissions varies on a somewhat species-specific basis. The optimal pattern of intromissions for some species has been called the "vaginal code" (Diamond, 1970). Under natural conditions, female rats control the pacing of reproductive activities to match closely the physical stimuli necessary for optimal reproductive efficiency. Female rats can adapt to the typical mating arena provided in most behavioral endocrinology studies, in which the pace of mating is faster than the physiological optimum. However, they may produce less progesterone during these behavioral assessments, and thus produce fewer offspring than females mating in naturalistic settings. Providing a seminatural environment to rats results in a slower pace of mating behaviors (McClintock, 1987). The reason for this reduction in mating pace is not certain, but the animals appear to interact with the environment and also to move farther away from one another during mating. The running and chasing observed during rodent mating bouts conducted in seminatural enclosures is often qualitatively and quantitatively different from what is observed during typical laboratory mating tests. In many species for which both laboratory and field hormonal data have been collected, hormone concentrations vary substantially between the two situations.

Not only the physical environment, but also the social environment of rodents is artificially simplified in laboratory studies of hormonal effects on reproductive behavior. Typical studies with laboratory rats pair a single male with a single female and record the resulting behavior. However, rats in nature do not necessarily mate in pairs; several males and females may mate in a group. Sperm competition studies suggest that the male having the most ejaculations with a female, or the last ejaculation during her series of copulations, usually sires the most offspring. Presumably, strategies have evolved for males to compete for copulations and to time their copulatory acts to maximize their chances of fertilizing a female. One interesting advantage for rats mating in groups (a panogamous mating system) is that because each sex can take turns mating with different partners, each sex can mate at a different "optimal" pace for fulfilling their respective neuroendocrine stimulus requirements (Figure 5.20; McClintock, 1984; see also Chapter 6).

The stimulus value of the female is another variable that may influence the outcome of behavioral endocrine investigations of male sexual behavior. Males have different mating responses to females in naturally occurring estrus than to females that are in artificially primed estrus (Hardy and Debold, 1971). Males also respond differentially to females brought into estrus with different hormonal treatments. For example, male rats with corticomedial amygdala lesions responded slowly to estrogen-injected females in one intriguing study. However, there was no difference in the rate of copulation between lesioned and intact males when the female was brought into estrus with both estrogen and progesterone (Perkins et al., 1980). Perhaps the additional hormonal treatment provided females with enhanced stimulus value that overcame the effects of the brain lesion. Additional studies are required to understand the effect of the hormonal condition of estrous females on male mating behaviors.

The presence of female rodents, especially novel females, induces an elevation in blood plasma testosterone concentrations in male rodents during mating (Bronson and Desjardins, 1982a; Purvis and Haynes, 1974). Prior to mating, sensory cues associated with females can cause a rapid increase in circulating LH and testosterone concentrations in sexually experienced male mice (Batty, 1978). This response can be classically conditioned to previously neutral stimuli (Graham and Desjardins, 1980). A natural stimulus, normally referred to as the unconditioned stimulus, normally causes some reflexive response, called an unconditioned

**5.20  Copulatory sequence of rats mating in groups.** In this example, three estrous females (left) are copulating with two males (right). A mating event is signified by either an open circle (intromission) or a star (ejaculation); the female and male participating in a given event are indicated by a horizontal line. The first mating event occurs when male 1 intromits with female 3; then female 2 receives an intromission from male 1, followed by male 1 intromitting female 3, then female 2 again. Thus, the inter-intromission interval (III) is different for female 2 than for male 1; in a more typical paired mating test, the III would be identical for each partner. Similarly, the post-ejaculatory interval (PEI) for female 1 is different than the PEI for male 2, but would be identical in a standard paired mating situation. Laboratory assessment of mating behavior in groups more closely approximates field conditions and thus provides data with more ecological validity than that obtained in paired mating tests. The time line indicates the order and relative temporal relationship of mating events, but does not reflect actual temporal intervals. Source: McClintock, 1984.

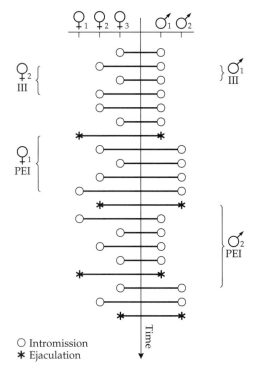

response. In Pavlov's famous studies, food in the mouth, the unconditioned stimulus, naturally caused a dog to increase salivation, the unconditioned response. If a previously neutral stimulus, one that normally does not cause the biological response, is paired repeatedly with the unconditioned stimulus, then the neutral stimulus, now called the conditioned stimulus, can cause the salivation, or conditioned response, in the absence of the food.

Female presence causes a rise in blood LH and testosterone concentrations in the CF-1 strain of male house mice. Exposure to the odor of wintergreen normally has no endocrine effects in mice. If female exposure is repeatedly paired with wintergreen odor, however, eventually the odor will evoke increased plasma LH and testosterone concentrations in the male mice in the absence of a female. In other words, the males will "learn" to increase their hormonal concentrations whenever they experience the odor of wintergreen (Figure 5.21). The sights and sounds associated with estrous females may promote endocrine changes prior to the onset of mating because of previous associations between these stimuli and mating behavior. The role of learning in mating and pre-mating elevations in reproductive hormones, and thus in mediating copulatory

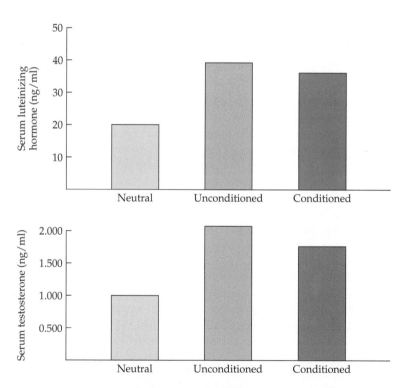

**5.21   LH secretion can be modified by classical conditioning.** Upon the first presentation of a neutral stimulus (in this case, wintergreen odor), there was no change in serum hormone concentrations (Neutral). Male house mice were then repeatedly exposed to the wintergreen odor paired with the presentation of a female. After training, conditioned males showed increased LH and testosterone secretion in response to the odor alone (Conditioned), at levels close to those shown by unconditioned males in response to a female (Unconditioned). Source: Graham and Desjardins, 1980.

behaviors, is not yet well understood, but this is one possible mechanism by which experience may interact with the endocrine system to preserve hormone-dependent behaviors in the absence of the hormone.

Also not well understood is the observation, initially reported by Steinach (1936) and verified by Folman and Drori (1966), that socially isolated castrated males display a post-castration reduction in reproductive organ mass faster than that of heterosexually reared males. Social isolation is stressful for many mammalian species, and stress could mediate the reproductive effects reported in these studies (see Chapter 11). Again, social influences on reproductive physiology, morphology, and behavior are potent, but are unfortunately often ignored in the study of hormone–behavior interactions.

### Individual Differences in Male Mating Behavior

Vast individual differences exist in the amount of sex drive and sexual performance observed among individuals of many species. That is, the sexual behavior of males falls along a continuum between hyposexual and hypersexual activity. If male rats are tested in typical time-limited mating tests, some may mate several times within the time constraints, but others will not mate at all. An early hypothesis proposed to account for individual differences in mating behavior was that animals with high sex drive had higher circulating testosterone concentrations than animals with low sex drive. This hypothesis was tested initially on guinea pigs prior to the availability of direct assays of circulating steroid hormones (Grunt and Young, 1952, 1953). Males were pre-screened for sexual activity and categorized as high, medium, or low sex drive males based on their number of ejaculations during a time-limited mating test. All the males were then castrated, and their copulatory behavior was tested during the following weeks (Figure 5.22). Low sex drive males stopped mating first, followed by the medium and high sex drive animals. After 16 weeks, all the males had completely stopped displaying mating behavior. They were then injected with low (50 µg/day) doses of testosterone propionate, and each male returned to his pre-castration level of sexual behavior. A similar study examining high and low rates of sexual activity in rats yielded similar results (Larsson, 1966). The results of these studies indicate that animals do not differ in their mating behavior because of different concentrations of hormones. More likely, differences exist in the target tissues that mediate reproductive behaviors.

With technological advances in hormone measurement, it is possible to address the question of hormone concentrations directly. When such a study was conducted on laboratory rats, its outcome was in agreement with the earlier study by Grunt and Young on guinea pigs: differences in blood hormone concentrations did not account for the differences observed in the frequency of sexual behaviors. Males were identified as copulators or noncopulators, and blood plasma testosterone was assayed for all the animals. All the males in this study had testosterone concentrations between 2 and 3 ng/ml of plasma. The known copulators were then castrated, and testosterone-filled Silastic capsules of different lengths were implanted in them, resulting in different blood concentrations of testosterone. However, normal sexual behavior was restored in most of the males, even those with very low testosterone concentrations. Seventy-two percent of the males ejaculated normally with only a 2 mm capsule, yet the concentrations of their plasma testosterone were *much* lower than normal values (Figure 5.23; Damassa et al., 1977).

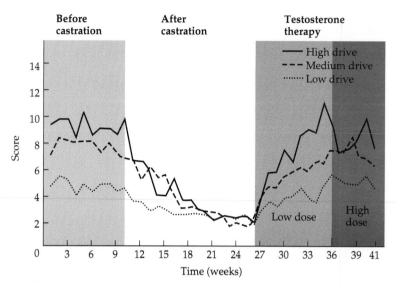

**5.22  Individual differences in sex drive** are retained following castration and restoration therapy. Guinea pigs that were classified as having high, medium, or low sex drives based on behavioral assessments were castrated. After castration, the sexual behavior score eventually dropped to an equal baseline for all three groups. Both low-dose and high-dose testosterone therapy restored copulatory behavior in the castrated males, and the differences in sexual behavior among the groups was still observed. This study demonstrated that differences in blood androgen concentrations do not correspond closely to individual differences in sexual behavior, which are more likely due to variation in target tissue sensitivity to androgens. Source: Grunt and Young, 1952.

This study demonstrates that very low concentrations of circulating testosterone can maintain sexual behavior. Why, then, do males have circulating androgen concentrations an order of magnitude higher than necessary to maintain sexual behavior? Probably because local testis androgen concentrations must be very high to support spermatogenesis, and mating behavior has evolved to depend on the diluted concentrations of androgens in the general circulation. Thus, large variations in circulating concentrations of testosterone (of even an order of magnitude) will presumably not affect behavior. High androgen concentrations are also important in aggression and in maintenance of other male traits. Indeed, high androgen levels support secondary sex characters that are often the criteria by which females choose mates (Andersson, 1994).

Differences among genetic strains in reproductive behavioral responsiveness to hormones have also been noted. In one study, for example, several strains of mice were examined for male copulatory behavior, and a strain was eventually discovered in which males continued to copulate for 2 years after castration (McGill, 1962, 1977). Usually mice, like rats, stop mating soon after castration, so genotype appears to be one of the most salient factors underlying the dependency of male sexual behavior upon hormones in mice. But how does the genotype code for behavioral responsiveness to hormones? The answer to this question specifically, and the answer to the question of how genotype codes for any behavior generally, must be obtained in order to make the link between molecular biol-

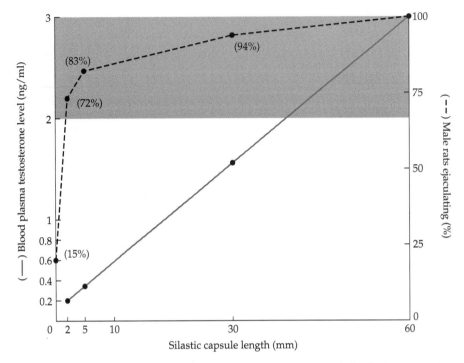

**5.23    Clinically low testosterone concentrations can restore mating behavior** in castrated rats. Rats that were known copulators and had plasma testosterone concentrations of 2–3 ng/ml (shaded area) were castrated. Most of the rats exhibited normal ejaculatory behavior after implantation with a 2 mm Silastic testosterone capsule, even though the capsule treatment resulted in plasma testosterone concentrations that were much lower than those found in intact rats. Source: Damassa et al., 1977.

ogy and organismal analyses of hormone–behavior interactions. Probably, a constellation of strain-specific traits accounts for the individual differences.

Reproductive performance and competence decline as mammals, including humans, pass the midpoint of their life expectancy (Bishop, 1970; Vom Saal and Finch, 1988). Reduced reproductive behavior may be due to age-related changes in sexual motivation, perceptual capabilities, attractiveness to the opposite sex, physical prowess, or some combination of these factors. Reductions in the frequency of sexual behavior may or may not correlate with changes in reproductive physiology or morphology. Aged mice (30 months old) have reduced gonadal mass and rates of spermatogenesis, and average blood plasma LH and testosterone concentrations compared with 6-month-old mice (Bronson and Desjardins, 1982b). Numerous syndromes can be described in which various physiological systems change, leading to decreased reproductive competence. But the most interesting question vis-à-vis issues of aging is why some healthy male mice can mate at 30 months of age and others cannot, despite equivalent blood concentrations of testosterone.

We currently do not understand completely the physiological mechanisms underlying individual differences in reproductive activity. Uptake and metabolism of testosterone in the MPOA of the hypothalamus does not differ between sexually active and inactive rats. However, estrogen receptor numbers in the MPOA are significantly reduced in sexually nonresponsive male rats as compared with copulating males (Clark et al., 1985). Perhaps protein synthesis is differentially affected by hormones, causing changes in synthesis of hormones, receptors, or structural proteins necessary for dendritic spines. Rats with inherited insensitivity to androgens lack specific androgen receptors, but have normal estrogen receptors; testosterone causes less of an increase in their sexual behavior than in normal rats (Beach and Buehler, 1977). With the exception of receptor numbers in the MPOA, we cannot yet point to any structural difference between the brains of copulators and those of noncopulators. Further analyses are necessary to understand individual, strain, and species differences in reproductive drive and performance.

Individual differences in adult sexual behavior may reflect different experiences during development. For example, if pregnant rats are stressed by exposure to bright lights *and* consume alcohol, their male offspring fail to ejaculate as adults (I. L. Ward et al., 1996). Although their adult blood LH and testosterone concentrations are in the normal range, they can ejaculate only with pharmacological testosterone treatment. The effects of prenatal stress and alcohol exposure are maximal if they coincide with days 18 and 19 of gestation, a time when males normally secrete testosterone.

# Male Sexual Behavior in Primates

Despite the importance of sexual motivation in human behavior, the physiological components of human sex drive and performance have not been well studied, and with only a few notable exceptions, scientific descriptions of human sexual behavior are rare. The theoretical bases of sexual behavior across humans and nonhumans are rarely linked; investigators in each field have developed separate scientific literatures and rarely interact (Pfaus, 1996). The best descriptions of the power of sexual motivation among men are often provided by playwrights, poets, and novelists. In literature, however, descriptions of sex drive and performance are masked or presented under the guise of burning passions, emotional imperatives, or even a desperate desire to marry. For example, Shakespeare's Romeo is a classic tragic character because of his nearly obsessive desire for Juliet. Despite a number of obstructions, some social, others truly physical, Romeo is highly motivated to interact with Juliet, and we in the audience share his intense emotions as he risks everything for her. Their story is a great tragedy because the audience can see, although Romeo is blinded to it, the trajectory of his life as he attempts to overcome the obstructions in his path and obtain his goal of being with Juliet. Romeo's powerful sex drive, couched in terms of passion, overruns his life, and from the beginning of the story, we uneasily sense the sad end of the play. But to what extent does art reflect life, or in this case, hormones and behavior?

## *The Strength of the Sex Drive in Human Males*

In their classic book, *Patterns of Sexual Behavior,* Clellan Ford and Frank Beach (1951) combined information about sexual behavior from three major sources: (1) anthropological data on human sexual behavior from non-Western societies, (2) the Kinsey studies on the sexual habits and attitudes of married Americans (Kinsey et al., 1948), and (3) data about sexual behavior in nonhuman animals. This synthesis of knowledge about sexual behavior laid the foundation for much of the subsequent research in human sexual behavior. One striking observation in this book is how powerful the motivation to engage in sexual activities truly is among humans as well as nonhuman animals. For example, young people in every culture examined often participate in premarital sexual activities, despite threats in some societies of extremely severe disgrace and punishment if discovered. This is particularly true among sexually restrictive societies, including North America. In another sexually restricted society that inhabited the Pacific Gilbert Islands, a girl's chastity prior to marriage was required. If a sexual liaison was discovered, both parties were immediately put to death (Ford and Beach, 1951). Examples of instantaneous death sentences for unmarried couples who engage in sexual intercourse have been reported for many societies, both Western and non-Western. To engage in sexual activities, men often risk injury or death from a woman's disapproving relatives or husband. The lack of sexual restraint in the face of such drastic and immediate threats provides a striking and compelling indication of the power of the motivation driving the sexual behavior of men.

If instant death sentences are ineffective in controlling sex drive, then policymakers and educators may be naive in their belief that adolescents will curtail their sexual activities because of the vague possibility of an unwanted pregnancy or contracting a disease like AIDS that may not have any ill effects for years. To support this assertion, recall that 70 years ago the possibility of contracting a horrible venereal disease, namely, syphilis, did not really reduce sexual behavior. In fact, the "Roaring Twenties" were a time of sexual liberation in both North America and Europe (Quétel, 1990). There was no cure for syphilis prior to the development of antibiotics, and this disease often led eventually to blindness and severe neurological dysfunction prior to a painful death. Treatments of the day included cellular poisons such as mercury and arsenic, which, like AZT treatment of AIDS today, had debilitating side effects. Until antibiotics became generally available, sexual abstinence or the use of condoms provided the best protection against syphilis. However, many men and women have reported that during sexual arousal they were so motivated to engage in sex that the possible consequences of the act were forgotten.

Understanding the physiological bases of the human sex drive would seem very important if we hope to reduce the number of unwanted pregnancies or prevent the spread of sexually transmitted diseases like AIDS. There is something different and possibly unique about sexual motivation as compared with other motivated behaviors that impairs decision-making processes. Do hormones contribute to this "clouding of logic" many individuals experience during sexual arousal? Obviously, an understanding of the physiological mechanisms underlying typical human male sexual behavior is also required before we can understand undesirable behaviors such as rape or sexual molestation. But, as noted above, basic research on human sexual behavior is rare, and the physiological mechanisms of human sex drive remain obscure. The majority of human sex research has focused on performance, primarily emphasizing the physiology of erectile function (Sachs and Meisel, 1988; Tanagho et al., 1988). With very few exceptions, funding sources have been reluctant to provide money for basic research on human sexual behavior. Sex research currently being conducted on animal models may help us to understand the physiological bases of human sexual behavior as well as the basic processes and mechanisms underlying all reproductive behavior. Animal research, mainly on rats, provides most of our knowledge of the effects of hormone–behavior interactions. However, basic data on human behavior and physiology would be useful in making informed public policies. Given the fundamental importance of understanding human sexual behavior, remarkably little research is presently being conducted.

## Human Male Sexual Behavior: A Description

Prior to describing what is known about the physiological mechanisms underlying human sexual behavior, a brief description of human sexual behavior will be provided (see also Chapter 6). Scientific descriptions of human male sexual behavior are available, the best known of which come from the so-called Kinsey reports of the late 1940s (Kinsey et al., 1948; Masters and Johnson, 1966; Money, 1988), but their utility is somewhat limited. As you might have guessed, human sex researchers, with clipboards and stopwatches in hand, have not placed large numbers of couples in glass-enclosed rooms and recorded the ensuing sexual behaviors. Yet, the sorts of descriptive analyses that have been conducted on rodents are necessary before issues of causation can be addressed in humans. Like rodent mating behavior, sexual behavior in men can be divided into two components: (1) sex drive (appetitive), which is sometimes called sexual motivation or libido, and (2) sexual performance (consummatory) or potency. As we discovered in the discussion of rodent mating behavior, both components are required for normal sexual behavior, and one or both components can fail. Hormones appear to be crucial for maintaining both behavioral components, although much more research is needed to verify this claim.

There is no universal sexual position for humans. In contrast, if you see two dogs copulating at a distance, you can easily assign the sex of each participant with virtual certainty. If she is in estrus, the female stands relatively motionless, deflects her tail, and allows the male to mount her. The male mounts her from behind, clasps his forepaws around her sides, and repeatedly thrusts his hindquarters as he intromits (see Figure 5.6). This mating position, with the male mounting the female from the rear, is common among nearly all mammals, and few nonhuman examples of other mating positions exist. Aristotle reported in his *Historia Animalium* that hedgehogs (a European relative of porcupines) mated belly to belly. However, later observations proved Aristotle wrong. His notion that hedgehogs mated belly to belly was probably due to his disbelief that these beasts could manage to mate and avoid each other's sharp quills in any other fashion. But hedgehogs mate in the same position as dogs; that is, the male mounts the female from the rear and intromits (Reed, 1946). Many humans also copulate in this position, with the woman allowing the man to enter from behind. This position is not the dominant sexual position in any culture sampled, probably because of the lack of clitoral stimulation it affords (Ford and Beach, 1951; Kinsey et al., 1953). Copulation from behind is most commonly practiced lying side by side when the woman is pregnant or the couple is attempting discretion in crowded sleeping quarters.

Far from having a stereotyped mating posture, humans copulate in a variety of positions (Figure 5.24). Generally, one position for copulation is preferred and dominates in most societies, but other positions are also usually practiced. Most humans mate in face-to-face positions.* The most common sexual position among humans of all cultures appears to be some version of the woman sitting or squatting on the supine man. Of course, the most common sexual position among Europeans and North Americans is the face-to-face position with the man above the woman, sometimes derisively called the "missionary position."

The point of this shopping list of human sexual positions is that the mere description of human sexual behavior indicates that, in contrast to rodents, stereotyped mating sequences are not observed in humans. There are some basic constraints, but within these constraints many sexual positions exist among humans. Stereotyped mating postures like lordosis do not exist in women, and male copulatory behavior in men cannot be partitioned easily into mounting, intromissions, and ejaculations. The lack of stereotyped behaviors suggests that hormonal regulation of the muscle patterns underlying human sexual behavior is unlikely. Therefore, the hormonal regulation of human copulatory behavior must differ fundamentally from that of rodent mating behaviors, although hormonal control of human male sexual motivation and penile erection may be similar to that in rodents.

### Nonhuman Primate Male Sexual Behavior: A Description

In contrast to humans, the mating posture of all adult nonhuman primate species is virtually the same—and it is the position least preferred by women. Female nonhuman primates turn their backs to the male and bend at the waist to reveal their genitalia. The vaginae of all nonhuman primates are located more posteriorly than the vaginal opening of women, and thus entry from the front is nearly impossible. Typically, the male clasps the female around her waist and intromits as he remains standing (Figure 5.25). Nonhuman primates have occasionally been reported to employ unusual mating positions in zoos (usually a male sitting while a female backs into his erect penis), but nearly all observations of mating positions among natural populations of nonhuman primates have indicated that copulation occurs only with male entry from the rear. A few exceptions to this pattern have been observed. One great ape, the orangutan (*Pongo pygmaeus*), has been observed in nature mating face-to-face hanging upside down by their toes (Mitani, 1985)! Thus, the mating patterns of nonhuman primate males are less stereotyped than those of rodents or carnivores, but more programmed than those of humans.

The primary exception is provided by bonobos (*Pan paniscus*), also known as pygmy chimpanzees. These animals are very closely related to humans (about 98% gene homology), and primatologists have been impressed by their social interactions. Unlike the male-dominated, highly "political" and confrontational nature of common chimpanzee social life, bonobo society is best characterized by the phrase "make love, not war" (de Waal and Lanting, 1997). Bonobos use sexual interactions to resolve a wide range of social conflicts. Importantly, bonobos

*The Hebrew word for "knowing" someone and "copulating" with someone is the same; hence the term, "knowing someone in the Biblical sense." The reason for the two meanings of the word apparently arises from the observation that humans copulate face to face and, unlike other animals, "know" their partner.

**5.24  Human copulation is not constrained to stereotyped positions.**  This illustration from a 1940s manual used by physicians in marriage counseling depicts several possible coital postures, and well-known Eastern works such as the *Kama Sutra* describe many others. Because of the varied copulatory postures adopted by humans, it is unlikely that hormonal correlates or stereotyped muscle patterns associated with behaviors such as "mounting" will be discovered. Therefore, the hormonal regulation of human copulation must differ fundamentally from the hormonal regulation of rodent mating behavior, although the hormonal control of sexual motivation and penile erectile function may be similar. From Dickinson, 1949.

**5.25    The typical mating posture of nonhuman primates** is exhibited by copulating rhesus monkeys. In this posture, the female faces away from the male and bends from the waist to reveal her genitalia. The male usually clasps the female around the waist and intromits from the rear as he remains standing. The vaginae of nonhuman primates are located more posteriorly than the vaginal opening of women, making penile entry from the front virtually impossible in these species. Courtesy of Doug Meikle.

also have been observed to engage in numerous sexual postures, including the face-to-face position (Figure 5.26). In fact, most of the copulations observed in captivity (70.1% at the San Diego Zoo) (de Waal, 1987) are face to face. Face-to-face positions are also observed in the wild, but not as often as reported in captivity (29.1%) (Kano, 1992). One hypothesis for this difference is that the observers' presence in the wild disturbs bonobos and induces them to climb trees, where face-to-face copulation is more difficult. Importantly, the female genitalia in bonobos are situated more frontally than in other nonhuman primates, facilitating face-to-face copulations.

### Hormonal Correlates of Primate Male Sexual Behavior

Prepubescent boys do not engage in sexual activities outside of the context of play. After puberty, sexual behaviors are expressed. The average age of onset of masturbation among North American boys is about 13.5 years (Bancroft, 1978). The average age of first intercourse is 17. Frequency of sexual behavior usually peaks during the twenties and slowly declines thereafter throughout life (Figure 5.27). The general pattern of average androgen concentrations found in men of different ages corresponds to these average levels of sexual activity. Blood plasma concentrations of testosterone peak during the mid- and late teen years and remain high throughout much of the twenties. Testosterone concentrations typically diminish as men age, usually showing a sharp decline in the sixth or seventh decade of life. This decline in blood testosterone concentrations mirrors the pattern of male fecundity and sperm counts (Figure 5.28).

   All of these data suggest, but do not prove, that human sexual behavior is influenced by androgens. As you probably already have surmised, there is vast indi-

**5.26 Face-to-face mating in bonobos.** Courtesy of Frans de Waal.

vidual variation in the age of onset of human sexual activities, as well as in the lifelong frequency of sexual behaviors (Figure 5.29). Individual variation in the role of the testes in sexual behavior is also large among human males. The effects of castration on men's sexual behaviors vary from absolutely "no loss of sexual capacities and responsiveness" to a "decrease or total loss" (Money, 1961). In one study of men who were castrated for "treatment" or punishment of sex crimes, there appeared to be three classes of behavioral response. More than half of the men stopped exhibiting sexual behavior shortly after castration. In other words, they responded to castration like a rodent, with a rapid cessation of sexual behavior. The frequency of post-castration sexual behavior decreased more gradually in about one-quarter of the men; in some cases many years elapsed before sexual behavior had completely waned. In these men, castration appeared to hasten the

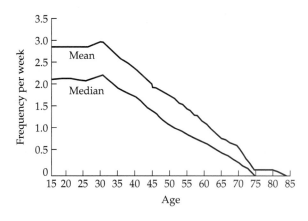

**5.27 The frequency of total male sexual outlet,** including heterosexual, homosexual, and autoerotic activities, peaks in the early 30s and declines thereafter, according to the Kinsey data. Although more recent surveys suggest that the peak frequency has shifted to the mid-20s, it is remarkable that human males continue to engage in sexual behaviors well into their 80s, when plasma levels of testosterone may have fallen substantially. Source: Kinsey et al., 1948.

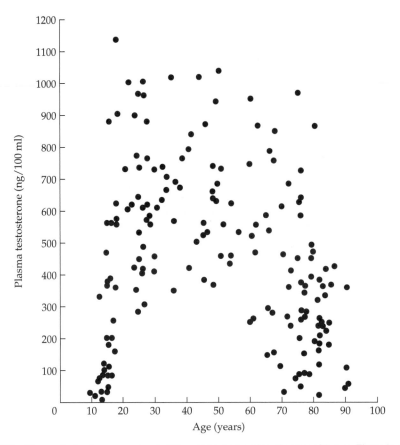

**5.28    Plasma testosterone concentrations in human males** change with age. There is great variation among men in plasma concentrations of testosterone, but the general trend is for testosterone levels to increase during the teens and 20s, stay generally stable until the 60s, and then gradually decrease to prepubertal levels into the 90s. Note, however, that 90-year-old individuals may have plasma testosterone levels comparable to those of many teenage males. Source: Vermeulen et al., 1972.

normal age-related decline in sexual behavior. The frequency of sexual behavior was unchanged after castration for about 10% of the men (Heim and Hursch, 1979). The age at castration accounted for some of the variation in behavioral response; older men appeared to show the greatest reduction in the frequency of post-castration sexual behavior. However, the variation in behavioral responsiveness to castration remains largely unexplained for all vertebrates thus far studied.

Very few studies have directly examined the role of hormones in the sexual behavior of men (Wang and Swerdloff, 1997). One of the best experiments was a double-blind study performed on hypogonadal men at the Stanford Medical Center. These men met the clinical definition of "hypogonadal" because their blood plasma testosterone values were less than 3 ng/ml (Davidson et al., 1982). In the Stanford study, six hypogonadal patients were injected with one of three different substances: (1) 100 mg of a long-lasting androgen called testosterone enanthate dissolved in oil, (2) 400 mg of testosterone enanthate in oil, or (3) the oil

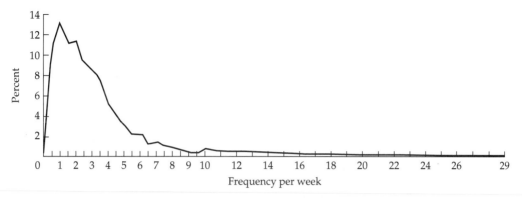

**5.29   Individual variation in weekly frequency of sexual outlet of men.** According to the Kinsey data, most North American men engage in 1–3 sexual acts per week, including heterosexual, homosexual, and autoerotic activities. Less than 1% of men engage in 12 or more sexual events per week. Source: Kinsey et al., 1948.

vehicle alone. Each patient received each of the three treatments in a different order; 6 weeks elapsed between treatments.* The low and high doses of androgens resulted in blood concentrations of about 6 and 15 ng/ml, respectively; the oil treatment did not change plasma testosterone concentrations from the pre-study average of approximately 1.5 ng/ml. The patients kept daily logs of their erotic thoughts, penile erections, and sexual activities. The researchers found that the incidence of erections depended on the dose and timing of androgen treatment. Peak numbers of erections occurred about 1 week after the onset of the high dose of testosterone enanthate (Davidson et al., 1982). Injections of oil alone did not influence sexual thoughts or behaviors. Low doses of testosterone enanthate caused intermediate behavioral effects (Figure 5.30).

Other studies have demonstrated a dose-dependent effect of androgens upon sexual fantasy and subsequent sexual arousal resulting from those erotic thoughts (O'Carroll et al., 1985). Interestingly, chronic monitoring of penile girth revealed that erections occurred normally among hypogonadal men in response to sexual fantasy or viewing erotic films (LaFerla et al., 1978). However, these men did not have spontaneous and nocturnal erections. This study suggests that, in contrast to rats, androgens in men appear to be unnecessary to increase the probability of a sexual response in the presence of the appropriate stimuli.

Does testosterone affect sexual behavior in humans directly, or does it serve as a prohormone, as it does in rodents? The answer is not clear. Testosterone and DHT were equally effective in ameliorating the reduction of sexual activities in

*This study is called "double-blind" because neither the patients nor the investigators knew which treatment the patients were receiving. Recall that Brown-Séquard knew that he was injecting an aqueous solution of testicular tissue into himself, and his beliefs about its potential effects probably influenced his reports of increased abilities. If someone else had injected Brown-Séquard either with androgens or with the inert vehicle in which the steroid hormone would have been dissolved, then the study would have been considered single-blind. That is, the patient would be ignorant of the treatment, but the investigator would be informed. In double-blind studies, neither the subjects nor the researchers are informed, so neither can unconsciously influence the outcome.

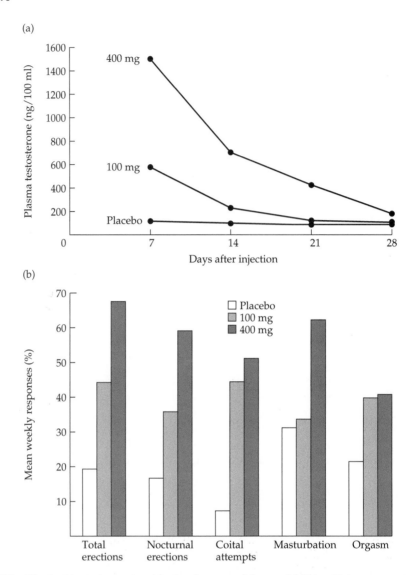

**5.30 Effects of testosterone treatment on hypogonadal men.** (a) Men with low concentrations of blood plasma testosterone (<3 ng/ml) received three injections, 6 weeks apart: a placebo, and low (100 mg) and high (400 mg) doses of testosterone enanthate, both of which temporarily increased plasma testosterone concentrations in a dose-dependent manner. (b) The patients' self-reports indicated that the incidence of erections and certain sexual behaviors also increased in a dose-dependent manner. Source: Davidson et al., 1979.

hypogonadal men. Neither blocking of estrogen receptors in normal men nor treating them with an aromatase inhibitor, a drug that blocks the conversion of androgens to estrogens, influenced their sexual behavior (Gooren, 1985). The results of additional studies have hinted that estrogens may influence sexual behavior in men receiving these steroids for treatment of a variety of diseases, but there has been no conclusive demonstration of an effect of estrogen on sexual behavior in normal human males (reviewed in Meisel and Sachs, 1994).

**TREATMENT OF PARAPHILIAS.**    Despite a lack of data, assertions of a strong link between blood androgen concentrations and human sexual behavior are common, as is the belief that removal of the source of these androgens will diminish human sexual behavior. This belief has found expression in some legal systems that sentence some sex offenders to "chemical castrations" in lieu of prison sentences (for example, State of Michigan v. Roger Gauntlett, 1984). The two most common chemical compounds used for these purposes are medroxyprogesterone acetate (MPA) and cyproterone acetate (CPA). Both substances are used for treatment of sex offenders in Western Europe, but only MPA is currently approved for treatment of aberrant sexual behavior in North America. They are primarily used to treat paraphiliac disorders, in which individuals exhibit atypical sexual behaviors such as heterosexual and homosexual pedophilia, sexual sadism, self-mutilation, self-strangulation (asphyxiophilia), lust homicide, voyeurism, exhibitionism, fetishism, transvestitism, and frotteurism (rubbing against persons or objects for sexual stimulation) (Lehne, 1988).

CPA is a potent anti-androgen that interferes with the binding of androgen to its receptors. MPA reduces plasma concentrations of testosterone in two ways. First, it reduces LH secretion, and decreased LH secretion leads to reduced secretion of testicular androgens. Second, MPA raises the level of specific enzymes in the liver that metabolize testosterone, accelerating its clearance from the blood (Gordon et al., 1970). Blood plasma testosterone concentrations are usually less than 1 ng/ml after 60 days of MPA administration (Meyer et al., 1985).

Many studies have suggested that MPA treatment is effective in reducing paraphiliac activities (Cooper, 1986). Most of these studies were based on self-reports from patients receiving MPA treatment, either voluntary or court-ordered; in other words, former sex offenders were asked whether they continued to engage in their inappropriate sexual behaviors, and, perhaps predictably, most reported in the surveys that they did not. Such studies typically did not use control groups. In one controlled, double-blind study, penile engorgement (measured by a device, called a plethysmograph, that monitors pressure changes) in response to erotic slides was not affected by MPA treatment, despite a 68% reduction in plasma testosterone values. Physiological arousal was similar in patients treated with MPA and with a placebo. However, the patient self-ratings of arousal in response to the erotic slides revealed a *reduction* in self-perceived arousal in response to provocative visual stimuli (Langevin et al., 1979). Most clinicians agree that MPA treatment does not actually "cure" paraphiliac behaviors, but rather reduces the frequency of paraphiliac fantasies. This reduction in fantasy seems to allow the individual to benefit from counseling therapy (Money and Bennett, 1981).

One study reported that blood plasma LH concentrations were higher in men viewing erotic films than in men viewing nature films (LaFerla et al., 1978). The elevated LH concentrations were positively correlated with self-reports of sexual arousal; that is, men who reported that they were highly aroused by the erotic movies had higher LH concentrations than men who reported less arousal.

In another study, rapists and nonrapists watched pornographic movie scenes, and both became sexually aroused when viewing depictions of consensual sex. Similarly, both groups of men became sexually aroused when watching scenes of simulated rape in which the women acted as if they were involuntarily experiencing pleasure. However, the rapists, but not the nonrapists, became sexually aroused when viewing rape scenes in which the women appeared to be experiencing displeasure, pain, or suffering. Thus, rapists and nonrapists do not appear to differ in what activates sexual arousal, but differ in what normally terminates sexual arousal (Abel et al., 1977; Malamuth et al., 1980). Rapists and nonrapists do not differ in their average blood concentrations of androgens, despite a tendency of violent men to have higher average blood values of testosterone than nonviolent men housed in prison (see Chapter 9).

Rapists are reported to be insensitive not only to the suffering of rape victims, but to the feelings of all women (Malamuth et al., 1980). Sexually aggressive men possessing these insensitive attitudes toward women may believe that neutral, or even negative, behaviors exhibited by women actually represent receptive or proceptive behaviors (see Chapter 6). Rapists often report that they believe their victims derive pleasure from a sexual assault (Malamuth et al., 1980). Although castration of rapists has been proposed as a punishment for sexual assaults, recall that this surgery is ineffective in curbing sexual activities in nearly half of the normal men who undergo it. The extent to which androgens permit males to discriminate between receptive and nonreceptive females has not been investigated in humans. Perhaps rapists differ from other men fundamentally, because of hormones, learning, or both, in how their brains process information about sexually receptive behavior in others.

**NONHUMAN PRIMATE STUDIES.**    Investigations of nonhuman primates have not yielded much more specific information about the hormonal regulation of sexual behavior in humans. This lack of progress is due, in part, to the fact that most of the primate species investigated, unlike humans, show large seasonal variations in reproductive function. For example, free-ranging rhesus monkeys exhibit seasonal covariation between sexual behavior and androgen-dependent secondary sex characters, such as scrotal sac color (Vandenbergh, 1969). Also, large, inadequately explained interexperimental variations have been reported in the extent of hormonal influences upon male nonhuman primate sexual behavior.

Generally, free-ranging castrated adult male rhesus monkeys exhibit fewer sexual behaviors than intact males (Wilson and Vessey, 1968). The effects of castration and testosterone replacement therapy on the sexual behavior of adult male rhesus monkeys have also been examined in captive animals. Prior to castration, all of the males exhibited at least one ejaculation during a mating test. Half of the animals ejaculated when tested 6 months after castration, and 30% ejaculated 1 year post-castration. Two of ten males failed to ejaculate after castration. Daily intramuscular injections of testosterone propionate (1 mg/kg) restored mating behaviors to pre-castration levels (Phoenix et al., 1973). This study demonstrates that the hormonal control of sexual behavior in nonhuman primates is similar to the regulation of human sexual behavior; that is, enormous individual variation exists in the extent to which males are dependent upon steroid hormones to initiate mating behaviors. Other studies on nonhuman primate male sexual behavior have revealed the same general outcome (reviewed in Eberhart, 1988).

### Brain Mechanisms of Primate Male Sexual Behavior

As stated previously, rodents have been the primary animal model used in studies of reproductive hormone–behavior relationships. However, rodents differ from humans in many important and fundamental ways. Therefore, experiments that are considered unethical to perform on humans have been performed on nonhuman primates, animals that presumably share more characteristics with humans than do rodents. Studies of the brain mechanisms underlying primate sexual behavior have relied almost exclusively on rhesus monkeys (*Macaca mulatta*) (Eberhart, 1988; Michael et al., 1992; Michael and Zumpe, 1996).

Lesions of the MPOA severely disrupt copulation in male rhesus monkeys. MPOA lesions in primates produce mating deficits that are superficially similar to those observed in MPOA-lesioned rodents, but additional descriptive analyses of the lesioned males revealed that they continue to masturbate, maintain erections, and ejaculate at the same rate as they did prior to the surgery (Slimp et al., 1978). Clearly, destruction of the MPOA in male rhesus monkeys does not abolish the physiological mechanisms underlying sexual arousal, or even possibly sexual performance, but these lesions severely interfere with their ability to copulate with estrous females. As in rodents, the primate MPOA integrates internal and external information relevant to mating behavior. Destruction of the MPOA disables this sensory integration and thus apparently blocks the generation of appropriate sexual behavior in the presence of the appropriate stimuli.

Electrical stimulation of the MPOA causes penile erection in socially isolated male rhesus monkeys (MacLean and Ploog, 1962). Remote electrical stimulation of different brain sites of males living alone and in heterosexual social groups produced various behavioral responses: (1) erections, (2) mounting, and (3) mounting with erections. Of 59 sites within the diencephalic and telencephalic regions of the brain, stimulation of 19 sites, including several hypothalamic areas, evoked erections, but did not affect, or in some instances actually decreased, the number of mounts. Stimulation of 8 sites produced mounting behavior in the absence of erections, whereas 9 sites produced both erections in social isolation and mounts with erections in social groups (Perachio, 1978; Perachio et al., 1973, 1979). Some of the stimulation sites that caused erections also produced behaviors not normally associated with sex, including eating and urination. This finding suggests that "sex centers" were not being activated by the electrical stimulation, but that possibly some general level of arousal was increased.

Chemosensory cues are not as important for successful mating in primates as they are in rodents. Removal of the olfactory bulbs has no effect on rhesus monkey mating behavior (Goldfoot et al., 1978). Lesions that interrupt the function of the amygdala have produced mixed results. The most consistent series of studies on the amygdala's influence upon sexual behavior arose from studies of the Klüver-Bucy syndrome in monkeys. Scientists became interested in the influences of the amygdala and temporal lobe on sexual behavior after reports of so-called hypersexuality in primates in which the temporal lobes had been surgically removed (Klüver and Bucy, 1939). Removal of the temporal lobes removes both the temporal lobe cortices and the underlying limbic structures, including the amygdala. Postoperatively, these monkeys became very docile and fearless. Inappropriate behaviors, including ingestion of inedible material and indiscriminate mounting behavior, were observed. Removal of only the temporal cortex did not produce the Klüver–Bucy syndrome, suggesting that deeper, limbic structures were involved in the hypersexuality (Eberhart, 1988).

Autoradiographic studies of steroid hormone binding in male primate brains have revealed that cells concentrating androgens, estrogens, and progestins are most abundant around the ventricles. That is, the hypothalamus, amygdala, and hippocampus, a bilateral forebrain limbic structure of the temporal lobe, show significant numbers of steroid hormone receptors (Eberhart, 1988; Michael et al., 1995). Thus, the pattern of steroid receptors in the male primate brain closely resembles the pattern found in rodents. In fact, the distribution of sex steroid hormone receptors is a rather conserved feature throughout the evolution of vertebrate brains (Balthazart and Ball, 1992). However, the location of steroid-metabolizing enzymes in neural tissue appears to have changed substantially during the evolution of vertebrates.

Because these initial studies of primates generally agreed with the results of steroid receptor and enzyme labeling studies in rodents, further data on adult primates were not obtained for several years, and subtle differences between primates and rodents may have been missed. For instance, the data for DHT binding came from a single male rhesus monkey (Sheridan et al., 1982), and the data for testosterone binding came from only two males (Bonsall et al., 1985). Although the economy of using the fewest possible animals should be applauded, the danger of this approach is that researchers may accept that steroid binding patterns are identical in disparate groups of animals when the brain regions regulating sexual behavior are only similar. More recent studies have confirmed the patterns of steroid hormone binding and have mapped out the development of these binding sites (for example, Bonsall and Michael, 1992; Michael et al., 1992).

Electrode recording during testosterone treatment of gonadally intact male rhesus monkeys revealed slow, synchronized electrical activity representing patterns of neural firing among groups of neurons in the anterior and posterior hypothalamus, as well as in the mammillary bodies, structures located just behind the hypothalamus. These wave forms appeared to spread to the amygdala and hippocampal regions during the recording session. Synchronization of neural activity in these brain regions was intensified and accelerated after castration (Mangat et al., 1978a,b). In other studies, androgens appeared to change the speed of neural transmission, as well as the pattern of neural firing (Eberhart, 1988).

### Social Influences on Male Sexual Behavior

As we have seen, behavior can feed back to affect hormone concentrations in rodents. Interactions with women can also affect hormone–behavior interactions in men. The scientist who we met in Chapter 1, presumably a little bored, maintained daily records of the weight of his beard trimmings in his electric razor (Anonymous, 1970). He noticed that his beard trimmings were heavier immediately prior to and during his visits to his fiancée than at other times. He attributed the increased beard weight to elevated androgen concentrations induced by sexual anticipation and sexual activity. This demonstration has many flaws as a scientific study, but the general concept that behavior can feed back to affect hormone concentrations has been observed experimentally in several other contexts. A few studies have directly measured androgens prior to, during, or immediately after sexual behavior in men. In one such study, blood plasma concentrations of testosterone increased immediately prior to and after ejaculation during copulation (Fox et al., 1972). In another study, testosterone, as well as DHT and androstenedione, were elevated following masturbation, suggesting that ejaculation per se stimulates steroid hormonal production in men (Purvis et al., 1976). But laboratory studies on steroid hormone–sexual behavior interactions in humans have produced mixed results. Many studies have found no hormonal changes after masturbation or coital ejaculation (for example, Lee et al., 1974; Lincoln, 1974; Stearns et al., 1973).

The endocrine effects of visual erotic stimuli in men were investigated in another study. Fifteen normal adult males viewed either erotic or sexually neutral films. Changes in penile girth, self-reports of arousal, and blood concentrations of testosterone, LH, prolactin, cortisol, ACTH, and β-endorphin were recorded. Sexual arousal, as indicated by both self-assessment and erectile function, was greater in all the men when viewing the erotic than when viewing the neutral films. However, no hormonal changes corresponding to the sexually aroused state were observed (Carani et al., 1990).

### Individual Variation and Aging

Men in their sixties start to show decreases in circulating blood concentrations of androgens (see Figure 5.28). However, approximately one-half of healthy men over 80 years of age have plasma testosterone concentrations in the normal range for men aged 25–59. (Tserotas and Merino, 1998) The mechanisms underlying the enormous variation in the sexual behavior of aging men are unknown. A small proportion of aging males with sexual dysfunction have hormonal deficiencies; however, most do not. If an elderly man complains of impotence, and his blood plasma testosterone concentrations are below 1 ng/ml, then three possible neuroendocrine problems may be responsible: (1) the hypothalamus may not release sufficient GnRH to start the endocrine cascade that normally stimulates testosterone production, (2) the anterior pituitary may not release sufficient gonadotropins, or (3) the Leydig cells may not produce sufficient androgens in response to gonadotropin stimulation. In most cases, men over the age of 60 exhibiting hypogonadal concentrations of androgens also have elevated plasma concentrations of LH, thus indicating a failure of the Leydig cells to produce sufficient steroid hormones to feed back and maintain normal blood concentrations of LH.

As we have seen, there is great individual variation among men in their dependence on steroid hormones for the maintenance of sexual behavior. It has been suggested that male animals are less dependent on hormones for sexual behavior the higher they are on the phylogenetic scale (Beach, 1947). If experiments on different species in which proven copulators are castrated and later examined for mating behavior are compared, the following observations can be made: (1) most rodents and birds show a decrease in sexual behavior immediately after castration, (2) cats also exhibit a striking decline in sexual behavior after castration, and (3) the post-castration sexual behavior of monkeys and humans is very dependent upon prior experience. Dogs typically show no behavioral effects on mating during the first 15 weeks post-castration. But again, the effect of gonadectomy is very dependent on experience even in so-called lower animals. For example, a sexually experienced cat or dog may continue to copulate for a long time after being neutered (Dunbar, 1975; Rosenblatt and Aronson, 1958). Adrenalectomized, castrated dogs may continue to display complete copulatory behavior for years after the surgery, indicating a lack of dependence on steroid hormones for mediation of sexual behavior (Beach, 1970). The extent of individual differences in post-castration mating behavior is great regardless of species; that is, the variation within species is generally as large as that between species in the reliance of sexual behavior on hormones (Hart, 1974).

There is no correlation between blood testosterone concentrations and frequency of sexual behaviors among human males (W. A. Brown et al., 1978). Variation in human masculine behaviors does not correlate with differences in blood androgen concentrations. As described in Chapter 4, there is no reliable difference in blood androgen concentrations between homosexual and heterosexual

---

## Box 5.4
# Sodefrin, a Female-attracting Pheromone in Newts

Recent evidence suggests that amphibians are decreasing in numbers throughout the world. Some suggest that environmental endocrine disruptors are involved, whereas others hypothesize that other types of toxins are affecting reproductive function in these animals. A fungus or other pathogen may also be involved in the declining numbers of amphibians. Whatever the cause of the decline in amphibian populations, it serves as an early warning signal of environmental degradation for humans. We must understand the reproductive physiology and behavior of amphibians in order to understand how they, and we, might be affected by environmental agents.

If given a choice, female newts and salamanders (urodele amphibians) appear to be attracted to water in which a male conspecific was recently courting a female. During courtship, male red-bellied newts (*Cynops pyrrhogaster*) fan the water with their tails. This action tends to move water from the male's cloacal opening to the snout of the female. Females follow these males, and keep their snouts in contact with the male's tail (see figure at top right). Upon close inspection, it was noted that courting males extend small tubules from the cloaca in the presence of females (Kikuyama et al., 1997). These tubules are connected to the abdominal glands. Males without abdominal glands are not successful at courting females (Malacarne et al., 1984). Electrophysiological

recordings of the olfactory nerve showed that the neuroepithelial cells of female crested newts (*Triturus cristatus*) were more active when exposed to male odors or extracts of the male abdominal glands (Cedrini and Fasolo, 1970). Taken together, the evidence suggested that male urodeles were emitting a chemical signal that attracted conspecific females.

In an elegant series of experiments, a team of researchers in Japan has isolated, characterized, localized, and quantified the female-attracting agent (pheromone) in male red-bellied newts (Kikuyama et al., 1995). Using reverse-phase HPLC, they isolated a decapeptide from the abdominal glands of males. This decapeptide, which had no sequence homology with any known peptide, was named sodefrin (Kikuyama et al., 1995).*

When small blocks of sponge were impregnated with sodefrin, the minimal effective concentration to attract females (in 3000 ml of water) was determined to be between 0.1 pM

*The name was derived from two Japanese words prominent in a well-known poem. Nukada (see figure at bottom right) was a famous and beautiful poet who married an emperor. One day, she went out with the emperor to the outskirts of the city, but the emperor's brother, who was once her lover, solicited her by waving (*furu*) his sleeves (*sode*). She responded to his unwanted advances with a poem that loosely translates, "Don't be so bold as to wave your sleeves to me. People will say that we are still in love" (Sakae Kikuyama, personal communication).

men, and it is unlikely that differences in male sexual orientation are due to blood androgen concentrations.

### Peptide Hormones and Male Sexual Behavior

Steroids are the predominant hormones involved in the endocrine regulation of sexual behavior, but other hormones, particularly peptide hormones, appear to modulate their effects (Box 5.4). For example, GnRH has subtle effects on ejacula-

Courtesy of Sakae Kikuyama

and 1.0 pM. A synthetic version was produced, and its effectiveness in attracting females was similar to that of the native peptide (Kikuyama et al., 1997). This peptide appeared to act through the female's olfactory system because females whose nostrils were plugged with cotton and petroleum jelly were not attracted to the sodefrin.

An antibody to sodefrin was made in rabbits, and immunohistochemical and radioimmunoassay techniques were used to locate and measure, respectively, sodefrin in male red-bellied newts (Kikuyama et al., 1997). Sodefrin was primarily located in secretory granules in the apical portion of epithelial cells in the abdominal glands. Castration and hypophysectomy reduced sodefrin concentrations substantially, and testosterone and prolactin replacement therapy prevented this reduction. Testosterone appears to play a more critical role than prolactin in mediating sodefrin concentrations (Toyoda et al., 1994).

This pheromone seems to show species specificity. Sodefrin did not serve as an attractant to female sword-tailed newts (*Cynops ensicauda*), a related species (Kikuyama et al., 1997), and it appears that another pheromone with a different amino acid sequence may act as a chemical attractant in congeneric (belonging to the same genus) species. The sodefrin studies were the first to identify an amphibian pheromone, and the first to discover a peptide pheromone among vertebrate animals (Kikuyama et al., 1995). Because of their diversity, and their potential for small changes in amino acid sequence, other peptides could easily serve as chemical signals conveying species-specific messages.

Courtesy of Sakae Kikuyama

tion latencies in rats (Moss et al., 1975; Myers and Baum, 1980). Elevated prolactin concentrations interfere with male reproductive behavior. Other peptides that have been reported to influence male sexual behavior include vasopressin, oxytocin, and the neurohormones neuropeptide Y and VIP (reviewed in Meisel and Sachs, 1994).

The most consistent reports of peptidergic influences on male reproductive behavior have involved endorphins. Providing male rats with naloxone, an antagonist to endorphins, typically enhances reproductive behavioral performance. If noncopulators, for example, are given either naloxone or saline injections, then nearly three-quarters of the naloxone-treated, but none of the saline-treated animals, mate to ejaculation in subsequent tests (Gessa et al., 1979). Thus, readiness to mate appears inversely correlated with the amount of endorphin receptors available. Recall that sexually inactive male rats are nonreactive to many stimuli and that a tail pinch is very effective in initiating copulatory behaviors (Meisel et al., 1980; Pfaus and Gorzalka, 1987). Opioids appear to affect the dopaminergic systems involved in the release of GnRH and thus subsequently suppress blood concentrations of LH and androgens (Pfaus and Gorzalka, 1987). Opioids, from endogenous or exogenous sources, tend to inhibit male sexual behavior in humans and nonhuman animals (reviewed in Pfaus and Gorzalka, 1987). Chronic heroin use, for example, suppresses plasma testosterone and LH concentrations. Chronic heroin use among human males throughout puberty does not affect later testosterone or LH blood concentrations after heroin use is discontinued (Mendelson and Mello, 1982). This and other studies suggest that a tolerance for opiates, in terms of sexual behavior, does not develop.

## Male Reproductive Behavior in Birds

Reproductive behavior in male birds, both appetitive and consummatory, is highly dependent upon androgens. Males of most avian species engage in some sort of ritualized courtship behavior, and castration eliminates this behavior. Since Berthold's findings regarding castration in roosters (see Chapter 1), many species of birds have been studied. In virtually all species, mating behavior wanes rapidly after castration, and treatment of castrated male birds with androgens restores courtship and mating behaviors (reviewed in Silver et al., 1979; Crews and Silver, 1985). Both testosterone and DHT restore mating behaviors to pre-castration levels in male birds (Adkins and Adler, 1972; Adkins and Nock, 1976; Beach and Inman, 1965; Cheng and Lehrman, 1973; Hutchison, 1970; Silver, 1977). In contrast, male pigeons that congenitally lack testes exhibit little sexual behavior as compared with normal males (Riddle, 1924/1925).

Birds have some minor disadvantages as animal models for the study of hormone–behavior interactions. Blood concentrations of androgens in birds covary with their breeding season; that is, androgen concentrations are typically highest at the beginning of the breeding season and lowest during the early winter (Wingfield and Farner, 1980). These changes in steroid concentrations are linked to seasonal fluctuations in day length (see Chapter 9). Additionally, unlike female rodents, which provide rather consistent behavioral stimuli to males, female birds do not exhibit such rigid consistency. Consequently, the behavior of the male may be less easy to separate from the behavior or responsiveness of the female.

The earliest, and arguably the best, descriptive studies linking testicular steroid hormones with avian reproductive behavior were conducted on ring doves (*Streptopelia risoria*) (Lehrman, 1965). Ring doves, however, may not be an ideal avian model because several features of the endocrine control of behavior may be unique to the species. One such unusual feature is the lack of photoperiodic (day length) effects on the reproductive behavior of male ring doves. Second, ring doves possess a crop sac, a highly specialized adaptation that requires unique hormonal stimulation. Most breeding behaviors in the ring dove have been linked to changes in hormone concentrations (Figure 5.31). However, there is a gradual shift from the aggressive courtship behavior observed early in the courtship sequence to the nest-oriented courtship observed later that does not reflect a change in hormones, but probably reflects testosterone-induced changes in aromatase activity. That is, testosterone directly mediates the aggressive courtship behaviors, but it must be converted in the brain to estrogen to mediate the nest-oriented courtship behaviors (Hutchison and Steimer, 1983).

Japanese quail (*Coturnix japonica*) have also been used as a model species to understand the hormonal control of male avian sexual behavior (Balthazart, 1989; Balthazart and Ball, 1992). These quail provide a useful animal model for investigating hormone–reproductive behavior interactions because they have been selectively bred to mate quickly, and their other reproductive behaviors have waned; for example, in the laboratory these birds no longer incubate their eggs. Consequently, hormonal effects on their sexual behavior can be separated from effects on other reproductive behaviors. When a sexually mature pair of quail is introduced into a neutral mating arena, copulation usually is initiated within 10 seconds. The male grabs the neck of the female, mounts her, and brings his cloacal area into contact with hers (Figure 5.32). The male typically ejaculates during this brief cloacal contact period. After copulation, the male struts around the arena, often with a wing lowered toward the female. He may vocalize or crow. Castration eliminates this copulatory behavior within days, and testosterone therapy restores copulation to pre-castration concentrations. DHT is ineffective in restoring reproductive behavior in castrated quail (Balthazart, 1989).

Studies of Japanese quail have found that testosterone must be converted to estrogen in the POA before it produces an effect on copulatory behavior (Adkins-Regan, 1996). Blocking aromatase activity or estrogen binding prevents androgens from restoring copulatory behavior to pre-castration rates (Adkins-Regan, 1987; Balthazart, 1989). When immunocytochemical techniques are used, the preoptic area, especially the preoptic medial nucleus (POM), which is analogous to the MPOA in mammals, stains positively for estrogen receptors, as well as for cells containing aromatase enzymes (Balthazart and Ball, 1993; Panzica et al., 1996), indicating that androgens are converted to estrogens in these or possibly adjacent cells (Figure 5.33). Other sites where this may occur include the nucleus taeniae, nucleus accumbens, nucleus septalis lateralis, paraventricular nuclei, supraoptic nuclei, inferior hypothalamic nucleus, infundibular hypothalamic nucleus, ventromedial nuclei, intercollicullar nucleus, and substantia grisea nucleus (Adkins-Regan, 1996). Taken together, these data suggest that estrogens might influence behavior by affecting neurotransmitter dynamics, although it remains possible that estrogens influence the growth of neural processes.

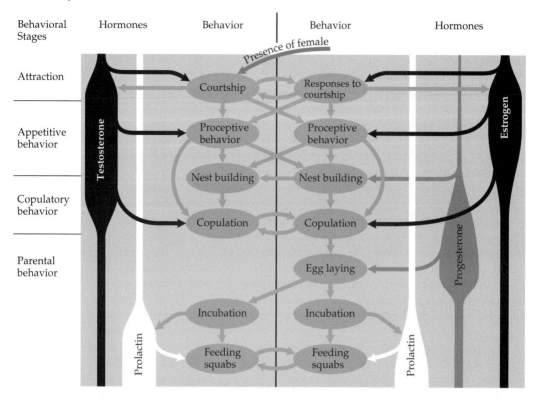

**5.31   Hormonal changes during the reproductive cycle of ring doves** follow a consistent pattern. In females (right), ovarian growth and estrogen secretion coincide with courtship behavior; ovulation and rising progesterone levels induce incubation behavior and suppress bowing and cooing courtship behaviors. Prolactin induces the formation of the crop sac and brood patch and also stimulates parental behaviors. In males (left), testosterone stimulates courtship behavior, and prolactin appears to be involved in incubation and other parental behavior. Testosterone levels decrease and courtship behavior is suppressed during incubation and paternal care. Progesterone does not appear to be involved in male ring dove reproductive behavior. As soon as one cycle is completed in the laboratory setting, a new cycle begins with the onset of courtship behavior. After Rosenzweig and Leiman, 1989.

In quail, as in roosters, crowing is an androgen-dependent behavior, and crowing and copulation occur in close temporal proximity to each other. If a castrated male or a female quail is injected with testosterone, crowing will ensue. Testosterone must be converted to DHT in order to have a behavioral effect on crowing (Adkins and Pniewski, 1978), but, as stated above, testosterone must be converted to estrogen prior to eliciting a copulatory behavioral response. The latter conversion appears to occur only in the brains of males: females injected with testosterone never show the mounting behaviors associated with male copulatory behavior (Adkins and Adler, 1972). Copulation is integrated in the POM, and as described above, the aromatase enzyme, which converts testosterone to estrogen, is present in that brain region. Vocalizations during courtship are probably regulated in the nucleus intercollicularis (ICo), a mesencephalic brain nucleus. This

**5.32   Copulation in Japanese quail** may take only 10 to 15 seconds. In a typical sequence, the male rushes at the female, mounts her, and positions his cloaca against hers. Because female birds do not exhibit rigid consistency from one test to the next, as do female rodents, it is difficult to separate factors associated with male behavior from those resulting from the behavior or responsiveness of the female. Courtesy of Jacques Balthazart.

area of the brain contains the enzyme 5α-reductase, which converts testosterone into 5α-DHT. Thus, the enzymes that produce the behaviorally active metabolites of testosterone responsible for copulatory behavior and for crowing are located in the brain regions that underlie these two separate, but linked, reproductive behaviors (Balthazart and Ball, 1993).

One report has suggested that castration does not affect copulatory behavior in white-crowned sparrows (Moore and Kranz, 1983). These birds breed in the spring when day lengths exceed 12 hours of light per day (see Chapter 9). If prepubescent male white-crowned sparrows are injected with testosterone while maintained under short-day light conditions, they will not mate with receptive females. Exposure to long day lengths appears to activate copulatory behavior in these sparrows permanently. If prepubertal males are castrated and then exposed to long days, they will continue to mate despite a complete lack of assayable testosterone in their blood (Moore and Kranz, 1983). The extent to which male mating behavior in other avian species may be divorced from hormonal control requires further investigation. Other species of sparrows appear to require androgens to elicit copulatory behavior (Balthazart, 1989). The extent to which species or individuals vary in their dependence upon hormones for the maintenance of mating behavior does not seem to have any evident systematic organization.

## Male Reproductive Behavior in Reptiles

Like birds, most male reptiles stop mating after castration (Crews and Silver, 1985). One notable exception is the red-sided garter snake (*Thamnophis sirtalis parietalis*), found on the midwestern Canadian prairies (Mason, 1987). Males of this species emerge from their winter hibernacula several weeks earlier than females, and

(a)

(b)

**5.33 Aromatase and estrogen receptors in the quail brain** shown in camera lucida drawings of sections double-labeled for aromatase and estrogen. Each panel shows an enlarged area of the brain, the location of which is indicated by the insets. (a) Sections of the preoptic area (POA), where only a small proportion of cells expressed both aromatase and estrogen receptor activity. Top left, middle part of the medial preoptic nucleus (POM); top right, POM at the level of the anterior commissure; bottom, caudal POA and septum at the level of the nucleus striae terminalis. (b) One section in the caudal hypothalamus at the level of the nucleus inferioris hypothalami. Solid circles = cells labeled for estrogen receptors; open stars = cells labeled for aromatase; solid stars = cells double-labeled for estrogen receptors and aromatase. From Balthazart et al., 1991.

attempt to mate with females as they emerge. Many males court a single female as she moves out of the hibernaculum (Figure 5.34). Females are much larger than males in this species. The male has two hemi-penes that are inserted into the female's two vaginae. Other males stop courting the female as soon as one male achieves an intromission. Apparently, a chemosensory signal is expressed by the copulating female that inhibits courtship behavior in the other males (Mason et al., 1989); the exact chemical identity of this substance is currently unknown.

Most male animals have an **associated reproductive pattern**. That is, during the breeding season, mating behavior coincides with maximal testis size, as well as maximal androgen concentrations and sperm production. The red-sided garter snake, however, exhibits a **dissociated reproductive pattern** (Crews, 1984, 1991). When the snakes are mating, the testes remain regressed; no sperm or androgens are being produced. The males inseminate females in the spring with sperm stored from the previous autumn. The testes begin to develop, produce androgens, and make sperm *after* all mating behavior has stopped (Figure 5.35). The testes then regress again, and the animal enters hibernation. The sperm are stored in a special organ until the following spring. Thus, copulation normally occurs in the complete absence of circulating steroids. Predictably, castration has no effect on subsequent mating behavior in this species. Removal of the adrenals, another potential source of androgens, or even the pituitary gland also has no effect on mating behavior in these snakes (Camazine et al., 1980; Crews et al., 1984). Neither treatment with steroid hormones nor treatment with gonadotropins affects copulation in this species (Crews, 1984). However, destruction of the MPOA (Krohmer and Crews, 1987) or removal of the pineal gland (Crews et al., 1988b; Nelson et al., 1987) eliminates mating behavior, probably because these two brain regions integrate the environmental information that allows the snakes to ascer-

**5.34  A "mating ball" of male red-sided garter snakes** forms when great numbers of males attempt to court and mate with females, which emerge from the winter hibernaculum several weeks after the males. As soon as one male successfully intromits, the female expresses a chemosignal that disperses the unmated suitors. Courtesy of David Crews.

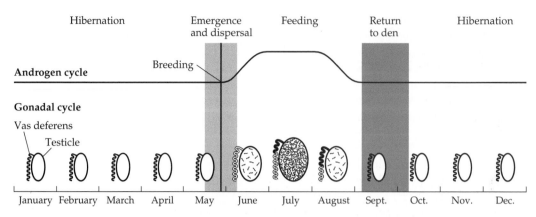

**5.35   Red-sided garter snakes display a dissociated reproductive pattern.** Male red-sided garter snakes emerge from hibernation and mate with females in the spring; however, the testes and vas deferens are regressed during the mating period, and the testes are not producing sperm or androgens. In midsummer, the testes develop and begin producing androgens and sperm. The gonads regress prior to hibernation in the fall, and sperm produced in summer is stored for the mating period in the following spring. After Crews and Gartska, 1982; © 1982 by Scientific American, Inc. All rights reserved.

tain the appropriate season of the year for mating (see Chapter 9). The finding that mating behavior is divorced from hormonal control among these snakes shows that brain size is not a perfect indicator of the independence of sexual behavior from direct hormonal control (cf. Beach, 1947).

Male whiptail lizards of the genus *Cnemidophorus* rely on androgens to regulate their reproductive behavior. Courtship is highly ritualized in this species. The male approaches the female from the rear, climbs onto her back, bites her back or foreleg, then brings his tail underneath her to bring their respective cloacal areas together, forming a so-called "doughnut" posture (Figure 5.36; Crews and Fitzgerald, 1980). The male dismounts after about 10 minutes and leaves the scene.

Some species within the genus *Cnemidophorus* are parthenogenetic; that is, all the members of these species are triploid females, which lay unfertilized eggs that all develop into daughters. These species evolved from hybrids of two sexually reproducing species. Interestingly, the occurrence of "male-like" *behavior* persists in at least five all-female *Cnemidophorus* species. Captive female *C. uniparens* alternate during the breeding season between displaying male-like "pseudosexual" behavior and female behavior. Female "receptive" behavior is observed before ovulation, when estrogen concentrations are relatively high (see Chapter 6); at this time, females allow other females to mount them. Male-like behavior is observed after ovulation, when blood concentrations of progesterone are elevated (Figure 5.37; Crews, 1987); postovulatory females court, mount, and form the doughnut mating posture with periovulatory females. Ovariectomized females injected with progesterone show male-like pseudosexual behavior, and those injected with estradiol show female pseudosexual behavior. Thus progesterone, rather than androgens, apparently mediates male-like behavior in these species.

Why do these parthenogenetic lizards engage in pseudosexual behavior (Crews, 1997)? Functionally, females that undergo mounting and pseudosexual

**5.36 Copulatory behavior in sexual and asexual species of whiptail lizards** is similar. (Left, top to bottom) The copulatory sequence in *Cnemidophorus inornatus,* a sexually reproducing whiptail lizard. The male mounts the female, tucks his hindquarters under the female, and finally bites the female's back and intromits, forming the so-called doughnut posture. (Right, top to bottom) Pseudosexual behavior in *C. uniparens,* a parthenogenetic whiptail species that developed from hybrids of species that reproduce sexually. Although both participants are females, the copulatory sequence closely resembles that of the sexual whiptail species, including the performance of the doughnut posture. This behavior has been found to be necessary to maximize ovulation. From Crews and Fitzgerald, 1980.

mating behavior produce more offspring than females that do not engage in this behavior. Apparently, the act of pseudomating stimulates the release of additional ova. The reciprocal alternation between male-like and female behavior facilitates breeding in these species (Crews, 1987). This seemingly altruistic behavior is to be expected when we recall that asexually reproducing animals share virtually all of their genes in common, so that an individual who helps other females to increase their production of offspring also enhances her own inclusive fitness. These unusual lizards provide a wonderful demonstration that the *structures* of

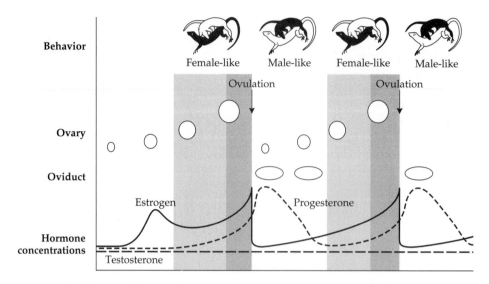

**5.37 Hormones mediate male-like behavior in parthenogenetic whiptail lizards.** Females in parthenogenetic whiptail species alternate in performing the male role during pseudocopulation, and this alternation has clear hormonal correlates. The bottom portion of the figure shows the hormone profile and events in the ovary and oviduct in relation to a hypothetical female alternating between female and male-like behavior (top; black lizard). In the preovulatory state, when estrogen levels are increasing, the female behaves in a female-typical fashion. After ovulation, when her oviducts are full of eggs, blood progesterone levels increase, estrogen levels decrease, and she exhibits male-like pseudosexual behavior. This cycle repeats itself throughout the breeding season. Note that this behavioral alteration has no relation to testosterone levels, which remain constant throughout the cycle, despite the importance of this steroid hormone in mediating male behavior in sexually reproducing whiptail species. The neural substrates of male-like courtship and copulatory behavior have apparently been retained in the parthenogenetic species, but are mediated by progesterone. After Crews, 1987.

hormones do not evolve very much, but rather, new *functions* for the hormones evolve in hormone–behavior interactions (Crews, 1997).

## Conclusions

How do hormones affect male sexual behavior? Based on our discussions of different species, a few generalizations can be made. Sex steroid hormones clearly do not act as a "switch" to activate sexual behavior. The presence of testosterone does not automatically stimulate mating behavior; rather, testosterone, or its metabolites, increases the probability that a sexual behavior will occur in the presence of appropriate stimuli. In both mammals and birds, sex steroid hormones appear to affect sensory input and central nervous system processing, as well as behavioral output. For example, androgens amplify chemosensory information associated with estrous females in the male rodent's brain, allowing further processing of that incoming information (Pfaff and Pfaffmann, 1969; Stern, 1990; Wood, 1997). Steroid hormones are, in turn, affected by environmental stimuli. Peptide hormones also appear to modulate the effects of steroid hormones on sexual behavior. Overall, hormones affect male sexual behavior in many interacting and complicated ways. Several physiological and behavioral systems integrate information in order to enhance the probability of an individual male's reproductive success.

## Summary

• Male sexual behavior consists of all behaviors necessary and sufficient to deliver male gametes to ova. Male sexual behavior can be divided into two phases: the appetitive phase (courtship) and the consummatory phase (copulation).

• Sex drive, the motivation to seek sexual contact, becomes extremely powerful and overtly expressed in males after puberty, when the testes begin to secrete androgens. Sexual performance and copulatory ability increase after puberty as well. Many male animals with seasonal breeding cycles exhibit sexual behavior coincident with maximal testicular secretion of steroid hormones.

• Castration reduces sexual behavior in some proportion of individuals of virtually all vertebrate species examined. However, there is great individual and species variation in the extent to which sexual behavior is regulated by hormones. Testosterone treatment generally reverses the decreased frequency of male sexual behavior observed after castration. More testosterone is necessary to restore sexual behavior in castrated males after it has ceased than is required to maintain male sexual behavior.

• There are three components of male rodent sexual behavior: mounting, intromission, and ejaculation. Corresponding penile responses—erections, flips, and cupping—can be elicited from animals independently from higher brain influences. Testosterone does not seem to regulate sexual behavior or penile reflexes directly, but rather acts as a prohormone; metabolic products of testosterone, namely, estrogens and dihydrotestosterone (DHT), appear to be important in mediating copulatory behaviors and penile sensitivity, respectively.

• An intact chemosensory system is necessary for the proper function of sexual behavior in rodents. Lesions along the neural circuit that mediates olfactory information, from the olfactory bulbs to the amygdala to the medial preoptic area of the hypothalamus (MPOA), result in diminished sexual behavior. Electrical stimulation along this circuit increases the frequency of sexual behavior in male rodents.

• The MPOA appears to be crucial for integrating sensory and internal stimuli in order for normal copulation to occur. Destruction of the MPOA eliminates copulatory behaviors in virtually all vertebrate males. Implantation of minute amounts of testosterone into the MPOA restores mating behavior in castrated males. Testosterone must be converted to estrogen in order to have a behavioral effect; DHT implanted into the brain does not stimulate copulation. Mapping the distribution of steroid hormone receptors and aromatase activity has helped to pinpoint exactly where in the brain hormones act to regulate male sexual behavior. The use of mice with targeted deletions of specific genes has yielded some novel, and in some cases, contradictory, information about hormone–behavior interactions underlying male sexual behavior.

- Females can affect hormone concentrations in males, and can also affect the frequency and timing of their copulatory behaviors. The Coolidge effect is one well-known example in which novel females have substantial effects on the reproductive behavior of males. Plasma concentrations of LH and testosterone increase in males after exposure to females. This elevation in hormone concentrations can be classically conditioned.

- Individual differences exist in the frequency of sexual behavior exhibited by males. This difference in sexual activity does not appear to correlate with blood androgen concentrations.

- The sexual behavior of men does not seem to be as dependent upon blood androgen concentrations as in some other taxa. However, there is great variation in the frequency of post-castration sexual activities among men. Hypogonadal men treated with a long-lasting androgen showed increases in several sexual behaviors and thoughts, indicating that androgens can affect sexual behavior in humans.

- The copulatory behaviors of men cannot be classified according to muscular reflexes as in other animals. Other male primates exhibit stereotyped mating positions. Androgens are important in maintaining nonhuman male primate mating behavior.

- The same brain regions underlying rodent sexual behavior appear to be involved in the hormonal mediation of primate sexual behavior, with the exception of the olfactory system.

- Female primates, like female rodents, affect sexual behavior and hormone concentrations in males, but systematic studies comparable to the experiments with rodents are, for the most part, lacking.

- Opioids appear to inhibit sexual behavior, especially with chronic exposure, whereas treatment with opioid antagonists appears to facilitate the expression of sexual behavior.

- Birds, like rodents, appear to require androgens to maintain sexual behavior. Androgens are converted to estrogens in the preoptic medial nucleus (POM) to mediate copulatory behavior, or to DHT in other regions to mediate vocalizations.

- Most male reptiles stop breeding after castration, and mating behavior is restored by androgen replacement therapy. Red-sided garter snakes, however, engage in copulatory behavior when the testes are regressed and no circulating androgens can be detected. The independence of male copulatory behavior from hormone levels in these snakes provides strong evidence that not only animals with a highly developed brain copulate without the presence of androgens.

- Individuals of female parthenogenetic lizard species engage in male-like behavior in order to increase the number of ova shed during ovulation. Although male copulatory behaviors in related sexual species are regulated by androgens, similar behaviors are mediated by progesterone in the all-female species.

## Questions for Discussion

1. Discuss the following assertion: "Hormones play a lesser role in the mediation of male sexual behavior in primates than they do in rodents."

2. Androgens cause sexual behavior in males. Is this statement really true? Defend your answer.

3. Should the goal of studying human or nonhuman sexual behavior be to gain control of human sexual behavior?

4. If you were put in charge of a large study to examine hormonal influences on the sexual behavior of men, how would you design your study? What would you measure?

5. What is sexual behavior? What behaviors do you think can reasonably be called sexual behavior in the following species: male rats, ring doves, and humans?

## Suggested Readings

Adkins-Regan, E. 1996. Neuroanatomy of sexual behavior in the male Japanese quail from top to bottom. *Poultry and Avian Biology Reviews,* 7: 193–204.

Bullough, Vern L. 1994. *Science in the bedroom: A history of sex research.* Basic Books, New York.

Crews, D., and Silver, R. 1985. Reproductive physiology and behavior interactions in nonmammalian vertebrates. In N. T. Adler, D. Pfaff, and R. W. Goy (eds.), *Handbook of Behavioral Neurobiology,* Vol. 7, *Reproduction,* pp. 101–182. Plenum Press, New York.

Hull, E. M., Du, J., Lorrain, S., and Matuszewich, L. 1997. Testosterone, preoptic dopamine and copulation in male rats. *Brain Research Bulletin,* 44: 327–333.

Meisel, R. L., and Sachs, B. D. 1994. The physiology of male sexual behavior. In E. Knobil and J. D. Neill et al. (eds.), *The Physiology of Reproduction,* Vol. 2, pp. 3–105. Raven Press, New York.

Michael, R. P. and Zumpe, D. 1996. Biological factors in the organization and expression of sexual behaviour. In I. Rosen (ed.), *Sexual Deviation,* pp. 452–287. Oxford University Press, Oxford.

Sachs, B. D. 1995b. Placing erection in context: The reflexogenic-psychogenic dichotomy reconsidered. *Neuroscience and Biobehavioral Reviews,* 19: 211–224.

Stone, C. P. 1922. The congenital sexual behavior of the young male albino rat. *Journal of Comparative Psychology,* 2: 95–153.

# 6

# Female Reproductive Behavior

My wife's family owns a beautiful Chesapeake Bay retriever named Molly. Nowadays, Molly is an ideal pet; she is quiet, well-behaved, and obeys commands. But she had once exhibited behavior that was unusual—even somewhat frenzied. She routinely whimpered, barked, and howled. When she was inside the house, she frequently tried to bolt outside whenever a door was opened. If she was left in the yard unattended, she continually tried to leap over the fence. If she was in the yard with her owners and they opened the gate, Molly raced away, ignoring their pleas and commands. When Molly escaped the confines of her yard, she always headed west, toward the home of a male dog that lived in the neighborhood, instead of her preferred route toward the bay. Molly's atypical behavior had been the result of her being in "heat," or

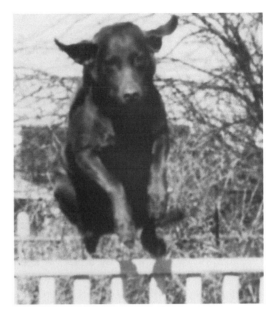

**6.1    Estrous females are motivated to seek males.**
High circulating estrogen concentrations increase the motivation of females to engage in sexual behavior. This estrous Chesapeake Bay retriever is shown jumping a fence to visit a neighboring male dog; she does not behave in this manner when not in estrus. Courtesy of Brigid DeVries.

**estrus**. The word *estrus* comes from the Latin word *oestrus*, which loosely translates, "in a frenzy, or possessed by the gadfly" (Feder, 1981). Many pet owners have experienced a dog or cat in "heat" and are often surprised by the intensity of effort displayed by their pets to mate (Figure 6.1). In a laboratory setting, an estrous rat will cross a highly charged electrified floor to gain physical access to a male (Warner, 1927); female rats in estrus will also diligently depress a lever or poke their noses through an opening many times in order to gain access to a male (Bermant, 1961; Matthews et al., 1997). Female rats (or dogs) that are not in estrus will not sustain pain or exert much effort to interact with males. The ovaries are involved in the expression of estrous behavior in rats and dogs. Since she was spayed (ovariectomized) last year, Molly no longer displays estrous behavior.

Other differences between estrous and **anestrous** (not in estrus) females are striking. First, a female in estrus will seek out males, initiate copulation, and prefer to remain in close proximity to males; the same female will not engage in these behaviors when not in estrus. Second, estrous females are more attractive to males than anestrous females; that is, conspecific males prefer to visit, and exert more effort to maintain close proximity to, estrous rather than anestrous females. Third, males mount estrous females preferentially as compared with anestrous females. Finally, only estrous females will permit mating to occur. Anestrous females will not tolerate male mounting behavior; in fact, anestrous females of many mammalian species will inflict serious injuries upon persistent male suitors.

What physiological changes are occurring to evoke these dramatic changes in a female's behavior as she cycles between an estrous and an anestrous state? Briefly, the hormones associated with maturation of her ova (eggs) have also evolved to affect her nervous system in a number of ways. The resulting neural changes influence her behavior in such a way that the probability of mating, and ultimately the successful production of offspring, is increased. Thus, mating behavior is tightly coupled in time with ovulation, and it occurs when successful fertilization of ova is most likely. Although analyses of the evolution of hormonal regulation of female sexual behavior are intriguing, the focus of this chapter will be the proximate endocrine mechanisms underlying sexual behavior in females.

As we have seen in the case of males, reproductive hormones do not "turn on" sexual behavior per se; rather, hormones change the probability that specific stimuli will elicit particular behaviors that lead to successful copulation. Hormones affect the input systems: the acuity, sensitivity, and efficiency of the sensory systems are enhanced by reproductive hormones. Consequently, estrous females are better able than anestrous females to detect and respond to conspecific males. The central nervous system is also affected by the endocrine changes associated with estrus. Females' motivation, attention, and perception change as sex steroid levels fluctuate. Finally, because effectors are also affected by hormones, the way that a female moves and reacts to stimuli also changes. Her behavior, as well as the stimuli she emits (for example, chemosensory agents or auditory signals), affects the way males behave; the males' behavior may also feed back to alter the endocrine state of the female further.

As described previously, sexual behavior is behavior that has evolved to bring the two gamete types together. Female sexual behavior is defined as all behaviors necessary and sufficient to achieve fertilization of female gametes (ova) by sperm. Sex drive provides a powerful motivational force urging females to seek sexual union, just as it does in males. Until recently, however, sexual motivation was not emphasized in studies of female mating behavior. Although male sexual behavior has been the subject of research for much longer than female sexual behavior, in some ways a more detailed understanding of the hormonal correlates and neural bases of sexual behavior has been achieved for females (Blaustein, 1996). For example, most of the neural circuitry underlying one female reproductive behavior—namely, lordosis, the reflexive mating posture of female rats—as well as the specific effects of hormones on this circuit have been elucidated (Pfaff et al., 1994; Micevych et al., 1997).

Female reproduction typically occurs in cycles. Mammalian female reproduction has six components: courtship, mating, ovulation, pregnancy, parturition, and lactation (Everett, 1961). This chapter will be limited to behavior associated with the first three components of female reproduction; the latter three components will be reviewed in Chapter 7, which discusses parental care. In common with the studies on males presented in Chapter 5, most of what we know about the physiological mechanisms underlying female sexual behavior has been gained through studies on nonhuman animals, especially rodents, and examples of such studies will be described below. But first, efforts to understand female sexual behavior will be presented from a historical perspective, and then female sexual behavior and reproductive cycles will be described. The last part of the chapter is devoted to experimental and correlational data relating hormones and female sexual behavior.

## Early Discoveries about Female Sexual Behavior

Remarkably little progress was made in the study of female sexual behavior until the 20th century. It is difficult to discern whether this lack of progress was due to the inherent complexity of female sexual behavior or merely reflected a lack of interest on the part of a predominantly male research community that assumed that females are passive participants in copulation (but see Beach, 1976). A possible practical impediment to research is that ovariectomy is a difficult operation compared with removal of the testes.* In any event, prior to 1900, there were relatively few studies on the effects of female gonadectomy on behavior, in contrast to the wealth of information already available regarding the behavioral effects of male castration. However, in all the early studies, as well as in most subsequent ones, the results were quite consistent: most adult female mammals stop mating behaviors immediately after the removal of the ovaries (reviewed in Beach, 1948).[†] The development of ideas and methodologies associated with studies of hormonal correlates of female sexual behavior paralleled the studies on male sexual behavior presented in the previous chapter.

A major complicating factor in understanding the physiological mechanisms underlying female sexual behavior is the cyclic nature of such behavior. Adult males are generally able to mate any time they encounter an estrous female during the breeding season, but females of many mammalian species, especially those commonly used in laboratory research, enter and leave estrus on a regular basis. For instance, if a female Syrian hamster (*Mesocricetus auratus*) is placed in a cage with a vasectomized male for a short period each night, she will allow copulation every fourth night. Her **estrous cycle** is thus said to be 4 days in length. If the male were not vasectomized and copulation continued until ejaculation, her eggs would be fertilized, and she would not display estrous behavior again for 16 days, until immediately postpartum (that is, after giving birth). Sustained copulation, even with a vasectomized male, would activate the formation of specific ovarian structures that would also disrupt the display of 4-day estrous cycles. The nature of this disruption, termed pseudopregnancy, will be described later in this chapter.

### The Development of the Vaginal Cytological Assay

Because estrous cycles stop after ovariectomy, it was surmised that the cycles in estrous behavior reflected cycles in ovarian function, but at the turn of the 20th century, it was difficult to discern these cyclic ovarian changes without surgical intervention. In most cases, after behavioral observations were made, the ovaries were removed and histologically fixed for microscopic examination, and the behavior was correlated with the presence or absence of different ovarian structures, such as follicles or corpora lutea (see Chapter 2). Only limited data could be obtained in this manner. Repeated behavioral tests could not be performed in the same animals because the behavior in question stopped after ovariectomy. Consequently, the first breakthrough in understanding the cyclicity of female sexual behavior was the technical development of noninvasive external markers that reliably reflected ovarian activity. The demonstration by Stockard and Papanicolaou (1917) that changes in vaginal cytology (cell types) could be closely correlated with changes in ovarian function in guinea pigs was an extremely important advance in the study of female reproductive behavior and physiology.

---

*In the context of females, the terms ovariectomy, gonadectomy, and castration all mean removal of the ovaries.

[†]Humans and rhesus monkeys are exceptions to this general rule, as we will see below.

This technique was soon extended to mice (Allen, 1922) and rats (Long and Evans, 1922), and eventually to hundreds of species (Asdell, 1964; Rowlands and Weir, 1984). This powerful tool allowed researchers to correlate mating behavior with vaginal cell types, and thus with ovarian function, without direct surgical examination of the ovaries.

The technique for assessing changes in vaginal cytology is rapid and straightforward. A modified version of this histological test, in which cells from the cervix (instead of the vaginal lumen, or opening) are obtained and examined, is part of every woman's annual medical examination and is commonly called the Pap test, after Dr. Papanicolaou. In rodents, the procedure consists of swabbing cells from the vaginal lumen after lavage (sterile wash), then examining these cells microscopically. When applied to rats, this method reveals changes in the cellular contents of the vaginal lumen that recur every 4 or 5 days (Figure 6.2; Long and Evans, 1922).* At one point in the cycle "cornified" epithelial cells are present; these cells look like cornflakes under the microscope. This stage, which lasts about 36 hours, is arbitrarily considered the first stage of the cycle and is called **vaginal estrus**. Vaginal estrus is followed by a period during which cornified cells become reduced in number, and leukocytes (white blood cells), as well as a few nucleated epithelial cells, appear. This stage is called **vaginal diestrus**, and has a duration of approximately 48 hours. The first day of diestrus is referred to as diestrus I, and the second day is often called diestrus II.[†] The next phase is characterized by the presence of many nucleated epithelial cells, as well as a dramatic reduction in the number of leukocytes. This final stage is called **vaginal proestrus**, and lasts for about 12 hours. An obvious external marker of vaginal proestrus is that the thin vaginal membrane disappears, revealing a patent (open) vaginal canal. This external marker coincides with the onset of mating behavior.

These changes in vaginal cell types were soon correlated with ovarian changes (Figure 6.3; see also Figure 2.13). When researchers took vaginal smears from rats, then removed the ovaries from the same individuals, fixed them histologically, and examined them under a microscope, they found that the following correlations between changes in vaginal cell types and ovarian activity could be made (Boling et al., 1941; Feder, 1981):

1. Vaginal estrus is correlated with the presence of recently ruptured follicles following ovulation. Also, tertiary follicles begin to develop from secondary follicles at this time. The next wave of ova released by the ovaries will eventually appear from these tertiary follicles after they fully develop. The antrum of each tertiary follicle is small at this stage. The granulosa cells, the epithelial cells surrounding the follicle, induce the formation of a distinct layer of connective tissue called the theca interna.

2. As the vaginal smear becomes diestrous, the tertiary follicles become larger and the granulosa cells become more numerous. Also, the antrum begins to fill with a clear fluid called the liquor folliculi. The

---

*For the sake of simplicity only 4-day cycles will be considered here, but it is important to note that among rats there are either 4-day or 5-day cycles, but no 4.5-day cycles (see below).

[†]Older studies sometimes refer to diestrus I as "metestrus." The 5-day rat estrous cycle includes an additional 24 hours of diestrus, called diestrus III.

**6.2 Cyclic changes in vaginal cell types** can be observed in the vaginal wall and in cells obtained from daily vaginal lavage. During vaginal estrus, cornified epithelial cells are present for about 36 hours. Vaginal estrus is followed by vaginal diestrus, which lasts for about 48 hours in females displaying 4-day estrous cycles; this stage is marked by the appearance of leukocytes and a few nucleated epithelial cells, as well as a decrease in the number of cornified cells. The first day of diestrus is called diestrus I, and the second is called diestrus II. The final stage of the estrous cycle is called vaginal proestrus and lasts about 12 hours. Vaginal proestrus is characterized by an increase in the number of nucleated epithelial cells, as well as a sharp decrease in the number of leukocytes. After Wang, 1923; Feder, 1981; Ganong, 1995; Norris, 1996. Photomicrographs courtesy of Deborah Drazen.

rupture sites where previous ovulations occurred have been repaired, and endocrine luteal cells surround the fluid-filled cavities of the former follicles to form corpora lutea.

3. By diestrus II, the layer of connective tissue surrounding the theca interna differentiates into a layer of spindle-shaped cells called the theca externa. The enlarging tertiary follicles are now referred to as Graafian follicles. The corpora lutea are fully formed; the inner cavity has been filled with endocrine luteal cells and their supporting blood and connective tissues.

4. As the vaginal cell cycle becomes proestrous, a growth spurt occurs in the Graafian follicles destined to ovulate (preovulatory swelling). Other follicles that are not going to ovulate regress. The corpora lutea also regress unless specific vaginal stimuli associated with intromission are experienced by the female.

When ovulation occurs, the cycle begins anew—unless the female mates. If she receives sufficient vaginal stimulation through copulation or simulated copulatory stimuli, then the corpora lutea do not regress. If the mating is fertile and the female becomes pregnant, then the corpora lutea remain large throughout most of the pregnancy. If the mating is sterile and the female does not become pregnant, then the corpora lutea remain large for approximately 14 days before regressing. Because it causes a number of physiological changes that resemble those of pregnancy, this state of sustained corpora luteal function is called pseudopregnancy (see below). The estrous cycles are suspended during pregnancy or pseudopregnancy.

| Time of day | 1400 | 1400 | 1400 | 1400–1800 |
|---|---|---|---|---|
| Hours after ovulation | 12 | 36 | 60 | 84–88 |
| | Estrus | Diestrus I | Diestrus II | Proestrus |
| Vaginal lavage | | | | |
| | Primary corpus luteum | Primary follicle | Secondary follicle | Graafian follicle |
| Follicular development | | | | |
| Sexual behavior | — | — | — | + |

**6.3 Cyclic changes in ovarian structure** have been correlated with cyclic changes in vaginal cytology. Vaginal estrus occurs after ovulation and corresponds with the formation of corpora lutea. Luteal function wanes rapidly in the absence of stimuli associated with mating, and the corpora lutea regress. New follicles begin to develop during diestrus I and diestrus II. Vaginal proestrus coincides with maximal follicular development; behavioral estrus and mating occur during vaginal proestrus. After Feder, 1981.

The linkage of vaginal cytology to ovarian structural changes enabled researchers to make a very good guess about ovarian function simply by observing cells obtained from the vaginal lumen. As these studies continued, other research was proceeding that linked mating behavior with vaginal cell type changes (see Figure 6.3). A classic monograph by Long and Evans (1922) provided an excellent description and partial quantification of the sexual behavior of female rats correlated with vaginal cytology. Long and Evans found that mating behavior is observed only when the vaginal smear shows many nucleated epithelial cells; in other words, as noted above, behavioral estrus coincides with vaginal *proestrus*. Female rats generally stop mating by the time *vaginal estrus* occurs. This unfortunate duplicity of terms has confused students for decades. Remember that behavioral estrus coincides with vaginal proestrus; vaginal estrus follows behavioral estrus.

As a result of these studies, vaginal cycles in cell types could be correlated with cycles of estrous behavior, and thus, logically, estrous behavior could be correlated with ovarian function through observations of vaginal cytology. Because both the cycles of vaginal cytology and of estrous behavior stop after ovariectomy, researchers reasoned that the ovaries must produce a cyclic signal that drives the changes in both vaginal cell types and behavior. Because the cycles continue if the ovaries are denervated, it was reasoned that hormones must be mediating the cyclic signal. The next part of the puzzle involved understanding the endocrine products associated with the various ovarian structural changes. Relating these endocrine changes to behavioral alterations provided the framework for the modern era of female sex research (Beach, 1981).

### Research in the "Modern Era"

The two ovarian structures that were considered most likely to be producing hormones that influenced estrous behavior were the follicles and corpora lutea. Researchers tested these hypotheses by injecting laboratory animals with extracts from ovaries obtained from slaughterhouses. When chemical extracts derived from the follicles of hog ovaries were injected into ovariectomized mice, they caused four physiological changes that are normally observed in estrous female rodents: hyperemia (vascular development) of the reproductive tract, uterine growth, hypersecretion in the genital tract, and growth of the mammary glands (Allen and Doisy, 1923). Mating behavior was also observed in ovariectomized mice injected with the chemical extract from ovarian follicles. These four physiological changes, as well as the presence of mating behavior, served as important bioassays in the attempts to isolate and identify endocrine products from the ovarian follicles.

The substance in the follicles that produced these effects was called an estrogen, a generic term for "estrus-generating substances." Estrogens were the first steroid hormones to be chemically isolated when Doisy and co-workers (1929) and Butenandt (1929) independently succeeded in crystallizing the first known estrogenic material, now known as estrone, from the urine of pregnant women. Isolation of estrogens directly from ovarian tissue occurred a few years later (Doisy and MacCorquodale, 1936), using hormone isolation techniques that are quite crude by today's standards. For example, MacCorquodale obtained approximately 12 milligrams of relatively pure estradiol-17β by processing over 3800 kg

(4 tons) of sows' ovaries! However, the availability of even small amounts of these relatively pure hormones ushered in a new era for behavioral endocrinology and allowed the first direct correlations to be made between hormones and behavior.

Researchers soon established the role of estrogens in stimulating female sexual behavior. It was found that the fluid within the Graafian follicles is rich in estrogenic hormones, which are secreted into the general blood circulation. Rapidly increasing estrogen concentrations during the day of proestrus induce behavioral estrus, as well as cornification of vaginal epithelial cells. These findings were originally reported in mice (Allen and Doisy, 1923; Allen et al., 1924; Wiesner and Mirskaia, 1930), rats (Boling and Blandau, 1939), and guinea pigs (Dempsey et al., 1936). However, although estrogen injections induced estrous behavior in most ovariectomized rodents, in all these early studies a substantial minority (approximately 40%) of ovariectomized females failed to mate after estrogen treatment, regardless of dosage (Ring, 1944). It should be noted that the doses of estrogen provided in these studies were typically in a pharmacological, rather than physiological, range. The observation that many animals did not mate even after receiving large doses of estrogen prompted several researchers to suggest that a supplemental factor might be working in concert with estrogen to induce behavioral estrus (Wiesner and Mirskaia, 1930).

When chemical extracts from corpora lutea, also obtained from slaughterhouses, were injected into ovariectomized rabbits, it was found that they effectively prepared the uterus for pregnancy and maintained pregnancy (Corner and Allen, 1929). The luteal steroid hormone responsible for these effects was called progesterone, so named because it produced a progestational condition (i.e., supportive of pregnancy) in the uterus. Progesterone was identified and isolated from ovarian tissue in the mid-1930s (Turner and Bagnara, 1971). It was not identified initially in urine because pregnanediol, the urinary metabolite of progesterone, is biologically inactive and thus difficult to quantify with bioassays.

Progesterone was discovered to be the supplemental factor that operates in concert with estrogen to induce behavioral estrus. In a series of papers, Young and his collaborators (for example, Dempsey et al., 1936; Young et al., 1935, 1938, 1939) demonstrated that estrogen alone was insufficient to produce behavioral estrus in guinea pigs. Because one of the ovarian changes associated with the onset of estrus is preovulatory swelling, and because injections of luteinizing hormone (LH) cause preovulatory swelling, Young and his associates reasoned initially that LH was the substance acting in concert with estrogen to cause estrus. However, subsequent experimentation revealed that LH does not act directly with estrogen to cause behavioral estrus. Rather, LH causes the formation of corpora lutea; in turn, the developing corpora lutea secrete progesterone, which acts synergistically with estrogen to cause behavioral estrus (Dempsey et al., 1936).

Progesterone exerts biphasic effects on sexual behaviors, and these biphasic effects appear to differ among species. Initially, studies reported that progesterone was important, although not required, for causing behavioral estrus in rats (Boling and Blandau, 1939) and a number of other species as well (Ring, 1944). Subsequently, progesterone has been discovered to be important in mediating estrous behavior during natural estrus in rats (Feder, 1981). However, Ball (1941) reported that progesterone administered to estrogen-primed, ovariectomized monkeys decreased sexual behavior. This counterintuitive finding was explained when it was eventually discovered that progesterone has biphasic actions on female mating behavior. First, progesterone, in concert with estradiol, initiates female sexual behavior in rats. This preovulatory progesterone comes from the Graafian follicles. As the cycle continues after copulation and estrogen concentrations fall, the corpora lutea secrete larger amounts of progesterone, and elevated concentrations of progesterone in the blood inhibit female sexual behavior. The importance of progesterone in sexual behavior varies among species, as we will see below.

In rats and certain other rodent species, elevated estrogen secretion accompanies follicular development during diestrus II and proestrus, and stimulates cornification of vaginal epithelial cells as well as estrous behavior. As just described, progesterone is also needed for the full expression of female sexual behavior in many species. In several rodent species, including rats, mice, guinea pigs, and hamsters, progesterone concentrations increase abruptly prior to ovulation to induce mating behavior. After ovulation, the corpora lutea secrete progesterone at high rates, which often serves to terminate estrous behavior. The neural and endocrine events that drive this cycle of estrogen and progesterone secretion, and thus drive the cycle of estrous behavior, will be described later in the chapter. But first, a description of female mating behavior, as observed in the laboratory, will be presented.

## Mammalian Female Mating Behavior: A Description

### Rodents

If an adult female rat is placed with an adult vasectomized male in a typical laboratory cage for 30 minutes every evening, a very consistent behavioral pattern will emerge (Long and Evans, 1922). Every fourth (or fifth) night, the female will be in behavioral estrus. The most prominent aspect of her estrous behavior is the assumption of the mating posture called **lordosis** (Figure 6.4), a name derived from a medical term that refers to curvature of the spine. When touched on or near the flanks, an estrous female rat will arch her back, deflect her tail, and stand completely immobile to aid the male's penile insertion. In the absence of lordosis, intromission and ejaculation are impossible (Figure 6.5; Diakow, 1974; Pfaff et al., 1978). In order to initiate or maintain mounting behavior by the male, she may approach him, then dart away. Hopping a short distance away, waiting, moving back, and wiggling the ears (actually, moving the head rapidly makes the ears appear to wiggle) are all behaviors that male rats find very attractive, and males are motivated to follow and usually mount a female performing these behaviors (Figure 6.6). After an intromission, the female will leave the mating posture, groom herself or the male, walk about the test arena, or perhaps rest.

Mice, hamsters, voles, lemmings, and many other rodent species display patterns of female copulatory behavior similar to those of rats . However, guinea pigs differ strikingly from other laboratory rodents in the latency to ejaculation (Young et al., 1938, 1939). Male guinea pigs mount females, intromit, and ejaculate immediately; there is no pelvic thrusting (see Chapter 5). Consequently, it is not necessary for female guinea pigs to display lordosis for sustained periods of time, although they may maintain the lordosis posture for over 4 seconds in response to

(a)

(b)

**6.4   Lordosis,** the characteristic mating posture of estrous female rodents, as seen in (a) rats and (b) Syrian hamsters. Lordosis occurs in response to tactile stimulation of the flanks and anogenital region, usually provided by a mounting male; in (b), the female exhibits lordosis in response to the male's investigation of her anogenital region, and his previous tactile stimulation of her flanks. During lordosis, the female arches her back and deflects her tail to allow a male to gain intromission; in the absence of this posture, a male can not copulate successfully. The female will maintain the lordosis posture for some time after a male has dismounted. Photograph in (a) courtesy of Robert Meisel; (b) courtesy of Robert E. Johnston.

male mounting behavior in the laboratory, and if stimulated by manual palpation, may maintain lordosis for 10–20 seconds (Goy and Young, 1956/1957).

### Canines

Female mammals in estrus have often been portrayed as "out of control" because they appear to be indiscriminate about their mating partners, but part of this portrayal results from the laboratory testing situations used, especially for rodents. Dogs, and many other mammalian species (especially primates), display substantial selectivity when in estrus (LeBoeuf, 1967). An estrous dog may absolutely refuse to mate with a male to whom she is not attracted, and there is substantial individual variation among female dogs in mate choice. Females may or may not

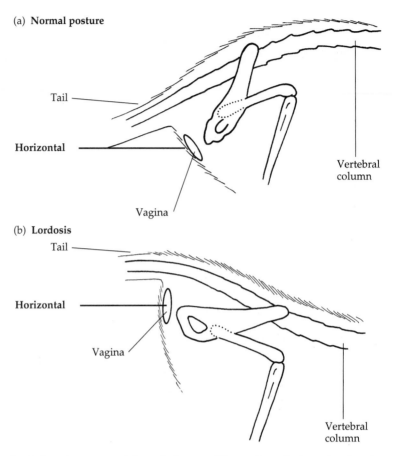

(a) **Normal posture**

Tail

**Horizontal**

Vertebral column

Vagina

(b) **Lordosis**

Tail

**Horizontal**

Vagina

Vertebral column

**6.5 Lordosis makes successful copulation possible,** as shown in these drawings based on x-ray images of female rats. (a) When the female is standing in her normal posture, it is impossible for the male to intromit, but during lordosis (b), the vaginal opening is accessible and the vagina is horizontal. Because rats have no manual dexterity, this precise postural adjustment on the part of the female is necessary for the male to successfully intromit. After Pfaff et al., 1978.

choose their mates by rank in the pack; the alpha males of domestic canine packs do not appear to possess mating advantages over lower-ranked dogs (Beach and LeBoeuf, 1967).

An estrous dog is likely to seek out males to whom she is attracted. Male dogs are likely to seek out estrous females because a chemosensory cue in the urine of estrous females is very attractive to them (Beach and Gilmore, 1949). When an estrous female and a male meet, she will orient her hindquarters toward his muzzle and deflect her tail. The male will lick her vulva, sometimes so vigorously that he lifts her hindquarters off the ground (Beach and LeBoeuf, 1967). The male then mounts the female and presses his erect penis into her vagina; the female may assist the male by backing into him as he thrusts. She may also compensate for missed intromissions by changing her position slightly. After a brief series of intromissions, the male ejaculates and dismounts. The two animals are

**Full solicitations**

**Partial solicitations**

**Interception**

**6.6 Female initiation of sexual interactions** in rats often involves solicitational behaviors. In so-called full solicitations, a female rat will dart toward the male and run or hop away; the male often follows. During partial solicitations, the female may pause in front of the male (touchback) or run past (runby) the male. In mating situations involving multiple animals, interceptions may occur, whereby a female darts in front of a male that is following another female and distracts him. After McClintock, 1984.

locked together for some minutes as seminal fluid is transferred to the female (see Chapter 5). An anestrous female dog will not allow a male to mount. She will sit down, try to move away, or growl and snap at the male.

The estrous cycle of canines is about 7–8 months in duration, but recurs more frequently in unmated females (Asdell, 1964). Estrus persists for a week or 10 days. Termination of estrus is signaled when the female refuses to be mounted by males. Estrus is followed by about 2.5 months of diestrus, during which corpora lutea persist. After the corpora lutea regress, the female enters anestrus, which continues for about 4 or 5 months. The follicles begin to grow and secrete estrogens during proestrus, which lasts about 10 days. Vaginal bleeding is often observed during proestrus; the female will not mate during this time. The onset of estrus coincides with the female's acceptance of a male.

## Primates

Research conducted at the first Yerkes primate center in Florida provided a very complete quantification of the sexual behavior of chimpanzees in a laboratory setting (Yerkes and Elder, 1936). This description of chimp copulatory behavior was quite lively:

What happens when a male and female meet, under the conditions of our experiment, has been found to depend upon individuality, physiological status, social relations, and environmental circumstance. . . . [Various] postures and gestures [by the male] evidently are intended as appeals for sexual contact. If perchance the female does not respond to his solicitations, the male goes to her, usually examines her genitalia, and thereupon either attempts to copulate or turns away. Ordinarily, however, she responds instantly, when she sees the male . . . by running quickly to him and crouching low or even flat upon the ground, with limbs flexed and genitalia directed toward him. To this female presentation [the male] bends over her back, with his hands on her shoulders or sides, or touching the floor. In this posture, he presses forward against her genital swelling and forces the long slender penis into the vagina. . . . Insertion is followed by pelvic thrusts [which] may vary from as few as four or five to as many as twenty or thirty in our observation. Successful and mutually satisfactory copulation may be followed by manual, oral, or olfactory self- or mutual examination of the genitalia, and by grooming.

Obviously, some of the researchers' remarks, including "mutually satisfactory copulation" were inferences, but on the whole, their description is very accurate.

The mating posture of the female chimpanzee is rather stereotyped; there is little variation among females of this species. In contrast, as noted in Chapter 5, humans often seek variety in copulatory postures (Masters and Johnson, 1966). Variation in the sexual posture of some other nonhuman female primates has also been noted; for example, the ventral–ventral, or "face-to-face" position associated with humans has been observed in gorillas and orangutans (Nadler, 1976, 1988). Thus, among primates, there are species in which female sexual behavior is highly stereotyped (for example, chimpanzee and marmoset) and other species (human, gorilla, bonobo, and orangutan) that tend not to exhibit stereotyped female copulatory patterns.

Some primates, such as marmosets, have clearly defined estrous cycles, and mating behavior is limited to estrus. Other female primates, including rhesus monkeys, bonobos, and humans, do not limit sexual activity to a particular time and thus do not possess an estrous cycle per se (de Waal, 1995). There has been recurring controversy about the extent to which copulatory behavior in female humans and other so-called higher primates is regulated by ovarian hormones. Some investigators contend that because higher primates can copulate at any time during the ovarian cycle or even after ovariectomy, hormones are not involved in mediating female sexual behavior. Others have noted that under the appropriate circumstances, female primate sexual behavior shows a clear reliance on gonadal hormones. The controversy remains unresolved. It is also possible that androgens, possibly of adrenal origins, could be involved; this possibility is discussed later in the chapter.

## Are Females Active Participants in Sexual Behavior?

Prior to the mid-1970s the consensus among sex researchers, especially laboratory researchers, was that females were more or less passive recipients of male sexual attention. Although this perspective continues to dominate bird sexual research (cf. Cheng, 1992; van Tienhoven, 1983), Beach (1976) addressed this issue in mammals by noting that females often initiate sexual activities. We now know that females indeed take a very active role in initiating sexual activities, and in many species virtually always act as the initiators of copulation (reviewed in Erskine, 1989; Wallen, 1990). The sex drive of females may equal or even exceed that of male conspecifics, but may be expressed only in very specific spatial, temporal, or social contexts. Recall that the number of offspring a female can produce in her lifetime is limited, as compared with males, who can potentially sire a large number of offspring. Thus, females generally have evolved to provide more resources to their offspring than males because they have a larger stake in the successful outcome of each breeding effort than males, who typically invest little in each reproductive effort (Clutton-Brock, 1991). Consequently, females exhibit much greater selectivity than males in their choice of mating partners. This choosiness, which can easily be explained at an ultimate, evolutionary level of analysis, should not be invoked at the proximate level to suggest that females have less sex drive than males. Rather, the sex drive of females has evolved to maximize the reproductive success of each individual.

In retrospect, it may seem surprising that sex researchers "forgot" that *estrus* means "in a frenzy." And it may also seem surprising that they failed to notice the highly motivated behavior of pets like Molly in their attempts to copulate. Of course, the behavior of pets provides only anecdotal evidence at best, but there were many scientific reports, from field settings, of females that were highly motivated to engage in sex. For example, one study of a seminatural population of chimpanzees revealed that females risked physical attack whenever they approached males. Nevertheless, in most cases females were the initiators of copulation (Carpenter, 1942b; emphasis added):

> During her receptive period, her social status in the group shifts and she becomes a sexual incentive for the group's males. She actively approaches males and must overcome their *usual resistance* to close association, hence she becomes an object of attacks by them. Even other females attack her as a result of her shifted social status. . . . Females 49, 105, 126, 144, "f.n." and 109 were all severely wounded during their estrous periods. Female 105 lost parts of both ears, was cut severely on the arm and received a network of wounds over her face and muzzle. Female 144 had a leg wound which compelled her to walk on three legs for several days. Female 145 was deeply cut on the thighs. Female "f.n." had a badly bruised nose while female 109 had a long, deep gash and her infant was wounded so severely that it died.

This account indicates that these females initiated copulation despite the threat of severe physical punishment and social disruption. Even the earliest laboratory accounts of primate mating (Ball and Hartman, 1935; Yerkes and Elder, 1936) indicated that females were highly motivated to copulate:

> Under the conditions which we have specified, copulation is determined and controlled almost entirely by the female. The male is suitor and servitor, not lord and dictator. There may be no suggestion of compulsion. The female ignores his solicitations if she sees fit; terminates the sexual union when she will—and that may be before orgasm and completion of ejaculation. (Yerkes and Elder, 1936, 10)

What accounted for the failure of subsequent laboratory researchers to note the initiatives of females in copulation? As noted in Chapter 1, observer bias can adversely affect behavioral observations. Because feminine sexuality was widely assumed to be of a passive nature, it is possible that cultural constraints limited the interpretations of feminine sexual behavior observed in the laboratory. And in all fairness to those earlier sex researchers, the most striking aspect of female rodent sexual behavior in the laboratory test situation is the adoption of the rigid mating posture, lordosis. Maintaining immobility during copulation does indeed appear passive. It is also likely that sex researchers were victims of their own methods, born of their desire to control as many variables as possible during behavioral tests. Fieldwork produces highly valid results, but it is difficult, expensive, and occurs under uncontrolled conditions. Moving sex research into the laboratory permitted a high level of experimental control, but inadvertently removed important environmental and social variables that mediate female sexual behavior in nature. For example, pairing a single female with a single male has been the most common testing situation used in studies of rodents and primates, but it completely ignores the social reality of these animals. When a female is confined in a small space with a single male, her behavior may appear more passive than it would be if she could control the pacing of mating behavior or choose her mating partner, as is often the case in nature (see below).

## Components of Female Sexual Behavior

The knowledge that estrogens and progestins influence feminine sexual behavior is important, but is insufficient for students of behavioral endocrinology. In order to understand in greater detail how these hormones relate to behavior, researchers have been conceptually partitioning female sexual behavior into smaller and smaller component parts. Beach (1976) proposed the concept of dividing female sexual behavior into three components: (1) attractivity, (2) proceptivity, and (3) receptivity. **Attractivity** is the stimulus value of a female for a given male, a hypothetical construct that must be inferred by observation of a conspecific's behavior, and must always be measured in relational terms. If a male will expend effort to sit next to a particular female, then she is more attractive than something else; perhaps she is more attractive to the male than being alone, an empty box, food, or another female. **Proceptivity** is the extent to which a female initiates copulation. It reflects her overt behavior, as well as her underlying motivational state. **Receptivity** reflects the stimulus value of the female for eliciting an intravaginal ejaculation from a male conspecific; in other words, receptivity is her state of responsiveness to the sexual initiation of another individual (Beach, 1976).

Proceptivity and receptivity overlap conceptually, as well as in practice. For example, a proceptive female rodent may initiate copulation by assuming the lordosis posture; this mating posture would also indicate her receptivity. The conceptual separation of proceptive behavior from receptive behavior was an important means of clarifying and operationalizing observations of female sexual behavior. Prior to Beach's classification scheme, hormonal effects on female "receptive" behavior, from assumption of the lordosis posture in rats to solicitation of copulation by rhesus monkeys, appeared to vary immensely. In retrospect, it is not surprising that few general principles arose relating hormonal influences to such poorly defined female sexual behavior. Beach's scheme of separating female sexual behavior into these three components has (1) contributed to the acknowledgment of female sexual initiation, (2) facilitated the study of female sexual behavior, (3) provided a conceptual framework that equalizes the sexes in terms of sexual motivation and responsiveness, and thus (4) facilitated the identification of hormone–behavior relationships in female sexuality. Sex steroid hormones, especially estrogens, affect all three components of female sexual behavior (Figure 6.7). Sorting out the degree to which hormones affect attractivity, procep-

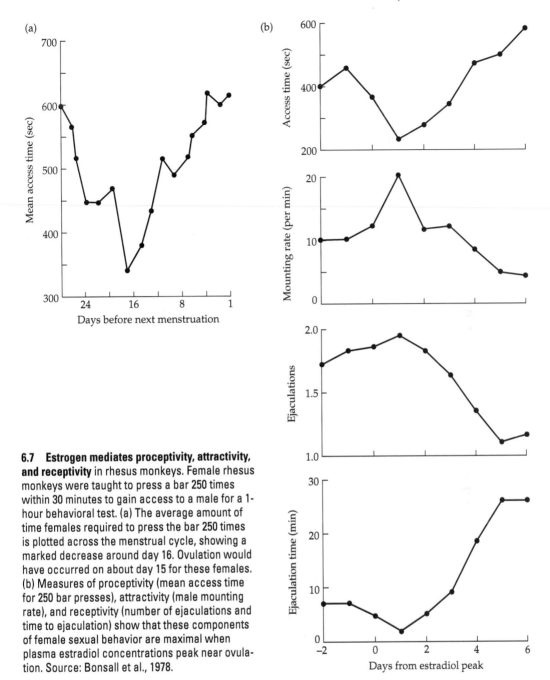

**6.7    Estrogen mediates proceptivity, attractivity, and receptivity** in rhesus monkeys. Female rhesus monkeys were taught to press a bar 250 times within 30 minutes to gain access to a male for a 1-hour behavioral test. (a) The average amount of time females required to press the bar 250 times is plotted across the menstrual cycle, showing a marked decrease around day 16. Ovulation would have occurred on about day 15 for these females. (b) Measures of proceptivity (mean access time for 250 bar presses), attractivity (male mounting rate), and receptivity (number of ejaculations and time to ejaculation) show that these components of female sexual behavior are maximal when plasma estradiol concentrations peak near ovulation. Source: Bonsall et al., 1978.

tivity, and receptivity has led to an increased understanding of the complex interactions between hormones and behavior and has also provided clues about the underlying physiological mechanisms.

Other researchers have divided female sexual behavior into two phases: the precopulatory phase and the copulatory phase (Madlafousek and Hlinak, 1977).

The precopulatory phase roughly corresponds to proceptive behavior in Beach's scheme. The precopulatory phase also corresponds to the appetitive phase described earlier for males, and may also be called courtship. The precopulatory phase involves all of the behaviors that allow a female to attract a male and initiate copulation. Behaviors as diverse as searching for males, emitting a chemical attractant, or assuming a mating posture and soliciting copulation may occur during courtship. Courtship functions as a communication opportunity during which information about species, readiness to mate, resources, and genetic endowment is shared. As with males, the precopulatory phase lasts much longer than the second phase, copulatory behavior, which corresponds roughly to receptive behavior in Beach's scheme. Although this dichotomy, like any other classification scheme, may artificially divide a unified behavioral program, such partitioning can be valuable for elucidating the hormonal bases of female reproductive behavior, and possibly for discriminating the underlying neural mechanisms. As in males, sexual motivation, as represented by proceptive behaviors, may be regulated in females by different hormones—or to a different extent—than sexual performance, as represented by receptive behaviors.

Recently, a third classification system has been proposed for female sexual behavior. A strong argument has been made that the term "female sexual initiation" should be used for any feminine behavior that facilitates mating, and "female sexual motivation" should be used for the state underlying sexual initiation or accommodation (Wallen, 1990; Zehr et al., 1998). Under this nomenclature, behaviors such as lordosis that facilitate copulation would be separated from solicitational behaviors that indicate sexual motivation. Hormones could affect these two components of female sexual behavior in the same way, or differently. For example, female rodents differ from some female primates in their reliance on hormones for the expression of sexual behavior. Under laboratory conditions, female rodents appear to require ovarian hormones to maintain both facilitatory and motivational behaviors. In contrast, many primates appear to require hormones only for maintenance of female sexual motivation. Sex steroid hormones allow the expression of lordosis among female rodents in response to male tactile stimulation during mounting. As we have seen, lordosis is necessary for copulation because penile insertion is impossible unless the female stands immobile. Because of their manual dexterity, primates do not require the female to maintain a rigid mating posture in order for successful copulation to occur. Female primates may permit copulation at all times during their ovarian cycle, but this copulation may not reflect their sexual motivation because female primates, especially those confined in the laboratory with a male, may copulate for a variety of reasons. Thus, the only valid measure of primate sexual behavior would be female-initiated mating, because primate facilitatory behaviors are somewhat unnecessary. While this argument is valid and helps to sharpen researchers' definitions and interpretations of behavior, especially the behavior of primates, Beach's nomenclature will be used in this chapter because of its descriptive strengths.

### Attractivity

Remember that bringing the two sexes together (attraction) when both are potentially fertile is the primary function of sexual behavior. Therefore, it should not be surprising that hormones associated with ovulation also mediate attractivity in females. In general, estrogens enhance attractivity. One way to test the attractiveness of females is to confine them separately and measure how much time a male spends with each of them. The assumption is that the duration of visitation by the male reflects the attractiveness of the female; the amount of time spent in close proximity to a female is called the PROX score (Phoenix, 1973). In this situation, males always spend more time in close proximity to estrous than anestrous females (reviewed in Beach, 1976). Ovariectomized females are rarely attractive to males. However, their attractivity is greatly enhanced by estradiol treatment. When spayed female dogs were injected with estradiol, the average duration of visits by males was increased sixfold (Beach and Merari, 1970). Similarly, ovariectomized monkeys are rarely mounted by males (Figure 6.8). However, if ovariectomized female monkeys are injected with estradiol, then they are mounted at a much higher frequency by males (Wallen, 1990).

In nature, high blood estradiol concentrations correspond with the time of maximal fertility. From an evolutionary perspective, it is predictable that females would be considered most attractive by male conspecifics when they are maximally fertile. Attracting males in order to mate is especially important for solitary animals such as cats or hamsters, which must signal their fertile condition to males over great distances. In a number of species, estradiol-induced attractivity is reduced or abolished by progesterone treatment, which is also predictable because high concentrations of progesterone are often associated with pregnancy or other nonfertile (from the male's perspective) states.

What exactly is attractivity? Both nonbehavioral and behavioral components sum together to form the stimulus bases of attractivity (Beach, 1976). Female attractivity is usually measured in terms of preference; that is, the extent to which a male prefers to be near one female as compared with others (Figure 6.9). As indicated in Chapter 5, the stimulus basis of male attractivity remains for the most part unspecified. As for females, nonbehavioral bases of attractivity include morphological changes that coincide with ovulation. For example, female primates in estrus experience a swelling of the peri-genital skin. The visual stimulation provided by this conspicuous swelling attracts male attention (Carpenter, 1942b). Subordinate males in a troop of primates may not be permitted to get

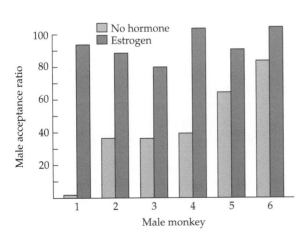

**6.8   Estrogen increases attractivity** in ovariectomized rhesus monkeys. The proportion of solicitations by a female monkey that result in male mounting behavior is called the male acceptance ratio. Males are more likely to mount an ovariectomized female after she is injected with estrogen (dark bars) than after she is injected with a biologically inert substance (light bars). Note the enormous individual differences in mounting behavior among males, and thus in the test female's attractivity to specific males. Male 1 rarely mounted the female in the absence of estrogen, but male 6 regularly mounted this female regardless of her hormonal condition. Source: Dixson et al., 1973.

**6.9   A three-chamber preference test** is used to determine attractivity. All three chambers contain food and water. Females are tethered in the outer two chambers, and a male is free to move among all three chambers. He will spend the majority of the test period with the female to which he is most attracted. Courtesy of Sabra Klein.

sufficiently close to females to have a real opportunity to mate, but even these males spend more time looking at estrous females than at anestrous females (Dixson et al., 1973).

Chemical cues are also important in forming the stimulus bases of female attractivity throughout the animal kingdom. For instance, chemosensory cues emanate from the urinary and vaginal secretions of estrous females (Box 6.1).

---

Box 6.1

# Chemosignals and Courtship in the Red-sided Garter Snake

An interesting twist to the story of chemical signals in courtship is provided by the red-sided garter snake (*Thamnophis sirtalis parietalis*) described in Chapter 5. Recall that the males of this species emerge from their winter hibernacula earlier than females, and attempt to mate with females as they emerge several weeks later. Females emerge one at a time, so many males court a single female as she leaves the hibernaculum, forming a large, writhing mating ball of snakes (see Figure 5.34).

How does a courting male identify the female in such a tangle of snakes? One possibility is that males discriminate by size; females are larger than males of this species. But size is not the primary cue male snakes use. They mainly rely on chemosensory information. Males produce one type of chemical signal, a squalene, that acts to identify them as males. Females produce another type of chemosensory signal, a methyl ketone, that males find very attractive. When males are courting, they flick their tongues along the scales of the female. As their

sensory systems are stimulated by the female "attractive" cue, they begin to rub their chins on the female until one male gains intromission. As soon as an intromission occurs, the female expresses another chemical cue that immediately "turns off" the courtship behavior of the other males. Thus, female attractiveness is mediated directly by chemical factors: males are attracted to females emitting one chemosignal indicating readiness to mate, and repelled by females emitting another chemical cue signaling that mating has already occurred (Mason et al., 1989). Estrogen is necessary for the production of the "attractiveness" chemical; however, injection of estrogen into adult males does not cause them to be courted by other males. In other words, estrogen alone is not the basis of female attractiveness in snakes.

In nature, however, about 15% of the males in a mating ball are courted by other males; that is, other males are observed slithering along their scales, tongue-flicking and chin-rubbing.

Males sniff and lick females' external genitalia and vagina prior to copulation in many species of mammals, and males are much more likely to engage in this behavior with estrous than with anestrous females (Beach and Merari, 1968). Males of many mammalian species, especially carnivores, ungulates, and rodents, discriminate estrous from anestrous females on the basis of chemosensory signals that are processed through the vomeronasal organ (see Chapter 5). Male ungulates commonly display a **flehmen response** when sexually excited, extending the neck and curling the upper lip to reveal the upper gums (Figure 6.10), which allows the female chemosignal to be delivered to the vomeronasal organ (see Figure 5.13; Wysocki, 1979). The vomeronasal organ is reduced or absent in higher primates, and humans are notoriously poor among mammals in their olfactory abilities. For example, most farmers who raise cattle do so by artificial insemination: sperm is obtained from a bull by electrically induced ejaculation, and is introduced into estrous cows. However, discerning when a cow is in estrus has not been an easy task for cattle farmers, so dogs have been trained to discriminate estrous from anestrous cows. The dogs' chemosensory ability aids the farmers in knowing when artificial insemination will "take," although new electronic sensors have recently been developed to replace the dogs (Lane and Wathes, 1998).

What causes these males to be attractive objects of courtship? The courted males might have picked up the chemical attractant from a female that they were courting. But when researchers wiped off courted males with a chemical solvent and released them into a mating arena, this treatment did not reduce the incidence of courtship behavior directed at them (Mason, 1987). Chemical analyses of the skin secretions of courted males revealed that they produce the same attractant chemical that females do and none of the male-identifier chemosignal. These so-called "she-males" have higher testosterone-to-estrogen ratios than typical males (blood plasma testosterone levels about 2.5 times higher than those of "he-males" and more than 3000 times higher than those of females), and also have very high concentrations of aromatase, the enzyme that converts testosterone to estradiol, in their skin. These differences may account for the she-males producing the female attractant chemosignal.

But why have male snakes that are attractive to other males evolved, and how are they maintained in the population? The answer appears to be that these she-male snakes pursue an alternative reproductive tactic. In mating competition tests, in which one she-male was placed with twenty he-males, the she-male obtained significantly more matings than the typical males (see figure; Mason et al., 1989). Apparently, the she-males confuse the other males, which waste time and energy courting the wrong animal in the mating ball. This provides the she-males with a competitive advantage during mating. Thus, in this species, some males exploit the "attractive" signals produced by females to gain a reproductive advantage over rival males.

**6.10    The flehmen response,** seen here in a male red deer, is common in many male mammals, especially carnivores, ungulates, and rodents. In response to chemosignals obtained during anogenital investigation, the male extends the neck, curls the upper lip to reveal the gums, and usually presses the tongue against the roof of the mouth to force the chemosignals into the vomeronasal organ. Courtesy of Fiona Guinness.

In addition to physiological and morphological stimuli, various types of behavior may also increase the attractiveness of females. For example, females that actively solicit copulations have a higher stimulus value for males than females that do not. As noted above, females of many nonhuman primates present their genitalia to males by backing their hindquarters toward the males (Figure 6.11); males spend more time with females that engage in this presentation behavior than with females that do not present (Dixson et al., 1973). Female rats also solicit mounts from males as described above by darting, hopping, and crouching behaviors and by running away from and returning to the male. As we will see below, in seminatural or natural settings, these female behaviors set the pace of the copulatory sequence, because virtually all male mounts follow a female solicitation (Erskine, 1989; Coopersmith et al., 1996).

All of these factors associated with attractivity, both behavioral and nonbehavioral, appear to involve sex steroid hormones. However, there are also nonhormonal factors that affect attractivity. Individual preferences exist among many species. For example, even when several ovariectomized female dogs are treated with equal amounts of estradiol, some consistently evoke more sexual responses from males than others (Beach and Merari, 1970; LeBoeuf, 1967). There is also sexual "favoritism" among male monkeys, apes, and humans (Herbert, 1970; Michael

**6.11   Female rhesus monkey presenting to male.** One measure of proceptivity among nonhuman primates is the number of solicitations made prior to sexual contact. Solicitations take the form of assuming the mating posture or standing in front of a male and exhibiting genitalia. Virtually all social contacts between males and females prior to copulation in nonhuman primates are initiated by females. Courtesy of Kim Wallen.

et al., 1972). A female may be very attractive to one male, but unattractive to another. This variation is consistently observed in the "Coolidge effect" (see Chapter 5), in which the stimulus value of a female is reduced for a male that has already copulated with her several times. She remains attractive to other males that have not just mated with her, but she has temporarily lost her stimulus value for the first male.

Understanding the stimuli underlying attractivity in various animal species is an extremely daunting task. To get some idea of the complexity involved, think about the various components of individuals to whom you are attracted. Even though you can use language and can describe the features important in forming an attraction, it is very difficult to assign values to each feature. To some individuals, honesty may be a very important characteristic; to others, a clear complexion is important. How do you assign weight to each characteristic? Ask your friends to describe attractive people. How do you account for the vast differences among individuals in attraction? There is no reason to assume that the stimulus basis for attractiveness is any less complicated in nonhuman animals.

## Proceptivity

Proceptive behavior comprises all of the appetitive activities shown by females. In other words, proceptivity is indicated by sexually solicitous behaviors that initiate sexual union, but is not copulatory behavior per se. Proceptivity reflects a female's underlying motivational state in much the same way libido or sex drive reflects a male's motivational state (see Chapter 5). Molly's escapes from her yard and visits to her male neighbor indicated proceptivity (see Figure 6.1). Estrous females, as well as being the most attractive to males, are also the most attracted to males.

Several behavioral measures have been used to assess proceptivity in females. The most common assay of proceptivity has been assessment of affiliative behaviors—efforts by females to establish and maintain proximity to males, which is a universal response of proceptive females. Female rhesus monkeys rarely interact with males except to initiate mating (Carpenter, 1942a,b). In one study, more than 80% of all proximate social interaction between male and female monkeys was initiated by females prior to mating (Cochran, 1979; Wallen et al., 1984). Another behavioral measure of proceptivity is the number of solicitations made before sexual contact; in other words, assumptions of the mating posture or presentations of the genitalia to the male (reviewed in Wallen, 1990) (see Figure 6.11). Such solicitations are commonly observed in primates, but are also observed in many disparate taxa, including birds, reptiles, and fishes. Vocalizations and head bobbing are also observed among monkeys that are soliciting copulations (Ball and Hartman, 1935; Carpenter, 1942a; Michael, 1972). Finally, a study of rhesus females was conducted during the nonbreeding season, when males are not responsive to females. Estradiol treatment during this time increased female sexual initiation among ovariectomized rhesus monkeys despite the lack of behavioral feedback from males (Zehr et al., 1998) (Figure 6.12).

Another female behavior that is highly proceptive is alternating approaches and withdrawals. This pattern is commonly observed in rodents, and is also part of ungulate, canine, and primate copulation sequences. The female approaches the male, and if he follows her, she may pseudo-retreat, but eventually she allows him to investigate her. If the male does not follow her, then she approaches him again. This pattern of approach and withdrawal is very stimulating to most conspecific males and is in no way indicative of nonreceptivity or disinterest on the part of the female. Females may also initiate physical contact by investigating the male's anogenital region. Occasionally, mounting by females is observed by highly proceptive females (Beach, 1968). Females may mount males or other females, and these mounts are accompanied by thrusting pelvic movements (Beach, 1942d). In fact, ovulation may result from female–female mounting behavior among rabbits (Fee and Parkes, 1930). After being mounted by a female several times, the male often mounts the female in turn.

A final determinant of female proceptivity is the attractiveness of the male mating partner. As noted above, females do not initiate copulation with males to whom they are not attracted. Castrated male rhesus monkeys, dogs, and hamsters elicit fewer approach responses by females than gonadally intact males in two-choice tests (reviewed in Beach, 1976). Female proceptivity is especially critical in species such as gorillas and rhesus monkeys because most copulation is

**6.12 Estradiol enhances proceptivity in the absence of male interest.** Estradiol treatment of ovariectomized rhesus monkeys during the nonbreeding season, when males are not responsive to females, increased the frequency of female sexual initiation. Source: Zehr et al., 1998.

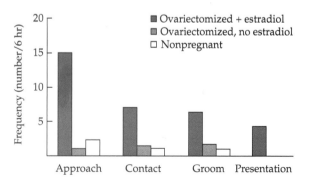

due to the females' initiative and mate selection (Cochran, 1979; Pomerantz and Goy, 1983; Wallen et al., 1984) (see Figure 6.11). Beach (1976) maintained that presentation to males by females is highest during midcycle, when ovulation occurs. This observation was based on laboratory, zoo, and natural populations of animals. In all species examined, high concentrations of estrogens facilitate proceptive behavior.

## *Receptivity*

Receptivity is the consummatory phase of mating behavior, and can be defined as those female reactions that are necessary and sufficient for fertile copulation with a potent male. As Beach (1976) said, "*Sexual receptivity* is distinguished equally by the ubiquity of its usage and the infrequency of its definition." Prior to the development of Beach's classification scheme, behavioral measures of either receptivity or proceptivity were taken as evidence of receptivity.

Receptivity is indicated by a species-specific mating posture in all nonprimate mammals examined. For example, sows tread backward during copulation to help the boar gain intromission. Female rodents display the lordosis posture in response to tactile stimulation by the male. Females of several primate species back into males and literally seize the penis (reviewed in Wallen, 1990). Virtually all nonmammalian species also have a characteristic female mating posture (Crews and Silver, 1985). Most behavioral measures of receptivity are expressed in terms of ratios between the male's attempts to mate with a female and his success in doing so. This ratio is expressed in rats as a lordosis quotient (LQ), in dogs as a rejection coefficient, or in primates as an acceptance ratio (AR).

It has been proposed that female ring doves initiate their own receptive behavior by hearing themselves cooing. Cooing is usually performed by females in response to behavioral stimuli provided by males (Lehrman, 1961). It was first thought that the male induced receptivity in the female. However, the male actually induces the female to emit cooing vocalizations, and *her* behavior feeds back to affect her endocrine state and to initiate receptivity (Cheng, 1986; Cheng et al., 1998). If females are induced to coo in the absence of males, their follicles develop and secrete estrogens, and if females are devocalized by any of several means, including brain lesions, their ovaries do not develop in response to male stimulation. If the females' cooing vocalizations are recorded prior to devocalization and played back to them, *even in the absence of males,* the follicles develop and estrogens are secreted, inducing further receptive behavior (Cheng, 1992). Thus, ring doves present an interesting case of behavior in one individual inducing a behavioral change in the receiving animal that stimulates hormonal changes that cause further behavioral changes. In fact, part of the circuitry involved, from the midbrain vocal nucleus, thalamus, and neuroendocrine hypothalamus, has been identified (Cheng and Zuo, 1994). Specific hypothalamic neurons have been identified that respond to the female nesting coo and induce the secretion of LH (Cheng et al., 1998). Although the ring dove is the first species for which this sort of interactive feedback has been demonstrated, these sorts of complex social–behavioral–hormonal interactions are probably common and awaiting discovery.

There is abundant evidence that estrogen stimulation is very important in receptivity. For example, the display of the mating posture disappears in ovariectomized females of virtually all species examined. As noted above, lordosis can be induced in rodents by injections of estradiol and progesterone or sometimes estradiol alone (Feder, 1981). Rabbits, as well as rhesus monkeys and women, are maximally sensitive to tactile stimulation when the stimulation is concurrent with high blood concentrations of estrogen, but individuals of all these species will permit copulation at all stages of their ovarian cycle. These findings have led to confusion regarding the endocrine bases of female sexual receptivity among primates (Wallen, 1990).

**FEMALE CONTROL OF COPULATION.**    Much has been made of the so-called constant receptivity reported for humans and other primates. Their ability to copulate at any time during the ovarian cycle, or even in the complete absence of ovarian steroid hormones, caused many sex researchers to conclude that the sexual behavior of many primate species is not under hormonal control. However, as suggested above, the behavior of a female primate accepting copulation may not reflect the same motivational state as the behavior of a female rodent accepting copulation. A male rodent or canine cannot successfully copulate without female cooperation; the female must maintain a rigid posture. Primates do not exhibit this constraint, and copulation is mechanically possible without the female's cooperation. Although forced copulation is rare among most nonhuman primates, it has been consistently observed among orangutans (Mitani, 1985). In a traditional laboratory test of paired partners, female primates require little sexual motivation to copulate. Frankly, there is little else to do. A male is provided in a small room, and there are no other animals with which to interact. Under these test conditions, a female primate's sexual behavior is unrelated to her ovarian cycle or endocrine state (Wallen, 1990). If animals are tested in more complex social conditions—that is, in the presence of multiple males and females—then females risk aggression from other females when they actively solicit males for sexual contact, especially if they are low-ranking females (Carpenter, 1942b; Wallen et al., 1984). Presumably, attacks by other females are aversive, and sexual motivation must be high to overcome this aversiveness. When female primates are tested in such group settings, copulatory behavior is tightly coupled to endocrine state (Figure 6.13; Wallen, 1990).

Is the sexual receptivity (or proceptivity) of women affected by hormones? This question has not been adequately answered, in part because the definitions of receptivity and proceptivity have become entangled and in part because social factors are not appropriately considered. Virtually all studies of human sexual behavior involve self-reports by couples in long-established, usually marriage, relationships. Under these circumstances there is little change in the frequency of copulation over the ovarian cycle (Adams et al., 1978; Udry and Morris, 1968), although some studies have revealed a peak in human female sexual activity around the time of ovulation. Ovulation is said to be "hidden" in women, by which it is meant that few women, and presumably fewer men, know precisely when ovulation occurs; however, the validity of this assumption remains unknown. Diaries of erotic thoughts or autosexual activities by women show a peak around the time of ovulation, suggesting an endocrine effect on sexual motivation (Adams et al., 1978). Studies that report a peak in sexual behavior among married couples around the time of ovulation usually have not controlled for the possibility that males find periovulatory females more attractive, and hence, that men may initiate more sexual contacts around the time of ovulation. One study controlled for this

**6.13   Endocrine control of receptivity can be affected by social factors.** If female rhesus monkeys are tested with one male in a small area, there is no close relationship between estrogen concentration and receptivity (as measured by the number of tests with ejaculations); however, a clear relationship between receptivity and estrogen concentration emerges when females are tested in mixed social groups in a large area. Source: Wallen, 1990.

possible confounding variable by examining the frequency of sexual activities among lesbian couples (Matteo and Rissman, 1984). This study reported a small peak in sexual activity around the time of ovulation, along with a secondary, perimenstrual peak. Other studies of heterosexual couples have also suggested a secondary perimenstrual peak in sexual behavior (for example, Sherwin, 1988a,b; Van Goozen et al., 1997; Harvey, 1987; Slob et al., 1991, 1996). A study of sexual arousability over the menstrual cycle used both subjective self-reports and objective (labium minor temperature) measures to discover cycles in erotic responsiveness (Slob et al., 1996). This study revealed that the order of testing (i.e., whether the test was first administered during the luteal or the follicular phase) could affect subjective reports of erotic arousal. Thus, caution must be exercised when gathering self-reports to make certain that multiple cycles are followed.

As indicated at the beginning of this chapter, female dogs will not accept males unless they are in estrus, or have been treated with estrogens. However, while sex steroid hormones are necessary for receptive behavior in dogs, they are not sufficient. For example, beagle females reject certain males, even when in estrus (LeBoeuf, 1967). Under natural conditions, nonanthropoid primate females are receptive only during the time of their cycle when estradiol blood concentrations are high, but even then they discriminate among males with which to mate (Clutton-Brock, 1991). In virtually all nonmammalian species examined, females' blood concentrations of estrogens are elevated from some basal concentration coincident with the time when they mate with males (reviewed in Crews and Silver, 1985).

**FEMALE PACING OF COPULATION.**    Sex steroid hormones are necessary and sufficient for normal sexual behavior among female rodents in the laboratory. There does not seem to be much selectivity of mating partners among estrous female rats when they are tested in the typical laboratory apparatus with a single male. Under these conditions, an estrous rat will mate with virtually any adult male with which she is paired. But estrous rats do not normally mate with a single male in an enclosed space. Wild rats and mice typically live in small breeding units, called demes, consisting of one or two adult males, several females, and their offspring (Figure 6.14; see also Figure 5.20). The animals often mate in groups, and the pacing of mating behavior is usually under the control of the females. Group-living females often come into estrus together (see below), and two or more estrous females may compete to copulate with two or more attendant males (Bronson, 1979; Calhoun, 1962a; McClintock and Adler, 1978). Because the first and last

**6.14    A breeding deme,** the typical social organization of wild rats, consists of a small group of animals that includes a few adult males, several adult females, and many subadults. In this social setting, the females may undergo estrous cycles synchronously and mate with several males simultaneously. The burrows and runway systems in the rats' natural habitat promote a slower mating pace than is typical in a laboratory setting. From McClintock, 1987.

males to ejaculate with a female in a group mating situation sire proportionally more of her offspring than other ejaculating males, a female can to some degree choose the sires of her offspring by her choice of males for these roles.

When researchers tested groups of rats in a seminatural setting in which female rats could control the pace of mating behavior, the temporal pattern of rat copulatory behavior began to emerge (McClintock, 1987; McClintock and Adler, 1978). The natural pace of mating can also be simulated in a single-pair mating test by using a setting that allows the female to escape from the male between mating events (Erskine, 1985). Under conditions that allow females to pace copulation, the intervals between intromissions are longer than those observed in more typical artificial settings (Erskine, 1985; McClintock and Adler, 1978). In group mating tests in a natural setting, the female retires to her burrow or moves behind some barrier for approximately 3 minutes after each intromission. In contrast, the average inter-intromission interval during standard paired rat mating tests is less than 1 minute. Females paired with a single male in a standard mating arena, but able to escape, also show differential timing as compared with females in nonpaced tests: females in paced paired tests retire away from the male for a longer time after an ejaculation than after an intromission, demonstrating that they are able to discriminate the type of vaginal stimulation they have received (see Yang and Clemens, 1996). Anesthesia of the perianal region disrupts this discriminative ability (Figure 6.15; Bermant and Westbrook, 1966).

The larger size of the mating arena in natural (Calhoun, 1962a) or seminatural (McClintock and Adler, 1978) settings permits the full expression of female solicitation behaviors, including approach and withdrawal behavior, that are often missing or altered in standard mating test situations (Erskine, 1989). Approach and withdrawal behavior appears as the hopping and darting behaviors observed in typical laboratory settings. This behavior is an important component of normal rat sexual behavior and precedes 90% of intromissions in natural or seminatural settings. In contrast, only 3% of male-initiated contacts result in intromissions (McClintock, 1987).

The temporal pattern of copulatory events has a very important role in rodent reproduction; namely, the induction of corpora luteal function. In Chapter 5, a variety of rodent copulatory patterns were presented. In some species, such as the guinea pig, males ejaculate on the first intromission, and there is no pelvic

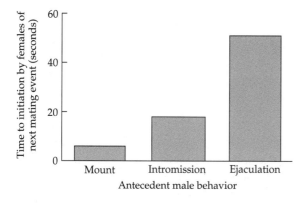

**6.15   Female pacing of copulation.** Female rats in paced paired mating tests, in which they are provided with an "escape" area away from the male, return to the male more slowly following an ejaculation than after an intromission or mount, indicating that they can discriminate among different types of vaginal stimulation. Source: Erskine, 1985.

thrusting. In rats and mice, males mount a number of times, and there are multiple intromissions before ejaculation. Why have multiple intromissions? Physiologically, multiple intromissions stimulate sperm transport after ejaculation. But there are other important coadaptations between the physiology of females and the behavior of male conspecifics. If no mating stimuli, or insufficient stimuli, are received, a female undergoes recurrent estrous cycles of 4 or 5 days. The corpora lutea regress soon after being formed and do not secrete sufficient progesterone to build up the uterine endometrium to support pregnancy. Multiple intromissions maintain luteal function so that the fertilized ova can implant in the uterine wall. The sensory input from the multiple intromissions stimulates secretion of prolactin from the anterior pituitary in a characteristic twice-daily pulse. The secretion of prolactin in this manner supports the corpora lutea for about 10–12 days (Gunnet and Freeman, 1983). The corpora lutea then persist until the end of pregnancy without further prolactin support. Unlike a female guinea pig, a female rat cannot become pregnant with just a single intromission and ejaculation—unless corpora luteal function has been activated by artificial vaginal stimulation.

The female's pacing of copulation may be a means of ensuring that she receives a pattern of stimulation as close as possible to the "vaginal code"—the so-called optimal pattern of stimulation for producing offspring—for her species (see Chapter 5). In standard nonpaced mating tests, approximately ten intromissions are required to induce luteal function and ensure successful pregnancy. In a paced mating test in which the female controls the timing and duration of the copulatory activity, only five intromissions are necessary to induce corpora luteal function, and more females are impregnated after five intromissions than after ten intromissions (Figure 6.16). Males also need fewer intromissions to ejaculate in paced as compared with standard laboratory mating tests (Erskine, 1985). Presumably, his interaction with a female displaying the approach and withdrawal

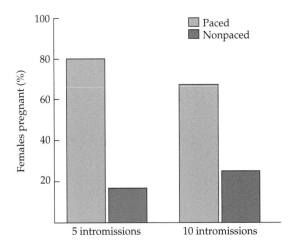

**6.16   Paced mating enhances reproduction.** The slower mating pace seen in female-paced mating tests optimizes reproduction: in this study, five male intromissions in a paced test resulted in more successful pregnancies than did ten intromissions, and both paced tests resulted in more pregnancies than did the nonpaced tests. Source: Erskine, 1985.

behavior pattern increases the male's arousal so that fewer intromissions are required prior to ejaculation (Erskine, 1989). It appears that the number, rather than the timing, of prior intromissions affects subsequent mating behavior and termination of estrus in rats (Coopersmith et al., 1996). Furthermore, paced mating appears to be more effective than nonpaced mating in inducing the expression of c-*fos* genes in neurons that are part of the neural circuitry underlying female sexual behavior (Erskine and Hanrahan, 1997). The role of proper pacing of mating behavior in other species has not been specified. "Pacing" is unnecessary in guinea pigs. Male guinea pigs ejaculate on the first intromission, but female guinea pigs have spontaneous corpora luteal activity, so multiple intromissions are unnecessary. Such co-adaptation between male and female copulatory behavior and reproductive physiology is a fundamental characteristic defining a species.

## Female Reproductive Cycles

The duration of estrus and the interval between estrous periods vary from species to species (Table 6.1). Rats, as we have seen, come into estrus every 4 or 5 days. For some species, like the golden-mantled ground squirrel (*Spermophilus lateralis*), the estrous period may last only a few hours per year during a single morning. In other species, such as rabbits, females will permit mating at any time during the breeding season. Female mammalian reproductive cycles can be classified into several types based on how and when ovulation and pseudopregnancy occur. Although these types will be presented here as if they were discrete categories, keep in mind that reproductive cycles actually vary along a continuum. The description of reproductive cycles that follows is largely based on the classification system put forth by Conaway (1971).

Table 6.1
**Typical length of the estrous cycle of several common species when living under optimal conditions**

| Common name | Taxonomic name | Cycle length (days) |
| --- | --- | --- |
| Laboratory rat | *Rattus norvegicus* | 4–5 |
| House mouse | *Mus musculus* | 4–6 |
| Guinea pig | *Cavia porcellus* | 16 |
| Golden hamster | *Mesocricetus auratus* | 4 |
| Deer mouse | *Peromyscus maniculatus* | 4–5 |
| Cotton rat | *Sigmodon hispidus* | 4–20 |
| Domestic cat | *Felis catus* | 9–10, 2/year |
| Domestic dog | *Canis familiaris* | 10, 2/year |
| Sheep | *Ovis aries* | 16 |
| Goat | *Capra hircus* | 21 |
| Cow | *Bos taurus* | 21 |
| Pig | *Sus scrofa* | 22 |

*Source:* Asdell, 1964.

### Types of Reproductive Cycles

The follicular phase of an ovarian cycle occurs prior to ovulation, when the follicles are developing. The luteal phase is that part of the cycle after ovulation during which the corpora lutea are active and producing progesterone. Successful fertilization usually occurs in the fallopian tubes, as the egg travels from the ovary to the uterus. Progesterone—the "progestational" hormone—normally induces the buildup of the uterine endometrium in preparation for the implantation of a blastocyst, the small mass of dividing cells that develops into an embryo, and supports the uterus during pregnancy. If a luteal phase occurs during a cycle when no mating, or a sterile mating, has taken place, then a pseudopregnancy will occur as the uterus is prepared for blastocyst implantation. The estrous cycles are suspended during pregnancy, pseudopregnancy, and lactation. Pseudopregnancy is considered spontaneous if the formation of functional corpora lutea always follows ovulation; if the occurrence of functional corpora lutea does not automatically follow ovulation, but requires some sort of additional stimulus, as in rats, pseudopregnancy is considered induced. In Conaway's classification system (Table 6.2), **pseudopregnancy** is defined as "the occurrence of any functional luteal phase in a non-pregnant cycle" (Everett, 1961). Although the "luteal phase" of the ovarian cycle and "pseudopregnancy" are endocrinologically identical, the term luteal phase is reserved mainly for describing primate ovarian cycles. Exceptions include guinea pigs and sheep, which both display spontaneous luteal phases.

The reproductive cycles of female anthropoid primates, including humans, are not technically estrous cycles because, as described above, mating behavior

**Table 6.2**
**Types of female reproductive cycles in mammals**

| Cycle | Length | Features | Examples |
|---|---|---|---|
| **Type 1** | | | |
| Subtype 1.1.A | 2–5 weeks | Spontaneous ovulation and pseudopregnancy; copulation limited to periovulatory period | Guinea pigs/other histricomorph rodents |
| Subtype 1.1.B | 2–5 weeks | Spontaneous ovulation and pseudopregnancy; copulation may occur throughout cycle | Great apes, including humans |
| Subtype 1.2 | >5 weeks | Spontaneous ovulation and pseudopregnancy; copulation limited to periovulatory period | Dogs and other canids |
| **Type 2** | | | |
| Subtype 2.1 | 3–5 weeks | Induced ovulation, but spontaneous pseudopregnancy | Rabbits and hares; lemmings and voles |
| Subtype 2.2 | >5 weeks | Induced ovulation, but spontaneous pseudopregnancy | Cats, minks, ferrets, and skunks |
| **Type 3** | <1 week | Spontaneous ovulation, but induced pseudopregnancy | Rats, mice, and hamsters |

Source: Conaway, 1971.

is not confined to a particular phase of the ovarian cycle. Women and females of a few other primate species may copulate on any day of the cycle (Wallen, 1990). The ovarian cycle displayed by most primates is called the **menstrual** ("moon") **cycle** because of the recurring period of menstruation (sloughing off of the uterine endometrium) that typically occurs during each cycle, about once a month in humans (Figure 6.17). Dogs and some other mammals discharge blood from the vagina prior to estrus, but this discharge is fundamentally different from menstrual bleeding. Menstruation occurs when blood concentrations of estrogens and progesterone are basal. The endometrial layer of the uterus, no longer supported by the sex steroid hormones, is shed, and the corkscrew-shaped blood vessels that remain leak blood into the uterine lumen. The blood discharged by proestrous or estrous dogs, on the other hand, results from estrogen-induced stimulation of the uterine wall (hyperemia), which causes rapid growth of the endometrium and many tears in the supporting blood vessels. Thus, vaginal bleeding in canines results from steroid stimulation, whereas menstrual bleeding in primates results from steroid hormone deprivation.

### *The Ecology of Reproductive Cycles*

Table 6.2 describes the several different kinds of reproductive cycles in mammals. The type 3 reproductive cycle was once considered to be the pattern most typical of mammals because of the enormous amount of research that was conducted on species—typically rodents—that exhibit it. However, the actual number of mammalian species with type 3 reproductive cycles is probably quite low. Mammals with type 3 cycles do not have functional luteal phases if they do not mate; this ensures a rapid return to estrus. In nature, nonpregnant cycles are a rarity because most animals with type 3 cycles mate and become pregnant during a spontaneous postpartum estrus, and thus gestate a new litter while nursing the previous one.

What are there so many different types of reproductive cycles? From an ecological perspective, each species' cyclic pattern can be seen as an adaptation for increasing its reproductive success. The cyclic pattern increases the probability that mating will occur when the female is fertile and that offspring will be produced and survive. Keep in mind that female mammals in the wild are typically pregnant, lactating, or in seasonal diestrus; that is, reproductively quiescent. Repeated estrous cycles are laboratory artifacts that occur infrequently in free-ranging mammals. Also, sterile copulation is probably very rare in nature (Nalbandov, 1976). Repeated, sterile estrous cycles represent an abnormal state, a pathological luxury that cannot be afforded by a female in the wild (Conaway, 1971).

What are the relative advantages of the various reproductive cycle types? One correlation that is immediately apparent is that small, short-lived prey species (for example, rodents and lagomorphs [rabbits and hares]) display either type 2.1 or type 3 reproductive cycles, which minimize the time spent in a nonpregnant condition. Animals that live longer, such as predators, do not require as many adaptations to reduce nonpregnant intervals, and can focus more effort on rearing fewer offspring successfully. Another loose correlation occurs between induced ovulation and solitary living. Many of the solitary carnivores are induced ovulators; this ensures that ovulation occurs only when males are present. In other species of induced ovulators, *behavioral* estrus is also induced by the presence of male conspecifics.

**6.17  The human menstrual cycle.** After menstrual bleeding has ceased, blood concentrations of LH and FSH increase gradually, stimulating the development of estrogen-secreting follicles. When estrogen concentrations are high, a positive feedback response occurs, causing a surge of gonadotropins that induces ovulation. After ovulation, negative feedback returns gonadotropin concentrations to baseline values, and estrogen concentrations wane. Corpora lutea are formed and secrete progesterone. If a woman is not pregnant, the corpora lutea regress, progesterone concentrations sharply decrease, and menstruation begins.

In many species of lagomorphs, behavioral estrus is induced by synchronized courtship displays by the males in the population (Conaway and Wight, 1962). In this case, group synchrony in mating probably confers individual advantages because births will be synchronized, and the chance of any one offspring becoming the victim of predation will be much less than if births were randomly timed throughout the breeding season. In contrast, many large group-living mammals are spontaneous ovulators. A social organization such as a herd probably guarantees that males will be present whenever a female comes into estrus.

Female prairie voles (*Microtus ochrogaster*) do not display regular estrous cycles, but are induced into behavioral estrus by the presence of a conspecific, fertile male or exposure to his urine (Richmond and Stehn, 1976). Undisturbed, isolated female prairie voles never display the cycles in vaginal cell types or opening observed in mice and rats. When a male is present, the female may ingest a few drops of his urine during mutual anogenital investigation. The urine is delivered to the vomeronasal organ (reviewed in Wysocki, 1979; Wysocki and Lepri, 1991). As described in Chapter 5, this chemosensory organ connects with the accessory olfactory bulb of the brain via the vomeronasal nerves. In many rodent species, the cell bodies of neurons that secrete GnRH are found in the olfactory bulb (Dluzen and Ramirez, 1983); these neurons project to the median eminence of the hypothalamus. The delivery of male urine to the vomeronasal organ of the female stimulates a cascade of endocrine events. Within an hour, GnRH is released from the olfactory bulb, which stimulates LH, and probably FSH, secretion from the anterior pituitary gland (Dluzen et al., 1981). The secretion of gonadotropins results in follicular development and subsequent production of estrogen. Elevated estrogen concentrations cause estrous behavior within 24 hours (Carter et al., 1986). Ovulation occurs approximately 12 hours after mating and is induced by copulation.

The behavior of a female prairie vole directly influences her endocrine state. If the female does not engage in anogenital investigation, she will not be induced into estrus. When females are housed with their fathers or brothers, they do not engage in anogenital investigation, are not induced into estrus, and thereby avoid incestuous mating (Carter et al., 1980). Because the ovaries are quiescent prior to the induction of estrus, proceptive behavior (anogenital investigation) is not mediated by ovarian steroid hormones in this species (Moffatt and Nelson, 1994).

In nature, the first estrus of the breeding season in prairie voles is induced by males, but subsequent matings occur during a spontaneous postpartum estrus (Nelson, 1985; Richmond and Conaway, 1969). Most pregnancies among natural populations of rodents are the result of mating during postpartum estrus. Rats ovulate about 3–6 hours after delivery of their young, and postpartum estrus occurs within 24 hours of the onset of parturition. The hormonal milieu of parturition is similar to the endocrine state associated with ovulation during an estrous cycle (Connor and Davis, 1980a,b). A female in postpartum estrus is attractive and signals males to mate with her (Greef and Merkx, 1982). Typically, she becomes pregnant again within a day after giving birth, and gestates a new litter while nursing the previous one. At about the time the current litter of pups is weaned, a new litter arrives, the female again enters estrus, and the sequence is repeated until the end of the breeding season (see Chapter 9). Thus, this reproductive pattern decreases the interval between successive litters and effectively doubles reproductive output. If a female fails to become pregnant during postpartum estrus, she enters a lactational diestrus and does not enter estrus again until her young are weaned 25–30 days later. This type of reproductive pattern is common among many mammalian groups, including marsupials, mustelids (mink, ferrets, skunks), and rodents. Despite the preponderance of pregnancies in the wild that arise from postpartum matings, little is known about the physiology of, or behavioral changes associated with, postpartum estrus (Blandau and Soderwall, 1941; Connor and Davis, 1980a,b; Everett, 1961; Greef and Merkx, 1982; Lu et al., 1976).

Why have estrous cycles evolved? Estrous cycles are probably best considered to be an adaptation that allows a female to enter reproductive condition at the beginning of the breeding season or reenter estrus after a failed reproductive attempt. If nutritional availability wanes, or some other disruption of reproduction occurs, the estrous cycle returns the female to reproductive condition as soon as possible when conditions improve.

### Social and Environmental Effects on Reproductive Cycles

Social conditions and environmental factors can dramatically affect female reproductive cycles, as several of the examples in the previous section demonstrate. Several effects of the social environment on reproductive cycles have been observed in laboratory studies. For example, female house mice (*Mus musculus*; type 3 cycle) that are housed together in groups of four or more often enter a period of anestrus. If a male conspecific, or his odor, is introduced into such a group, the females ovulate synchronously 3 or 4 days later (van der Lee and Boot, 1955; Whitten, 1956b). Thus, the organization of estrus among house mice can resemble that of prairie voles under the appropriate social conditions, and these effects appear to be mediated by chemosensory cues. Four such effects that have been observed in the laboratory are described below.

THE LEE–BOOT EFFECT.    One of the first demonstrations that the social environment of a female could influence reproductive cycles was made by van der Lee and Boot (1955). As briefly described above, these investigators showed that female mice, when housed four per cage with no males present, displayed estrous cycles of extended length; this increase in cycle length was always due to the lengthening of the diestrous stage. In other words, the regular 4- or 5-day periodicity of the estrous cycle in these mice was interrupted by prolonged diestrous periods. These longer cycles were considered comparable to the pseudopregnancies induced by sterile matings because growth of the uterine lining was sometimes observed. Also, if the uterine lining was scratched slightly by the experimenters, the uterus responded as it would to a blastocyst and produced a small vascular structure called a deciduomata. This process, called the decidual reaction, indicates that the corpora lutea are producing sufficient progesterone to support implantation of blastocysts, and provides additional evidence of pseudopregnancy. The cues that suspend estrous cycles appear to be chemosensory in nature.

THE WHITTEN EFFECT.    Another well-known reproductive phenomenon, the Whitten effect, involves estrus induction and synchronization and suppression of estrus. Initially, Whitten (1956b, 1957) observed that mating behavior by female mice did not occur with equal frequency during the first four nights after their initial placement with a male. One might expect that 20–25% of the mice in a laboratory colony would mate on each night if they were undergoing regular 4- to

5-day estrous cycles. However, fewer than the expected number of females mated on the first, second, and fourth nights, whereas mating on the third night exceeded statistical expectations, with about 50% of the females mating on that night. Mating occurred more frequently on the first night after pairing if the male had been housed in a small basket within the females' cage for 2 days previously. The incidence of mating on the first night was also increased by placing females in a cage in which a male had previously been housed 48 hours before pairing. In short, many of the females came into estrus on the third night after exposure to a male or his odor. The substance responsible for estrus induction is present in the urine of males and is androgen dependent. This was demonstrated by applying urine from castrated and intact males to the nares (nostrils) of individually housed females and observing the effects on their estrous cycle length.

The second part of the Whitten effect is similar to the Lee–Boot effect, but is more extreme. In Whitten's laboratory, mice were maintained in large colony cages, with 20–30 females housed together. When females are housed individually, the majority show regular estrous cycles. However, when females are caged together in large numbers, estrus and ovulation occur infrequently. Because the uteri of such mice fail to respond to uterine trauma by forming deciduomata, this reaction to group living conditions appears different from the pseudopregnancy responses of mice housed four per cage, the Lee–Boot effect. These qualitative differences may be due to quantitative differences in one or more pheromone(s) produced by adult female mice. The group living situation actually mimics living conditions in the wild, where females exposed to a male, or his odor, come into estrus together, get pregnant, and give birth at the same time. Copulation is synchronized among female mice that have been raised in a large group to occur on the third night after exposure to a male. As in rabbits, the synchronization of estrus, mating, and subsequent births may be adaptive for individual female mice because of the protection afforded by the reduced odds of any one of their offspring becoming a victim of predation.

**THE BRUCE EFFECT.**   Perhaps the most striking effect of social conditions on reproductive cycles has been termed the Bruce effect. In the course of studying the effects of progestins during the development of the birth control pill, Hilda Bruce placed pregnant mice receiving progestin treatments with males that were not their original mates, and noted that many such pairings resulted in termination of the pregnancy (Bruce, 1959). This caused some concern, because spontaneous abortion by women who became pregnant while using oral contraceptives would be a highly undesirable side effect. Further studies demonstrated that the female mice aborted or resorbed their fetuses even when there was no hormone treatment; this result indicated that something about the interaction with a strange male ended the pregnancy. Bruce also noted that the failed pregnancy was always followed by subsequent mating with the new male within 3 to 6 days.

Albino mice were used as breeding pairs in a follow-up study (Bruce, 1960), in which the stud male was removed after observation of mating. When another male mouse of the same strain (strange male) was introduced into the female's cage, her pregnancy was terminated approximately 25% of the time. When the second male was a wild-type male (alien male), pregnancies were blocked in 70–80% of the cases. Females required 48 hours of exposure to the strange male for the maximum number of pregnancy blocks to occur; however, mice were observed to return to estrus within 12 hours after exposure to an alien male. Females can easily discriminate among males, because reunion with the original mate after a 24-hour separation never resulted in terminated pregnancies. Pregnancy block also did not occur if a new male was introduced while the stud male remained in attendance. Castrated or juvenile males did not terminate pregnancies, nor did other females. The pregnancy block phenomenon has been demonstrated in many rodent species (reviewed in Heske and Nelson, 1984).

Several theories have been proposed to account for this phenomenon (Labov, 1981; Schwagmeyer, 1979). From the perspective of the male, blocking a pregnancy sired by another male brings the female into estrus and permits her to mate with the new male, a result that has direct and obvious fitness consequences. From the female's perspective, it may seem hard to imagine an adaptive advantage to pregnancy interruption, but novel males often attack and consume a newborn litter of young that they did not sire (see Chapter 7). The female may be able to recoup some of her investment in the current litter by resorbing the fetuses and mating with the new male, rather than bearing young to feed the novel male.

**THE VANDENBERGH EFFECT.**    In the late 1960s and early 1970s it was discovered that the social environment also affects the rate of sexual maturation in rodents. This phenomenon will be referred to here as the Vandenbergh effect (Vandenbergh, 1967, 1983, 1994).

Previous work had indicated that female rat pups that were handled daily by researchers displayed estrus earlier than unhandled pups; that is, handled females underwent puberty sooner than their unhandled peers. Furthermore, handled females that were housed with males attained puberty earlier than females housed without males. Female albino mouse pups exposed to adult males also matured earlier than those exposed to adult females. Exposure to an adult male for 20 days after weaning was more effective in accelerating puberty than exposure to an adult male 20 days before weaning. In these studies, maturation, or puberty, was measured by the age of vaginal opening, first vaginal estrus, and first mating. When males are absent in a laboratory environment, puberty occurs at about 60 days of age in female house mice. Overall, maturation rate was increased by about 15–20 days in female pups exposed to adult males. A similar phenomenon has been observed in other rodent species (Vandenbergh, 1994).

A second part of the Vandenbergh effect is that a pheromone emitted by female rodents can delay sexual maturation in female conspecifics (Vandenbergh, 1994); isolated female mice attain puberty sooner than females reared in all-female groups. A similar phenomenon has been reported in tamarins (*Saguinus oedipus*), a monogamous primate species, in which reproductive development is suppressed in females living in their natal group. First ovulation was later in females that were exposed to the odors of their natal families than in females exposed to a control odor (Savage et al., 1988). Visual, olfactory, and auditory contact with strange males initiated ovulation in otherwise suppressed female tamarins (Widowski et al., 1992). These studies suggest that chemosensory and social cues can affect reproductive function in primates.

**THE ROLE OF PHEROMONES.**    As we have seen, social effects on mammalian reproductive cycles appear to be mediated by chemosensory cues. There appear to be two pheromones that are responsible for these effects. One of these chemical signals comes from females and tends to suppress ovarian function. Depending on the reproductive condition of the recipient animals (prepubertal or cycling) and the strength of the stimuli, exposure to the female chemosignal either inhibits puberty or suspends estrus. This chemosignal probably acts by suppressing gonadotropin release from the anterior pituitary. The other chemical signal is emitted by males and, depending on the reproductive condition of the recipient female (prepubertal, suspended estrous cycling, or pregnant), accelerates puberty, induces estrus, or interrupts pregnancy. The male chemosignal appears to induce an abrupt release of LH, which stimulates follicular growth. Prolactin appears to interfere with the induction of LH release; for example, lactating females that become pregnant during postpartum estrus are protected against pregnancy block due to male chemosignals (Komisaruk et al., 1981).

From where do these chemical signals emanate? The entire body can, in theory, provide a multitude of chemical signals, but probably the most important source of chemical signals in rodents is the urine and feces. The source of the pheromone emitted by females has not been identified, but there are strong indications that it is excreted in urine. There is, however, good evidence that the male primer pheromones are androgen-based components of urine; urine from castrated or prepubertal males is not very effective in producing estrus in females.

The effects of social factors on ovarian cycles are not limited to rodents. Women who live together for extended periods of time eventually begin to synchronize their menstrual cycles (McClintock, 1971). Records of menstrual cycles obtained from undergraduate women attending Radcliffe College showed that menstrual synchronization was more likely among roommates than among women who lived in the same dormitory building, and that approximately 7 or 8 months of cohabitation is required before menstrual cycles become synchronized. This phenomenon may be mediated by chemosensory signals, but the experiments necessary to determine this cannot be conducted on humans. Analogous studies have, however, been conducted on rats, showing that rats living in groups show a similar estrus-synchronizing phenomenon, with chemosensory cues providing the stimuli allowing synchronization of the estrous cycles (McClintock, 1978). Olfaction is probably a very important component of normal human sexual behavior, but it has rarely been studied until recently (but see Doty, 1986) (Box 6.2). Clinical reports on women with congenital absence of the olfactory bulbs revealed a markedly increased incidence of ovarian hypoplasia (nondevelopment) (Schwanzel-Fukuda et al., 1989), but this probably reflects the lack of GnRH neuronal migration rather than the loss of olfactory ability.

**ENVIRONMENTAL EFFECTS.**    Environmental factors have an enormous influence on ovarian cycles. Lack of proper nutrition, stress, or lack of appropriate habitat can adversely affect ovarian cycles (Wade et al., 1997; Schneider et al., 1998). Stressful events ranging from starting college to imprisonment can suspend menstrual cycles in women (Bachman and Kemmann, 1982; Bass, 1947). One study found that premenopausal women awaiting their execution on death row were not experiencing any menstrual cycles (Pettersson et al., 1973)(see Chapter 11).

Estrous cycles occur only during the breeding season for most mammals. The breeding season represents the "temporal fit" among many selective forces—including food availability, thermoregulatory pressures, climatic factors, and the species' mating system and gestation length—that best ensures reproductive success. The environmental factors that turn the ovaries on and off at the beginning

## Box 6.2
# Human Pheromones

Although there have been many claims of the existence of human pheromones—chemical signals that are released by an individual and travel through the air or water to affect the physiology or behavior of another individual—until recently there was no solid evidence of such substances. Despite the lack of scientific evidence, one can buy perfumes, bearing such provocative names as Lure, Scent, and Instinct Pheromone, purported to contain human pheromones specifically formulated to attract the men or women of one's choice. The best part of these sales pitches (if you were the "naked emperor" selling these fragrances) is that the pheromones are essentially odorless (buyers can mix them into their favorite perfume or cologne) and affect the behavior of recipients without their conscious awareness. One such product claims to have 50 "known" human pheromones as ingredients. Despite these widespread claims for their existence, no human pheromones have been isolated and characterized, and until very recently, their existence was unproven (Stern and McClintock, 1998).

A recent study established the existence of two human pheromones in women, one produced prior to ovulation during the follicular phase, which shortens the ovarian cycle in recipients, and a second one produced around the time of ovulation, which lengthens the ovarian cycle in recipients. These pheromones mediated a specific neuroendocrine response in women without the recipients' conscious awareness (Stern and McClintock, 1998). Women between the ages of 20 and 35 were used in the study. Nine of these women provided chemosensory samples during different times of their menstrual cycles by wearing absorbent

pads under their arms for at least 8 hours daily. The pads were quartered and stored frozen until tested on other women. The pads were wiped under the noses of the recipient women. Pads obtained from donor women during their follicular phase accelerated the periovulatory surge of LH and shortened the menstrual cycles of the recipient women by 1–14 days over two menstral cycles (see figure) (Stern and McClintock, 1998). Pads obtained from donor women around the time of ovulation delayed the periovulatory LH surge and lengthened the menstrual cycle of recipient women by 1–12 days. Approximately 70% of the recipient women responded to the pheromones. Because the same donors provided all the chemosensory samples, this study demonstrated that the timing of ovulation in women could be manipulated and provided the first definitive evidence of human pheromones. This work opens the door to a more "natural" way of manipulating the timing of ovulation, which could help in birth control and fertility treatments.

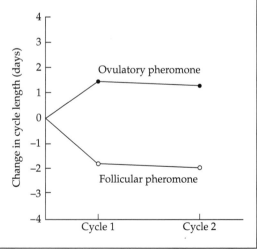

and the end of the breeding season will be discussed in Chapter 10. As indicated in Chapter 3, perinatal events can also affect subsequent estrous cyclicity. Recall that proximity to brothers in the uterine horn during gestation increased estrous cycle length and reduced attractiveness in female rats and mice as compared with individuals gestated between two sisters (vom Saal and Bronson, 1980). Illness can also affect female sexual behavior (Box 6.3).

## Experimental Analyses of Female Sexual Behavior

By now you have noted that a tremendous amount is known about estrous cycles. The research efforts aimed at understanding the temporal characteristics, physiological mechanisms, and adaptive functions of estrous cycles have been enormous. However, as the previous discussion has revealed, most laboratory studies examining female reproductive physiology and behavior have been conducted on females undergoing repeated estrous cycles. Although a strong case was made above that the chronic estrous cycles observed and studied in the laboratory are merely artifacts, a great deal of valuable information has been gained by studying those cycles: virtually all that we know about the regulation of female sexual behavior has been derived from studying cycling female rodents. The development of oral contraceptives for human use was accomplished by understanding the endocrinology of cycling rodents and nonhuman primates; all of our understanding of the relationships among the nervous system, hormones, and female sexual behavior has been achieved by studying cycling rodents and nonhuman primates. Therefore, despite their lack of ecological validity, laboratory studies of estrous cycles have been valuable. The final sections of this chapter detail the endocrine–neural interactions underlying female sexual behavior that have been revealed by such studies.

Attempts to localize the neural bases of female sexual behavior have followed, in many cases, the same sequence as attempts at localization in males. However, it is much easier to quantify receptivity in females in the form of lordosis than it is to quantify "receptivity" in males in the form of appetitive behavior. As is the case for males, there have been two major lines of research dealing with the interaction of female sexual behavior and hormones. The physiological line of research has attempted to determine the sources of the signals generating sexual behavior; that is, to discover the loci of the interaction between sex hormones and behavior (for example, Bard, 1936; Beach, 1944b; Brookhart et al., 1941). As with males, early research established that the interaction does not take place at the level of the gonads; consequently, much of the subsequent work has focused on the central nervous system. The second line of research has considered sexual "motivation." The strength of the female sex drive has been tested and quantified using a variety of motivational tests (for example, Nissen, 1929), and in some cases, the neural bases of female sexual motivation have been discovered inadvertently during studies of receptivity. Pioneering sex researchers faced social pressures against positing a sex drive for females, as opposed to the

## Box 6.3
# Illness Suppresses Female Sexual Behavior

Physical condition, including body mass and blood concentrations of specific metabolic fuels, has dramatic effects on female sexual physiology and behavior. Females with low energy, or otherwise in poor condition, are usually not receptive or proceptive toward males, and males are generally less attracted to females in poor condition than to females in good condition. Similarly, females that are ill are generally less receptive, proceptive, and attractive than females that are not ill.

The behavioral cues associated with illness are probably well known to you. An entire constellation of so-called "sickness behaviors," which occur in response to systemic diseases or localized infections, has been documented in humans and several other mammalian species. Obvious behavioral changes observed in sick individuals include lethargy, hypersomnia, malaise, anorexia, loss of interest, and reduction in goal-directed behaviors (Hart, 1988). To induce "sickness behaviors" experimentally, animals are treated with endotoxin (which consists of heat-inactivated shells of *E. coli*) or lipopolysaccharide (LPS, which is the major molecular component of the cell walls of *E. coli*); both treatments activate the immune system, but do not give the animals a replicating infection.

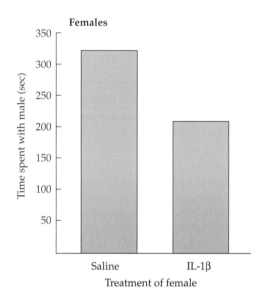

Activation of the immune system is communicated to the neuroendocrine system by chemical messengers called cytokines. Cytokines are released by activated macrophages during immunological responses to infections. Several of these chemical messengers, including interleukin-1β (IL-1β), interleukin-6 (IL-6), and tumor necrosis factor-α (TNF-α), affect neuroendocrine processes in the hypothalamus and

"obvious" sex drive manifested by males. Then, as today, sexual behavior was a politically charged scientific topic. More recently, female sexual motivation has been quantified in terms of proceptive behavior (Erskine, 1989; Wallen, 1990).

This section will review the hormonal events associated with female ovarian cycles in rats and rhesus monkeys. The final section will present the neural bases of female sexual behavior.

### *Hormonal Correlates of Female Reproductive Cycles*

Recall from Chapter 2 that there is a dynamic relationship among the gonadal sex steroid hormones, the gonadotropins, and the hypothalamic releasing hormones. Basically, this relationship is one of reciprocal inhibition. The hypothalamus secretes pulses of releasing hormones, which stimulate the release of gonadotropins from the anterior pituitary. Pulses of gonadotropins drive the pituitary (Segreti et al., 1997). For example, administration of IL-1β causes fever, hypersomnia, and slow-wave sleep, as well as reductions in locomotor activity, exploratory behaviors,

**Males**

food intake, and social contact (Yirmiya et al., 1995; Avitsur et al., 1997a,b). IL-1β treatment also inhibits GnRH gene expression in the hypothalamus, decreases GnRH release in rats on the afternoon of proestrus, and decreases circulating LH concentrations in ovariectomized rats and monkeys, as well as inhibiting steroid hormone synthesis in the ovaries and testes (Rivest and Rivier, 1993; Yirmiya et al., 1995).

Administration of IL-1β to female rats significantly reduced their sexual receptivity and proceptivity (Yirmiya et al., 1995). IL-1β–treated females also lost their preference for sexually active male rats. Surprisingly, IL-1β treatment of males did not diminish their sexual behavior. Both males and females displayed reduced locomotor activity after receiving IL-1β, which suggests that the sex difference in responsiveness to IL-1β is limited to sexual behavior. IL-1β also affected attractivity of female, but not male, rats. When males had a choice between estrogen-treated, ovariectomized females injected with either IL-1β or with saline, males preferred saline-injected females (Avitsur et al., 1998); that is, IL-1β reduced attractiveness in females (see figure, opposite ). In contrast, when presented with a choice of males that had been injected either with IL-1β or with saline, females did not discriminate between these males except at high doses (see figure at left).

Taken together, these studies suggest that cytokines have direct and dramatic effects on behavior. Furthermore, the effect of IL-1β on sexual behavior shows a clear sex difference. The ultimate cause of this sex difference probably reflects the differential effects of illness on the reproductive success of males and females. As these studies show, the interactions between the immune and endocrine systems that affect behavior are becoming a rapidly expanding area of research.

release of sex steroid hormones by the gonads. Negative feedback works in the following way: as sex steroid hormone concentrations increase, secretion of gonadotropins is reduced, which stimulates decreases in gonadotropin-stimulated steroid hormone synthesis. Removal of the ovaries causes the well-known **castration response**: the removal of the source of steroid hormones removes the negative feedback that regulates gonadotropin secretion, resulting in sustained elevated gonadotropin concentrations, as well as elevated releasing hormone secretion. The simplified version of the relationship between gonadal sex steroid hormones and the gonadotropins is reflected in the metaphor of a seesaw (Figure 6.18; Moore and Price, 1932).

**THE OVARIAN CYCLE IN RODENTS.**    Gonadotropin-releasing hormone (GnRH) is released by the hypothalamus in brief pulses. These pulses of GnRH stimulate cells in the anterior pituitary to release follicle-stimulating hormone (FSH) and

**6.18    The castration response.** Normally, the gonadotropins and sex steroid hormones exhibit a so-called seesaw profile. For example, increasing LH concentrations stimulate increased estradiol secretion until high concentrations of estradiol inhibit LH through negative feedback, which in turn lowers estradiol concentrations. After ovariectomy, estradiol concentrations decline, and LH concentrations continue to rise, unchecked by negative feedback.

luteinizing hormone (LH) (Figure 6.19). FSH, as its name implies, causes the follicles of the ovaries to grow. As the follicles develop, they produce estrogens and progestins. During the diestrous and proestrous periods of the rat estrous cycle, the follicles are stimulated to produce sex steroid hormones in increasing concentrations. On the afternoon of proestrus, the pulse amplitude and pulse frequency of GnRH release, and subsequently the pulse amplitude and pulse frequency of LH and FSH release, increase. Under these conditions, negative feedback fails momentarily, and the follicles release a large surge of estrogen and, soon thereafter, a smaller surge of progesterone. This preovulatory LH surge stimulates ovulation, reflecting the positive feedback feature of the hypothalamic–hypophyseal–gonadal control mechanism (see Chapter 3). The elevated estrogen and progesterone blood concentrations also stimulate estrous behavior. Estrogen concentrations fall back to baseline rapidly, but the blood progesterone concentration remains high for many hours if no mating occurs, or for many days if mating does occur. The elevated progesterone concentrations act eventually to terminate estrous behavior (Goy and Young, 1956/1957; Zucker, 1966, 1968).

The tonic release of GnRH throughout most of the estrous cycle is mediated by the medial basal hypothalamus, as it is in males. The release of increasingly higher pulses of GnRH is mediated by this so-called pulse generator. A neuronal pathway made up of neurons located in the anterior hypothalamus, preoptic area, and suprachiasmatic nucleus regions, as well as the arcuate nucleus, is involved in providing a daily signal for ovulation if the appropriate endocrine milieu is present. This surge generator normally transmits every afternoon; that is why there are 4- *or* 5-day estrous cycles in rats, but no 4.5-day cycles. Experimental disruption of the surge generator pathway or anesthesia during the afternoon of proestrus prevents transmission of the signal and delays estrus for another 24 hours. Only when the daily signal for a large surge of GnRH is coincident with

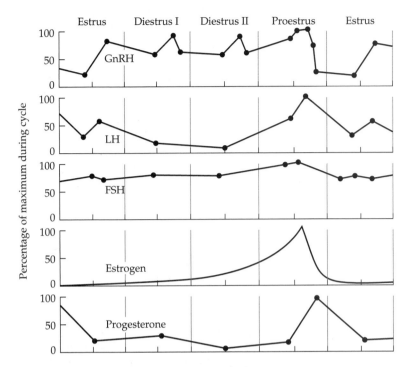

**6.19   The ovarian cycle in rats.** GnRH stimulates the secretion of LH and FSH, which cause a steady increase of estrogen until the afternoon of proestrus. Then the pulse amplitude and frequency of GnRH-release increase, causing a rapid increase in LH and FSH concentrations, and a corresponding surge of estrogen and progesterone that leads to ovulation and estrous behavior. Estrogen concentrations decline rapidly at vaginal estrus, but progesterone concentrations decline more gradually, especially if mating has occurred. Source: Ganong, 1995.

previous estrogen priming will the positive feedback mechanism be engaged. Soon after ovulation, the negative feedback mechanism is restored, and low concentrations of GnRH, gonadotropins, and steroid hormones are secreted during early diestrus. The cycle resumes when pulses of GnRH stimulate brief pulses of gonadotropins, which stimulate follicular development anew. The 2 days of diestrus and 1 day of proestrus can be considered the follicular phase of the rat estrous cycle because follicular development occurs in anticipation of ovulation. Because the corpora lutea are not maintained after ovulation in unmated rats, there is no luteal phase. Thus, natural estrous behavior is the result of prolonged, high concentrations of estrogen followed by high concentrations of progesterone. Behavioral estrus can be induced in ovariectomized rats and guinea pigs with appropriately timed injections of estradiol and progesterone (Feder, 1981; Pfaff et al., 1994; Blaustein, 1996). In other species, such as Old World primates, a preovulatory GnRH and LH surge also occurs, but is not necessary for ovulation.

Although the sequential elevation of estradiol and progesterone is necessary to induce full estrous behavior in rats and guinea pigs, the sequential presence of progesterone and estradiol is necessary to induce estrus in sheep (Robinson, 1954). In other species, such as prairie voles (*Microtus ochrogaster*) and Siberian hamsters (*Phodopus campbelli*), progesterone is unnecessary for the expression of estrous behaviors (Carter et al., 1987; Wynne-Edwards et al., 1987). Female musk shrews (*Suncus murinus*) secrete testosterone from their ovaries around the time of ovulation. The testosterone enters the blood circulation and is aromatized to estradiol in neurons located in the preoptic area and in the hypothalamus. The intracellular interaction of estradiol with its receptors produces behavioral estrus (Rissman, 1991). Testosterone and other androgens have been shown to be important in mediating female sexual behavior in several vertebrate species (Staub and De Beer, 1997). Thus, most female mammals require ovarian steroid hormones associated with ovulation to evoke behavioral estrus. However, the pattern of steroid hormone secretion is species-specific (Blaustein, 1996).

**THE OVARIAN CYCLE IN PRIMATES.**   The ovarian cycle of rhesus monkeys is virtually identical to that of humans. In women and rhesus monkeys, only one follicle usually develops during each cycle. The corpus luteum is maintained after each ovulation (type 1.1B cycle) and persists for about 14 days in a nonpregnant cycle. The endometrial lining of the uterine wall develops in anticipation of blastocyst implantation. If the ovulated ovum is not fertilized in the fallopian tube and there is no blastocyst to implant, the endometrial lining is shed, and menstrual bleeding occurs. The follicular phase is more variable among individuals, and ranges between 10 and 20 days. Variation in menstrual cycle length is almost always due to variation in the length of the follicular phase.

If a female rhesus monkey has a 28-day cycle, then the following endocrine profile occurs (Table 6.3) (Knobil and Hotchkiss, 1988): Blood plasma concentrations of FSH and LH slowly increase for approximately 10 days following the end of menstrual bleeding. Under the stimulation of FSH, the primary ovarian follicle secretes estrogen. Estrogen concentrations (primarily estradiol) increase gradually during the first week after the onset of menstrual bleeding, and increase sharply during the following week. Estrogen concentrations display a periovulatory surge, which stimulates a surge of LH and a lesser surge of FSH release from the anterior pituitary. The gonadotropin surge stimulates ovulation of the ripe ovum. After ovulation, plasma estrogen concentrations plummet to basal concentrations, and gonadotropin concentrations also diminish. As the corpus luteum

Table 6.3

**Daily production rates of sex steroid hormones in women at different phases of the menstrual cycle**

| Hormone | Menstrual phase | | |
| --- | --- | --- | --- |
| | Early follicular | Preovulatory | Midluteal |
| Progesterone (mg) | 1.0 | 4.0 | 25.0 |
| 17-Hydroxyprogesterone (mg) | 0.5 | 4.0 | 4.0 |
| Dehydroepiandrosterone (mg) | 7.0 | 7.0 | 7.0 |
| Androstenedione (mg) | 2.6 | 4.7 | 3.4 |
| Testosterone (μg) | 144.0 | 171.0 | 126.0 |
| Estrone (μg) | 50.0 | 350.0 | 250.0 |
| Estradiol (μg) | 36.0 | 380.0 | 250.0 |

*Source:* After Yen and Jaffe, 1991.

begins to function, plasma concentrations of progesterone increase. In a non-pregnant cycle, the corpus luteum begins to regress and progesterone concentrations fall back to baseline approximately 10–12 days after ovulation. The low progesterone concentrations evoke menstruation, and the cycle recurs. This cycle is similar to the human menstrual cycle (see Figure 6.17).

Androgens seem to be critical in mediating sexual behavior in women. The source of androgens in females appears to be the ovaries and adrenal glands. Blood concentrations of these androgens fluctuate during the menstrual cycle. In a study that assayed plasma concentrations of free estradiol, testosterone, and progesterone at weekly intervals, it was discovered that only free testosterone correlated positively with sexual desire, sexual thoughts, and anticipation of sexual activity (Alexander and Sherwin, 1993). Treatment of surgically induced menopausal (ovariectomized) women with several steroid hormones in double-blind studies revealed that androgen treatment was most effective in restoring sexual desire (Sherwin, 1988a; Sherwin and Gelfand, 1988; Sherwin et al., 1985). These results are reminiscent of the effects of androgens on sexual motivation among hypogonadal men (see Chapter 5; Davidson et al., 1979).

As in hypogonadal men, hormone concentrations above a certain threshold that maintains sexual behavior do not further increase the frequency of sexual behavior in ovariectomized women (Sherwin, 1988b). One study compared several aspects of sexual behavior in women using oral contraceptives and in nonusers (Alexander et al., 1990). Nonusers exhibited lower blood plasma concentrations of testosterone than oral contraceptive users, and they also displayed perimenstrual decreases in plasma testosterone concentrations, which was associated with a reported drop in the level of sexual desire. There was no significant difference reported in the frequency of autosexual activities, but users of oral contraceptives reported more frequent and more satisfying sexual experiences than nonusers (Alexander et al., 1990). Of course, these results may reflect a relaxation of pregnancy fears rather than endocrine events. Taken together, these findings suggest that androgens induce sexual motivation, receptivity, and satisfaction in women (Bancroft et al., 1991a,b; Sherwin and Gelfand, 1988). Androgens appear to enhance receptive and proceptive behaviors in female rhesus monkeys as well (e.g., Everitt and Herbert, 1971; Herbert and Trimble, 1967; Wallen and Goy, 1977).

The fluctuating concentrations of gonadal, pituitary, and hypothalamic hormones in female mammals complicate somewhat the understanding of hormone–behavior interactions. Generally, slowly rising concentrations of estrogen seem necessary to prime mammalian females for the subsequent elevated progestin concentrations that induce behavioral estrus. As the ratio of estrogen to progesterone in the blood is reversed, progesterone often acts to stop estrous behavior. The hormonal correlates of the estrous cycle of rodents and of the menstrual cycle of primates differ in a few important ways. Ovulation and peak estrogen concentrations coincide in both rats and primates. However, rats display a periovulatory progesterone peak that is reduced or absent in primates. In rodents, and probably other nonprimate species, both sexual motivation and sexual performance are mediated by sex steroid hormones; copulation does not occur unless there are high blood concentrations of estrogen. In contrast, the ability to copulate is not linked to hormones in primates, but motivation to copulate in primates appears to be linked to a periovulatory peak in androgen concentrations. The following section reviews how these fluctuating hormones affect neurons directly to change female behavior.

### Neural Mechanisms Mediating Female Sexual Behavior

Virtually everything that is known about the endocrine effects on neural tissue that mediate female sexual behavior has come from studies on the neural and endocrine control of lordosis in rats. As we have seen, lordosis is a receptive behavior, a sexual reflex observed in female rats. This behavior is primed with estrogen and progesterone, and occurs in response to tactile sensory information normally provided by a copulating male. Thus, sensory input is one aspect of the behavior on which hormones can be predicted to act.

How does sensory information get to the hypothalamus? Relevant sensory input enters the female rat's nervous system during mating via cutaneous receptors on the flanks, rump, and perineum. Information from the stimulated skin receptors and from pressure-responsive sensory neurons enters the spinal cord, where the motoneurons controlling the muscles involved in lordosis are located, and is sent to the medullary reticular formation (Figure 6.20a; Pfaff and Schwartz-Giblin, 1988). This pathway to the brain stem is necessary, but not sufficient, for lordosis to occur.

Hormones can also be predicted to act on the central brain mechanisms integrating the endocrine, social, and environmental stimuli coincident with mating. Several brain sites have been discovered to mediate lordosis (Figure 6.20b). Researchers found that lesions of the ventromedial nuclei of the hypothalamus (VMN) or destruction of their afferent and efferent fibers typically reduced the frequency of lordosis (Clark et al., 1981; Kennedy, 1964; Yamanouchi, 1980; but see Emery and Moss, 1984), demonstrating that the VMN are critical to the lordosis response. In order to map the neural circuit involved in lordosis, the incoming and outgoing fibers then had to be traced. Certain fibers leaving the VMN via a sweeping lateral–posterior pathway were found to be necessary for lordosis, whereas other exiting fibers were less critical. (Pfaff et al., 1994). The essential axons descend to the midbrain central gray region; lesions of this region were found to reduce lordosis (Sakuma and Pfaff, 1979). Destruction of the midbrain ascending ventral noradrenergic bundle (VNAB) completely abolished the appearance of lordosis (Hansen et al., 1980, 1981). Neurons in the midbrain central gray region project axons to the medullary reticular formation in the brain stem. This region of the hindbrain controls motoneurons for axial muscles, especially the deep back muscles, which are critical for lordosis (see Figure 6.20a; Pfaff and Schwartz-Giblin, 1988). The connection of this brain stem region with the descending fibers from the midbrain central gray region permits lordosis only when sex steroid hormones are available to neurons in the midbrain or to cells in the VMN. Figure 6.21 is a detailed diagram of these neural circuits.

What is the mechanism of action of estrogens and progestins on these brain regions? The steroid hormone receptors found in the brain are chemically similar to those found in the uterus. As described in Chapter 2, steroids can stimulate production of their own receptors as well as production of other steroid receptor types. Because all the steroid hormones are structurally similar, elevated estrogen concentrations can stimulate the production of both estrogen and progestin receptors in the cytosol of neurons throughout the nervous system. Thus, high concentrations of estradiol (injected by an experimenter, for example) can induce the production of progesterone receptors. This is the likely explanation for how estrogen alone induces estrous behavior in ovariectomized female rats. Anti-steroids—that is, substances that occupy steroid receptors without producing any biological effect—block the occurrence of lordosis (Pfaff, 1980; Pfaff et al., 1994; Delville and Blaustein, 1991; Blaustein and Olster, 1989).

Cells that concentrate estradiol and progesterone have been discovered throughout the vertebrate brain. These target cells show virtually the same distribution regardless of taxon, and correspond closely with the distribution of receptors for androgens (see Figure 5.17). The areas with the highest density of

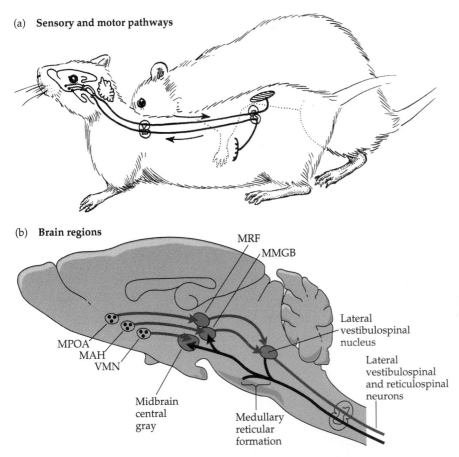

**6.20   The neural basis of lordosis.** (a) Male mounting behavior causes activation of pressure receptors in the female's flanks; axons from these receptors form a sensory nerve that projects to the dorsal root of the ganglion of the spinal cord. From the spinal cord, the sensory signals travel to the reticular formation in the hindbrain and the midbrain central gray area (lower arrow). When estrogen concentrations are high, various brain regions activate the spinal motoneurons innvervating the deep back muscles (upper arrow), resulting in the characteristic postural changes of lordosis. (b) Brain regions activated by estrogen and involved in lordosis include the ventromedial nucleus of the hypothalamus (VMN), the medial preoptic area (MPOA), and the medial anterior hypothalamus (MAH). Signals from these regions reach the midbrain central gray, medullary reticular formation (MRF), and medial geniculate body (MMGB); the MRF and MMGB ultimately activate the spinal motoneurons innervating the back muscles involved in lordosis behavior. After Pfaff et al., 1994.

estradiol- and progesterone-concentrating cells are located in the forebrain, including the medial preoptic area, the anterior hypothalamus, and the ventro-medial–ventrolateral hypothalamus, as well as the amygdala and midbrain central gray area (Figure 6.22) (Pfaff and Conrad, 1978; Blaustein, 1996). Many lesion studies and electrical stimulation studies have revealed that these regions are involved in the regulation of female sexual behavior.

There are hormone manipulations that can mimic the hormonal profile of natural estrus. One way to bring an ovariectomized mouse or hamster into estrus is

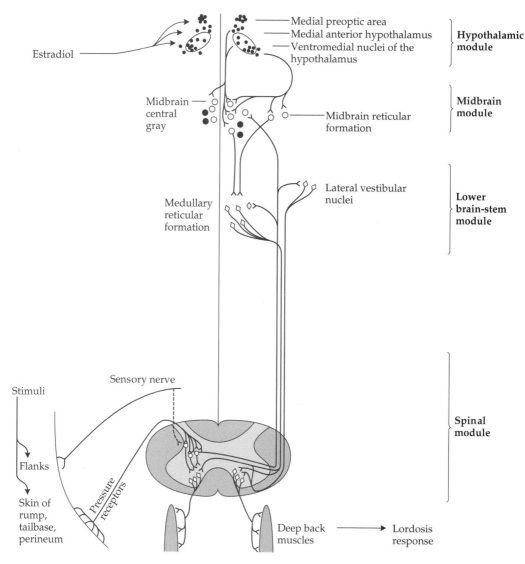

**6.21   A detailed view of the neural circuitry mediating lordosis** in rats. The neural circuits outlined in Figure 6.20, separated into structural and functional neural modules. After Pfaff et al., 1994.

**6.22    Estrogen receptor immunoreactivity** shows that neurons in the hypothalamus have estrogen receptors (shown here with dark staining) in all parts of the cell (i.e., cytosol, nucleus, cellular processes). Courtesy of Jeff Blaustein.

to inject her with estradiol early one morning and inject her with progesterone about 6 to 8 hours later. In about 12 hours, the female will display lordosis in response to the appropriate tactile stimulation. To bring female rats into estrus, estradiol is injected, then progesterone is injected 24–48 hours later. Behavioral estrus is observed approximately 4 hours after the progesterone injection. Another way to bring an ovariectomized rat into estrus is to implant a Silastic capsule of estradiol under her skin, which will secrete estradiol at a constant rate that varies with the length of the capsule. If the female is then injected with progesterone about 12 hours prior to her pairing with a male, estrous behavior will ensue when the male is present.

Several experiments have demonstrated that estrogens must prime the CNS for further estrogen and progesterone exposure in order for estrous behavior to be exhibited. Implants of crystalline estradiol into the VMN induce lordosis in ovariectomized rats (Barfield and Chen, 1977; Lisk, 1962), but this lordotic behavior is relatively weak and infrequent compared with that observed among female rats in natural estrus. However, if crystalline estradiol is implanted into the VMN and the animal is then injected systemically with progesterone (or if crystalline progesterone is implanted into the VMN and the animal is then injected systemically with estradiol), virtually all females display lordosis that resembles that observed in females in natural estrus (Rubin and Barfield, 1983). A variety of techniques, including microimplants of protein synthesis inhibitors, transcription inhibitors, and anti-estrogens, have demonstrated that the ventromedial nucleus of the hypothalamus is critical for estradiol priming in rats (Blaustein and Olster, 1989). Thus, it can be concluded that estrogen treatment primes the CNS for subsequent estrogen or estrogen/progestin treatment (Parsons et al., 1979; Walker and Feder, 1977, 1979). Estrogen priming requires about 24 hours unless doses are vey high, in which case the first lordosis response occurs in about 18–20 hours.

Progesterone facilitates estrus. Occupied progesterone receptors in relevant neurons mediate many of the behavioral effects of progesterone by serving as gene transcription factors (Blaustein, 1996) (see below). In many species, including rats and guinea pigs, progesterone initially facilitates estrous behavior, but eventually a refractory period occurs. In other species, especially reptiles, progesterone inhibits female receptive behavior (Godwin et al., 1996). The physiological explanation for the termination of estrous behavior is the down-regulation of progesterone receptors (see Chapter 2).

What is the mechanism of estrogen priming? One possibility is that receptor dynamics are affected by estrogen treatment; that is, estrogen secretion might induce the production of estrogen and progestin receptors in the CNS. This is a reasonable hypothesis, but in some studies no changes in steroid hormone receptor numbers were detected after estrogen priming (e.g., Parsons et al., 1979). Other studies have indicated that receptor numbers do change, but well after estrogen priming (reviewed in Pfaff et al., 1994). Interestingly, the behavioral changes first occur well after all bound estrogen has been metabolized by the liver, as shown by one study in which radioactive estradiol was given to ovariectomized rats. It was observed that peak binding of estrogen to nuclear receptors in the hypothalamus occurred 1 to 2 hours after injection; estrogen binding had returned to basal concentrations by 12 hours post-injection (McEwen et al., 1975).

Once estrogen binds to nuclear receptors in the hypothalamus and elsewhere, the estrogen–receptor complex attaches to the nuclear DNA and serves as a gene transcription factor. Thus gene transcription and translation are either activated or, in some cases, decreased by estrogen treatment. Predictably, protein synthesis inhibitors block the effects of steroid hormones on estrous behavior. Over the course of the next few hours, estrogen causes electrophysiological changes in the pattern and frequency of firing rates of neurons in the VMN, especially in slow-firing neurons in this region (Pfaff and Schwartz-Giblin, 1988). These changes alone cannot account for behavioral changes, because no lordosis is observed if only this part of the brain is exposed to estrogen priming. Electron microscopy studies have revealed that estrogen binding and subsequent DNA transcription promotes RNA synthesis. Growthlike processes occur in and around the VMN in response to estrogen treatment, which is consistent with the observed increases in RNA and structural protein synthesis after estrogen exposure. Conversely, treatment of the hypothalamus with protein synthesis inhibitors eliminates lordosis (Meisel and Pfaff, 1984). Thus electrophysiological and structural changes occur in the VMN in response to estrogen priming, and continued exposure to high estradiol or progesterone concentrations induces the expression of lordosis in response to appropriate sensory input. Furthermore, intermittent exposure to estrogens is sufficient to prime ovariectomized rats and guinea pigs behaviorally to progestins (Clark and Roy, 1983; Olster and Blaustein, 1988).

Many neurotransmitters have been implicated in the neural mediation of hormone-induced estrous behavior. For example, there is evidence that norepinephrine, dopamine, acetylcholine, serotonin, and GABA (each acting through their own specific receptor subtypes), as well as GnRH, prolactin, oxytocin, and substance P, facilitate estrous behavior (Blaustein, 1996). Serotonin (acting through the 5-HT$_{1A}$ receptor), dopamine, β-endorphin, and CRH may inhibit lordosis. The effects of hormones probably affect these and other neurotransmitters. Estradiol mediates many neurotransmitters that facilitate female sexual behavior (McCarthy and Pfaus, 1996); for example, estradiol evokes oxytocin and enkephalin gene expression and increases the numbers of many types of postsynaptic neurotransmitter receptors (Flanagan-Cato and Fluharty, 1997). However, no clear pattern of neurotransmitter and steroid hormone receptor co-localization has been found in the brain. That is, knowing that a particular neuron has estrogen or progestin receptors does not tell us the type of neurotransmitter used by the neuron in question. However, recent work suggests that there can be "cross talk" between certain neurotransmitters (e.g., dopamine) and steroid hormone receptors (e.g., progestin). A dopamine D$_1$ receptor agonist, but not a dopamine D$_2$ receptor agonist, mimicked the effects of progesterone in facilitating sexual behavior in female rats (Mani et al., 1995). If the rats were treated with a progesterone antagonist, then the facilitatory effects of dopamine were blocked. These results suggest that neurotransmitters may affect in vivo gene expression and behavior by means of cross talk with steroid hormone receptors in the brain (Mani et al., 1995; Auger et al., 1996).

Two primary hypotheses regarding the role of estrogen in promoting lordosis have been proposed: the trigger hypothesis and the maintenance hypothesis (Pfaff et al., 1994) (Box 6.4). The former hypothesis states that one brief pulse of estrogen sets off a chain of events that, once triggered, continues to the end of the program with the display of lordosis. This hypothesis was generated in response to data indicating that a relatively brief exposure (approximately 30 minutes) to estrogen could result in lordosis (e.g., Bullock, 1970; Johnston and Davidson, 1979). However, the esterified estrogens used in these studies have relatively slow clearance rates and probably stayed in the blood and affected neural tissue for much longer than 30 minutes (Clemens and Weaver, 1985). The maintenance hypothesis contends that estrogen must be present continuously from the beginning of estrogen treatment throughout the behavioral test in order for lordosis to be displayed. However, tests using estradiol implants that could be inserted and removed rapidly revealed that two discontinuous exposures to estrogen could facilitate progesterone-evoked lordosis (Södersten et al., 1981). Using a variety of temporal schedules of estradiol exposure, it was reported that only 2 hours of total estrogen treatment were sufficient to increase progesterone receptor numbers in the hypothalamus, as well as to permit lordosis. The second estrogen treatment had to begin at least 4 hours after the end of the initial estrogen exposure, but not more than 13 hours later (Parsons et al., 1982).

More recently, a cascade hypothesis has been proposed to explain the endocrine events underlying lordosis. According to this hypothesis, (1) specific and discrete events occur within the nerve cells of the VMN as a result of initial estrogen–receptor binding, and (2) these events are required for later estrogen-dependent events to occur. This hypothesis differs from the maintenance hypothesis because continuous estrogen receptor occupation is not required; rather, estrogen must occupy receptors at specific, critical times in order for lordosis to be expressed (Pfaff and Schwartz-Giblin, 1988). When the two-pulse experiment described above was replicated, it was found that anesthesia (Roy et al., 1985) or protein synthesis inhibition (Meisel and Pfaff, 1984; Roy et al., 1985) prior to either

Box 6.4

# Nongenomic Behavioral Effects of Steroid Hormones

Traditionally, the behavioral effects of steroid hormones have been assumed to be mediated via intracellular receptor–ligand interactions that ultimately affect gene transcription (Flanagan-Cato and Fluharty, 1997). However, an alternative mechanism of steroid action has recently emerged (Moore and Orchinik, 1994). It was reported that corticosterone administration could rapidly interfere with mating behavior in a species of newt (*Taricha granulosa*) (Orchinik et al., 1991; Moore and Orchinik, 1994). Membrane-bound corticosterone receptors have been located in neuronal membrane fractions from these newts (Moore et al., 1995). The discovery of the membrane-bound steroid receptors and the rapidity of the response suggested that the genetic machinery could not have been engaged, and it was hypothesized that a nongenomic mechanism must mediate this rapid behavioral effect of steroid hormones.

Additional evidence for the existence of nongenomic effects of steroid hormones on behavior has been provided in mammals. For example, rapid onset of sexual receptivity can be induced in estrogen-primed female golden hamsters (*Mesocricetus auratus*) by providing

progesterone that has been conjugated with a protein that presumably prevents the steroid from entering cells and interacting with intracellular receptors (DeBold and Frye, 1994; Frye and Debold, 1993; Frye et al., 1992).

Other research has demonstrated that estradiol evokes rapid electrophysiological effects in the CA1 neurons of the hippocampus, and that the rapid effects of estradiol on hippocampal neurons can be blocked by interfering with protein kinase A or with G protein receptors (Wong and Moss, 1992; Gu and Moss, 1996; Wong et al., 1996).

Steroid hormones also bind to the GABA receptor–chloride ion channel complex (Majewska et al., 1986) as well as other membrane-bound receptors (Ke and Ramirez, 1990) to affect neurotransmission (Becker, 1990). Taken together, these findings suggest that steroid hormones can affect behavior both through traditional genomic actions and via alternative membrane-bound receptors. It appears that both mechanisms could act in concert to increase or decrease the likelihood of a particular behavior in a specific context (Frye et al., 1996).

pulse of estrogen (Parsons et al., 1982) or between the two pulses interfered with the facilitation of lordosis. These results suggest that electrophysiological events (suppressed by anesthesia), new protein synthesis, and incoming sensory information are all critical components of a cascade of events that begins with the initial exposure to estrogen and ends with the onset of the lordosis response. The cascade hypothesis is reminiscent of the organizational/activational hypothesis presented in Chapter 3 to explain sex differences in neural function. Recall that sex steroid hormones organize neural structures perinatally in a masculine or feminine pattern, and that subsequent postpubertal hormonal stimulation activates these previously organized neural circuits, resulting in sexually differentiated behaviors. The cascade hypothesis put forth to explain endocrine effects on lordosis is fundamentally the same as the organizational/activational hypothesis. There is a much shorter time course between the organizing effects of the initial estrogen exposure—late during diestrus II in the rat—and the activating effects of estrogen and progestin during late proestrus, but the principles are the same. The cascade hypothesis, along with the wonderfully detailed data on cellular and subcellular mechanisms now available (Pfaff et al., 1994), suggests that the organizational/activational principles proposed in 1959 may be the fundamental principles underlying all hormone–behavior interactions.

### Genetic Knockouts

As noted in previous chapters, studies of mice that have had specific genes deleted (knocked out) can be very useful in hormone–behavior studies. In most cases studied, production of progesterone receptors is induced when estradiol interacts with estrogen receptors. Thus, many of the effects of progesterone on reproductive physiology and behavior could actually be due to a combination of progestins and estrogens. To separate out the effects of these two steroids, mice were created that lacked functional progesterone receptors (PR–/–) (Lydon et al., 1996). Both male and female PR–/– mice develop to adulthood; males are fertile, but females are sterile. Female PR–/– mice display uterine hyperplasia and minimal mammary gland development, and are anovulatory even when stimulated with exogenous gonadotropins (Lydon et al., 1996; Mani et al., 1997). When ovariectomized, neither PR–/– mice nor PR+/+ mice displayed lordosis after treatment with estradiol. However, treatment with progesterone induced lordosis in virtually all of the estrogen-primed PR+/+ mice, but none of the PR–/– females (Figure 6.23) (Lydon et al., 1996). This work with PR knockout mice supports previous work in which lordosis could not be elicited in estrogen-primed rats that received infusions of PR antisense into the ventromedial nucleus of the hypothalamus (Ogawa et al., 1994).

Estrogen receptor knockout mice (ER–/– ) have also been developed (Lubahn et al., 1993; Ogawa et al., 1996a,b; Rissman et al., 1997a). When ER–/– and ER+/+ female mice were ovariectomized, then given equivalent doses of 17β-estradiol, only the ER+/+ mice displayed lordosis when tested with a wild-type male in a neutral arena (Rissman et al., 1997a). Progesterone treatment did not facilitate lordosis in ER–/– females (Rissman et al., 1997b). When these ER–/– females were given foster pups, the induced maternal behavior was also impaired (Ogawa et al., 1996a).

Males mounted both ER–/– and ER+/+ females, suggesting that mice of both genotypes were attractive to males. When tested in a three-chamber preference apparatus, males spent equivalent amounts of time with ER–/– and ER+/+ females (Rissman et al., 1997b). If the conditions under which the female ER–/– mice were tested were changed, however, then a different pattern of results emerged (Ogawa et al., 1996a,b). When ovary-intact ER–/– mice were tested in mating tests in the males' home cages, then some lordosis was observed. However, males often responded with aggressive attacks against the ER–/– females (suggesting that they were not particularly attractive to them). Males responded to male intruders into their home cages with similar aggressiveness, but never responded to ER+/+ females in this manner.

Taken together, the results of these behavioral analyses of steroid receptor knockout mice suggest that the presence of a functional estrogen receptor is necessary for female-typical reproductive behavior. Recently, a novel estrogen receptor type (ER$_\beta$) was discovered; the original estrogen receptor was therefore named ER$_\alpha$ (Couse et al., 1997). Each of these two isoforms of estrogen receptors (as well

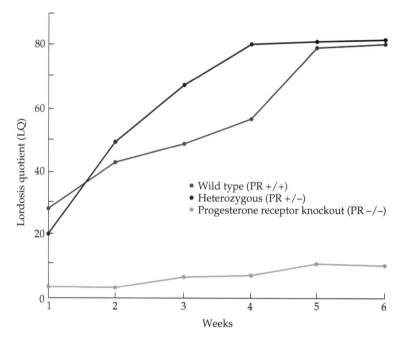

**6.23    Lordosis does not occur in progesterone receptor knockout (PRKO) mice.** Treatment with progesterone induced lordosis in virtually all of the estrogen-primed wild-type progesterone receptor (PR+/+) mice, but none of the progesterone receptor knockout (PR–/–) females. After Lydon et al., 1996.

as possible as yet unidentified isoforms) may play specific roles in the mediation of female sexual behavior, as well as in other behavioral functions (e.g., learning or maternal behavior).

## *A Neural Model of Lordosis*

Pfaff and Schwartz-Giblin (1988) have modeled the neural regulation of lordosis. Their comprehensive and extraordinarily detailed model is based on the idea that several neural modules (specific subsections of the nervous system) function together to mediate the lordosis response. This model should be celebrated as the first complete circuitry map of a mammalian hormone–behavior interaction. Pfaff and colleagues mapped the sensory input, central integration, and effector pathways involved in lordosis and documented their interactions with hormones. Five modules are described by the model: the spinal cord module, lower brain stem module, midbrain module, hypothalamic module, and forebrain module. A brief synopsis of the role of each module is provided below (Figure 6.24; refer to Pfaff et al. [1994] for more details).

**SPINAL CORD MODULE.**    The spinal cord module receives the majority of somatosensory information during copulation. As mentioned above, lordosis is triggered by sensory input from the rump, flanks, and perianal region of the female. Light touch or pressure between 40 and 450 millibars elicits the lordosis response. The receptive fields of sensory neurons increase in size in estrogen-treated females

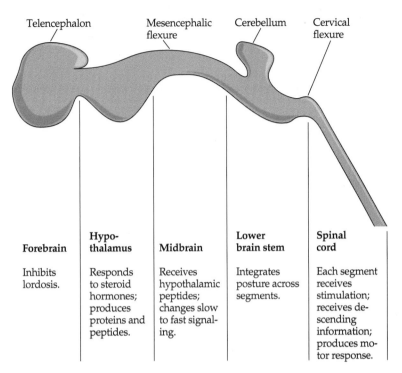

| Forebrain | Hypo-thalamus | Midbrain | Lower brain stem | Spinal cord |
|---|---|---|---|---|
| Inhibits lordosis. | Responds to steroid hormones; produces proteins and peptides. | Receives hypothalamic peptides; changes slow to fast signaling. | Integrates posture across segments. | Each segment receives stimulation; receives descending information; produces motor response. |

**6.24  Five neural modules that mediate lordosis.**  The components of the nervous system that mediate lordosis in rats can be separated into five component parts. The forebrain normally inhibits lordosis, but estrogen plus tactile stimulation disinhibits the behavior, as do lesions of the forebrain. Nuclei of the hypothalamus are either inhibited (the MPOA) or activated (the VMN) by estrogens, and produce proteins and other peptidergic hormones that interact with the midbrain, which serves to transduce these relatively slow endocrine changes into fast neural signals. The lower brain stem is critical for the postural changes involved in lordosis, and the spinal cord is responsible for moving sensory information associated with male mounting behavior to the brain and bringing motor signals from the brain to the deep back muscles that directly cause lordosis. After Pfaff et al., 1994.

(Figure 6.25; Kow et al., 1979). In addition to initially processing the sensory input, the spinal cord module generates the motoneuronal output that results in lordosis. Although the behavioral program of sensory input and motor output is located in the spinal cord, female rats differ from males in that the sexual response will not occur without input from the brain (Meisel and Sachs, 1994). Thus, female rats with transected spinal cords will not display lordosis.

**LOWER BRAIN STEM MODULE.**   Integration of information about posture and moment-to-moment corrections to posture are mediated in the lower brain stem module. Input from the vestibular organs and from proprioceptors throughout the body is necessary for maintaining a rigid posture and making corrections to maintain the weight of the mounting male.

**MIDBRAIN MODULE.**   The midbrain module receives input from the hypothalamus and elsewhere in the brain, and translates and integrates these signals to mediate firing rates in the reticulospinal neurons in the lower brain stem mod-

(a)

(b)

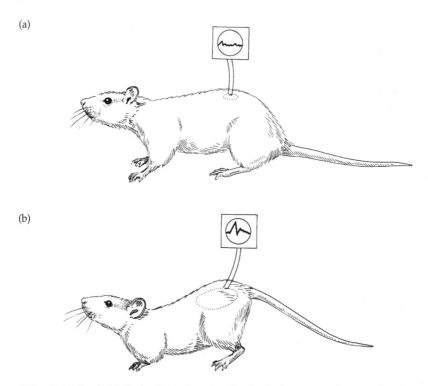

**6.25 Receptive fields in the flanks increase in size during estrus.** By recording from sensory nerves, the area of the skin that causes increased sensory nerve firing can be mapped during light tactile stimulation. (a) Relative size of a flank receptive field in an anestrous rat. (b) Relative size of receptive field in an estrous rat; the receptive fields of the flank sensory neurons expand under the influence of estrogen.

ule. Peptides are transmitted from the hypothalamus to the central gray area of the midbrain module, where these typically slow neuroendocrine signals (on the order of hours) are transduced to neural signals. If the midbrain module is not activated by peptidergic information from the hypothalamus *and* by steroid hormones, lordosis will not occur. Lordosis is steroid-dependent, and it is the midbrain module and, even more extensively, the hypothalamic module where the action of steroids is critical.

**HYPOTHALAMIC MODULE.**   The effects of estradiol and progesterone on the electrophysiological properties of neurons, RNA transcription, and the synthesis of new structural and other proteins are primarily mediated in the hypothalamic module.

**FOREBRAIN MODULE.**   The forebrain module exerts primarily inhibitory effects on lordosis. Large frontal cortical lesions, as well as lesions to the olfactory bulbs or septum, facilitate lordosis.

According to this model, sex steroid hormones, as well as several peptide hormones, including GnRH, prolactin, β-endorphin, and substance P, modulate lordosis by acting on one or more of the neural modules during normal or experimentally induced estrus. When females with estrogen concentrations insufficient to evoke lordosis by themselves are primed with GnRH, prolactin, or substance P, lordosis results. GnRH is transported to the midbrain central gray area along axons from the medial basal hypothalamus, and in the presence of estrogen, stimulates excitatory responses in central gray neurons (Moss and McCann, 1973). Experimental treatment with GnRH antibody in the central gray region caused reductions in lordosis responding in rats (Sakuma and Pfaff, 1980). Application of CRH or β-endorphin to the central gray area also leads to decreased lordosis responding (Pfaff and Schwartz-Giblin, 1988).

In contrast to this comprehensive model of receptive behavior, the neural loci mediating proceptive behavior have been only partially identified. Because lordosis is such a prominent feature of female rat mating behavior, the vast majority of brain lesion studies and hormone implant studies have used the presence or absence of lordosis as a behavioral assay in much the same way that mounting and intromission have been employed in studies of the neural bases of male copulatory behavior. However, during the course of behavioral analyses of brain-altered females, changes in proceptive behaviors have occasionally been reported (Erskine, 1989).

As described above, implants of estradiol alone into the VMN induced lordosis in ovariectomized rats, but at a low frequency. Proceptive behaviors were never observed during mating tests under these conditions (Rubin and Barfield, 1983). However, a full complement of proceptive behaviors, including hopping, darting, and ear wiggling, was observed among estrogen-injected, ovariectomized female rats that received progesterone brain implants into the VMN, but not in those that received implants into the preoptic area of the hypothalamus (POA), midbrain central gray region, hippocampus, or medullary reticular formation (Rubin and Barfield, 1983). Infusions of progesterone into the VMN facilitated lordosis in less than 2 hours, suggesting that changes in electrophysiological parameters, rather than structural changes or protein synthesis, mediate the effects of progesterone (Glaser et al., 1983; McGinnis et al., 1981). The ventromedial nuclei of the hypothalamus are involved in the mediation of female sexual behavior across a wide range of taxa, including parthenogenetic whiptail lizards (*Cnemidophorus uniparens*) (see Chapter 5) (Kendrick et al., 1993).

Lesions of the VMN, or destruction of their afferent and efferent fibers, typically reduce the frequency of lordosis. Proceptive behaviors also appear to be affected by VMN lesions. As described above, projections from the VMN to the midbrain are important parts of the neural circuitry mediating lordosis (Kow and Pfaff, 1998). However, the midbrain appears to be less involved in the mediation of proceptive behaviors (Erskine, 1989). In fact, proceptive behaviors remain intact, or in some instances are enhanced, after destruction of the ascending ventral noradrenergic bundle (VNAB), a procedure that completely abolishes the appearance of lordosis (Hansen et al., 1980, 1981). Thus, different brain regions may mediate receptive and proceptive behaviors. This possibility suggests that different neural substrates underlie sexual motivation and sexual performance in both males and females.

To summarize, hormones affect female sexual behavior by affecting the input, central integration, and output functions of the central nervous system. Estrogen affects sensory input by increasing the receptive field size in sensory cells (Kow et al., 1979). Estrogen affects protein synthesis, the electrophysiological responses of neurons, and the appearance of growthlike processes on neurons (Pfaff and Schwartz-Giblin, 1988). Finally, estrogen affects the muscular output that results in lordosis, as well as chemosensory stimuli important in attracting a mating partner (Beach and Gilmore, 1949).

## Summary

• Copulatory behavior in females usually coincides with ovulation. Because females ovulate periodically, copulatory behavior is observed in cycles called estrous cycles. Female mammals are said to be in estrus when they permit copulation.

• Female sexual behavior has been the subject of formal study for much less time than male sexual behavior. Despite this disparity, much is known about the mechanisms underlying the hormone–behavior interactions involved in the regulation of female copulatory behavior. Ovariectomy consistently results in decreased sexual behavior in females from all vertebrate taxa.

• Cyclic changes in vaginal cytology have been correlated with changes in ovarian structure and subsequently with behavior. In rats, the vaginal estrous cycle consists of 2 or 3 days of diestrus, followed by a 12–18-hour proestrous phase, and then a 24–36-hour estrous period. Behavioral estrus and mating occur near the end of proestrus and end as the vaginal smear becomes estrous. Ovulation occurs near the beginning of vaginal estrus.

• Mating behavior coincides with the preovulatory follicle; chemical extraction of this ovarian structure led to the discovery of the estrogen class of steroids. Mating behavior often stops with the onset of corpora luteal activity; chemical extraction of this ovarian structure led to the discovery of progesterone. These steroid hormones were purified, and replacement studies using these purified steroids on ovariectomized animals demonstrated that estrogens and progestins were required for mating behavior in guinea pigs, mice, rats, and many other species. In most species, in order to stimulate behavioral estrus, ovariectomized individuals had to be "primed" with estradiol, an estrogen, for about 24 hours, then progesterone had to be provided 4–8 hours prior to the display of the behavior. This injection paradigm mimicked closely the endocrine environment of natural estrus.

• Females of most vertebrate taxa display species-specific mating postures. In rodents, the characteristic mating posture is called lordosis. Females in lordosis arch their backs, deflect their tails, and remain immobile to allow male intromission. Female dogs, cats, and many other mammalian species deflect the tail and display a virtually rigid mating posture. With the notable exception of rhesus monkeys, primates typically do not display stereotypical mating postures.

• Females have historically been portrayed as passive recipients of male sexual attention. However, in many species, especially primates, females initiate virtually all sexual interactions. In an attempt to reduce variation in behavioral tests, researchers have traditionally studied female copulatory behavior in single-pair tests. In this context, females appear rather passive. However, when they are tested in social groups that simulate natural conditions, females' initiation and control of copulatory activities become evident.

• Female sexual behavior can be divided into three components: (1) attractivity, (2) proceptivity, and (3) receptivity. Attractivity is the stimulus value of the female for a given male. Proceptivity is the extent to which females initiate copulation, and reflects overt behavior as well as the underlying motivational state. Receptivity reflects the stimulus value of the female for eliciting an intravaginal ejaculation from a male conspecific; in other words, receptivity is the state of responsiveness to the sexual behaviors of another individual. Proceptivity and receptivity overlap conceptually, as well as in practice. Generally, estrogens enhance attractivity, proceptivity, and receptivity, and progestins reduce these parameters. Female receptivity and control of copulation vary among species; some females copulate even when not in estrus, and others reject certain males even when in estrus. Pacing of copulatory behavior by female rats has important physiological consequences for induction of corpora luteal function and subsequent maintenance of pregnancy.

• Female reproductive cycles have been categorized into three basic types. In type 1 cycles, ovulation and pseudopregnancy are spontaneous. Humans and other primates display type 1 cycles. In type 2 cycles, ovulation is induced by copulation or other vaginal stimulation, but pseudopregnancy is spontaneous. Cats and ferrets display type 2 ovarian cycles. Both ovulation and corpora luteal formation are spontaneous in animals with type 3 cycles, but pseudopregnancy is induced via the release of prolactin following copulation. Mammals with type 3 cycles do not have functional luteal phases in nonpregnant cycles. Rats, mice, and hamsters have type 3 ovarian cycles.

• Reproductive cycles have evolved so as to maximize reproductive output, and thus vary with the ecology of the species. Repeated estrous cycles are laboratory artifacts and occur infrequently in free-ranging mammals. Females in nature are typically pregnant, lactating, or in seasonal diestrus. Most pregnancies in nature are the result of mating during postpartum estrus.

• Reproductive cycles can be influenced by a number of social and environmental factors. Four examples of social effects on murine estrous cycles are the Lee–Boot, Whitten, Bruce, and Vandenbergh effects. The Lee–Boot effect is the interruption of regular estrous cycles in mice by prolonged diestrous periods when females are housed in groups. The Whitten effect involves two different effects of conspecific females on one another: estrus induction and synchronization, and suppression of estrus. The ability of a strange male to interrupt pregnancy and cause a return to estrus is the basis of the Bruce effect. The Vandenbergh effect reflects the retardation of first estrus in female mice housed in the presence of adult females and the acceleration of first estrus in female mice housed with adult males. All of these effects on estrus are mediated by chemosensory factors.

• The effects of social factors on ovarian cycles are not limited to rodents. Women who live together for extended periods of time also may synchronize their menstrual cycles.

• Ovulation and peak estradiol concentrations coincide in both rats and primates. However, rats exhibit a periovulatory peak in progesterone that is reduced or absent in primates. Primates of many species, including humans, often display periovulatory peaks in androgen concentrations. Both sexual motivation and performance are mediated by sex steroid hormones in rodents, and probably other nonprimate species as well; in these species copulation does not occur in the absence of high blood concentrations of estrogen. In contrast, the ability to copulate is not linked to hormones among primates. Motivation to copulate appears to coincide with blood concentrations of androgens in primates.

• Several brain sites are necessary for lordosis. Lesions of the ventromedial nuclei of the hypothalamus (VMN) or destruction of their afferent and efferent fibers reduces the frequency of lordosis. Lesions of the central gray region also reduce lordosis behavior. Destruction of the midbrain ascending ventral noradrenergic bundle (VNAB) completely abolishes lordosis. The medullary reticular formation in the brain stem controls motoneurons for axial muscles, especially the deep back muscles that are critical for lordosis.

• Sensory input enters the female rat's nervous system during mating via cutaneous receptors on the flanks, rump, and perineum. Information from these skin receptors and from pressure-responsive neurons enters the spinal cord and is sent to the medullary reticular formation. Interaction of these ascending sensory messages with descending fibers from the midbrain central gray, which carries information from the VMN, will permit lordosis only when sex steroid hormones are available to these cells in the central gray and to cells in the VMN.

• Estrogen promotes estrogen and progesterone receptor formation in the VMN, as well as stimulating RNA transcription, protein synthesis, electrophysiological changes in neurons, and delivery of peptides to the midbrain central gray region. According to the cascade hypothesis, estrogen induces these changes over several hours, or "primes the nervous system" for subsequent estrogenic facilitation of lordosis. Although there is a large difference in the temporal gap between the first and subsequent endocrine events, the cascade hypothesis is similar to the organizational/activational model of sexual differentiation; hormones affect subsequent behavior by causing structural changes prior to evoking electrophysiological or other fast-acting changes.

• A comprehensive model of the regulation of lordosis behavior has been proposed, based on five neural modules (specific subsections of the nervous system)—namely, the spinal cord module, lower brain stem module, midbrain module, hypothalamic module, and forebrain module—that function together to mediate the lordosis response. Sex steroid hormones, as well as several peptide hormones, modulate lordosis behavior by acting on one or more of these neural modules.

• The neural and endocrine bases of proceptive behaviors are different from those of lordosis, a receptive behavior. Males and females are similar in that sexual motivation and sexual performance are organized separately in the nervous system.

## Questions for Discussion

1. Discuss the proposition that a female mammal can be sexually receptive without being sexually attractive. Also provide examples of a female that is attractive, but not receptive. Would such observations negate a role for hormones in the mediation of attractivity and receptivity?

2. Document the following assertion: "Hormones play a lesser role in mediating sexual behavior in female primates than in female rodents." Is it reasonable to state that the sexual behavior of women is unaffected by sex steroid hormones?

3. Given the number of fundamental differences between rodents and primates, is it useful to study hormone–behavior interactions in rodents? Defend your answer.

4. Discuss the implications of the following quote in terms of the study of female sexual behavior: "It is an unfortunate accident that studies of reproductive physiology and behavior have been limited to a few domesticated species because our conceptual limits in the understanding of the regulation of female reproductive processes have become compressed and distorted."

5. Activation of female sexual behavior often requires both estrogen and progestins. If you discovered that a female rodent exhibited a type 2.1 reproductive cycle, would you predict that progesterone would be necessary for the expression of estrous behavior in this species? Why or why not?

## Suggested Readings

Bancroft, J., Sherwin, B. B., Alexander, G. M., Davidson, D. W., and Walker, A. 1991. Oral contraceptives, androgens, and the sexuality of young women: The role of androgens. *Archives of Sexual Behavior, 20*: 121–135.

Beach, F. A. 1976. Sexual attractivity, proceptivity, and receptivity in female mammals. *Hormones and Behavior, 7*: 105–138.

Erskine, M. S. 1989. Solicitation behavior in the estrous female rat: A review. *Hormones and Behavior, 23*: 473–502.

Kow, L. M., and Pfaff, D. W. 1998. Mapping of neural and signal transduction pathways for lordosis in the search for estrogen actions on the central nervous system. *Behavioral Brain Research, 92*: 169–180.

Mani, S. K., Blaustein, J. D., and O'Malley, B. W. 1997. Progesterone receptor function from a behavioral perspective. *Hormones and Behavior, 31*: 244–255.

McMillan, H. J., and Wynne-Edwards, K. E. 1998. Evolutionary change in the endocrinology of behavioral receptivity: Divergent roles for progesterone and prolactin within the genus *Phodopus*. *Biology of Reproduction, 59*: 30–38.

Pfaff, D. W., Schwartz-Giblin, S., McCarthy, M. M., and Kow, L.-M. 1994. Cellular and molecular mechanisms of female reproductive behaviors. In E. Knobil and J. Neill (eds.), *The Physiology of Reproduction*. Vol. 2, pp. 107–220. Raven Press, New York.

Wallen, K. 1990. Desire and ability: Hormones and the regulation of female sexual behavior. *Neuroscience & Biobehavioral Reviews, 14*: 233–241.

# 7

# Parental Behavior

**T**hus far we have focused on the interactions between hormones and mating behavior. Mating behavior is critical for reproductive success because it brings the two sexes together in order to combine their respective genetic material. However, successful mating is insufficient if reproduction is to be judged successful. From an evolutionary perspective, the only currency of reproductive success is the production of successful offspring; that is, offspring that themselves manage to survive and produce descendants. The offspring of many animal species require assistance from one or both parents in order to attain maturity and reproduce themselves.

The amount of assistance parents provide varies widely both among and within species, and reflects an optimal evolutionary strategy for maximizing fitness. The strategy for each parent is to provide sufficient care, but no more than is absolutely necessary, to produce successful offspring. **Parental investment**, the extent to which parents compromise their ability to produce additional offspring in order to assist current offspring, may result in a conflict of interest between parents and young. At one end of the parental care continuum are the numerous vertebrate species that provide absolutely no parental care. Females of many fish species, for example, simply release hundreds or even thousands of eggs from their bodies to be fertilized and leave them to face the vagaries of the cold, harsh world on their own. Females of most reptilian species merely cover their newly deposited eggs with dirt and other debris, and provide no additional parental assistance. These young must fend for themselves immediately upon hatching. Parental care, ranging from rudimentary to complex, is observed among invertebrate animals, mainly in the form of nest defense or provisioning the young with food (Box 7.1). Parents of many other vertebrate species go further, providing food, shelter, and protection from harm as their offspring mature (Figure 7.1). Humans represent the other termi-

---

Box 7.1
# Parental Care among Insects

Compared with the enormous amount of research conducted on the ecology of invertebrate parental behavior, few studies have focused on the physiological bases of parental care among invertebrate animals. Although a wide range of parental behaviors are observed among invertebrates, most studies of the hormonal bases of invertebrate parental care have focused on insect species that carry young and build nests (see figure below) (Trumbo, 1996).

Photograph © Mark Moffett/Minden Pictures.

The best examples of species that carry young are provided by cockroaches, which, depending on the species, are either oviparous (egg-laying), viviparous (give birth to live young), or ovoviviparous (eggs hatch internally). A rich "milk" is secreted from the walls of the brood sac in the viviparous species *Diploptera punctata*. Essentially, juvenile hormone (JH), the primary insect gonadotropin, which is secreted from the corpora allata, is inhibited throughout the cockroach's "pregnancy." With the onset of parturition and the termination of care, JH concentrations rise in preparation for the next brood (Rankin and Stay, 1985).

Many variations of the mother–offspring relationship exist among cockroaches. Displays of long-term association between mother and offspring occur in the Australian burrowing roach (*Macropanesthia*) and the woodroach (*Cryptocercus*) (e.g., Matsumoto, 1992; Ruegg and Rose, 1991). Young of the ovoviviparous cockroach *Leucophaea maderae* are reported to join in on their mother's nus of the parental care continuum, providing substantial care and resources to their children for decades.

## What Is Parental Behavior?

**Parental behavior** can be broadly defined as any behavior performed in relation to one's offspring (Rosenblatt et al., 1985), but more specifically, parental behavior is any behavior that contributes directly to the survival of fertilized eggs or offspring that have left the body of the female. If a father performs parental behavior, then a more specific term, **paternal behavior**, is typically used; similarly, parental behavior performed by mothers is called **maternal behavior**.

Why is parental care an important topic to study? Parental care is critical for infant survival among many species, including humans, and hence is critical for the reproductive success of the individual parent(s). Parental care plays an impor-

---

foraging excursions soon after birth, as Mom presumably "shows them the ropes" (Trumbo, 1996). Little is known about the hormonal bases of these associations; clearly much more research needs to be conducted on these fascinating creatures.

Another parental behavior that has been studied among invertebrates is nest building. The proximate mechanisms underlying nest building have been well characterized in earwigs (Dermaptera). As in *Diploptera*, JH levels rise prior to oviposition (either egg laying or giving birth), then remain low during most phases of parental care (Rankin et al., 1995). If the clutch of eggs is removed on the first day of the "parental phase," then JH concentrations increase, presumably to prepare for a new cycle of egg laying. If the eggs are returned within 24 hours, most females accept them. If mothers are separated from their eggs for 48 hours, then only 36% of mothers accept the eggs, and no mothers accept eggs after 72 hours of separation (Vancassel et al., 1984). These results suggest that high JH levels are incompatible with parental care in these insects.

A slight variation in JH profile is observed in the biparental burying beetle (*Nicrophorus orbicollis*; see figure). These fascinating insects breed only when they locate a small vertebrate carcass, a somewhat rare resource that is necessary for the success of their offspring

(Trumbo, 1997). Within 10 minutes of locating a carcass, JH concentrations double and ovarian mass increases dramatically (Trumbo, 1996). Neither feeding on the carcass nor mating per se induces the rapid increases in JH concentrations; rather, the beetle's evaluation of the carcass and sensory feedback seem to trigger the endocrine changes (Trumbo et al., 1995; Trumbo, 1997). The burying beetles inject antibiotic secretions into the carcass to delay decomposition during its preparation as a nest. After oviposition, JH concentrations decline, but remain elevated relative to those prior to the discovery of the carcass. When the young hatch out, about 5 days after the discovery of the carcass, a secondary peak of JH secretion is observed. At this time, the parents increase their locomotor activity and nest-maintaining behavior, as well as regurgitating liquified carrion for the young (Trumbo, 1996). As the young become more independent, the parents' activities wane, and their primary parental duties consist of predator defense. Tissue fluid JH concentrations decline during this latter part of the parental cycle, but rise again when the parents leave the nest to find a new carcass (Trumbo, 1996). All of these studies indicate that the hormone–behavior interactions underlying parental behavior are complex and environmentally mediated in insects, just as they are in vertebrate animals.

(a)

(b)

**7.1 Some species provide little or no parental care.** (a) Female salmon shed large numbers of eggs into the water to be fertilized by a courting male. The eggs remain where they fall, and no parental care is provided. The sheer number of eggs released ensures that some offspring will survive despite the absence of parental protection. (b) Female Nile crocodiles protect their newly hatched young by gently carrying them to the water in their mouths. Aside from nest building, this is the extent of parental care in this species; males make no parental contribution.

tant role in the evolution of competition for mates because individuals may seek mates that can best provide care for their offspring; the intensity of mate competition within each sex influences the selection pressures operating upon behavior, physiology, and morphology (Clutton-Brock, 1991). Parental care influences the course of physical and psychological development of offspring, and is also important among many species in the socialization of young. Individual humans display a wide range of parenting skills; it would be useful to discover any endocrine correlates of poor parenting because poor parenting is associated with numerous social problems in the offspring. The importance of mothers as nurturers of new life has been an inspiration to artists for eons (Figure 7.2).

As you will see, there is a wide diversity of parental care strategies among vertebrates. Some of this diversity is due to variations in the developmental maturity of the offspring when they are produced. Two broad categories of off-

**7.2 Women's ability to produce and nurture new life is accorded great respect in many African societies,** as demonstrated by this mother and child wood carving from Mali, West Africa. The carving celebrates the nurturant power of women, while depicting a nearly universal image of human maternal behavior. Photograph courtesy of the Kinsey Institute.

spring production are found among vertebrates. In the first, females produce large numbers of immature and helpless, or **altricial**, young. Females that engage in this reproductive strategy may or may not display parental care. In the second, females produce a few **precocial** offspring that are well developed and may be able to survive with little or no parental intervention. There are trade-offs between these two strategies. If we consider the costs and benefits of producing precocial or altricial young for similar-sized individuals, precocial young require a greater *initial* investment per individual offspring, as the female must invest more energy in their development before birth or hatching, but less parental investment is usually required after birth. Altricial young require less prenatal investment, but if parental care is given, a greater amount is needed. Some species, rather than giving parental care to their altricial offspring, rely on the production of large numbers of offspring to ensure that at least a few will survive. Other species, including humans, produce semiprecocial young that always demand significant parental care at birth, but can thermoregulate and cling to the mother.

In those animals that display parental care, the behaviors must be performed correctly, with little margin for error; they initially must be performed without previous experience; and they must usually begin immediately after the hatching or birth of the offspring. Given these constraints, the onset of parental behavior is often remarkable for its precision and suitability. For instance, the confidence with which first-time mother dogs attend to their newly arrived pups is impressive. A day or two prior to giving birth, a pregnant dog builds a nest (often using only the best shirts, towels, or sweaters available) into which her puppies will be delivered. The pups are born about 20 to 60 minutes apart. As each pup is born, the mother behaves solicitously toward it, licking off the amniotic fluid and membranes, and also vigorously licking the anogenital region to stimulate the elimination of wastes and other physiological processes. After consuming the placentas, she lies on her side so the pups can attach to her nipples to nurse (Figure 7.3). The altricial puppies are blind and partially deaf, their coats are not completely established, and their thermoregulatory and locomotory abilities are not fully developed. During the first days of their lives, the mother continues to groom her pups as they nurse, and she also keeps them warm. She will retrieve pups by the scruff of the neck should they wander too far from the nest, and may move the entire litter if there are too many disturbances. If another dog, a well-known human acquaintance, or even the father of the litter comes too close to the pups, the mother may act very aggressively and can inflict serious damage on the intruder. The ferocity of this **maternal aggression** in previously docile animals can be surprising and dangerous to unsuspecting pet owners.

The parental competence exhibited by dogs and other nonhuman animals can lead to a powerful impression among human observers that nonhuman par-

**7.3   Females of many species provide their offspring with food, shelter, and protection from harm.**   Mammals, such as this female dog, have evolved to provide a specialized secretion, milk, to feed the young. Because male mammals do not lactate, only females can meet the nutritional demands of the young. In some mammalian species, the male contributes by feeding the female while she nurses. In very rare cases, male mammals participate more fully in parental care.

ents always perform parental behavior perfectly, and it is perhaps for this reason that comparatively few studies have examined the development of parental behavior. In all fairness to human parents, however, the "decisiveness" with which dogs and other nonhuman mothers seem to perform their parental behaviors is often an illusion. Upon close observation, it can be seen that errors are committed by inexperienced mothers and that trial-and-error learning often occurs during the onset of maternal behavior. Parental "instinct" is not completely "hardwired," and one can observe variation from parent to parent within the same species. With that said, the behavioral patterns of parents within a species share much in common.

Ordinarily, female dogs do not act in a solicitous and protective manner in the presence of newborn puppies; however, female dogs that have just delivered their own pups virtually always behave maternally. What triggers the set of maternal behaviors in dogs? While one might suppose that the stimuli, neural or otherwise, associated with the birth process initiate the onset of parental behavior, this hypothesis can be dismissed because dogs that give birth by cesarean section also behave maternally toward their puppies as soon as they recover from anesthesia. Indeed, many correlational studies in dogs, rabbits, and other mammals, especially rats, have demonstrated that it is the hormones associated with pregnancy and lactation that regulate the onset of mammalian parental behavior. In other vertebrate orders, hormones involved in egg production, nest building, egg laying, and incubation may activate parental behavior. In any case, hormones affect motivation to engage in parental care.

The hormones that trigger parental behavior wane soon after the arrival of the young. What factors serve to maintain parental behavior? If you observe mother dogs as their puppies mature, you will note that their maternal behaviors change over time. Nest building and pup retrieval behaviors wane, and the duration of nursing and play behaviors increases. Many maternal behaviors, including nursing, completely disappear after a few additional weeks. How are these changes in parental behavior coordinated with changes in the pups? What role, if any, do hormones play in the maintenance and termination of parental behavior? These questions will be answered in detail in this chapter.

## Sex Differences in Parental Behavior

With the exception of most bird and some fish species, paternal behavior is rather rare in the animal kingdom; maternal care is much more common. Why does this sex difference exist? As described in Chapter 3, the two sexes produce different types of gametes. Females produce relatively few, large, immobile, resource-rich gametes (eggs), whereas males produce large numbers of small, mobile gametes containing few or no resources (sperm). One male can produce enough sperm to fertilize many more eggs than one female can produce. For example, 5 ml of human semen (the average volume of a single ejaculation) contains sufficient sperm, in theory, to fertilize all the women in North America. In contrast, a woman produces only a few hundred eggs in her lifetime. Because of this difference, males and females differ fundamentally in how they can best achieve reproductive success.

Reproductive effort can be divided into mating effort and parental effort (Trivers, 1972). Males tend to concentrate their reproductive effort on mating because locating and fertilizing as many different females as possible is the best way for males to achieve maximal reproductive success. Females tend to put the majority of their reproductive effort into parental care because each offspring represents a substantial lifetime investment of time and resources. A female can best increase her reproductive success by turning food into eggs or offspring at a faster rate. Mating with additional males while pregnant or lactating typically does nothing to increase her reproductive success. Consider human females. Pregnancy lasts 9 months, and lactation-induced infertility may delay further reproductive efforts for another year or two. During this same time a human male could potentially fertilize hundreds of other women.

The various factors limiting male and female reproductive success were first documented experimentally by Bateman (1948). He put equal numbers of male and female fruit flies in a large bottle and scored the number of matings and the number of offspring produced by each individual. Bateman was able to use specific genetic markers to assign parentage. He found that some males fertilized many females, while others never fathered offspring; however, all the females fared about equally well. The reproductive success of a male depended on the number of females he fertilized, while the females achieved maximal reproductive success, in most cases, with a single copulation.

A male forgoing additional mating opportunities in order to assist in the rearing of his offspring is typically at an evolutionary disadvantage relative to a nonparental conspecific male. The reproductive success of the nonparental male will be higher than that of the parental male—that is, unless the offspring cannot survive without parental assistance from two adults. Only in those situations in which two adults are required to guarantee the survival of the young, as is the case for many avian species, will parental males achieve higher reproductive success than nonparental males. Given these theoretical considerations, it is not surprising that paternal care is rare. Animals that have pursued existing reproductive strategies have been more successful than animals that have not. Importantly, it is not necessary for these strategies to be consciously directed, even among humans, to be successful. By analogy, birds do not require a conscious understanding of aerodynamic theories to fly. But birds that *behave* as if they do understand the theories of flight increase their reproductive success.

This chapter describes patterns of parental behavior in various species, the hormonal correlates of parental behavior, and the cues that are necessary and sufficient to elicit parental care. In addition, what is currently known about the neural foundations of parental behavior will be reviewed. As you will see, there is an enormous variety of parental behaviors among vertebrate taxa. But although parental care has been well studied in numerous species, little is known about its endocrine mechanisms in any but a few well-studied species. The vast majority of research addressing the hormonal correlates of parental behavior has been conducted on ring doves, sheep, and laboratory rats. Parental behaviors in birds are described first, followed by a description of the hormone–behavior interactions underlying them. Birds are interesting to study for a variety of reasons, including the fact that more is known about the endocrine correlates of paternal behavior in birds than in mammals. A discussion of parental behavior in mammals follows.

# Parental Behavior in Birds

Birds show enormous diversity in parental behavior. Some avian species are nest parasites that never engage in parental behavior. Female cuckoos and cowbirds deposit their eggs secretly into the nests of other birds, and the unknowing "adoptive" parents provide parental care for their "guests," incubating the eggs and feeding and protecting the hatchlings. In other avian species, such as chickens and ducks, only the female provides parental care. In some rare cases, only the male provides parental care. Mallee fowl and jacana males build and maintain nests and incubate the eggs deposited in them. The females compete with one another to lay eggs in different males' nests. Such instances of sex role reversal are interesting to study because they provide clues about the selective pressures driving the evolution of parental care. Biparental care, in which both male and female birds provide virtually equivalent parental care, is the most common pattern of avian parental care (Figure 7.4). Nearly 90% of avian species are putatively monogamous, and in contrast to mammals, paternal care is a common avian trait.

Parental behavior in birds typically includes nest building, incubating the eggs, brooding the newly hatched nestlings, and taking care of the young until

**7.4   Biparental care is common in birds.**  In most bird species, both parents make approximately equal parental investments in the form of nest building, incubation, feeding, and protection of the young. Immature birds require nearly continuous food intake to survive and develop successfully, and in most cases two parents are required to meet their needs.

they are ready to live independently. The extent to which the young are cared for depends on their developmental state at hatching. Altricial young are generally helpless after hatching and require substantial attention, feeding, brooding, and protection, whereas precocial young generally require only supervision. Many fowl, including chickens, pheasants, and ducks, produce precocial young. Maternal care in chickens involves nest building, incubation, and broody behavior, which consists of clucking and hovering over the chicks and nest. The hen may stimulate the chicks to feed by pecking at grains herself; she calls attention to the potential food by emitting a species-specific sound. But generally, the chicks are fully capable of feeding themselves after a day or two. If the chicks are threatened by an intruder, a broody hen will chase it with her wings extended and emit loud squawking sounds. Birds that produce altricial young, such as robins and starlings, also build nests and incubate eggs, but they must provide their newly hatched young with food for several weeks. Regardless of whether altricial or precocial young are produced, many birds (sometimes both sexes) develop a brood patch on the breast, which loses feathers and becomes highly vascularized during incubation, facilitating heat transfer from the parent to the egg.

Males contribute some parental care in approximately 60% of avian subfamilies; in 20% of these subfamilies, the males provide virtually all of the parental care (Buntin, 1996). Males of some avian species, such as roosters, provide little or no paternal care. Males of other species, such as flycatchers, tits, pigeons, and doves, are more or less equal partners in rearing their offspring. Male spotted sandpipers and Wilson's phalaropes, like male jacanas and mallee fowl, provide all the parental care to their young. Males may assist in one, several, or all of the parental tasks (Silver et al., 1985).

Why is paternal care common among birds? At an ultimate level of causation, as we have seen, males care for their offspring when they can better increase their own reproductive success by continuing to invest in those offspring, rather than by seeking additional mates and fathering additional offspring. Most young birds are helpless at hatching and require constant food and warmth to develop sufficiently in just a few weeks to leave the nest. If males did not help to feed them, the hatchlings would die, and the males' fitness would suffer. In most cases, male birds are as capable as females of providing parental care in the form of nest construction, incubation of the eggs, and feeding of the young. This ability of avian fathers to feed their young—usually by regurgitating the results of recent foraging trips—contrasts sharply with most mammalian species, in which only the mother can meet the nutritional demands of the infants.

In some avian species, care of nestlings is provided by several male parental assistants, called **alloparents** or "helpers at the nest" (Emlen, 1978; Skutch, 1935), as well as by the parents. These helpers are usually elder brothers that are unable to set up their own breeding territories because of scarce resources, and they increase their reproductive fitness indirectly by helping their younger siblings.

Behavioral endocrinologists have focused their studies on two groups of birds, namely, the Galliformes (e.g., chickens) and the Columbiformes (e.g., pigeons and doves), that are probably the two most atypical representatives of the class Aves (Buntin, 1996). Chickens have been studied because of their economic value, even though galliform birds are highly unusual in that only the mother provides any care. The pattern of avian parental behavior on which most endocrine investigations have focused, however, is one of the rarest: a unique mode of providing food to the young observed only among members of the family Columbidae. In this family, both sexes engage in full parental care. The male brings nest material to the female, who does most of the nest construction. Both parents incubate the eggs, and both help feed the young, which are called squab, after they hatch. So far, this pattern of behavior is not unusual among birds. What makes the pigeons and doves unique is that both parents produce crop milk, which is fed to the young. The crop milk, which resembles small-curd cottage cheese, is produced in a specialized exocrine gland called the crop sac, from which it is regurgitated to feed the squab (Figure 7.5) (Horseman and Buntin, 1995). Immediately after hatching, the squab are fed crop milk exclusively, but a mixture of seeds, insects, and crop milk is provided by the parents as the squab grow older. This unique avian adaptation of providing the young with "milk" is sufficiently similar to mammalian behavior to suggest that common underlying physiological mechanisms may be involved. Thus, pigeons and doves have proved to be attractive avian animal models in which to study hormonal effects on parental behavior.

### Endocrine Correlates of Avian Parental Behavior

Parental behavior, often performed by both mothers and fathers, is extensive among birds. The hormonal correlates of avian parental behavior are described in the following sections.

**AVIAN MATERNAL BEHAVIOR.**   Which hormones mediate maternal behavior in birds? Hens exhibit maternal behavior, or broodiness, by making "clucking" vocalizations and by persistent incubation or "nesting" (Figure 7.6). The term *broodi-*

**7.5   A young wood pigeon feeds on crop milk,** which is produced by both males and females in response to stimulation by prolactin. As the squab get older, a greater and greater proportion of the adult diet of seeds and insects is mixed with the crop milk until eventually only the adult diet is consumed, and parental crop milk production wanes.

**7.6 An extreme example of broodiness.** After maternal behavior has been initiated by hormones, virtually any contact comfort, even when provided by the young of another species, is sufficient to maintain normal broody behavior in the hen.

*ness* can refer either to sitting on eggs in a nest, or, more commonly, to protecting, covering, and warming the young under the wing. When hens become broody, they stop laying eggs, so there has been much research among poultry scientists aimed at preventing broodiness in order to increase egg production. Over 70 years ago, it was discovered that blood serum from a broody hen could induce a nonincubating hen to sit on a clutch of eggs (Leinhart, 1927). Oscar Riddle and his colleagues provided compelling evidence that prolactin induces broodiness in pigeons and chickens (Riddle et al., 1935a,b). Increased blood concentrations of prolactin are associated with broodiness in all female birds studied (Figure 7.7; see Goldsmith, 1983; Riddle et al., 1935b; Silverin and Goldsmith, 1983). Even in nest parasite species such as cowbirds, which never show broodiness or any other parental behavior, blood titers of prolactin are increased after egg laying (Rissman and Wingfield, 1984). Because the parental behavior of cowbirds differs substantially from that of other birds despite the similar hormonal profile, it is plausible to suggest that these behavioral differences are due to differences in the sensitivity of the central nervous system to hormones; experimental evidence supporting this proposition will be presented below.

The vast majority of studies on endocrine correlates of avian maternal behavior have been done on ring doves (*Streptopelia risoria*). Female ring doves, which were studied extensively by researcher Daniel S. Lehrman (Box 7.2), undergo a stereotyped sequence of mutually exclusive behaviors during their reproductive cycle (Lehrman, 1965). The cycle begins with courtship, which is followed by nest

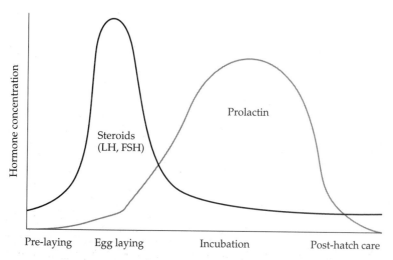

**7.7    Generalized endocrine profile of north temperate zone birds.** While individual birds in a population may display different concentrations of reproductive hormones on any given sampling date, if these blood samples are arranged according to reproductive activity, a clear pattern of hormone concentration and reproductive function is observed. Sex steroid hormones usually increase coincident with the onset of courtship behavior, peak during the time of egg laying (oviposition), and rapidly decrease to baseline prior to incubation. Prolactin concentrations begin to increase at the time of egg laying, remain high during incubation, then drop off gradually to baseline concentrations during post-hatching care. Source: Ball, 1991.

building, incubation, feeding the young, and finally resumption of courtship behavior. Changes in hormone concentrations have been found to correlate with the different stages of this cycle. Incubation is initially evoked by progesterone (against a background of high estradiol concentrations), but around mid-incubation, it is sustained by prolactin, which is secreted in response to ventrum (belly) stimulation from contact with the eggs. Ovariectomy eliminates nest building and incubation behavior. Injections of either estradiol or progesterone fail to restore nest building or incubation behavior, but treatment with both steroid hormones restores these behaviors to normal levels (Cheng and Silver, 1975). Prolactin is critical for stimulating brooding and development of the crop sac in ring doves (Figure 7.8) (Silver, 1978). Prolactin secretion wanes by the time the squab are 20 days old, at which time the mother no longer participates in the feeding of her brood. Although the female and male begin to court and build a new nest at this time, the male continues to secrete prolactin and provide crop milk to the squab. Thus the onset, maintenance, and termination of parental behavior in pigeons and doves appear to depend primarily upon prolactin concentrations.

**AVIAN PATERNAL BEHAVIOR.**    Despite the wide variety of parenting patterns found among male birds that provide parental care, there have been few studies of the endocrine correlates of avian paternal behavior in noncolumbid birds. Early research on the endocrine bases of parental behavior focused on sex differences in the expression of parental care in species in which males normally do not provide any paternal assistance. Roosters typically do not exhibit paternal care, but a castrated rooster, or capon, becomes broody almost to the same extent as a hen

Box 7.2

# Daniel S. Lehrman

Daniel S. Lehrman made major contributions to behavioral endocrinology, particularly by untangling the complex interactions among social, psychological, and hormonal stimuli that control courtship behavior in ring doves (e.g., Lehrman, 1965). An avid birdwatcher, Lehrman worked as a volunteer research assistant at the American Museum of Natural History for Dr. G. K. Noble while completing his undergraduate education at the City College of New York. At the Museum, he was encouraged by Frank Beach and Ernst Mayr to study animal behavior. After completing Army duties, he returned to the Museum in 1946 and met Theodore C. Schneirla, a well-known comparative psychologist, with whom he completed a doctoral degree in 1954. Lehrman joined the faculty at Rutgers University and founded the Institute of Animal Behavior in 1958; the Institute has been an important research establishment and home to many prominent behavioral endocrinologists.

Despite his seminal work in behavioral endocrinology, Lehrman was probably most widely known for firing a major salvo at the European ethologists in 1953, in the form of his "A Critique of Konrad Lorenz's Theory of Instinctive Behavior." Ethologists focused on "instinctual" behaviors, whereas comparative psychologists focused on learning. Although the publication of this biting attack on Lorenz's notions of "hard-wired" behavioral programs

initially caused a number of caustic debates between North American comparative psychologists and European ethologists, the net effect of the paper was to bring the two schools together, setting up an eventual synthesis between the two scientific disciplines (Dewsbury, 1984).

Lehrman was a member of the National Academy of Sciences and is remembered by his students for his outstanding ability to communicate his ideas to scientists and nonscientists alike: he was famous for jumping onto tabletops and performing enthusiastic imitations of courting ring doves bowing and cooing.

Daniel S. Lehrman (1919–1972)

when provided with foster chicks (Goodale, 1918). Tom turkeys also do not display paternal care, but males restrained so that they are forced to sit upon a clutch of eggs eventually show incubation behavior (Taibell, 1928).

Generally, nest building and incubation behaviors by male passerine (i.e., perching) birds are observed after courtship and mating and correspond with a sharp decline in blood concentrations of androgens and sometimes progesterone; prolactin concentrations generally increase at the onset of incubation behavior (Ball, 1991; Silverin, 1990). However, in field populations of sparrows, which may sire multiple broods, paternal behavior is observed while the birds maintain inter-

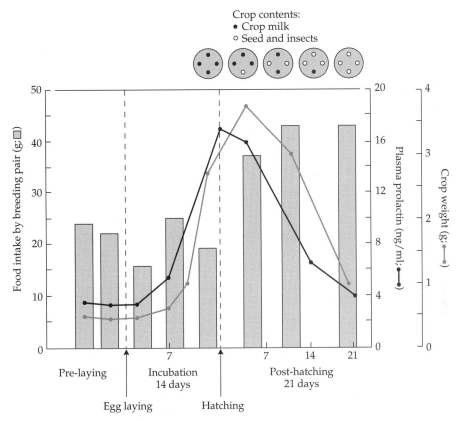

**7.8  Plasma prolactin, crop development, crop contents, and parental food intake are related in ring doves.** Plasma prolactin concentrations increase post-hatching and are associated with elevated food consumption by the breeding pair, presumably to support foraging for insects for the squab. As prolactin begins to fall 10–14 days post-hatching, the crop mixture changes from crop milk to mainly seeds and insects. After Horseman and Buntin, 1995.

mediate, and occasionally high, blood concentrations of testosterone (Wingfield and Moore, 1987). These elevated androgen concentrations are necessary to maintain the territorial defense behaviors required for successful rearing of the young. Males of species that display reversal of sex roles, such as the spotted sandpiper (*Actitis macularia*) and Wilson's phalarope (*Phalaropus tricolor*), exhibit the typical pattern of reduced steroid and increased prolactin concentrations; usually their prolactin concentrations exceed those of female conspecifics (Oring et al., 1986a,b).

As with maternal care, most of the work on hormonal correlates of avian paternal behavior has been accomplished on ring doves in laboratory settings (Buntin, 1996). During the reproductive cycle, male ring doves first exhibit courting behavior; after copulation, they engage in nest building. After the eggs are laid, males begin to incubate them, and after the squab hatch, males assist in feeding them for the first 3 weeks or so of their lives (Lehrman, 1965). These behaviors occur sequentially (see Figure 7.8), and hormones are important in the transition from one behavior to the next.

Although testosterone is required for courtship, this steroid hormone is not necessary for the onset of nest-building behavior in male ring doves. Castrated males treated with daily injections of testosterone either courted females or built nests; which behavior they chose was solely dependent upon the behavior of the females (Silver, 1978). Thus, in contrast to females, maintenance of male nest-building behavior is independent of hormonal status. This example makes the interesting point that virtually identical behaviors can have markedly different physiological bases in the two sexes. Apparently, stimuli from the female, rather than hormonal changes, induce the male to begin incubation behavior as well (Silver, 1978). In both sexes, prolactin is required to stimulate broody behavior and production of crop milk (Lehrman and Brody, 1961). Testosterone, but not progesterone, appears necessary for incubation behavior in castrated male doves (Ramos and Silver, 1992; Lea et al., 1986).

The endocrine correlates, if any, of alloparenting by siblings have not been discovered. Presumably, similar parental behavior performed by mother, father, and brothers could have very different endocrine correlates.

**NEURAL REGIONS ASSOCIATED WITH AVIAN PARENTAL BEHAVIOR.**    Very few studies have investigated the neural substrates of avian parental behavior. However, in the few studies performed, a consistent pattern has emerged indicating that the preoptic area anterior to the hypothalamus is essential for the expression of parental behavior (Erikson and Hutchison, 1977; Komisaruk, 1967; Slawski and Buntin, 1995). Most of these studies have involved making lesions to the preoptic area and observing the resulting behavioral deficits (Buntin, 1996). Lesions of the posterior medial hypothalamus of male ring doves significantly reduced courtship behavior in the presence of females (Bernstein et al., 1993). If lesioned males were housed continuously with females, their courtship behaviors recovered; however, if they were housed individually and then introduced to females, the deficits in their courtship behavior were sustained. These findings suggest that the social environment can affect behavioral recovery from specific brain lesions. The neural circuitry underlying incubation behavior remains unknown (Buntin, 1996).

Another approach that has been useful in understanding the neural substrates of avian parental behavior has employed comparisons of prolactin receptors in the brains of bird species that differ in their parental behavior. This comparative approach has yielded data suggesting that differences in parental care are mediated not by differences in hormones per se, but by differences in brain receptor numbers. For example, prolactin binding sites were compared in the brains of female cowbirds, red-winged blackbirds, and European starlings. Recall that cowbirds do not show parental care, but exhibit prolactin profiles similar to those of other birds. The pattern of prolactin binding was similar among all three species; however, the cowbirds displayed reduced binding in the preoptic area compared with the species that exhibit parental care (Ball, 1991). Thus, it seems reasonable to conclude that species differences in parental care may be mediated by differences in target tissue sensitivity, rather than differences in blood concentrations of hormones.

One important question regarding the hormone–brain relationship in avian parental behavior is how prolactin, a relatively large protein hormone, crosses the blood–brain barrier to interact with prolactin receptors on neurons. Short-term studies using intravenous injections of radiolabeled prolactin into the blood of ring doves revealed that somehow prolactin does cross the blood–brain barrier and accumulates in brain neurons that have prolactin receptors (Buntin et al., 1993). Presumably, some sort of transport system exists to move prolactin into the brain, where it interacts with receptors on the surfaces of neurons in the hypothalamus and preoptic area (Buntin, 1996).

## Parental Behavior in Mammals

Mammals have evolved specializations for taking care of their young (Bridges, 1990). The development of mammary glands, which provide nourishment to the young after they are born, makes mammals unique among vertebrates. Parental care, specifically maternal care, is a particularly important mammalian characteristic.

**MAMMALIAN MATERNAL BEHAVIOR.**   Among the mammals, species exist that produce offspring at virtually every developmental stage. The **marsupials** have specialized in the production of altricial young. These mammals have a pouch that contains the mammary glands and also serves as a receptacle for the young. Most marsupials, including wallabies and kangaroos, have temporary or permanent pouches in which the embryonic young are carried for several months. When the young reach a certain species-specific age, they leave the pouch, but return to the mother to nurse. Other marsupial species, such as opossums and koalas, bear young that cling to the mother's fur outside of the pouch and are carried in this manner as the mother forages for food (Figure 7.9). These patterns of maternal care are adaptations based on the mothers' need to remain mobile, both to obtain food in their usually barren habitats and to escape predators (Sharman, 1970; Tyndale-Biscoe and Renfree, 1987). The young, in turn, are adapted to remain attached to the mother, either in the pouch or outside of it; should they become dislodged, the mother does not attempt to reattach them, and they invariably perish. Thus, marsupials do not invest in gestation, but instead invest in postpartum maternal *care*, which does not include extensive maternal *behavior*. Their unreliable habitat favors this arrangement because maternal marsupials can jettison a pregnancy, or even their young, if conditions turn bad. Because of the short gestation period, they can replace these young quickly when conditions improve.

Another group of mammals, the **monotremes**, produce young that are born at an even earlier developmental stage than those of the marsupials: as eggs. These odd creatures are considered to be modern representatives of very ancient forms of mammals that have retained the reptilian egg-laying trait (oviparity). In terms of maternal behavior, monotremes represent a transitional stage between reptiles, which lay eggs and may or may not bury them, and the more solicitous behavior common among modern mammalian species (Burghardt, 1988). As with the marsupials, there are two basic patterns of maternal care among the monotremes (Nowak and Paradiso, 1983; Rosenblatt et al., 1985). The first is evident in the duck-billed platypus (*Ornithorhynchus anatinus*). The female of this species constructs a grass-lined burrow in which she lays her eggs. She then remains with the eggs and incubates them until they hatch. In the sealed burrow containing the nest, she cares for the young and provides them with milk, which drips from the hair surrounding her mammary glands. Females of this species do not develop a

(a)

**7.9 Maternal behavior in marsupials.** Marsupials have specialized in the production of altricial young, and have developed means for the mother to stay mobile and forage while the young are nursing. (a) Marsupials such as kangaroos have a pouch in which the mammary glands are located, and which also serves as a carrier for the young. (b) In other species of marsupials, such as opossums and koalas, the young stay in the pouch only briefly and are carried by the mother, clinging to her fur, until they are weaned.

(b)

pouch. The second pattern is seen in the spiny anteaters (*Tachyglossus aculeatus* and *Zaglossus bruijni*), which produce a single egg and carry it in a special pouch that develops at the time of egg delivery. The offspring, when it hatches, lives in the pouch and obtains milk from a milk-secreting gland that lacks a nipple.

The widest variety of maternal care patterns has evolved among the **eutherian** (*eu* = true; *therion* = beast) mammals, which have placentas during pregnancy. There are three basic patterns of maternal care among eutherian mammals, which are related to several characteristics of the species, but mainly reflect the developmental status of the newborn. These patterns were initially described by Rosenblatt et al. (1985). Eutherian mammals, in contrast to the marsupials and monotremes, live and reproduce in more stable and reliable habitats, and therefore have invested in relatively long gestations, which allow for greater development of the young before birth. Mechanisms have evolved in all mammalian species to provide parental care regardless of whether or not maternal behavior is present.

In the first pattern of maternal care, the mother provides offspring with food, care, and shelter. This pattern is characteristic of dogs, as was described above (see Figure 7.3), as well as other carnivores, rats and most other rodent species, and insectivores (such as shrews).

Females exhibiting this pattern of maternal care give birth to altricial young, which require a great deal of care: the mother must build a nest and deposit the young there. She must visit the offspring frequently to feed them and protect them from predators.* Recall that mother dogs usually choose a site for the nest and construct it before the young are born. After parturition, she eats the placenta (this also occurs in other mammalian species; see, e.g., Figure 7.21) and licks the amniotic fluid off the puppies. In dogs, the mother's cleaning of the pups is crucial for maternal acceptance of the newborns, and this is probably true of other animals as well: if pups are removed from the nest immediately after birth, washed, and returned to the mother, she will reject them and will not provide any maternal care (Abitbol and Inglis, 1997). A mother dog also nurses the young (Figure 7.10) and continues to lick them to stimulate various physiological processes (see Box 7.4).

In dogs and many other mammalian species, the mother will retrieve the young if they wander from the nest, but this is not always the case. Rabbit and hare mothers, for example, will not retrieve young that leave the nest. Also, mammalian mothers that follow this pattern often exhibit maternal aggression, attacking any animal that approaches her nest or young.

The many maternal behaviors described above can be classified according to whether or not a particular behavior is directed toward pups (Bridges, 1996). In this scheme, nest building, consumption of the placenta, and defense of pups are classified as non-pup-directed; pup-directed behaviors include grouping the pups together in the nest, huddling with them to provide warmth, retrieving them if they wander, licking their anogenital regions, or providing other forms of tactile stimulation. There may be different mechanisms underlying pup-directed versus non-pup-directed behaviors.

In a second pattern of mammalian maternal care, females bear precocial young that are capable of a high degree of independent activity when they are born, though they may be confined to a nest at birth and for a few days afterward. Some hoofed mammals, such as white-tailed deer, cows, and Thomson's gazelles, give birth to one or two precocial offspring. These species are characterized as **hider-type** animals because the young remain hidden at the nest site for 7–10 days (Geist, 1971). The mother spends most of her time away from the nest foraging for food, but visits her offspring to nurse them. Hider-type offspring eventually grow mature enough to leave the nest and follow the mother about. Other hoofed and non-hoofed species, including sheep, goats, elephants, and many species of

---

*Rabbits and hares show a similar pattern, except that they typically visit their litters only once daily to nurse the young; the rest of the day is spent foraging for food.

**7.10 Rat maternal care has three major components.** As with mother dogs, rat mothers ("dams") must engage in three behaviors in order for their altricial offspring to survive. First, they must lick their pups after birth to clean off the amniotic fluid and to stimulate elimination of wastes. They must adopt a nursing posture, huddling above the pups to allow access to the ventrum and to provide warmth and protection. They must also bring the pups back to the nest if they wander away. After Alberts and Gubernick, 1990.

whales, have offspring that follow the mother about from birth; these species are characterized as **follower-type** animals (Figure 7.11). The mother nurses her young and maintains constant vigilance, leading them away from danger and protecting them from predators.

Maternal care in many species that bear precocial young is noted for the exclusive bond that forms between the mother and her offspring (Gubernick and Klopfer, 1981). This bonding occurs soon after birth, which takes place in a secluded location away from the social group. Sheep and goat mothers that have just given birth emit characteristic low-pitched bleats in the presence of the newborn, which appear to attract the lamb to the ewe. In these species, the mother initially licks her offspring and allows them access to her udders. If the mother is separated from her newborn offspring, the maternal bond does not form with that specific lamb. She continues to behave maternally for about 24 hours and is nonexclusive about which lambs are permitted to nurse. There appear to be two distinct processes in sheep maternal behavior: (1) maternal responsiveness and (2) maternal selectivity (Lévy et al., 1996). Both processes are dependent on cues from the lamb; however, anosmia interferes with the ewe's selective responses to her individual lambs, but not with maternal responsiveness to lambs in general (Poindron and Le Neindre, 1980).

Many other mammalian species bear young that are neither precisely precocial nor precisely altricial; such offspring are usually described as **semi-precocial**. The offspring of humans and several other primate species are essentially helpless at

(a)

(b)

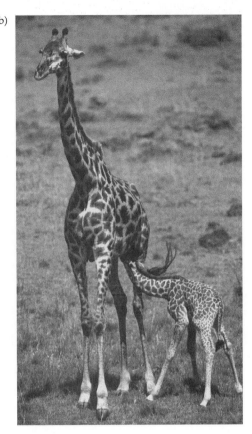

**7.11   Some mammalian species bear precocial off-spring.** Unlike dogs and rats, some mammals bear young that are quite well developed. In most mammalian species that bear precocial offspring, an exclusive bond forms between mother and young. (a) Hider-type young, such as white-tailed deer, are born in a nest and may be sequestered there for a few days. Hider-type young eventually leave the nest and follow their mothers about. (b) Follower-type young follow their mothers about from birth. Mother giraffes nurse their offspring and watch for danger, leading the young away from impending trouble.

birth, but they can cling to the mother in order to move about with her. In some species, mothers alternate between carrying the young and placing them in a nest or crib; in other species, the mother may deposit her young in a tree nest, where they remain during their early development. Galagos hide their young while foraging during the day and return to carry them during the night (Figure 7.12).

**MAMMALIAN PATERNAL BEHAVIOR.**   Among mammals, paternal care is relatively uncommon, but it is occasionally observed in certain carnivore, rodent, and primate species (Kleiman and Malcolm, 1981). If it is assumed that paternal behavior occurs when it increases male reproductive success, then there should be obvious and compelling selective factors among the species displaying paternal care. Thus far, no such generalities have emerged, except the assumption that females would be unable to rear offspring successfully without the additional support of the male. Another supposition is that certainty of paternity must be very high in order for paternal care to occur (Werren et al., 1980). It could also be argued that continued proximity to the female after mating improves the males's chances of paternity and is a factor in fostering paternal care (Gowaty, 1996).

**7.12   Many primate species produce semi-precocial young.** The offspring of several primate species are neither precocial nor altricial. These young are virtually helpless at birth, but can cling to the mother as she moves about. Female galagos, small secretive primates, sequester their offspring in a hidden nest as they forage during the day, but return at night to nurse and carry them.

Males clearly would not increase their reproductive success by relinquishing the opportunity for additional matings in favor of rearing the offspring of other males. Therefore, paternal behavior should be observed only in species that have a high degree of mating exclusivity between males and females.

Historically, paternal care was reported in fewer than 6% of rodent genera, and even in those relatively rare cases, the behavior was poorly documented with small sample sizes (for example, one or two individuals) in artificial laboratory environments (Gubernick and Alberts, 1987). This led some to question how often, if ever, paternal behavior is actually exhibited among mammals. Although it remains clear that paternal care is rare among mammals, recent studies have convincingly demonstrated paternal behavior in a number of species. Among rodents, paternal care has been documented in laboratory studies of several species of deer mice (*Peromyscus*) (Gubernick and Alberts, 1987; Hatton and Meyer, 1973; McCarty and Southwick, 1977), golden hamsters (*Mesocricetus auratus*) (Marques and Valenstein, 1976), house mice (*Mus musculus*) (Priestnall and Young, 1978), grasshopper mice (*Onychomys torridus*), and two vole species (*Microtus ochrogaster, M. pinetorum*) (Gruder-Adams and Getz, 1985; Hartung and Dewsbury, 1979; Oliveras and Novak, 1986; Thomas and Birney, 1979; see Elwood, 1983 for review). California mice (*Peromyscus californicus*) exhibit a biparental system of parental care. These animals form long-term pair bonds in the wild and in the laboratory and remain together throughout both the breeding and nonbreeding seasons (Ribble and Salvioni, 1990). Furthermore, these animals are exclusively monogamous (Ribble, 1990). Males and females exhibit the same parental behaviors to the same extent, with the obvious exception of lactation (Figure 7.13). Males spend as much time in the nest as females, help build nests, and carry young. Males also groom the pups and lick the anogenital regions of the pups to stimulate urination (Gubernick and Alberts, 1987).

Another well-studied biparental species is the marmoset (*Callithrix jacchus*), a New World primate that also displays a monogamous mating system. The male assists during birth, chews food for the babies, and except during nursing sessions, he always carries the young (Hampton et al., 1966). Other nonhuman primates, including tamarins (*Leontocebus midas*), Japanese macaques (*Maccaca fuscata*), gibbons (*Hylobates lar*), and siamangs (*Symphalangus syndactylus*), also show paternal involvement in the care of the young (Yogman, 1990). In the limited confines of the laboratory setting, many species of rodents and primates

**7.13    Male california deer mice display paternal behavior.** With the exception of lactation, males of this species exhibit the same parental behaviors as females, and to the same extent: males spend as much time with the pups as females, help build nests, carry young, groom pups, and lick the pups to stimulate urination. This species is reported to be monogamous in both the laboratory and the field. Courtesy of David Gubernick.

exhibit paternal behavior even though they never display these behaviors in nature (Elwood, 1983; Redican and Taub, 1981; Suomi, 1977).

### Endocrine Correlates of Mammalian Parental Behavior

The endocrine correlates of the onset, maintenance, and termination of maternal behavior in rats are probably the best understood of any species. Because the onset of maternal behavior coincides with the birth of the young, the hormones associated with pregnancy and lactation were historically considered likely candidates for causing maternal behavior. In many respects, lactation is the key to mammalian maternal behavior, but it is just one element in a complex system. Because prolactin and lactation are closely linked, prolactin was initially considered to be the critical hormone underlying maternal behavior (Riddle et al., 1935a), but a number of endocrine manipulations have since revealed that several additional hormones are involved; namely, oxytocin, β-endorphin, cholecystokinin, prostaglandins, relaxin, progesterone, and several estrogens (Bridges, 1996; Nelson and Panksepp, 1998). Pituitary prolactin and placental lactogen (a prolactin-like hormone) play leading roles in maternal behavior, but how they are related to other hormones has not yet been specified (Rosenblatt, 1990). Although some straightforward relationships between hormone concentrations and behavior have been found, there are many subtle endocrine interactions as well. For example, the generation of maternal behavior seems to be dependent on hormones, yet some components of maternal behavior are virtually independent of hormonal influences.

     **SENSITIZATION OR PUP INDUCTION.**    An experimental paradigm often used to explore the occurrence and hormonal correlates of rat parental behavior is the presentation of foster pups. Researchers present pups of differing ages (typically between 1–10 days of age) to adult females (and males) in different endocrine states and observe whether, and how quickly, the adults begin to behave parentally toward them. During the first day of exposure to pups, castrated or intact male rats normally ignore them, or in some cases attack them. Adult females that are not pregnant or pseudopregnant also ignore or attack the pups initially. Pregnant females, however, soon begin to behave maternally toward foster pups if they are first exposed to them during the last few days of their pregnancy (typically starting on day 16 to 18 of the 22-day pregnancy) (Figure 7.14). Pseudopregnant rats may also show a rapid onset of maternal behavior at the end of their 12–13 day pseudopregnancy. Once a female rat has weaned pups of her own, she retains an enhanced sensitivity to rat pups and will show a reduced latency to behave maternally in future tests (Bridges, 1990).

If foster pups are presented to an adult female rat that has never been pregnant (a nulliparous female) for several hours each day, she begins to behave maternally after 5 or 6 days. This phenomenon is called **concaveation** (Rosenblatt, 1967; Wiesner and Sheard, 1933), **sensitization** (LeBlond, 1938), or **pup-induced parental behavior** (Fleming et al., 1996). All the behaviors, except maternal aggression in defense of the nest, that are typically observed in a rat that has just given birth are observed in these "sensitized" females; they even adopt a nursing posture, albeit an imperfect one in the absence of suckling pups (of course, they do not lactate without the proper hormonal priming). Remarkably, male rats also show this response to exposure to rat pups, although they take more time to achieve the level of maternal behavior observed in females, and the behavior is less consistent than that shown by females (Lubin et al., 1972; Mayer et al., 1979). Sensitization appears to have little or nothing to do with hormone concentrations, because the effect persists after the removal of the gonads, pituitary, or adrenal

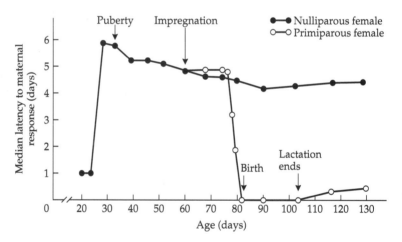

**7.14 Latency to maternal behavior in rats.** Prior to puberty, rats behave maternally on the first day of exposure to foster pups. After puberty, 5–6 daily exposures to novel pups are required to elicit maternal behavior; that value gradually drops to about 4 days as rats age. Pregnant rats do not show maternal behavior during most of the gestation period, but during the last 2–3 days of pregnancy there is a rapid drop in the latency to display maternal behavior in response to pups. This sensitivity to pups remains high for some weeks after weaning. Source: Bridges, 1990.

glands; the behavioral changes appear to be induced by the mere presence of the pups (Rosenblatt, 1967).

Mother rats, or dams, on the other hand, behave maternally toward their own pups as soon as they are born, and this rapid onset of maternal behavior is hormonally mediated. Normally, adult rats are fearful of pups; they approach them very tentatively, sniff them, and withdraw quickly. One way in which the hormones associated with pregnancy and lactation predispose the new mother to behave maternally is by reducing the fear associated with the presence of rat pups (Fleming, 1986; Fleming and Luebke, 1981, and see below). Continued exposure to her pups also appears to allow the dam to overcome her initial fear of newborns as she becomes accustomed to them. Consistent with the hypothesis that anxiety or fear blocks the onset of maternal behavior is the observation that the onset of maternal behavior is facilitated in female rats that are treated with tranquilizers such as benzodiazepines (Hansen et al., 1985).

Males may require longer exposure to pups than females to behave maternally in sensitization tests because, as open field tests and other evaluations have shown, males are generally more timid than females (Gray and Lalljee, 1974). As noted above for dogs, rats that give birth by cesarean section (C-section) typically behave maternally toward their pups as soon as they recover from anesthesia if they receive some time with the pups. However, if C-sectioned or normally parturient mother rats are not permitted this initial interaction with their pups, maternal responsiveness to pups wanes during the first week after birth (Bridges, 1977; Orpen and Fleming, 1987). By the tenth day postpartum, dams show the same latencies to respond to foster pups as nulliparous females.

**EXPERIENTIAL INFLUENCES ON MATERNAL BEHAVIOR.**    The effects of various hormones and neuropeptides on maternal behavior change as a function of experience. In general, experienced mothers are "better" mothers. Females that have given birth previously display maternal care toward foster pups within 1 day regardless of hormone status (Bridges, 1996). Furthermore, rats undergoing their second pregnancy respond to pups with maternal care within 1 day during midgestation, in contrast to primiparous (pregnant for the first time) rats, which require 7 to 8 days (Bridges, 1978). Even hypophysectomy appears to have little effect on the maintenance of maternal behavior (Erskine et al., 1980a). Thus, hormones appear to be important to prime first-time mothers to behave maternally at the end of their pregnancy. Subsequently, experiential factors appear to mediate maternal care for future offspring (Bridges, 1996).

It seems that a "maternal memory" that depends upon experience with pups is normally formed immediately postpartum, and that this memory serves to reduce the latency to display maternal behavior (Bridges, 1975). Alison Fleming and her colleagues tested this hypothesis by administering cycloheximide, a protein synthesis inhibitor that interferes with memory formation in other contexts, to mother rats immediately before or after allowing them a 2-hour postnatal maternal experience with their pups. They found that cycloheximide blocks the expression of later maternal behavior toward foster pups (Fleming et al., 1990a). Cycloheximide apparently blocks the formation of a rat dam's memory of her early experiences with her pups by preventing the consolidation of new information (Davis and Squire, 1984). Precisely what new information is normally being consolidated is not known, although there are many hypotheses. Most likely, an association between stimuli correlated with the pups and the maternal response is stored during normal attachment. We know that protein synthesis is necessary for the formation of new memories. This protein synthesis may represent new growth of neural processes or an increase in neurotransmitter or receptor production. Thus, the protein synthesis inhibitor might prevent the consolidation of information by blocking either structural changes in or the enhancement of the efficacy of certain neurons. Based on chemical lesion studies, intracerebroventricular injections, microdialysis, and gene manipulations, researchers believe that the neurotransmitters involved in maternal behavior include dopamine, norepinephrine, and serotonin (Bridges, 1996; Thomas and Palmiter, 1997; Nelson and Panksepp, 1998).

**THE ONSET OF MATERNAL BEHAVIOR.**    The natural endocrine profile of late pregnancy and pseudopregnancy in rats includes a precipitous drop in blood plasma concentrations of progesterone after a dramatic increase throughout pregnancy; a steady, gradual increase in blood estradiol concentrations; and an increase in prolactin concentrations at the end of pregnancy and immediately postpartum (Figure 7.15a; Bridges, 1990). This endocrine pattern is also evident in near-term pregnant mice (McCormack and Greenwald, 1974), rabbits (Challis et al., 1973), and sheep (Chamley et al., 1973). In contrast, pregnancy in Old World primates, including humans, is characterized by high concentrations of both estradiol and progesterone throughout pregnancy, followed by a precipitous drop in the concentrations of both steroids at parturition (Figure 7.15b; Coe, 1990; Warren and Shortle, 1990). Oxytocin and endorphins increase around the time of parturition; oxytocin is important in the smooth muscle contractions necessary for giving birth (Bridges, 1996). The role of opioids remains controversial; they may reduce pain during childbirth, and they may be involved in the mediation of maternal behavior. Both stimulatory and inhibitory roles of β-endorphin in maternal behavior have been reported (reviewed in Bridges, 1996). Primates also show increases in concentrations of ACTH and cortisol throughout gestation. The elevation of cortisol concentrations may serve to lower progesterone concentrations in addition to suppressing immune reactions of the mother toward her fetus (Coe, 1990).

Research on the topic of endocrine induction of maternal behavior in rats has fallen into two general categories. One approach has attempted to induce maternal behavior in nulliparous females via the administration or removal of hormones associated with pregnancy and lactation. Techniques used in such endocrine induction studies have included hormone replacement therapy and the transfusion of blood between pregnant and nonpregnant animals. This approach has also been used in other mammals. The other type of study has attempted to induce maternal behavior by terminating pregnancy at various stages. The logic behind these pregnancy termination studies is that (1) hormones change during pregnancy, (2) maternal behavior is caused by the hormones associated with pregnancy, and (3) because pregnancy termination leads to the rapid onset of maternal behavior before its normal onset at parturition, correlating the onset of maternal behavior with the coincident endocrine profile will reveal the hormonal cause of these behaviors.

Over 70 years ago, Calvin P. Stone exchanged the blood of a female rat that was behaving maternally with the blood of one that was not by connecting their circulatory systems in what is called a parabiotic preparation. In this manner,

(a) **Rat hormone profile**

(b) **Human hormone profile**

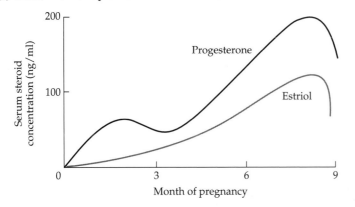

**7.15   Hormone profile during pregnancy in rats and humans.** (a) In rats, after blastocyst implantation, which occurs about 5 days after insemination, blood concentrations of progesterone begin to rise, peaking on days 15 and 16, then drop precipitously at the end of gestation. Blood estradiol concentrations remain stable during the first part of pregnancy, then rise dramatically at the end. Prolactin concentrations are high during the first half of pregnancy due to daily pulses of this hormone, but then decrease until the end of pregnancy, when they rise again; this hormone is necessary to support lactation and is important in mediating some maternal behaviors. Placental lactogen (rPL), secreted from the placenta, has actions similar to prolactin and growth hormone, supporting fetal growth and mammary gland development. (b) In humans, prolactin concentrations (not shown) increase gradually until parturition, and stay elevated until nursing is completed. Concentrations of progesterone increase dramatically during the first trimester, then continue to increase until just prior to parturition. Estriol concentrations show a slow, continuous rise until the last few weeks of pregnancy, then quickly drop prior to parturition. Source: Rosenblatt et al., 1979.

Stone attempted to induce maternal behavior in the nonmaternal rat, but he was unsuccessful (Stone, 1925). Many years later, Terkel and Rosenblatt (1968, 1972) set up a transfusion system whereby the blood of one female could be exchanged with that of another while they were free to walk around, appearing to behave normally (Figure 7.16). In one such experiment, the blood of a female that had just delivered a litter was exchanged with that of a nulliparous female. Virtually complete maternal behavior was observed in the nulliparous female within 24 hours of her receiving blood from the mother rat. This study demonstrated conclusively that a blood-borne factor is important in the induction of maternal behavior in rats.

The vast majority of work on the effects of pregnancy termination on the onset of maternal behavior has been conducted by Jay Rosenblatt and his colleagues (e.g., Bridges et al., 1978a; Rosenblatt and Siegel, 1975; Siegel and Rosenblatt, 1975, 1978). Female rats normally do not behave maternally toward foster pups at the beginning or middle of their pregnancies, but are intensely maternal at the end of pregnancy. The rationale behind these studies was to find out whether prematurely terminating pregnancy would induce the endocrine changes observed at birth and consequently induce maternal behavior. The researchers found that surgical removal of the uterus, fetuses, and placenta (hysterectomy) induces maternal behavior. Rats hysterectomized on day 16–19 of pregnancy respond rapidly with maternal behavior if they are presented with newborn foster pups 24–48 hours after surgery (Bridges et al., 1978b). Recall that nonpregnant female rats—with or without a uterus—require 5 or 6 days of periodic exposure to pups before they behave in a maternal manner.

Endocrinologically, the removal of the placenta is probably the main causative factor in the induction of maternal behavior in hysterectomized rats. The

**7.16   A blood-borne factor induces maternal behavior** in nulliparous rats. When the blood of a new mother was transfused into a nulliparous rat, the recipient showed maternal behavior within 24 hours. Normally, 4–6 days of sensitization are required to induce maternal behavior in nulliparous females. After Terkel and Rosenblatt, 1968.

removal of the placenta eliminates the source of a prolactin-like hormone, called placental lactogen, that supports the corpora lutea during mid- to late pregnancy in rats. Consequently, removal of the placenta during hysterectomy leads to rapid regression of the corpora lutea and subsequent reductions of blood concentrations of progesterone. The rat placenta is also the source of a gonadotropin that typically suppresses ovarian estrogen production until very late in pregnancy. Removal of this source of estrogen inhibition results in a rapid pulse of estrogen secretion, which normally results in postpartum estrus. Thus, mid- to late pregnancy termination via hysterectomy results in an endocrine profile resembling that found in a normal rat immediately prior to parturition.

In other studies of the hormonal bases of maternal behavior, attempts have been made to mimic the endocrine patterns of pregnancy in ovariectomized females by injecting them with different hormones in various sequences (Moltz et al., 1970; Zarrow et al., 1971; Bridges, 1990, 1996; Rosenblatt et al., 1998). Two of these early studies will be described in detail.

In one study, nulliparous rabbits that were injected with estradiol for 18 days and received progesterone injections on days 2 through 15 inclusive exhibited maternal nest building (Zarrow et al., 1963; reviewed in González-Mariscal and Rosenblatt, 1996). Maternal behavior is relatively difficult to assess in rabbits because of its brevity. The energetic demands on a lactating rabbit doe are enormous, and foraging demands virtually all of her time. Consequently, rabbit does do not engage in as much maternal behavior as other species that produce altricial young; for instance, a mother rabbit nurses her litter for only about 3–4 minutes once per day (Ross et al., 1959; Zarrow et al., 1965). Thus, the maternal behavior of rabbits that is most commonly assayed in the laboratory is nest building. Near the time of birth, the pregnant doe builds a nest of grass and lines it with her own fur, which loosens progressively throughout pregnancy so that it can be easily removed at this time. This fur loosening is dependent on hormonal changes. The increased estrogen/progesterone ratio at the end of pregnancy probably stimulates the release of prolactin from the anterior pituitary, as it does in rats and sheep. Treatment of pregnant rabbits with dopamine agonists (for example, ergot compounds), which block prolactin release, suppresses nest building; concurrent treatment with prolactin reverses the suppression (Zarrow et al., 1971). Thus, the maternal nest building observed at the end of pregnancy in rabbits correlates with an increased estrogen/progesterone ratio in the blood, as well as with elevated prolactin titers. In contrast to rabbits, house mice and golden hamsters build nests during early or mid-pregnancy. High concentrations of both estrogens and progestins induce maternal nest building in these species (Lisk, 1971; Richards, 1969; reviewed in González-Mariscal and Rosenblatt, 1996). External factors interact with hormones in mediating maternal nest building in rabbits (González-Mariscal et al., 1998). The endocrine profile during pregnancy and parturition is very different from the endocrine profile during nursing. Yet, the quality (and perhaps quantity) of maternal care in rabbits remains constant. As in other mammalian species, maintenance of rabbit maternal behavior appears to require sensory stimulation (e.g., olfactory, tactile, acoustic, and visual) that is provided by the offspring (reviewed in González-Mariscal and Rosenblatt, 1996).

In another study, female rats were injected with estradiol for 11 consecutive days, progesterone on days 6 through 9, and prolactin on days 9 through 11

(Moltz et al., 1970). This pattern of hormone treatment caused full maternal behavior within 35 hours. Although the induction of complex maternal behavior with a certain pattern of hormone injections is impressive, normal maternal behavior begins at or immediately before parturition, not 35 hours later. There must be other factors, endocrine as well as nonendocrine, involved in the induction of normal postpartum maternal behavior, or else the presentation of the hormones via systemic injections was insufficient to engage the neural machinery underlying this behavior. Infusions of prolactin directly into the MPOA of steroid-primed rats induces maternal behavior very quickly (Bridges and Freemark, 1995; Bridges et al., 1996; Bridges, 1996).

Recent studies suggest that placental lactogen may mediate the rise in maternal behavior that occurs during pregnancy prior to parturition. Infusion of placental lactogen into the MPOA of steroid-primed rats was as effective as prolactin infusion in stimulating maternal behavior (Bridges et al., 1995, 1996). It appears that the conceptus (the fetus plus placenta) secretes placental lactogen, which can stimulate maternal behavior during and at the end of the pregnancy (Bridges et al., 1996). Thus, the endocrine communication between the developing conceptus and the mother ensures that maternal behavior will occur as soon as possible after birth (Bridges, 1996). This intriguing "manipulation" of maternal endocrine function is in the best interest of the fetus, but also benefits the mother's long-term fitness.

Other recent experiments have suggested a role for oxytocin in mediating the onset of rat maternal behavior. In all mammalian species that have been investigated, oxytocin concentrations increase during parturition (Fuchs and Dawood, 1980; Fuchs and Fuchs, 1984). Oxytocin causes the uterine and vaginal contractions of birth as well as milk letdown, processes that may induce other physiological changes leading to the onset of maternal behavior. If oxytocin is injected directly into the ventricles of the brain in estrogen-primed ovariectomized rats, maternal behavior is observed within 1 hour (Pedersen and Prange, 1979; C. A. Pedersen et al., 1982). However, rats are very sensitive to the testing environment, and differences in apparatus and test procedures may mask the effects of oxytocin on maternal behavior. Oxytocin appears to act as a neurotransmitter or neurohormone in the brain, because systemic injections of oxytocin into estrogen-primed ovariectomized rats do not induce maternal behavior (Insel, 1990a).

It is possible that vaginal stimulation during parturition causes oxytocin secretion, which in turn stimulates further contractions. To test this hypothesis, multiparous (having previously given birth several times), nonpregnant sheep were injected with a hormone regimen that included 12 days of progesterone followed by a large dose of estradiol, then were tested for maternal responsiveness to newborn lambs (Keverne et al., 1983). Half of the ewes received vaginal stimulation with a vibrator 5 minutes prior to the presentation of the lambs. Vaginal stimulation elevated oxytocin concentrations in the cerebrospinal fluid (Keverne and Kendrick, 1994). Only 20% of the nonstimulated ewes showed maternal behavior during a 1-hour test, but 80% of the stimulated ewes displayed maternal behavior. These results suggest that oxytocin is important in the induction of maternal behavior in sheep (Box 7.3).

A suite of hormones, neuropeptides, and neurotransmitters is responsible for the initiation and maintenance of parental care in mammals. In rats, the factors

## Box 7.3
# Maternal Behavior in Sheep

Research on sheep has been especially informative about the hormone–brain–behavior interactions associated with maternal behavior. Sheep are seasonal breeders, and most lambs are born early in the spring to coincide with the maximal availability of green vegetation for food. Sheep form feeding flocks and graze over a common home range (Lévy et al., 1996). When pregnant ewes are about to give birth, they seclude themselves away from the flock. After the birth of the highly precocial lamb, the mother and infant form a strong social bond within the first hour after birth. During this time, the mother learns to discriminate her lamb from the other lambs in the flock. This discrimination appears to be based on olfactory cues emitted by the lamb (Kendrick et al., 1992). Ewes normally permit only their own lambs to approach their udders and suckle. This discrimination is important from an evolutionary perspective because ewes that permitted other lambs to nurse would give up resources that could go to their offspring (Lévy et al., 1996). Such misdirected parental care would have strongly negative consequences on fitness if there were insufficient milk for the ewes' own lambs. In fact, ewes are highly rejecting of approaching lambs with which they have not formed a social bond (Lévy et al., 1996). Thus, the establishment of an exclusive bond during the first hour is a critical component of sheep maternal care.

Importantly, establishment of the exclusive bond is separate from *maternal responsiveness,* a suite of behaviors that is directed toward any lamb immediately after parturition. Olfactory cues are also important in making lambs attractive stimuli to ewes. Both maternal responsiveness and establishment of the exclusive social bond characterize maternal behavior in sheep (Lévy et al., 1996).

As in other species of mammals, parturition in sheep is preceded by an increase in the ratio of estradiol to progesterone in the blood circulation. If nulliparous ewes are hormonally primed with estradiol and progesterone to mimic the conditions of the last week of pregnancy and presented with newborn lambs, the ewes are either indifferent or aggressive toward them. However, nulliparous ewes hormonally primed and given vaginocervical stimulation display a rapid onset of maternal behavior. The vaginocervical stimulation simulates parturition and evokes the release of oxytocin (Keverne and Kendrick, 1994). In vivo microdialysis studies of stimulated ewes revealed that oxytocin concentrations were elevated in the cerebrospinal fluid (CSF), as well as in the olfactory bulbs, MPOA, PVN, and substania nigra (reviewed in Lévy et al., 1996), all brain areas that are important in sheep maternal behavior. When oxytocin is injected directly into the CSF of nonpregnant ewes, the full complement of maternal behaviors is observed (Keverne and Kendrick, 1994). These results suggest that oxytocin is important for both maternal acceptance and other maternally motivated behaviors in sheep. The relevance of these findings to humans is potentially great.

that appear to have the greatest effects on parental care are estrogens and lactogenic hormones (i.e., prolactin and placental lactogens) (Bridges, 1996). The supportive roles of prolactin, progesterone, oxytocin, CCK, and probably β-endorphins on maternal care are estrogen-dependent (Insel, 1990b; Bridges, 1996) (see Figure 7.15a). Several neurotransmitter systems are involved in the mediation of rat parental care, but the dopaminergic system seems particularly important. The dopaminergic system can be stimulated by lactogenic hormones and inhibited by endogenous opioids (Bridges, 1996). Further research must be conducted to determine the extent to which the regulatory mechanisms underlying rat maternal behavior also mediate parental care in other mammals, including humans.

**MATERNAL AGGRESSION.**    Protection of offspring from predators or infanticidal conspecifics is an important component of parental care. Maternal aggression is one mechanism by which female mammals protect their offspring. The onset of maternal aggression appears to be regulated by hormones. However, the hormonal control of maternal aggression appears to differ from the hormonal control of other components of maternal behavior. Maternal aggression is rarely observed in the absence of the offspring.

Most of the research on maternal aggression has been conducted on house mice—more specifically, maternal aggression by house mice directed toward a male conspecific intruder. However, substantial work on the interaction of hormones and the somatosensory aspects of maternal aggression has been conducted on rats. Laboratory strains of mice and rats are rather docile and do not usually attack conspecifics. However, beginning in the middle of gestation and peaking in intensity during the first week after birth, mouse dams react to an intruding male by displaying intense threat and biting behavior. Prior to parturition, progesterone appears to induce maternal aggression (Svare, 1990). Four converging lines of evidence point to a role for progesterone in mediating maternal aggression in pregnant mice. First, progesterone treatment elevates the rate of aggressive behavior in nulliparous mice (Mann et al., 1984). Second, pseudopregnant females become more aggressive as blood concentrations of progesterone increase (Barkley et al., 1979). Third, pregnant females begin to show signs of maternal aggression when peak concentrations of progesterone occur (Mann et al., 1984). Finally, surgical pregnancy termination, which dramatically reduces progesterone concentrations, eliminates maternal aggression when performed on the 15th day of pregnancy, and progesterone replacement therapy partially restores maternal aggressive behavior in hysterectomized individuals (Svare et al., 1986). However, other hormones are also probably involved in maternal aggression, because progesterone treatment alone never induces the level of aggression in nulliparous females that is observed in newly parturient mice. Furthermore, maternal aggression is very high at the time of birth, when progesterone concentrations are relatively low, suggesting that other factors mediate aggressive behavior after the birth of the young.

The results of other studies suggest that in mice, and less so in rats, suckling by the young stimulates postnatal maternal aggression (Svare and Gandelman, 1976). Intense maternal aggressive behaviors are observed in mice after 48 hours of suckling, and thelectomized (nipples surgically removed) mice display lower levels of maternal aggression than normal postpartum mice (Svare, 1990). Because suckling was found to be a critical stimulus for the expression of maternal aggression, it was logically suspected that prolactin is responsible for the induction of this behavior. However, this hypothesis was ruled out because neither postpartum hypophysectomy nor treatment with prolactin-inhibiting ergot compounds affect the occurrence of maternal aggression (Erskine et al., 1980b; Mann et al.,

1980; Svare et al., 1982). Furthermore, no relationship has been found between blood plasma concentrations of prolactin and the initiation, maintenance, or decline of maternal aggression in house mice (Broida et al., 1981). However, prolactin does mediate maternal aggression in white-footed mice (*Peromyscus leucopus*) (Gleason et al., 1981) and golden hamsters (Wise and Pryor, 1977).

Thus, ovarian hormones present during pregnancy appear to regulate maternal aggression in mice and rats in two ways. First, ovarian steroids directly promote aggressive behavior during gestation. Second, these hormones indirectly induce aggressive behavior by stimulating nipple development for attachment and suckling by the young. Whether ovarian hormones exert additional effects on postpartum aggressive behavior remains unresolved. Nursing-induced postpartum aggressive behavior coincides with elevated levels of serotonin, and treatment with a serotonin antagonist reduces maternal aggression (Ieni and Thurmond, 1985). Endorphins and oxytocin could also play a role in the mediation of maternal aggression.

Maternal aggression per se does not seem to be a component of human maternal care, but direct tests are lacking. Experiments on humans are rarely conducted because of ethical considerations; consequently, correlational studies are usually preferred. In one study, women with high concentrations of circulating prolactin due to prolactin-secreting tumors reported higher levels of hostility in paper-and-pencil tests than normal controls; treatment with prolactin-inhibiting ergot compounds reduce these high hostility scores (Buckman and Kellner, 1985; Fava et al., 1981). In another study, new mothers rated themselves as more hostile on day 7 postpartum than did control females (hospital employees) (Mastrogiacomo et al., 1982/1983).

One can imagine nonendocrine explanations for the increased hostility scores of newly parturient women, but studies on women differ fundamentally from the assessment of maternal aggression in other animals. Reliance on hostility scores, rather than on the aggressive behaviors themselves, reduces the likelihood that accurate information about endocrine correlates will be obtained. Paper-and-pencil tests of hostility are rarely validated to ascertain whether they truly correlate with the likelihood of agonistic behavior. As noted above, assessment of maternal aggression among nonhumans is always conducted in the presence of their offspring. Mouse dams, for instance, rarely display maternal aggression in the absence of their pups. Women, however, are generally separated from their babies during questionnaire testing. Direct tests of maternal aggressive *behavior* in the presence of their infants and concurrent measurements of hormone concentrations have not been performed on humans (but see Fleming, 1990).

**MAINTENANCE AND TERMINATION OF MATERNAL BEHAVIOR.**    Hormones are clearly necessary to trigger maternal behavior when the offspring are first born. Yet maternal behavior persists after parturition, and long after the high hormone concentrations of pregnancy have returned to baseline levels. Are hormones involved in maintaining maternal behavior? Also, mothers act less maternal as their offspring grow older (Figure 7.17). Are hormone concentrations changing, or are the young less effective in stimulating maternal care?

These questions have been addressed in rats, which display three stages of maternal behavior. It is important to emphasize that at each stage, the pups are trying to get food from their mothers, and the pups' suckling behavior induces

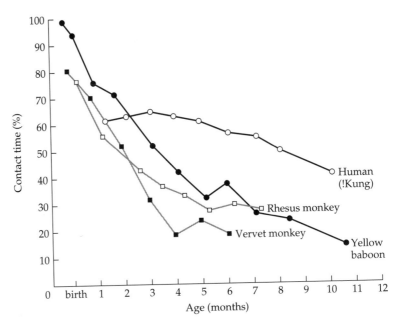

**7.17  Mother–infant contact decreases over time.** The percentage of time that mothers of four primate species and their young spent in close contact each day is plotted over the first year of the lives of the offspring. When the young are first born, virtually all of the mothers' day is spent in contact with them, but in nonhuman primate species, this value drops to 10–30% of the day after 6 months. At 10 months, approximately 40% of a human mother's time is spent in contact with her baby; this may reflect the slower maturation rate of humans or the increased solicitousness of human mothers. Source: Altmann, 1980.

maternal nursing behaviors. During the first stage, the majority of the maternal behavior is initiated by the mother. She builds the nest, delivers the young into it, and retrieves any pups that wander away from it. She huddles over her litter in the nursing posture. The pups must attach themselves to a nipple and stay attached, but the mother provides cues for the pups to promote the initial nipple attachment: she licks her vulva and ventrum during birth, spreading amniotic fluid across the front of her body, and the odor of the amniotic fluid attracts the newborn pups to the nipples. If the amniotic sacs of fetuses are injected with lemon oil during pregnancy, the pups are attracted to the odor of lemon oil after birth (Pedersen and Blass, 1982). As the pups age, the odor of their own saliva and their littermates' and that of their mother keeps attracting them back to the nipple. At an early age, nutritional state does not particularly influence the time it takes for pups to attach to a nipple, but as the pups age, the length of time since the last meal does influence the latency to reattach to a nipple.

In the second stage of rat maternal behavior, there is more mutually initiated contact. The mother may initiate care, but the pups often approach her for contact. Stimuli associated with the pups are critical for maintaining maternal care in ths stage (Box 7.4). If a mother rat is provided with new 4- or 5-day-old foster pups every few days, she continues to build nests and behave maternally (Sö-

Box 7.4

# Offspring Behavior
# and the Maintenance of Maternal Behavior

Research by Judith Stern has established the importance of somatosensory (tactile) feedback from pups for maintaining maternal care in rats (Stern, 1996). Most rat maternal behaviors, including nest construction, licking, and pup retrieval, involve the mouth. During the course of nuzzling or sniffing the pups, the female receives somatosensory input that stimulates further maternal behavior. Many maternal behaviors can be reduced or abolished by cutting or anesthetizing the nerves that innervate the area around the mouth (Stern, 1990). For example, a mother rat that has had her muzzle desensitized with a local anesthetic exhibits reductions in nest building, nest repair, pup retrieval, pup licking, and even biting of intruders.

Somatosensory information from the pups is also important for maintaining nursing behavior. Virtually all mammalian newborns arrive equipped with reflexes that allow them to find and attach to a nipple and ingest milk. Mothers' assistance of their offspring's nursing behavior ranges from the "passive tolerance" of marsupial mothers to the active participation in feeding seen in humans and other primate species (Stern and Johnson, 1990; Stern, 1990). In rats, ventral somatosensory information maintains the maternal nursing posture, an immobile, upright crouching posture in which the female stands over the pups. If the nipples are anesthetized or removed, then even an entire litter

cannot stimulate the female to exhibit a normal nursing posture (Stern et al., 1992). Similarly, if the mouths of the pups are anesthetized so that they no longer root up against the mother trying to locate her nipples, an unanesthetized dam will fail to adopt the nursing posture. Thus, tactile stimuli from the pups are important in maintaining nursing behaviors in mothers.

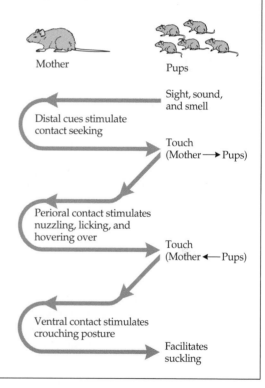

Mother                Pups

Sight, sound, and smell

Distal cues stimulate contact seeking

Touch (Mother → Pups)

Perioral contact stimulates nuzzling, licking, and hovering over

Touch (Mother ← Pups)

Ventral contact stimulates crouching posture

Facilitates suckling

dersten and Eneroth, 1984). This behavior is maintained by tactile and other sensory stimuli from the young pups. In the normal situation, however, maternal care eventually wanes as the pups mature.

Maternal rejection of the pups and subsequent separation from them constitutes the third stage of maternal behavior in rats. The mother makes herself less available to the pups by "hiding" her ventrum from them, by rejecting them, or by remaining out of their reach (Reisbick et al., 1975). What are the signals that reduce maternal care as the pups grow older?

One salient cue is the body temperature of the mother rat. As described above, rat pups are born blind, deaf, hairless, and unable to regulate their body temperatures. Rat pups are considered to be poikilothermic, like reptiles; the body temperature of an isolated rat pup is only slightly higher than the ambient temperature. However, although an individual pup cannot thermoregulate, a litter of pups can. After 4 hours of exposure to a 24°C ambient temperature, an individual pup possesses a body temperature of 26°C, while individuals in a huddle of four pups maintain a body temperature of 30°C (Alberts and Brunjes, 1978). Researchers examined the percentage of time that a rat pup spent on the outside of a huddle and found that there was considerable competition among littermates for inner and outer positions within the huddle. In one study, in which litters were culled to four, all four pups kept switching their positions within the litter. In another experiment (Alberts and Brunjes, 1978), one of the four pups in each litter was anesthetized, and the huddle was placed in either a hot or a cold environment (Figure 7.18). In the cold environment, the anesthetized pup spent up to 90% of the time exposed to the cold at the outer fringes of the huddle. In the hot environment, the anesthetized pup spent a considerable amount of time on the inside of the huddle.

Thermoregulation may play a major role in modulating mother–pup contact time during the third stage of rat maternal behavior, and hormones underlie the physiological orchestration of this behavior as well. The amount of time a mother rat spends with her litter decreases as the pups get older. The dam initially spends about 75% of the day in contact with her litter. The bouts of time she spends on the nest decline progressively during the first 2 weeks postpartum; that is, the number of nest bouts remains constant, but the length of each nest bout decreases.

(a)  **High temperatures**          (b)  **Low temperatures**

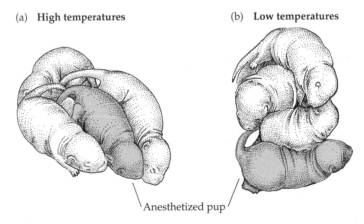

Anesthetized pup

**7.18    Thermoregulation in rat pups.**  An isolated rat pup's body temperature soon falls several degrees below the normal body temperature of 37°C, but pups in groups can maintain their temperatures at 37°C because individuals move in and out of the huddle to maintain their body temperature in an ideal range. This behavioral thermoregulation can be demonstrated by adding an anesthetized pup to the huddle. (a) At warm ambient temperatures, the pups maneuver so that the anesthetized pup is in the center of the huddle and becomes overheated. (b) At cool ambient temperatures, the anesthetized pup is shoved to the outside of the huddle. After Alberts and Brunjes, 1978.

Mother rats secrete progressively increasing amounts of prolactin during days 1–14 of lactation (Leon et al., 1990). When Adels and Leon (1986) treated mother rats with a drug, bromocryptine (an ergot compound), that blocks prolactin production and secretion, they found that nest time did not decrease during the first 2 weeks of lactation, but remained high. Adels and Leon suspected that prolactin was acting through another hormone, and in a series of endocrine gland ablation experiments, they showed that removal of the adrenal glands proved to be most effective in blocking the decrease in nest time. If the adrenal glands are removed, time on the nest does not show the normal decrease during days 1–14 of lactation, but removal of the adrenal medulla alone does not block the decline in nest time. Consequently, the researchers surmised that the decrease in nest time must be due to glucocorticoids (for example, corticosterone) rather than mineralocorticoids (for example, aldosterone). To discover which hormone would reverse the decline in nest time, adrenalectomized dams were injected with corticosterone, aldosterone, progesterone, or a control vehicle (the oil in which the injected steroids were dissolved—recall that steroids are not water soluble). By this means, corticosterone was eventually found to be the critical hormone responsible for the decline in nest time. Normally, ACTH increases during the first 2 weeks of lactation and induces increased concentrations of corticosterone in the blood; the increased blood concentrations of corticosterone in turn lead to a reduction in nest bout time.

How do these hormones influence nest bout time? One possibility is that hormones could affect the efficiency of milk transfer. Mothers might regulate the amount of milk that their pups receive by utilizing cues associated with milk delivery to regulate nest time; the pups might become more efficient with age and remove a given amount of milk in less time. Faster transfer of nutrients would allow more time for the mother rat to forage for food. But this hypothesis can be dismissed. The decline in nest bout time is also observed in animals with surgically closed nipples (Leon et al., 1978). Alternatively, the dams might monitor the pups' body temperatures and stay on the nest long enough to keep them warm. As the pups aged and began to thermoregulate on their own, she would need to spend less time with them. This hypothesis can also be rejected. The core temperature of the pups does not directly affect nest bout time (Leon et al., 1978).

Another possibility is that mother rats could monitor their own body temperature to decide when to leave the nest. Adrenal steroids increase the metabolic rate and thus chronically elevate the body temperatures of mother rats (Leon et al., 1990). They cannot dissipate their own body heat when crouching over a litter, so if they stay with the pups for too long, they are in danger of suffering hyperthermia and resultant brain damage. As the pups get older, they retain heat more efficiently, requiring dams to regulate their own body temperature by spending shorter bouts of time on the nest. When pups were experimentally heated or cooled, dams spent less time with hot pups than with cold pups (Woodside and Leon, 1980). When mother rats were shaved, they showed less of a decline in nest time than did furry mothers.

Thus, the suckling pups stimulate the secretion of prolactin by mother rats, which in turn stimulates increased corticosterone production. Elevated adrenal steroid concentrations increase the mother's basal metabolic rate, which causes a rise in her body temperature—more specifically, an acute rise in brain temperature: heating the medial preoptic area of dams directly induces immediate termination of a nursing session (Woodside et al., 1980). The dam's increased body temperature leads to a decline in time spent with the pups.

An alternative interpretation of these findings is that the overheated pups failed to induce nursing behavior in their mothers (Stern and Lonstein, 1996). It can be argued that the high temperatures used in these experiments, which rat mothers and pups do not normally experience in their natural habitats, had confounding effects. That is, hyperthermic pups usually do not suckle, and suckling is critical to inducing maternal behaviors. Because these studies were automated and assessed the time spent on the nest using photocells, no other behavioral changes were recorded. Another potential confounding variable is that the boxes in which the rat dams were tested at high temperatures were too small to allow them to adopt "heat-dissipating" nursing postures (Stern and Lonstein, 1996). Thus, the apparatus used in earlier studies might have altered the behavior under study in a manner reminiscent of female rat mating behavior that was constrained by the testing arena (e.g., Erskine, 1989).

The third stage of maternal care involves not only maternal rejection, but also separation initiated by the pups. Around day 16 of age, rat pups begin leaving the nest to feed on their own. How do they find their way back to the nest? They use odors. In home orientation tests using odor cues, pups orient to the nest during days 12–14 or so, then start orienting toward their mother. This switch from nest to mother is an important change that frees the pups from the nest. Beginning on day 15 or 16 of lactation and continuing through day 27, mother rats emit a chemosensory signal that pups find very attractive. Leon and Moltz (1972) tested the attractiveness of odors from nests of lactating dams compared with the nest odors of nulliparous females. They found that older pups have a stronger preference for the odors of lactating dams than do younger pups: 5-day-old pups showed no preference, but 15-day-old pups showed a strong preference. However, this preference is not specific to the odor of the pups' own mother (Leon, 1980).

What is the source of this attractive chemosensory signal? It is released in the anal excreta of mother rats—their urine does not attract pups. In addition to feces, rats excrete small pellets of partially digested food matter, called caecotrophs, that they usually reingest. Caecotrophs are distinguishable from feces in the caecum, and are the source of the mother rat's attractive odor. Young rats consume their mother's caecotrophs as an energy-saving measure. Also, a pup's digestive system is not very efficient, and it benefits from the bacteria found in caecotrophs in building its own internal gut fauna to aid in digestion, particularly digestion of cellulose (Moltz and Kilpatrick, 1978). Caecotrophs taken directly from the caecum of a lactating female attract young rats. Interestingly, caecotrophs taken from the caecum of a nulliparous female rat work almost as well as those of mothers in attracting pups. A nonlactating female, however, normally reingests all of her caecotrophs. A lactating female experiences an increase in appetite and food intake, stimulated by prolactin (Leon et al., 1990), and thus produces so many caecotrophs that some are left near the nest. Thus it is not a specific chemical agent found only in lactating females' caecotrophs, but the emission rate, that is responsible for attracting pups. If prolactin secretion is blocked in the mother rat, the attractiveness of her nest odor is decreased, probably because she then consumes all the caecotrophs she produces, just like a nonlactating female.

If nulliparous female rats are sensitized to pups so that they behave maternally, and are prevented from ingesting their caecotrophs, then eventually the caecotrophs from these females are attractive to other rat pups (Leon, 1992). It requires about 14 days after concaveation for there to be sufficient chemical stimuli to attract pups. As in mothers, the attractiveness of the caecotrophs to the pups increases as the pups age. Unlike those of lactating females, the blood prolactin concentrations of these rats do not change; again, it is the buildup of sufficient numbers of caecotrophs in the nest that makes the nest attractive to the pups, rather than a special chemical agent produced only by lactating females. The mechanism underlying this phenomenon in concaveated females is unknown. Pups lose interest in mothers' caecotrophs at about 28 days of age, when mothers reduce caecotroph production and the pups are about to be weaned.

**ENDOCRINE CORRELATES OF PRIMATE MATERNAL BEHAVIOR.**    The endocrine correlates of maternal behavior among primates generally, and humans specifically, remain largely unknown. The reasons for this are varied, but probably reflect an assumption by researchers that primate maternal care depends primarily upon experiential, not hormonal, factors (Figure 7.19). However, recent studies have indicated important roles for estradiol in nonhuman primate motivation to engage in maternal behavior, as well as for cortisol and the pattern of estradiol/progesterone secretion in mediating maternal behavior in women, and for prolactin and a decrease in testosterone concentrations in mediating paternal behavior in men.

**7.19  Maternal behavior in bonobos.** Female bonobos engage in extended maternal care of their semi-precocial offpsring. The female carries her infant and holds it to allow it to nurse. Photograph © Frans Lanting/Minden Pictures.

In one study, adult female rhesus monkeys were presented with an infant for 1 hour daily on 5 consecutive days. Some of the females were nulliparous; others had previously given birth to several offspring (multiparous females). Some of the multiparous females were bilaterally ovariectomized, others were intact, and others were aged, postmenopausal animals. Essentially, the nulliparous females avoided the infant, whereas the multiparous females, regardless of endocrine status, immediately accepted the baby rhesus (Holman and Goy, 1980). One possible conclusion from this study is that hormones are involved in the onset of maternal behaviors in first-time mother rhesus monkeys, but may not be necessary to stimulate maternal behavior in experienced females. The stimuli associated with primate infants, primarily visual, can trigger appropriate maternal behavior in multiparous females (Coe, 1990).

However, hormones associated with pregnancy and parturition can affect motivation to behave maternally in nonhuman primates (Pryce, 1996). In test situations in which primigravid (first-time pregnant) common marmosets (*Callithrix jacchus*) were able to press a bar to receive sensory stimuli associated with infants, the rate of bar pressing increased at the end of pregnancy in association with increasing estradiol concentrations. In the same study, the pregnant marmosets pressed the bar at high rates to turn off the recorded cries of an infant (Pryce et al., 1993). A high rate of bar pressing continues postpartum even though estradiol values are decreasing (Figure 7.20). This correlational study suggests that estradiol primes females to behave in an appropriately maternal manner. Administration of progesterone and estradiol to marmosets changed their rates of bar pressing (Pryce, 1996).

Among human mothers, it is assumed that hormonal factors facilitate the initial postpartum expression of maternal care, but data to support this assumption are minimal. In fact, hormones are neither necessary nor sufficient for the appearance of basic parental behaviors (Fleming, 1990). Adoptive parents, siblings, grandparents, other relatives, and caregivers can grow attached to infants during a process that appears identical in qualitative and temporal character to the process observed in the biological mother. Obviously, the endocrine profiles of biological parents, adoptive parents, and other caregivers will vary in the presence of virtually identical behavioral patterns. There may be parallels between concaveation and parental care in adoptive parents or caregivers.

Another issue in the study of endocrine correlates of human maternal behavior is that, in contrast to rats, humans have no clear-cut universal set of maternal behaviors. Human mothers typically provide most of the care for their infants, carry them, and nurse them, but this is by no means ubiquitous. There does not seem to be a single set of behaviors, or even attitudes, that characterize human maternal behavior. For example, consuming the placenta and umbilical cord after birth is virtually universal among nonhuman primates (Figure 7.21; Coe, 1990), but there is great variation in the occurrence of this behavior among human societies. (Placentophagia might be adaptive in that it reduces the likelihood of infection and hemorrhage in the infant.) Establishing hormonal correlates with human maternal behavior is difficult when the behavior itself eludes precise definition.

Information about human mothers' perceptions of their behaviors, attitudes, and feelings is typically collected on questionnaires; however, there has been no consensus about endocrine correlates of the attitudes observed in such studies

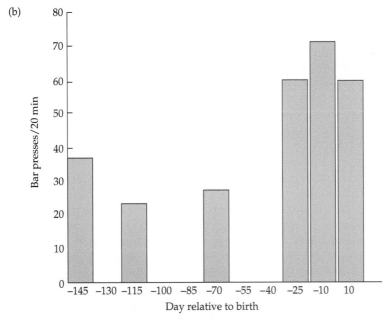

**7.20    During pregnancy, female marmosets increase bar pressing to receive infant sensory reinforcement.** (a) Plasma concentrations of estradiol (shaded line) and progesterone (solid line) over the course of pregnancy in common marmosets. (b) The number of bar presses made by females to gain infant sensory reinforcement. After Pryce et al., 1993.

**7.21　Placentophagia in the pigtailed macaque.** Eating of the placenta, or placentophagia, is an important component of maternal care among nonhuman primates. Females consume the placenta and umbilical cord up to the ventrum (belly) of the infant. Consuming the placenta and umbilical cord rids the nest of a source of infection for the parents and offspring. Courtesy of Leonard Rosenblum.

(reviewed in Krasnegor and Bridges, 1990). Items on questionnaires are usually designed so that the answers are marked on a five- or seven-point scale reflecting a range of beliefs from "strongly agree" to "strongly disagree" (Fleming, 1990). Blood samples are sometimes obtained, or correlations between obvious endocrine status (for example, midpregnancy or menstruation) and self-reports are made. However, as we have seen, associations between self-reports of attitudes and actual behaviors are not always evident, and experiments to test behavior itself are difficult to perform on humans. These difficulties seriously impair the ability of researchers to ascertain the endocrine correlates of human maternal behavior.

Self-report studies have found differences in attitudes and feelings between new mothers and non-mothers. For example, the hedonic values of a variety of infant-associated (e.g., general body, urine, feces) and non-infant-associated (e.g., cheese, spices, and lotions) odors were rated by individuals in four distinct experimental groups: (1) new mothers, (2) mothers that were one month postpartum, (3) non-parent women, and (4) non-parent men (Fleming et al., 1993). The odors were rated on a scale that ranged from "extremely pleasant" (+20.5) to "extremely unpleasant" (–20.5), and all of the participants completed several attitude questionnaires as well. In common with the results of studies on nonhuman animals (e.g., Poindron and Lévy, 1990; Lévy et al., 1996), new mothers rated infant-associated odors as more pleasant than nonmothers. New mothers also reported more nurturant attitudes and feelings (Fleming et al., 1993). Similar studies indicate that several postpartum factors, including hormone concentrations and learning, are important in the establishment of a mother's attraction to her newborn infant's odors (Fleming et al., 1993; Fleming and Corter, 1995; Schaal et al., 1980).

In another series of studies, new mothers were asked to identify, in a two-choice test, their own infant's tee shirt (Fleming et al., 1995). This task was easily performed by virtually all new mothers. Similarly, new mothers can identify their infants based on their cries (Formby, 1967) and tactile features (Kaitz, 1992). The ability of new mothers to discriminate their infants from others appears to rely primarily on experience with the infants, although hormones may potentiate or enhance the effect (e.g., Fleming et al., 1995). Also, both human mothers and fathers can discriminate the odors of two samples of amniotic fluid–either parent could identify the amniotic fluid associated with their own infants (Schaal and Marlier, 1998).

A series of elegant experiments by Alison Fleming and her collaborators (e.g., Fleming, 1990; Fleming et al., 1987, 1990b) examined the endocrine correlates of the behavior of human mothers as well as the endocrine correlates of maternal attitudes as expressed in self-report questionnaires. In one such study, behavioral responses of new mothers to their 3–4-day-old infants were recorded. Responses such as patting, cuddling, or kissing the baby were called affectionate behaviors; talking, singing, or cooing to the baby were considered vocal behaviors. Both affectionate and vocal behaviors were considered approach behaviors (Fleming, 1990). Basic caregiving activities, such as changing diapers and burping the infants, were also recorded. In these studies, no relationship between hormone concentrations and maternal responsiveness, as measured by attitude questionnaires, was found (Fleming, 1990). However, when *behavior*, rather than questionnaire responses, was compared with hormone concentrations, a different story emerged (Fleming et al., 1987). Blood plasma concentrations of cortisol were found to be positively associated with approach behaviors. In other words, women who had higher concentrations of blood cortisol, in samples obtained immediately before or after nursing, engaged in more physically affectionate behaviors and talked more often to their babies than mothers with lower concentrations of this steroid hormone. Additional analyses from this study revealed that the correlation was even greater for mothers that had reported positive maternal regard (feelings and attitudes) during gestation. In fact, nearly half of the variation in maternal behavior among women could be accounted for by cortisol concentrations and positive maternal attitudes during pregnancy (Fleming et al., 1987).

Presumably, cortisol does not induce maternal behaviors directly, but it may act indirectly on the quality of maternal care by evoking an increase in the mother's general level of arousal (Mason, 1968), and thus increasing her responsiveness to infant-generated cues (Fleming, 1990). For example, new mothers with high cortisol concentrations were also more attracted to their infant's odors, were superior in identifying their infants, and generally found cues from infants highly appealing (Figure 7.22) (Fleming et al., 1997b). Although there have been a few examples of glucocorticoid involvement in the onset of maternal care in nonhuman animals (e.g., Keverne and Kendrick, 1992), it is possible that cortisol might simply reflect other endocrine changes involving oxytocin, CRH, and opioids, all of which affect maternal responsiveness in nonhuman animals (Fleming et al., 1997b), and all of which are secreted in concert with the glucocorticoids. Perhaps not surprisingly, experiential factors also affect maternal responsiveness; experienced mothers find infants more attractive than do non-mothers and react to infant cues earlier in pregnancy than first-time mothers (Fleming et al., 1996). Moreover,

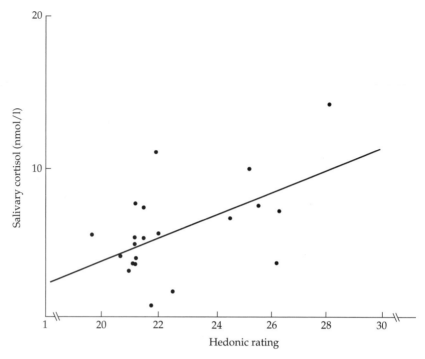

**7.22   Hedonic ratings of own infant's odors are positively correlated with cortisol levels.**
Saliva samples of cortisol from first-time mothers were compared with their hedonic ratings
(1–41) of their infant's tee-shirt odors. Mothers with higher cortisol concentrations found their
infant's odor more appealing than mothers with lower concentrations. After Fleming et al.,
1997b.

the relation between cortisol and attraction to infant odors is found only in first-
time mothers, in whom hormonal effects would presumably be most necessary.

Recent studies that examined both behavior and hormones in human maternal behavior have revealed more surprises. Mothers who displayed a positive
shift in the ratio of estradiol to progesterone during pregnancy were found to
have more positive attachment to their infants than mothers whose pregnancy
endocrine profile showed a negative shift (or no change) in the ratio of these two
steroid hormones during pregnancy (Figure 7.23) (Fleming et al., 1997a). Taken
together, the results of studies that examine endocrine correlates of human maternal behavior suggest that a greater emphasis on observing behavior in human
mothers is more likely to yield meaningful endocrine correlates than are scores
from questionnaires (Fleming et al., 1996). These studies, in common with studies described for sheep and rats, also emphasize the importance of early contact
between human mothers and infants at birth for optimal maternal behavior
(Klaus and Kennel, 1976).

**PATERNAL BEHAVIOR.**   Studies of the endocrine correlates of paternal behavior
in mammals that display this behavior in nature have been limited to a few
species, including California mice, dwarf hamsters, gerbils, tamarins, and marmosets. As described above, male California mice provide extensive paternal care
to their offspring. In one study (Gubernick and Nelson, 1989), the parental behav-

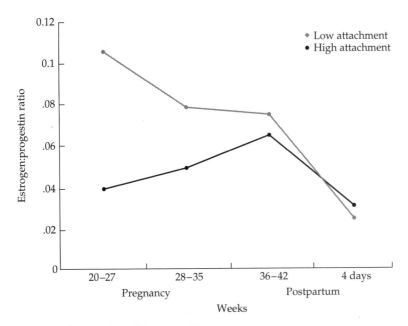

**7.23    Mothers with a positive shift in the ratio of estradiol to progesterone** during pregnancy (i.e., the ratio increases) show more positive attachment to their infants than mothers whose pregnancy endocrine profile shows a negative shift (or no change). After Fleming et al., 1997a.

ior of fathers, expectant fathers (males living with their pregnant partners), and unmated males was assessed. The males were exposed to a novel 1–3-day-old pup during a 10-minute test. Relatively few unmated males displayed parental behavior (19%) as compared with fathers (80%) or expectant fathers (56%). Plasma concentrations of prolactin were higher in fathers than in expectant fathers or unmated males (Figure 7.24). Assessment of oxytocin levels revealed an increase immediately post-copulation, but there were no detectable changes in oxytocin levels after the pups were born, when the males behaved paternally (Gubernick et al., 1995). Testosterone concentrations did not differ among the three groups of males. In contrast, examination of plasma concentrations of prolactin in male rats that had undergone pup induction revealed no relationship between prolactin concentrations and paternal behavior (Samuels and Bridges, 1983; Södersten and Eneroth, 1984; Tate-Ostroff and Bridges, 1985).

In male gerbils exposed to pregnant females or pups, prolactin values increased throughout pregnancy and remained elevated during the first 10 days after birth; plasma testosterone concentrations rose during pregnancy, then showed a steep decline in paternal males after their pups were born (Brown et al., 1995). However, there is substantial intraspecific variation in testosterone responses in gerbils; males seem to follow one of two reproductive tactics. Either testosterone remains elevated and males pursue additional copulations, or testosterone values decrease and males behave paternally (Clark et al., 1997). Studies on common marmosets have also found that males behaving paternally show a fivefold increase in blood concentrations of prolactin, and reductions in blood

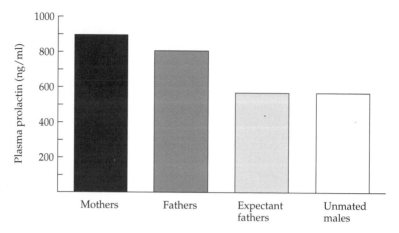

**7.24  California mouse fathers show increased prolactin concentrations.** Blood samples were obtained from California mouse mothers and fathers 2 days postpartum, from expectant fathers within 10 days of parturition, and from unmated males. Males of this species engage in virtually all aspects of parental care, and fathers show concentrations of blood prolactin comparable to mothers. Source: Gubernick and Nelson, 1989.

testosterone concentrations, compared with nonpaternal males (Dixson and George, 1982). Similar findings have been reported for paternal dwarf hamsters (*Phodopus campbelli*) (Reburn and Wynne-Edwards, 1998; Wynne-Edwards, 1998).

The hormonal correlates of human paternal behavior resemble the factors associated with paternal behavior in other mammals; namely, testosterone, prolactin, and cortisol. Plasma prolactin concentrations were elevated in fathers just prior to parturition (Storey et al., 1998). Men who responded physiologically to the sounds of babies crying also displayed elevated prolactin concentrations compared with men who did not respond to infant cries (Elwood and Mason, 1994; Storey et al., 1998). The dynamics of cortisol secretion are similar between men and women around the time of parturition (Storey et al., 1998). Recall that elevated cortisol levels in new mothers are linked with the establishment of social bonding between mothers and infants (Fleming et al., 1997b). Cortisol concentrations were highly correlated between men and women partners during pregnancy and birth (Storey et al., 1998). In common with other paternal mammals, men displayed depressed testosterone values (–33%) immediately postpartum (Storey et al., 1998). Women experience elevated testosterone levels near the end of pregnancy, but typically display a significant reduction in testosterone concentrations postpartum (Fleming et al., 1997a).

## Neural Changes Associated with Parental Behavior

The influences of hormones on the neural bases of parental care will be presented in this section. Again, most of the research on this topic has been done on maternal behavior in rats. There are very few studies addressing the neural control of parental behavior in nonmammalian species.

Michael Numan, Alison Fleming, and Judith Stern have recently provided much insight into the interactions among the nervous system, hormones, and

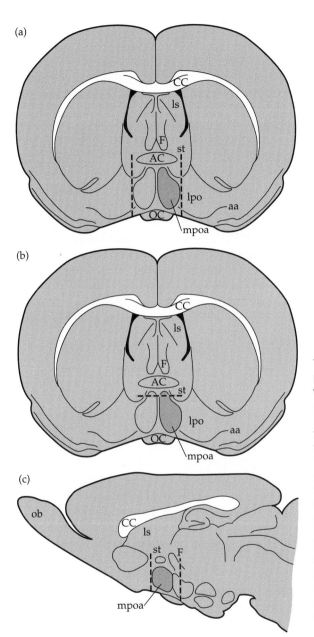

**7.25    Lateral projections from the medial preoptic area (MPOA) are critical in rat maternal behavior.** MPOA lesions severely disrupt the onset of maternal behavior in rats. (a) Coronal section of rat brain at the level of the MPOA, showing lesions (dashed lines) that sever the lateral connections of the MPOA to the rest of the brain. (b) Coronal section showing a lesion that severs the dorsal connections of the MPOA. (c) Sagittal section, showing that lesions cause anterior and posterior isolation. Only cuts severing the lateral connections interfere with maternal behavior. CC = corpus callosum; OC = optic chiasm; ob = olfactory bulb; mpoa= medial preoptic area; lpo = lateral preoptic area; aa = anterior amygdaloid nuclei; AC = anterior commissure; F = fornix; ls = lateral septum; st = bed nucleus of the stria terminalis. After Numan, 1990.

parental behavior. The first attempts to elucidate the neural bases of maternal behavior were made by Beach (1937) and Stone (1938c). Beach made multiple neocortical lesions in rats, and found that small lesions failed to disrupt the onset or maintenance of rat maternal behavior, but that larger lesions seriously interfered with the expression of most components of maternal care. Later, hypothalamic lesions were shown to seriously disrupt maternal behavior (Figure 7.25; Numan, 1990). Recently, several experiments have implicated the medial preoptic area (MPOA), just anterior to the hypothalamus, as a critical component of maternal behavior (Numan, 1988, 1990). Lesions of the MPOA eliminate maternal behavior in rats (Numan, 1974; Numan and Sheehan, 1997). Of course, the elimination of a behavior after the destruction of a brain region does not necessarily indicate that the destroyed brain area mediates the behavior in question. It is always possible that the destruction of axons of cell bodies originating outside of the lesioned area caused the change in observed behavior. One way to address this issue is to perform selective lesions of the neuronal cell bodies in a specific brain area. The excitotoxic N-methyl-DL-aspartic acid (NMA) is an amino acid that selectively kills neuronal cell bodies, but spares the axons that pass through them. When NMA was injected bilaterally into the MPOA of normally behaving mother rats 4 days postpartum, maternal behavior was severely curtailed. Bilateral NMA injections into the lateral preoptic area and adjoining regions, called the substantia innominata, also severely interfered with the display of maternal behavior (Numan et al., 1988). Estrogen implants into the MPOA stimulate maternal behavior in male rats (Rosenblatt et al., 1996; Rosenblatt and Ceus, 1998). Other brain areas are also involved in maternal behavior in rats. For instance, neurons in the lateral preoptic area contribute to pup retrieval, nest building, and nursing behavior (Numan, 1990). There are data suggesting that the preoptic area is also involved in mediating parental care in hamsters (Miceli and Malsbury, 1982b) and ring doves (Komisaruk, 1967).

Additional evidence supporting the importance of specific brain regions in maternal behavior has been provided by immunocytochemical visualization of the nuclear protein product (Fos) of the immediate early gene c-fos as an indication of neuronal activity. Several studies have reported an elevation in Fos production in the MPOA in maternal rats (e.g., Fleming et al., 1994; Fleming et al., 1996; Lonstein et al., 1998; Numan and Numan, 1994; Numan et al., 1998). For example, experienced and inexperienced female rats were allowed to interact with pups, then re-exposed to pups in a perforated box, to the box alone, or left in the home cage without further stimulation (Figure 7.26) (Fleming and Korsmit, 1996). Experienced rats showed increased Fos levels in the MPOA, the basolateral amygdala, the parietal cortex, and the prefrontal cortex (Fleming and Korsmit, 1996) in response to pup exposure. In another study using Fos as a marker for neural activity, dams were separated from their 5-day-old offspring for 48 hours to downregulate the c-fos gene. The dams were then reunited with pups that were capable or incapable (due to anesthetized snouts) of suckling. In a third group, dams were presented with pups housed in a double wire mesh box that they could see, smell, and hear, but not touch. Two additional control groups were also included in this study: one group of dams that was presented with the wire mesh box alone, and a group of females that had no further stimulation (Lonstein et al., 1998). Physical interaction with rat pups induced high Fos levels in the MPOA, regardless of whether or not the pups nursed (Lonstein et al., 1998). Expression of c-fos was relatively low in the three control groups.

As previously described, rats are quite neophobic—that is, they fear novel stimuli in their environment—and newly born pups are truly novel stimuli. Juvenile rats are often less neophobic than adults, and they readily perform parental tasks when presented with pups (Brunelli and Hofer, 1990). After an initial bout of sniffing the pups, adult nonpregnant female and male rats initially react to them in one of two ways. Most animals make a rapid retreat, then tend

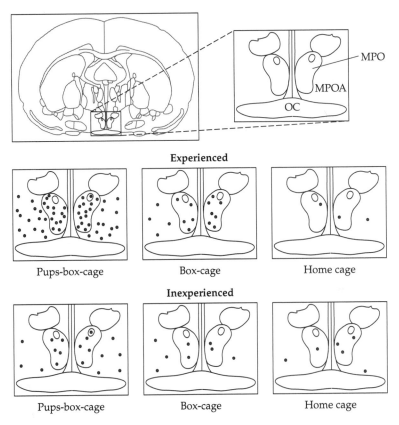

**7.26   Schematic drawing of Fos-labeled cells in the MPOA of female rats.** Each black dot represents 5 labeled cells. Experienced females showed increased Fos concentrations after exposure to pups. MPOA = medial preoptic area; MPO = medial preoptic nucleus; OC = optic chiasm. After Fleming and Korsmit, 1996.

to ignore and deliberately avoid the squeaking pups. Some animals are apparently so frightened that they attack the pups and may even cannibalize them. As we saw above, newly parturient rat dams overcome their timidity and behave solicitously toward their offspring. One function of hormones in mediating the onset of maternal behavior might be reduction of the fear associated with the newly arrived pups. In fact, hormones not only reduce the negative valence associated with the pups, but also separately increase the positive valence of the pups, thus drawing the mother into close contact with them. In other words, the pups become attractive stimuli, a phenomenon new human parents frequently report about their new babies.

A major component of the avoidance of pups is a chemosensory-based repulsion (Rosenblatt, 1990). The repulsiveness of the pups' odors appears to be overcome by exposure to maternal hormones or by repeated experience with pups during the process of concaveation. This repulsion can also be overridden by making nulliparous females anosmic. As described in Chapter 5, rats have two sets of chemosensory receptors, the olfactory receptors and the vomeronasal

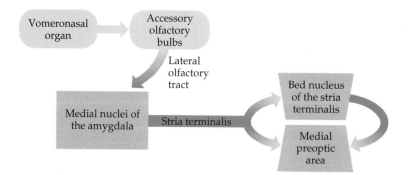

**7.27 The VNO–MPOA pathway.** Information from the vomeronasal organ travels directly to the accessory olfactory bulbs, then to the medial nuclei of the amygdala via the lateral olfactory tract. Via the stria terminalis, information from the VNO eventually reaches the bed nucleus of the stria terminalis or the MPOA. Information from the BNST is also relayed to the MPOA. Lesions anywhere along this pathway will interfere with chemosensory processing and will hasten the onset of maternal behavior in rats. After Numan, 1990.

organ. Chemosensory information from both inputs is relayed from the primary and accessory olfactory bulbs to the cortical and medial nuclei of the amygdala. The amygdala projects, via the stria terminalis, to both the bed nucleus of the stria terminalis (BNST) and the MPOA; the BNST also projects to the MPOA (Figure 7.27; Fleming and Rosenblatt, 1974). Lesioning both types of olfactory receptors with intranasal infusions of $ZnSO_4$ results in female nulliparous rats that do not avoid pups and which begin behaving maternally with a short latency.

The amygdala appears to inhibit maternal behavior in rats (Fleming et al., 1996). Lesions of the medial nucleus of the amygdala accelerate concaveation in nulliparous females (Fleming et al., 1980). Lesions anywhere along the pathway from the vomeronasal receptors to the amygdala also facilitate the onset of maternal behavior in nulliparous rats (Figure 7.28; Fleming and Rosenblatt, 1974; Fleming et al., 1979, 1980, 1983). Taken together, these results suggest that both olfactory and vomeronasal inputs to the MPOA normally inhibit maternal behavior in rats, and that maternal behavior occurs when the MPOA is released from this inhibition. Selective lesions along the vomeronasal organ–amygdala pathway disinhibit the MPOA and allow the expression of maternal behavior.

But let us return to the central question of this chapter: How do hormones stimulate the onset of maternal behavior? In light of the results described above, one possibility is that hormones act upon the MPOA to disinhibit maternal responsiveness. As noted above, in the presence of the appropriate hormonal priming, placement of small packets of estradiol in the MPOA triggers maternal behavior. Similar implants into other neural regions do not stimulate maternal behavior (Fahrbach and Pfaff, 1986). As one might expect, the number of estrogen receptors in the rat MPOA (Figure 7.29) increases during pregnancy (Giordano and Rosenblatt, 1986). The protein products produced by these cells in response to estrogen stimulation have yet to be discovered.

When the paraventricular nuclei (PVN) of rat dams were destroyed by a chemical (ibotenic acid) lesion, maternal aggression increased at day 5 postpartum, a time when maternal aggression is normally high (Giovenardi et al., 1998).

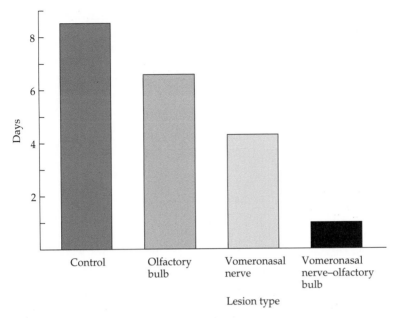

**7.28   Latency to maternal behavior is reduced after lesions to the chemosensory organs.** Adult female rats that cannot smell pups will behave maternally toward them almost as quickly as newly parturient mothers. Control rats began to behave maternally after about 8 days of exposure to pups. Lesions of the olfactory bulbs and vomeronasal nerve resulted in latencies of about 7 and 4.5 days, respectively. If both the olfactory bulbs and vomeronasal nerve are damaged, female rats will behave maternally after only 1 day of exposure to pups. These results suggest that the hormones associated with the onset of maternal behavior function by inhibiting chemosensory stimuli from the pups that adults usually find noxious. Source: Fleming et al., 1979.

Recall that the paraventricular nuclei of the hypothalamus are a source of oxytocin. To ascertain that oxytocin modulates maternal aggression, oxytocin antisense was infused into the PVN on the fifth day postpartum, and maternal aggression was elevated (Giovenardi et al., 1998). Oxytocin secretion in the PVN also appears to be important in the control of maternal behavior in sheep (Da-Costa et al., 1996).

There is also evidence that synapses in the hypothalamus are restructured during maternal behavior (Hatton and Ellisman, 1982; Modney and Hatton, 1990). Performing the electron microscopic technique of freeze-fracture analysis on the paraventricular nuclei (PVN) and supraoptic nuclei (SON) of the hypothalami of rats that had behaved maternally demonstrated the presence of a unique postsynaptic specialization in those animals. Restructuring of neural connections, as well as changes in the numbers of neurons and the types of neural connections and coupling mechanisms, have been reported in juvenile rats that have behaved maternally (Modney and Hatton, 1990). As described in Chapter 2, magnocellular neurons in the PVN produce vasopressin and oxytocin. Nearly all of the morphological changes in neural organization observed in maternal rats are reversed approximately 1 month after their pups are weaned. Probably, the secretion of

**7.29    Estradiol receptors in the rat POA.** In this schematic, magnified coronal section of a rat brain, each black circle represents a cell in the POA that binds estradiol and projects through or to the ventromedial midbrain. LPOA = lateral preoptic area; BNST = bed nucleus of the stria terminalis; MPOA = medial preoptic area; ot = optic tract; V = third ventricle. After Fahrbach et al., 1986.

oxytocin associated with parturition and lactation accounts for these changes in neuronal structure, but it remains possible that the change in postsynaptic specialization could reflect oxytocin-mediated effects upon maternal behavior, which in turn causes the neural changes. Presumably, progesterone and prolactin also affect neuronal structure or function underlying rat maternal behavior. The ultrastructural changes that are observed in the PVN and SON of mother rats are also observed in nonlactating, nulliparous females that behave maternally after undergoing concaveation (Modney and Hatton, 1990). Other studies of neurons in the SON have demonstrated that oxytocinergic neurons show a reduction in dendritic length because of decreased branching (approximately 40% reduction) during lactation (Stern and Armstrong, 1998). In contrast, SON neurons containing vasopressin show an approximate 50% increase in dendritic length during lactation (Stern and Armstrong, 1998).

Thus, merely *behaving* maternally causes structural changes in the brain independently from hormonal influences. Do similar structural brain changes occur in males that behave in a paternal manner? This question is best addressed in a species that normally shows paternal behavior. Perinatal exposure to androgens suppresses parental responsiveness in many species of rodents (Kinsley, 1990). As we have seen, androgens organize sex differences in anatomical structures in several brain areas of rodents and primates, including the MPOA (see Chapter 4). Are these structural differences in the organization of the MPOA, for instance, responsible for the sex difference in propensity to behave parentally? There is a sex difference in the size of the MPOA in California mice; the volume of the MPOA in virgin males is larger than in nulliparous females. Paternal behavior in California mice is associated with a decrease in the number of neurons in the MPOA (Alberts and Gubernick, 1990) and consequent shrinking of MPOA volume to approximately that of a female (Figure 7.30). There was no change in the size of the MPOA in females when they became mothers; this suggests that hormones act in females of this species, as in rats, to disinhibit maternal behaviors. The reduction in the number of neurons during paternal behavior suggests that the circuitry underlying this behavior is typically inhibited unless hormones activate some process leading to neuronal death, possibly by destroying the inhibitory neurons themselves. As noted above, the main endocrine correlates of paternal behavior thus far discovered are an increase in blood prolactin and a decrease in blood testosterone concentrations, but it has not been established whether prolactin or some other hormone causes the cell death associated with paternal behavior in this species.

You will recall from Chapter 1 that mice with a specific gene selectively disrupted are called knockout mice. Mice lacking the immediate early gene *fosB* display little maternal behavior (Brown et al., 1996). The lack of maternal behavior among *fosB* knockouts (*fosB*−/−) does not correspond to a lack of fertility or the ability to lactate. *FosB*−/−mothers appear to have endocrine profiles similar to those of wild-type (WT) dams (Brown et al., 1996), but they fail to display nest

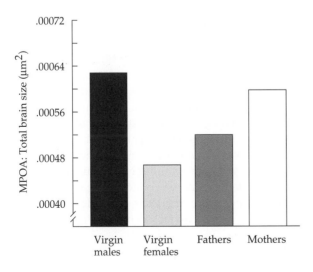

**7.30  Effects of parental behavior on MPOA volume in the California mouse.** There is a sex difference in the size of the MPOA in California mice: the volume of the MPOA of males without sexual experience is larger than that of nulliparous females. Paternal behavior caused the number of neurons in the MPOA to decrease and its overall size to diminish to approximately that found in females. The MPOA volume of females does not change significantly when they become mothers. After Alberts and Gubernick, 1990.

building, cleaning and retrieving pups, nursing, or protective crouching postures (Brown et al., 1996). It is not clear through what mechanism(s) the missing *fosB* gene affects maternal behavior.

As we saw above, oxytocin is an important mediator of maternal behavior. It was therefore surprising that in two studies, female oxytocin (OT) knockout mice (OT–/–) showed the full complement of normal maternal behaviors (Nishimori et al., 1996; DeVries et al., 1997). OT–/– females, however, failed to eject milk in response to suckling, so their pups had to be cross-fostered to WT mothers to survive. How do we interpret these data? Do we now believe that oxytocin is *not* involved in maternal behavior? Not necessarily. There are alternative explanations for the results of both studies of OT–/– animals. It appears that maternal behavior is easily induced in the particular strain of mouse used in the first study simply by brief exposure to pups (Young et al., 1997). Thus, knocking out the OT gene in rats might be a better test of the hypothesis that OT is necessary for maternal behavior. The other OT–/– mouse study also had problems; the OT gene was only partially deactivated in this knockout. Also, vasopressin concentrations were lower than normal because the neurophysin molecule was also damaged in this knockout (DeVries et al., 1997). Consequently, additional research must be conducted to clarify the role of oxytocin in maternal behavior.

In contrast to the disquieting results associated with the OT–/– mice, mice with the prolactin receptor (PRLR) gene deleted display defective maternal behavior, as expected (Lucas et al., 1998). Specifically, pup-induced maternal behaviors were disrupted in both PRLR–/– and PRLR+/– females, and primiparous PRL+/– females displayed dramatic deficiencies in maternal care of foster pups (Lucas et al., 1998). These studies clearly indicate that the prolactin receptor is critical in mediating maternal behavior.

One final example from knockout mice adds an evolutionary twist to the role of genes in maternal care. *Mest* (also known as *Peg1*) is an imprinted gene, meaning that it is expressed only from the paternal allele during development. *Mest*-deficient females displayed impaired maternal behavior and impaired placentophagia. These results provide evidence for the involvement of an imprinted gene from the father in the control of adult behavior of female offspring (Lefebvre et al., 1998).

These observations potentially open up a new area of inquiry into the mechanisms underlying hormonal mediation of maternal behavior. Behavioral studies of knockout mice may also evoke questions about established hormonal relationships. For example, the display of overtly normal maternal behavior in oxytocin knockout mice suggests that oxytocin may not be necessary for maternal behavior (Nishimori et al., 1996; DeVries et al., 1997). There may be subtle effects of missing genes on maternal behavior. Indeed, most knockout mice studied to date remain with their knockout mothers. The extent to which the altered behavior of knockout mice reflects atypical maternal behavior remains unknown (Caldji et al., 1998; Kinsley, 1994). Cross-fostering studies comparing the behavior of knockout mice reared with WT dams to that of knockout mice reared with knockout mothers will be critical in the future to further untangle the roles of extrinsic (environmental) and intrinsic (hormonal) factors in behavior.

# Conclusions

A good understanding of the manner in which parental behavior is affected by hormones has recently been gained in a few species, but the parental behaviors shown by individuals in the various orders and families of birds and mammals are extremely diverse. Are the underlying endocrine mechanisms and relevant hormones that are associated with them equally varied, or do just a few select hormones produce this diversity of parental responses? Too few species have been studied to answer this question at this time. However, it is reasonable to propose that a combination of common hormonal signals is paired with a variety of extrinsic cues to elicit the species-appropriate constellation of parental behaviors.

As with other behaviors we have examined, hormones affect parental behavior at the level of input, integration, and output systems. Sensory inputs related to the perception of rat pups appear to be changed by hormones in parturient rat dams. Nonparental rats fear pups, but hormones alter mothers' perception of their pups to make them attractive stimuli. Sensory input associated with nursing probably is perceived as rewarding via the actions of oxytocin and perhaps endogenous opiates. The effects of hormones on central processing have been well documented in rat maternal behavior. Restructuring of neural connections, as well as changes in the number of neurons and the types of neural connections and coupling mechanisms, has been reported in mother rats. Maternal behavior is integrated in the medial preoptic area and inhibited in the amygdala. Finally, hormones affect output systems to mediate maternal behavior. For instance, steroid hormones stimulate mammary gland development in mice; without mammary gland development, suckling stimuli could not trigger the onset of maternal aggression in this species. In birds, prolactin stimulates development of the brood patch, and feedback from this morphological feature encourages further incubation behavior.

Thus, parental behaviors are mediated by hormones via their effects on input, integration, and output systems, as well as the interactions of those systems with experiential factors. Although a great deal has been learned about this important topic, there is still a great deal left to learn. Parental care is fascinating to study because of its fundamental importance to the survival and reproductive success of individuals. The diversity of parental care patterns found in nature provides an opportunity for comparative studies that will reveal how different animals have evolved different solutions to the common problem of increasing the odds of offspring survival and reproductive success.

# Summary

• Parental behavior is any behavior that contributes directly to the survival of fertilized eggs or offspring that have left the body of the female.

• There are many patterns of mammalian parental care. The developmental status of the newborn is an important factor driving the type and quality of parental care in a species. Maternal care is much more common than paternal care.

- Birds show great diversity in parental care, ranging from nest-parasitic species that show absolutely no parental care to species in which both sexes build nests, incubate the eggs, and feed and protect the young.

- Most studies on hormonal correlates of avian parental behavior have been performed on ring doves, which share the parental chores more or less equally and also produce a protein-rich crop milk that is regurgitated and fed to the squab. Ovariectomy eliminates nest building and incubation behaviors in female ring doves. Estradiol and progesterone replacement restores these behaviors. Prolactin mediates brooding and stimulates development of the crop sac in both sexes. Gonadectomy does not affect nest building or incubation behaviors in male ring doves; behavioral cues from the female elicit these behaviors in males.

- The vast majority of research on the hormonal correlates of mammalian parental behavior has been conducted on rats. Rats bear altricial young, and mothers perform a cluster of stereotyped maternal behaviors, including nest building, crouching over the pups to allow nursing and to provide warmth, pup retrieval, and increased aggression directed at intruders.

- Sensitization of adult nonparental rodents to pups by daily exposure causes them to behave maternally, but several days are required in order for maternal behavior to be observed. This process is called concaveation.

- The onset of maternal behavior in rats is mediated by hormones. Several methods of study, including pregnancy termination, hormone removal and replacement therapy, as well as parabiotic blood exchange, have been used to determine the hormonal correlates of rat maternal behavior. A precipitous decline of blood concentrations of progesterone in late pregnancy after sustained high concentrations of this hormone, in combination with high concentrations of estradiol, and probably prolactin and oxytocin, induces female rats to behave maternally in the presence of pups. This pattern of hormones at parturition overrides the usual fear response of adult rats toward pups, and it permits the onset of maternal behavior.

- Laboratory strains of mice and rats are usually docile, but mothers can be quite aggressive toward animals that venture too close to their litter. Progesterone appears to be the primary hormone that induces this maternal aggression in rodents, but species differences exist. The role of maternal aggression in women's behavior has not been adequately described or tested.

- Female rats become less maternal as their pups mature, and spend less time with the pups during each nursing bout. Prolactin stimulates corticosterone secretion, which increases metabolic rate and subsequently raises the mother's body temperature. As the pups grow larger and produce more heat, they block the mother's ability to dissipate her own body heat. When her brain temperature rises acutely during nursing, she leaves the litter to reduce her heat load and avoid hyperthermia.

- Two- to three-week-old rat pups are attracted to the nest odors of lactating dams. The excess production of caecotrophs by lactating dams attracts the young back to the nest until they are fully weaned.

• With the exception of cortisol, few clear-cut endocrine correlates of human or other primate maternal behavior have been discovered. Behavior per se is rarely tested in humans; rather, responses to questionnaires or surveys are used to study hormone–behavior interactions. A further confounding variable is a lack of consistent or universal definitions of human maternal care.

• Elevated prolactin concentrations appear to mediate paternal behavior in the two best-studied mammalian species, the California mouse and the marmoset. Reduction in blood concentrations of testosterone is also associated with paternal behavior in marmosets.

• The medial preoptic area is critical for the expression of rat maternal behavior. The amygdala appears to inhibit the expression of maternal behavior. Lesions of the amygdala or afferent sensory pathways from the vomeronasal organ to the amygdala disinhibit the expression of maternal behavior. Hormones or concaveation probably act to disinhibit the amygdala, thus permitting the occurrence of maternal behavior.

• There is evidence that structural changes in neural organization occur during natural maternal and paternal behavior. These changes are reversible and also occur in animals exhibiting parental behavior after concaveation.

## Questions for Discussion

1. A common endocrine correlate of the onset of paternal behavior is a reduction of blood concentrations of androgens. Why do you think this is true?

2. Are studies of the hormonal correlates of paternal care in birds and mammals useful for understanding the mechanisms of paternal care in humans? Why or why not? Does the phenomenon of adoptive human fathers behaving paternally provide any insights?

3. What do the concaveation studies tell us, if anything, about the neural circuits mediating maternal behavior in rats?

4. If hormones are important in the onset of rat maternal behavior, then why do hormone replacement regimes require over 24 hours to induce maternal behavior in the presence of pups, as compared with natural conditions, in which fully developed maternal behavior appears as soon as the pups are encountered?

5. Defend or refute the following statement: "Differences in patterns of parental care reflect differences in receptor availability and distribution, rather than differences in circulating hormone concentrations."

## Suggested Readings

Bornstein, M. H. (ed.). 1995. *Biology and Ecology of Parenting*. L. Erlbaum Associates, New York.

Krasnegor, N. A., and Bridges, R. S. (eds.). 1990. *Mammalian Parenting*. Oxford University Press, Oxford.

Numan, M. 1994. Maternal behavior. In E. Knobil and J. D. Neill (eds.), *The Physiology of Reproduction*, Vol. 2, pp. 221–302. Raven, New York.

Rosenblatt, J. S., and Snowdon, C. T. (eds.). 1996. *Parental Care: Evolution, Mechanisms, and Adaptive Significance*. Academic Press, New York.

Rosenblatt, J. S., Mayer, A. D., and Siegel, H. I. 1985. Maternal behavior among the nonprimate mammals. In N. T. Adler, D. Pfaff and R. W. Goy (eds.), *Handbook of Behavioral Neurobiology*, pp. 229–298. Plenum, New York.

Silver, R. 1977. *Parental Behavior in Birds*. Dowden, Hutchinson and Ross, Stroudsburg, PA.

Stern, J. M. 1997. Offspring-induced nurturance: Animal-human parallels. *Developmental Psychobiology*, 31: 19–37.

Wiesner, B. P. and Sheard, N. M. 1933. *Maternal Behavior in Rats*. Oliver and Boyd, London.

# 8

# Affiliative and Aggressive Behavior

Social behavior involves interactions between individuals from which one or more of the individuals benefit (see Wilson, 1975). This definition is purposely very broad, and includes aggressive behavior, particularly in the context of territorial defense, as well as nonhostile interactions including affiliation, courtship, and parental behaviors. While the effects of hormones on courtship and parental behaviors were described in previous chapters, this chapter will emphasize the influence of hormones on affiliative and aggressive behaviors.

Animals display a wide range of social behaviors. Some animals are highly solitary and have few social interactions; in fact, after they have been weaned, their only social interactions may occur during mating. Other animals live together in large colonies where social interactions are frequent. Social behaviors that bring animals together are referred to as **affiliation** (Carter et al., 1997b). Social behavior that keeps animals apart is usually considered to be **territorial behavior** or **aggression**. Although these two types of social behaviors have the opposite effects on social interactions, the neural and endocrine mechanisms underlying affiliation and aggression do not have opposite effects on a single neural substrate; rather, they appear to involve different circuits. Scientific interest in affiliation has blossomed in the 1990s, whereas formal studies of aggression have been common since the 1920s.

## Affiliation

Affiliation is generally considered to have evolved from reproductive and parental behaviors (Crews, 1997). The same hormones that are important in promoting affiliative behaviors are also critical for reproductive success. The evolutionary importance of the relationship between hormones and affiliation is hinted at by the strong correlations among social systems (i.e., monogamy versus polygamy), blood testosterone concentrations, sperm production, and testicular size (Wingfield et al., 1997; Dixson, 1997). Males of polygamous species tend to have higher testosterone concentrations, higher sperm numbers, and larger testes than males of monogamous species. Formation of long-term pair bonds is critical for the reproductive success of some species, usually because both parents are required to rear the offspring. Because both parents have a 50% stake in the success of each offspring, they have evolved to cooperate because their offspring would die if either one abandoned the family. Hormones that evoke affiliation serve as the proximate means of bringing this about.

From the individual's perspective, the requirement for increased proximity during sexual reproduction may be potentially dangerous. Not only might the individual be attacked and maimed by a potential consort, but the potential for disease and parasite transmission increases during social gatherings (Crews, 1997). Mating behavior, like maternal behavior in rats, is a series of approach–avoidance behaviors. In order for laboratory rats to engage in successful maternal behavior, the inclination to flee from the frightening or aversive stimuli connected with pups must be suppressed, and the rats must approach the pups that previously elicited these aversive responses (Carter et al., 1997a). As noted in the previous chapter, neural–behavioral systems involving the medial amygdala have been implicated in avoidance behaviors, and neural–behavioral systems underlying approach include the medial preoptic area and the ventral portion of the bed nucleus of the stria terminalis (Newman and Newman, 1997).

Voles have been important animal models in studies of affiliation. Voles are rodents, sometimes referred to as "field mice," that are more closely related to lemmings than to laboratory mice (Figure 8.1). Voles inhabit much of the Northern Hemisphere, occupying a variety of habitat niches. Despite their similar habitats, different species of voles display very different types of social organization. For example, the prairie vole (*Microtus ochrogaster*), which inhabits grasslands throughout much of the midwestern United States, is socially monogamous. One closely related species, the meadow vole (*Microtus pennsylvanicus*), inhabits similar habitat throughout much of the eastern United States, but displays a highly polygamous social system (Klein and Nelson, 1998). Another closely related species, the montane vole (*Microtus montanus*), inhabits grasslands in the West, and is also

**8.1   Prairie voles are socially monogamous rodents.** Once a pair bond forms, the "couple" tends to stay together until death. Courtesy of Lowell L. Getz.

polygamous. Prairie voles are highly tolerant of other individuals, whereas meadow and montane voles are intolerant of other individuals during the breeding season, except to mate (Wolff, 1985). What are the endocrine bases of these differences in social organization?

One obvious hormonal candidate is testosterone. Males of polygamous species generally have larger testes and higher testosterone concentrations than males of monogamous species (Dixson, 1997; Klein and Nelson, 1998). Plasma testosterone concentrations in male prairie voles are about half of those in meadow or montane voles (Klein and Nelson, 1998). However, supplemental testosterone treatment of male prairie voles does not make them polygamous, and castration of male meadow or montane voles does not make them monogamous (Roberts et al., 1996; Gaines et al., 1985).

Oxytocin has been implicated in the mediation of several forms of affiliative behavior, including parental care, grooming, and sexual behavior (Carter et al., 1992, 1995). The locations of oxytocin receptors in the brains of monogamous prairie voles and polygamous montane voles have been characterized using in vitro receptor autoradiography (Insel and Shapiro, 1992). In the prairie voles, oxytocin receptor densities were highest in the prelimbic cortex, bed nucleus of the stria terminalis, nucleus accumbens, and the lateral aspects of the amygdala; oxytocin receptors were not evident in these brain regions in montane voles (Insel and Shapiro, 1992) (Figure 8.2). A similar pattern of social organization-dependent oxytocin receptor distribution was observed in the brains of monogamous (*Peromyscus californicus*) and polygamous mice (*Peromyscus maniculatus*) (Insel et al., 1991), as well as in the brains of monogamous pine voles (*Microtus pinetorum*) and polygamous meadow voles (*Microtus pennsylvanicus*) (Insel and Shapiro, 1992). The differences in oxytocin receptor distribution appear around the time of weaning (Wang and Young, 1997). Differences in the patterns of vasopressin receptor dis-

(a)

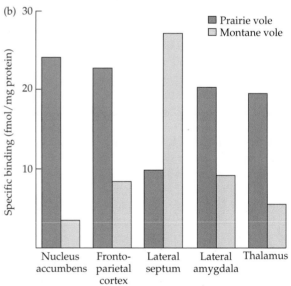

(b)

**8.2   The pattern of oxytocin binding differs between monogamous and polygamous male voles.** (a) In these autoradiograms, the dark regions represent $^{125}$I-oxytocin antagonist binding in saggital sections of the brains of a monogamous prairie vole (top) and a polygamous montane vole (bottom). In the prairie vole, oxytocin receptor densities are highest in the prelimbic cortex (PL), nucleus accumbens (NAcc), and the anterior olfactory nucleus (AOP); in the montane vole, receptors are not evident in these areas. LS =lateral septum; AOB = accessory olfactory bulb; VMN = ventromedial nucleus of the hypothalamus. (b) Levels of oxytocin binding in different brain regions of adult male prairie voles (dark bars) and montane voles (shaded bars). From Insel, 1997.

tribution in the brains of prairie and montane voles have also been reported (Insel et al., 1994).

The difference in adult affiliative behaviors is reflected in the response of infant prairie and montane voles to separation from their families (Shapiro and Insel, 1990). When prairie vole pups were isolated from their families for 5 minutes, they emitted about 314 distress vocalizations when they were 4–6 days old and 601 distress calls at 8–10 days of age. Plasma corticosterone concentrations were elevated fourfold to sixfold in isolated prairie vole pups. When montane vole pups were socially isolated, they did not emit any distress vocalizations, and there were no changes in their blood corticosterone concentrations (Shapiro and Insel, 1990). If montane vole pups were stressed by tail suspension or halothane (a gaseous anesthetic) vapors, they emitted distress vocalizations and showed elevated corticosterone concentrations. This latter observation indicates that the montane vole pups were capable of emitting distress vocalizations, but apparently did not find social isolation stressful (Shapiro and Insel, 1990).

Separation anxiety like that displayed by prairie vole pups is part of the phenomenon of infant attachment (Bowlby, 1969; Ainsworth, 1972), in which one individual (usually the infant) strives to maintain proximity to a specific other individual (usually the primary caregiver). Generally, attached individuals display distress if separation or loss is experienced, and are motivated to re-establish contact after separation (Mendoza and Mason, 1997). The concept of attachment was developed for human infant–parent interactions, but it has been applied to nonhuman animals as well. Social bonding occurs in many species and is particularly salient in parent–offspring interactions (Pedersen, 1997) (see Chapter 7). Even when all their physiological requirements are met—for example, with full stomachs in a warm, dry environment—young animals respond to social isolation promptly with characteristic distress vocalizations. In other words, babies cry when unattended (Kalin et al., 1988; Zimmerberg et al., 1994). The reaction of infants to social separation is fast and quite consistent across many disparate species (Panksepp et al., 1997).

A series of fascinating comparative studies of New World primates has provided new insights into the hormonal bases of attachment behavior. This research has focused on squirrel monkeys (*Saimiri sciureus*) and titi monkeys (*Callicebus moloch*), two South American arboreal, omnivorous primate species. Squirrel monkeys are polygynous and live in large social groups containing individuals of both sexes and all ages. With the exception of mother–infant interactions, squirrel monkeys typically interact within same-sex cohorts (Mendoza et al., 1991; Mendoza and Mason, 1997). Titi monkeys are socially monogamous; they live in small family groups, and the males provide substantial parental care (Mendoza and Mason, 1986). The infants spend more than 90% of their time riding on the backs of their fathers, transferring to their mothers only to nurse. Not surprisingly, then, titi infants form a very strong bond to their fathers (Figure 8.3).

If squirrel monkey mothers and infants are separated for 30–60 minutes, each individual shows a robust increase in cortisol concentrations (Coe et al., 1978). Because separating a mother and infant causes substantial commotion and distress among their cagemates, a control procedure was conducted in which all of the steps involved in separating the mother and infant were taken, but the pair was reunited within seconds. In this case, there was no increase in cortisol in either the mother or infant (Mendoza and Mason, 1997). Separation of pairs of adult animals, regardless of their relationship within the social group, did not influence their cortisol values, although cortisol concentrations were markedly decreased during the initial formation of female, but not male, pairs (Saltzman et al., 1991).

A different pattern of results was obtained in similar studies of the socially monogamous titi monkeys (Mendoza and Mason, 1997). Separation of titi infants from their fathers for 60 minutes caused a significant increase in cortisol concen-

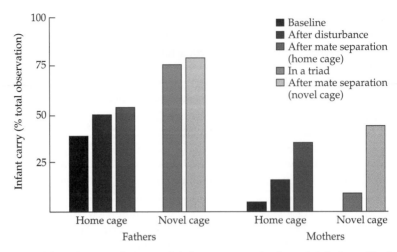

**8.3    Infant titi monkeys receive most of their contact comfort from their fathers.** The bars show the percentage of the observation time during which infants were carried by their fathers or their mothers under several conditions: at baseline, after a disturbance, and after mate separation in the home cage; and in a triad (infant, mother, and father) and after mate separation in a novel environment. Note that most of the time, fathers carried the offspring, even during times of stress. After Mendoza and Mason, 1986.

trations even if their mothers were present; separation from their mothers did not affect cortisol concentrations in the infant titi monkeys (Hoffman et al., 1996). Separation from the titi infant did not affect cortisol values in either parent. These different attachment patterns could contribute to the different social structures of these New World primate species (Mendoza and Mason, 1997), or they could be the result of these different social structures. These patterns may also serve to inform us about the different patterns of human social behavior.

The formation of social bonds has also been studied in socially monogamous prairie voles (Carter et al., 1995). Male and female prairie voles form long-term pair bonds, characterized by a social preference for a familiar partner, and in some cases selective aggression directed toward unfamiliar conspecifics (Getz and Carter, 1996; Winslow et al., 1993). In the laboratory, social preferences can develop when socially naive animals encounter and interact with strangers of the opposite sex (Carter et al., 1995). These partner preferences can be determined in the three-chamber apparatus described in Chapter 6. Social preferences for a familiar partner are not restricted to heterosexual pairs; partner preferences can form between animals of the same sex and animals of the opposite sex following nonsexual cohabitation (DeVries et al., 1995a). It is important to note that social preferences must remain stable during pair separation among monogamous species (Drickamer and Vessey, 1982; Wittenberger and Tilson, 1980). Partner preferences of heterosexual prairie vole pairs remain stable for up to 6 (males) or 8 (females) days (DeVries et al., 1995b). Typically, when socially naive prairie voles meet, they engage in a brief session of olfactory investigation, followed by prolonged periods of sitting in close proximity (Gavish et al., 1983; Moffatt, 1994). Separation by a wire screen barrier prevents the development of partner preferences, suggesting that physical contact or other forms of active interactions is critical for the development of social preferences (Shapiro et al., 1986).

Prairie voles have high basal corticosterone concentrations (600–1000 ng/ml) without any of the negative consequences normally associated with chronic glucocorticoid excess (Taymans et al., 1997). The resting corticosterone concentrations of prairie voles are 10–100 times higher than those of laboratory rats or mice (Taymans et al., 1997), and these concentrations can go up in stressed animals. Corticosterone appears to modulate partner preferences in prairie voles, but in a sex-specific manner (DeVries et al., 1996). In socially naive males, injections of corticosterone or the stress of swimming facilitated the development of partner preferences (Table 8.1). Adrenalectomized males did not form partner preferences unless injected with corticosterone (DeVries et al., 1996). In socially naive female prairie voles, adrenalectomy facilitated partner preference; partner preference was formed within 1 hour of cohabitation among adrenalectomized females (DeVries et al., 1995b). In contrast to males, corticosterone treatment or endogenous corticosterone elevation after swimming stress inhibited pair bond formation in females.

Sexual experience facilitates partner preference formation in both sexes (Carter et al., 1997a). Treatment with vasopressin, or vasopressin agonists, facilitates pair bonding in sexually experienced male voles; vasopressin also promotes the onset of aggression that is observed in male voles after mating (Winslow et al., 1993). Conversely, treatment with a V1 vasopressin antagonist (the most common type of vasopressin receptor) blocks the effects of vasopressin or sexual experience in facilitating pair bonding in males (Winslow et al., 1993). Unmated female prairie voles develop a partner preference following oxytocin infusions, but not after vasopressin or cerebrospinal fluid infusions. Females treated with a selective oxytocin antagonist displayed normal mating behavior, but did not establish a pair bond (Insel and Hulihan, 1995). Treatment with a vasopressin antagonist failed to block pair bond formation in sexually experienced females. These results suggest that oxytocin, released with mating, may be critical to the formation of a pair bond in female prairie voles; vasopressin appears to be more important for pair bonding in the male of this species. As noted in the previous chapter, oxytocin is important in the formation of the exclusive bond between mothers and offspring in several species (Keverne and Kendrick, 1992). Centrally administered oxytocin facilitates the onset of partner preferences in sexually naive female prairie voles; oxytocin antagonists reverse the behavioral effects of oxytocin infusion (Williams et al., 1994). The interaction between oxytocin/vasopressin and corticosterone in social bonding remains to be specified.

Table 8.1
**The effects of steroid hormones
on prairie vole partner preference**

| Treatment | Males | Females |
|---|---|---|
| Gonadal steroid hormones | 0 | 0 |
| Corticosterone | + | — |
| Stress | + | — |
| Adrenalectomy | — | + |

+ = increased partner preference; — = decreased partner preference; 0 = no change
*Source:* After Carter et al., 1997b.

Recent evidence suggests that dopamine, released in the medial nucleus accumbens, mediates the rewarding properties of many addictive drugs, including nicotine and cocaine. This same reward mechanism might drive social contact in prairie voles as well (Cascio et al., 1998). Oxytocin receptors are located on the surface of some neurons in the medial nucleus accumbens. Brain injections of dopamine agonists facilitated pair bond formation in female voles, whereas brain injections of dopamine antagonists blocked pair bond formation. When the natural production of dopamine was measured by microdialysis in the brains of prairie voles during mating, a dramatic elevation in the concentrations of this neurotransmitter was observed (Gingrich et al., 1998).

Other peptide hormones, particularly opioids, are involved in affiliative behaviors. Endogenous opioids mediate isolation-induced distress vocalizations, and social contact increases endogenous opioid concentrations (Panksepp et al., 1997). These conclusions were the logical outcome of two observations, namely, that endogenous opioids exist in the brain, and that there are remarkable similarities between narcotic addiction and the comfort of social contact. Narcotic addiction and social contact both involve strong emotional attachments, and both processes have characteristic psychological and physiological symptoms during withdrawal. Physiological symptoms common to withdrawal from narcotics and removal of the attachment figure include crying, depression, inability to eat or sleep, and general irritability (Panksepp et al., 1980b). These commonalities suggest a common physiological mediation.

If opioids mediate contact comfort, then treatment with naloxone or naltrexone, both opioid antagonists, should block the onset of comfort. In rodents, treatment with naltrexone blocks the effect of contact comfort in ameliorating the rate of distress vocalizations (Panksepp et al., 1980b). Young chickens display a characteristic sign of contact comfort when snuggled next to their mothers or cupped in a human hand: they rapidly close their eyes (Figure 8.4a). Treatment with naloxone reduces the effectiveness of contact comfort in causing chicks to close their eyes (Figure 8.4b; Panksepp et al., 1980a).

Opioids also mediate social grooming in rodents and primates. Social grooming is very important in maintaining social contact and serves to bond individuals. Treatment with opioid antagonists reduces the time primates spend in social grooming (Benton and Brain, 1988).

In sum, the mechanisms underlying hormone–behavior interactions during affiliation are similar to those underlying mating and parental behavior. Many of these hormones appear to blunt the "stress" or fear of social contact—animals' aversive responses—and allow them to come together and engage in social behavior or mating behavior.

## Aggression

A population of red deer (*Cervus elaphus*) has been studied on the island of Rhum, Scotland, since 1968 (Lincoln et al., 1972). The animals making up the main study population inhabit an area of about 12 square kilometers. During most of the year, the males live together in bachelor groups, grazing peacefully near the female herds. But beginning in late summer as their antlers come into hard horn, the males move to traditional rutting areas, usually located in large patches of grass-

(a)

(b)

**8.4  Contact comfort in chicks is mediated by opioids.** (a) When nestled next to a hen or held in a person's cupped hands, a chick will rapidly close its eyes. (b) The eye-closing response can be blocked by administration of the opioid antagonist naloxone. Source: Panksepp et al., 1980a. Photograph courtesy of Jaak Panksepp.

es and sedges. Males fight vigorously for control of these rutting locations throughout September and October. The battles are often fierce, with the males locking their antlers and attempting to inflict serious physical damage on one another (Figure 8.5). Nearly a quarter of the red deer stags on Rhum are wounded during the rutting season (Clutton-Brock et al., 1979); some animals may even die of their wounds. The social rank of a male and the size of the turf he controls are linked to his ability to win these battles. The oldest males, typically between 7 and 10 years old, are the most experienced fighters and sport fully developed antlers. Age and weaponry have their rewards: these senior males tend to hold the highest rank and win control of the largest rutting areas. After the rutting season has finished in late autumn, males shed their antlers, their levels of aggression are substantially reduced, and they return to a relatively peaceful coexistence in their bachelor herds.

(a)

(b)

(c)

**8.5   Male red deer fight vigorously for control of rutting areas.**  (a) Male red deer use their antlers to battle with one another during the rutting season, and attempt to wrestle their opponents to the ground (b). The loser of the aggressive encounter leaves the area (c), and the winner retains control of the rutting location and access to fertile females. Courtesy of Fiona Guinness.

What is the goal of the stags' aggressive behavior? What makes this real estate so valuable that they risk life-threatening injuries? The ultimate explanation is probably somewhat predictable to you. Like the elephant seals described in Chapter 5, these males are fighting for the opportunity to mate. Each male is apparently trying to control a large tract of pastureland in order to attract and eventually to mate with females. The females, which are called hinds, gather in the victors' rutting territories to feed on the grasses there. Each territorial male keeps other males away from his "harem." Stags can maintain large harems only if they manage to win control of sufficiently large patches of green vegetation to support females and their subsequent offspring. Otherwise, the hinds stray from the harem in search of better food and subsequently mate with other males (Figure 8.6).

Males have been selected to maximize the number of females that graze on their hard-won territories because most of the females come into estrus, or rutting condition, for just 3 weeks or so during October (Guinness et al., 1978). It is relatively easy to explain, on an adaptive level, why males behave in an aggressive manner prior to the onset of the females' estrous season. A stag impregnates most of the hinds in his harem. A large territory can support more hinds than a small one, and the more hinds that a stag has on his "property," the greater his reproductive fitness relative to males with access to fewer females (see Chapter 5). In many other cases, the adaptive, or ultimate, function of a seasonal cycle in aggressive behavior (such as that found in red deer stags) also appears to involve control of resources or mates to increase reproductive fitness. The remainder of this chapter, however, focuses on proximate causes, such as the physiological mechanisms underlying this remarkable transformation in social organization and

**8.6  A red deer stag with his harem.** The victor in the rutting battles controls an area of grassland upon which females graze. It is in the best interest of males to control as large a parcel of grassland as possible because it can support a large number of females, and the male mates with all the females grazing on his territory. It is in a female's best interest to choose a plot of grassland that is sufficient to support her and her offspring after it is born. Courtesy of Fiona Guinness.

behavior. This part of the chapter will also explore some of the ways in which hormones influence, regulate, and mediate aggression and other social interactions.

Aggression is overt behavior with the *intention* of inflicting damage or other unpleasantness upon another individual (Moyer, 1968, 1971). Intent is the key to differentiating aggressive behavior from other activities. For example, if you inadvertently kill hundreds of insects with your windshield while driving, your behavior could not be considered aggressive because your intent was merely to move at high speeds, and the death of the insects is an incidental occurrence. However, if you rampage through your apartment spraying insecticide after being bitten by a mosquito, your actions could be considered aggressive because of your intent to destroy insects. So different behaviors leading to the same outcome may or may not be considered aggressive, depending on the context in which the behavior appears. Of course, it can be tricky to attribute intention to animals, but by careful observation of the circumstances and outcomes of behaviors, the goals of animals' behaviors can be ascertained.

Aggression has been divided into various types for ease of classification (Moyer, 1968, 1971), and these different types of aggression appear to have different physiological causes. Maternal aggression and its underlying hormonal mediation have already been described in Chapter 7. Hormonal changes associated with production of offspring—especially the relationship among blood concentrations of estrogens, progestins, and prolactin—are correlated with the onset of maternal aggression. Steroid hormones also underlie other types of aggressive behavior. Intermale aggression and territorial aggression, as well as sex-related and rank-related aggression, all appear to be mediated by androgens (Bouissou, 1983). Predatory aggression is another type of aggressive behavior that is performed in the context of obtaining food. Hormones may be involved in this type of aggression, but few studies have examined this possibility.

Other types of aggression are most commonly evoked and studied in the laboratory. Learned aggression and irritable aggression are often studied in the form of restraint aggression, which results after an animal is held motionless. Another type of aggressive behavior commonly studied in the laboratory is fear-induced aggression. Many laboratory studies on aggression use albino house mice, which are normally quite docile. Consequently, the mice must be put into situations that promote aggression—for example, they are housed in isolation or given an electric shock. Female mice housed in groups will also attack a novel lactating female. Examples of these types of experiments will be provided below, but it is important to keep in mind that the hormonal control of aggression in these contrived situations is likely to differ from the endocrine correlates of natural expressions of aggressive behavior.

The possibility for aggressive behavior exists whenever the interests of two or more individuals are in conflict (Svare, 1983). Conflicts are most likely to arise over limited resources such as territories, food, and mates. A social interaction decides which animal gains access to the contested resource. In many cases, a submissive posture or gesture on the part of one animal avoids the necessity of actual combat over a resource. Animals may also participate in threat displays or ritualized combat in which dominance is determined, but no physical damage is inflicted. In order to facilitate the study of aggressive interactions, the term **agonistic** was adopted to describe the entire behavioral repertoire of both aggressive

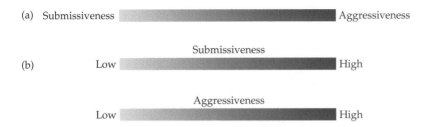

**8.7    Two models of agonistic behavior.** Aggressive and submissive behaviors can be seen as opposite ends of a single behavioral continuum (a), or they can be thought of as two separate aspects of an individual's behavior (b). Each model makes different predictions about how hormones might influence agonistic behavior.

and submissive actions within the context of a social interaction involving a conflict of interest (Scott and Fredericson, 1951). In the strict sense, however, submissive behaviors are not aggressive behaviors; consequently, hormonal mediation of the aggressive and the submissive components of an agonistic interaction may be different (Leshner and Moyer, 1975). Aggression and submission may represent the end points of a single behavioral continuum; alternatively, they may represent two independent, but interacting, dimensions of the behaving individual. This is not a trivial semantic issue, but rather a conceptual issue that influences the manner in which the neural and endocrine bases of agonistic behavior are studied (Figure 8.7; Schlinger and Callard, 1990).

There is overwhelming circumstantial evidence that androgenic steroid hormones mediate aggressive behavior. First, seasonal variations in blood plasma concentrations of testosterone and seasonal variations in aggression coincide. For instance, the incidence of aggressive behavior peaks for red deer stags in autumn, when their gonads are secreting large amounts of testosterone (see Figure 8.8). Second, aggressive behaviors increase at the time of puberty, when blood concentrations of androgens rise. Juvenile red deer do not participate in the fighting during the rutting season. Finally, in any given species, males are generally more aggressive than females. This is certainly true of red deer; relative to stags, red deer hinds rarely display aggressive behavior, and their rare aggressive acts are qualitatively different from the aggressive behavior of rutting males. There are some interesting exceptions to this general observation, however; these exceptions will be described later in this chapter.

## Seasonal Changes in Social Behavior

Animals that are preparing to mate, or have recently mated, and require resources for their offspring, are far more likely to behave aggressively than are nonbreeding individuals. Many animal species breed on a seasonal basis (see Chapter 9); consequently, a seasonal pattern of aggressive behavior is commonly observed. Recently, several experiments have been conducted to investigate seasonal changes in aggression and the role of androgens in this temporal variation. This section describes some of those studies by examining a number of animal species.

### *Aggression and the Breeding Cycle: Red Deer*

Red deer stags were the subject of one such experiment. Castration of stags during the winter caused them to plummet in social rank (Lincoln et al., 1972). The reduction in social status mainly reflected the loss of their weapons: castrated stags promptly cast their antlers and acquired so-called velvet horn (Figure 8.8). Normally, antlers develop throughout the summer. During the course of their development the new antlers are covered by a mossy, soft, and highly vascularized tissue called velvet; thus, the deer are said to be in "velvet horn" during antler development. The velvet is shed at the end of the summer, when high blood testosterone concentrations destroy the blood supply to the velvet tissue and it dies. The antlers gain their familiar bony appearance as the velvet is shed, and the animals are said to be in "hard horn." After rutting, the testes regress during the winter, and low blood concentrations of testosterone provoke the stags to cast their antlers. Thus, wintertime castration mimicked the normal vernal reduction in testosterone and caused the stags to cast their antlers prematurely. In this study, the gonadally intact males also shed their antlers at the end of the rut, and the castrated males regained some of their position in the dominance hierarchy at that time. However, they did not regain all of their former social rank.

Not only does the frequency of agonistic encounters change on a seasonal basis, but the quality of the encounters changes as well. Red deer stags use their antlers as both offensive and defensive weapons during the rutting season, but

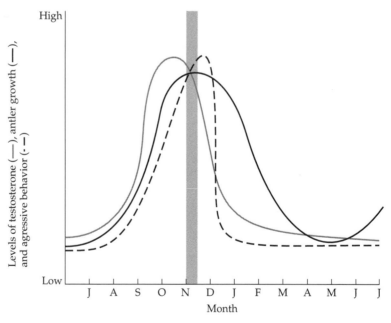

**8.8   Seasonal changes in red deer stags.** At the end of summer, testosterone levels (shaded line) begin to increase, and peak in mid-autumn. These rising androgen levels are accompanied by antler growth (solid line); the antlers come into hard horn in November, and the males begin to display aggressive behavior (dashed line). Mating behavior occurs for about two weeks in mid-autumn (shaded area). After mating, testosterone levels begin to diminish, aggressive behaviors wane, and the males engage in few agonistic interactions. When blood androgens reach low values in January and February, the antlers are cast.

aggressive behavior among nonbreeding males lacking antlers is mainly expressed by kicking with their forelegs. Females typically use their forelegs in agonistic interactions throughout the year.

Other castrated stags in the study were implanted with slow-release testosterone capsules either in the winter or in the summer (Lincoln et al., 1972). Winter-implanted males retained their antlers, were more aggressive than other males, and climbed in social rank throughout the spring and summer. Without antlers, the normal stags were easily intimidated by the antler-bearing, testosterone-treated stags. The continuous supply of testosterone across seasons permitted the stags to maintain their antlers and evoked aggressive behavior. However, not all androgen-dependent behaviors were supported by the chronic androgen exposure. For instance, the testosterone-treated males showed mating behavior only during the appropriate autumnal breeding season, suggesting either that estrous females generate a cue that normally stimulates mating behavior in stags or that the neural substrate controlling reproductive behavior in this species is responsive to androgens only at a particular time of year.

Stags implanted with testosterone in the summer began to climb in social rank even before the androgen could stimulate antler development, indicating that their aggressive behavior increased in response to androgen treatment even without the external morphological changes. In other words, these males behaved aggressively even in the absence of weapons to fulfill their threats. However, the antlers are the main factor controlling dominance behavior. Amputating the antlers of gonadally intact stags caused an immediate change in their social status without any change in endocrine state (Bouissou, 1983). Thus, steroid hormones affect social status in red deer stags in two ways: first, by acting directly on the brain to promote aggressiveness, and second, by acting on the antlers, the effectors of aggressive behavior. Males of other ungulate species differ from red deer; for example, castrated horses (Tyler, 1972) and reindeer (Espmark, 1964) may still dominate other male conspecifics. It is not yet known what accounts for this variation among species.

### Signals of Social Rank: Harris's Sparrows

There are other instances in which hormone concentrations appear to influence the perceived status of an individual through their effects on aggressiveness and morphological characters. Harris's sparrows (*Zonotrichia querula*) provide an elegant example of the endocrine mediation of social status. These birds set up individual territories and breed near the Arctic Circle during the summer. They migrate south to midwestern North America for the winter, where they form large mixed-sex and mixed-age, and even mixed-species, feeding flocks. The adaptive advantage of joining such a feeding flock probably arises from a "safety-in-numbers" strategy. Individuals compete for resources within the flock in the context of a social dominance hierarchy, or pecking order (see below). The membership of each winter flock is variable and changes frequently; consequently, these animals require an easily identifiable signal of social status. Such a signal would be advantageous to both subordinate and dominant birds because of the savings in time and energy; subordinate birds would benefit by avoiding potentially lethal fighting over resources with dominant birds, and dominant birds would benefit by avoiding many needless agonistic interactions (Rohwer and Rohwer, 1978).

Harris's sparrows apparently do have such a signal. Individual sparrows exhibit tremendous variation in winter plumage coloration, mainly in the number of dark or light feathers on the breast and head (Figure 8.9; Rohwer, 1975). The appearance of the sparrows is fixed for the winter during the autumnal molt. Birds with darker coloration invariably win contests over lighter-colored birds.

**8.9 Social dominance in Harris's sparrows is marked by plumage coloration,** with the darkest birds at the top and the lightest birds at the bottom of the "pecking order." (Top) Fourteen sparrows arranged in a dominance scale, from submissive (1) to dominant (14). (Bottom) Four individuals shown both with their natural coloration (left in each panel) and after their feathers were dyed (right). These birds' altered coloration did not allow them to rise in the social hierarchy. Courtesy of Sievert Rohwer.

Direct confrontations are rare, however, because of the extent to which the plumage signal is respected. In most cases, lighter birds simply leave a feeding area upon the approach of a darker bird (Rohwer and Rohwer, 1978; Rohwer and Wingfield, 1981).

Harris's sparrows with darker winter coloration have higher testosterone concentrations that lighter-colored birds. Males and females have similar coloration during the breeding season, with relatively dark heads and breasts. When they molt at the end of the breeding season, the variation in coloration becomes apparent, with males generally darker than females. Possibly, the concentration of circulating androgens during the autumnal molt is reflected in the number of pigmented feathers (Rohwer and Wingfield, 1981); however, some females are darker than some males within a given flock.

An experiment was conducted to determine the degree to which coloration dictated the aggressive prowess of Harris's sparrows (Rohwer, 1977). The throat and crown feathers of some dark birds were bleached, and these same anatomical areas were dyed black on some lightly colored sparrows. Neither group of altered sparrows fared well with their new social identity. Newly bleached, formerly dominant birds frequently engaged in fierce fighting because subordinate birds attempted to displace them on the feeding areas and the dominant birds refused to yield. These formerly dominant, newly bleached birds became outrageous bullies, picking fights far in excess of what was necessary or reasonable for merely obtaining foraging positions. They appeared to be trying to regain their former social status. On the other hand, newly dyed, formerly subordinate birds did not fare much better in their new social station. These dyed sparrows were persecuted by the true dominant individuals, which resulted in a quadrupling of attacks aimed at them. Many of the newly dyed birds left the relative safety of the winter flocks and fed alone. Apparently, the behavior of these sparrows did not match their artificial status signals, and their flockmates retaliated against this blatant social cheating. If, however, individuals were both dyed and implanted with testosterone capsules, they showed dramatic increases in social status (Rohwer and Rohwer, 1978). These testosterone-treated birds apparently behaved in a manner appropriate to their new coloration.

The altered plumage coloration caused great difficulties for Harris's sparrows because of the confusion that ensued: behavior did not match social signals. For these birds, as well as for red deer, androgens appear to modify both behavior and morphology. In some cases, it is possible that behavior feeds back to elevate steroid hormone concentrations further and stimulate greater development of androgen-dependent secondary sex characters, including behavior, as we will see below. There was no correlation, however, between natural winter blood androgen concentrations and dominance status among wintering Harris's sparrows (Rohwer and Wingfield, 1981).Thus the relationship between hormones and dominance is not apparent unless the hormone concentrations are monitored when the dominance hierarchy is being established.

Harris's sparrows, like many other migratory birds, must compete with resident birds for food and shelter in their winter habitat. Recent research with migratory redstarts (*Setophaga ruticilla*) demonstrated that the future reproductive success of migrants depends on the quality of the wintering habitat (Marra et al., 1998). At low latitudes, the resident birds are in reproductive condition during the winter and are extremely territorial. Although first reported as anomalous behavior, territoriality has recently been reported among wintering migrants and may be common among passerines (perching birds) that winter in the Neotropics (Greenberg, 1986; Marra et al., 1998). Wintering migrants are not in reproductive condition, and their gonads are not producing any measurable amounts of steroid hormones. The physiological mechanisms underlying territoriality or short-term site defense in these reproductively regressed nonresident migrants remain a mystery (Nelson et al., 1990). However, research on resident European robins (*Erithacus rubecula*) suggests that aggression during the winter may be testosterone-independent (Schwabl and Kriner, 1991), because when these birds are castrated during the winter, they continue to display aggressive behavior. Additional studies that rule out the adrenals or brain as sources of testosterone must be conducted to determine conclusively that winter aggression in these birds is truly testosterone-independent.

### Aggression and Winter Survival: Voles

Individuals of many rodent species shift from a highly territorial social strategy during the breeding season to a social, and highly interactive, existence during the winter. These species undergo reproductive regression at the end of the breeding season in response to short days (see Chapter 9); the resulting lower concentrations of androgens may enable this shift. There are adaptive benefits that accrue from changing social systems on a seasonal basis. During the breeding season, animals benefit from controlling resources to promote their own survival and that of their offspring, and they defend those resources aggressively. However, rodents may benefit from group living during the winter because this strategy conserves energy and enhances survival during this time of low temperatures and reduced food availability. Many species of rodents conserve energy during the winter by forming aggregations of huddling animals (West and Dublin, 1984). These aggregations, like winter feeding flocks of birds, may consist of different sexes and different rodent species (Madison, 1984).

Even in the absence of huddling behavior, animals may tolerate one another at close quarters during the winter, whereas interspecific commingling is not tolerated during the breeding season. For example, meadow voles (*Microtus pennsylvanicus*), as their name implies, occupy grasslands during their breeding season; the males are highly territorial at this time. Red-backed voles (*Clethrionomys gapperi*) prefer to breed in spruce forest habitats. But during the winter months, meadow voles move from open meadows into the forest habitats occupied by the red-backed voles, presumably to take advantage of the protective cover provided by the trees. In some cases, they occupy nests with other rodent species. Individual meadow voles, trapped during the winter then tested in paired encounters in a small neutral arena, exhibit less interspecific aggression than summer-trapped voles (Turner et al., 1975). The winter reduction in aggressiveness allows habitat sharing during harsh conditions. As the animals enter breeding condition in the spring, they once again establish mutually exclusive territories.

In another study, seasonal differences in social interactions between wild-caught adult and juvenile meadow voles were examined (Ferkin, 1988). Adults responded differently to juvenile male voles, but not to juvenile female voles, depending on the season. Adult male meadow voles were more aggressive toward juvenile males during the first part of the breeding season (May through August) than during the later months (Ferkin, 1988). In contrast, adult female voles were more aggressive toward juvenile males late in the breeding season than in the early portion of the breeding season. This seasonal shift in the aggressiveness of adult voles toward juvenile males may influence dispersal, and may also influence the formation of overwintering aggregations; overwintering groups of meadow voles typically include more females than males (Ferkin and Seamon, 1987).

Some individual male rodents do not undergo reproductive regression when exposed to short days; rather, these males maintain testicular function and produce sperm and androgens during simulated winter conditions (Nelson, 1987). Males capable of continuous breeding would appear to be superior in fitness to individuals whose reproductive apparatus regresses, because they are capable of siring offspring at any time of year. The obvious advantage of continuous mating ability must incur some hidden costs, however, because only a minority of individuals adopt that strategy. If there were no costs to a strategy of continuous breeding, continuous breeders would eventually replace the seasonally breeding animals. One possible cost is that nonregressed males, with their elevated androgen concentrations, may remain too aggressive during the winter to benefit from communal huddling, and thus may give up substantial energy savings relative to reproductively regressed males in order to be reproductively competent all year long. The high behavioral and energetic costs associated with maintenance of the reproductive system would compromise survival, and may explain why nonregressive types do not normally predominate in temperate or boreal zone populations of rodents (Nelson, 1987; Nelson et al., 1989).

A recent field experiment on the winter nesting behavior of prairie voles (*Microtus ochrogaster*) supports this contention (McShea, 1990). The majority of voles in the population were reproductively inactive during the winter and formed groups of huddling individuals. However, there were two males in the population that remained in breeding condition and were never observed to huddle with other animals. In pairwise tests of aggression, these reproductively competent males were much more aggressive than reproductively quiescent individuals. In a laboratory study, reproductive status influenced odor preferences of meadow voles maintained in simulated winter day lengths (Gorman et al., 1993). Males that retained reproductive function in winter day-length conditions preferred the odors of females that also failed to inhibit reproduction during short days. This preference may facilitate the sporadic occurrences of winter breeding frequently reported for this species (reviewed in Nelson, 1987).

In dusky-footed wood rats (*Neotoma fuscipes*), the levels of intermale aggression, both in laboratory and in field encounters, rise dramatically during the breeding season, which closely parallels the seasonal rise in testosterone concentrations (Caldwell et al., 1984). However, males castrated as adults also show the seasonal rise in aggression in laboratory encounters with castrated opponents, and show no decrement in fighting ability when paired with intact opponents (Caldwell et al., 1984). These results demonstrate the independence of seasonal aggression from the proximate modulating effects of testosterone in these wild wood rats.

In addition to the change in blood plasma androgen concentrations, seasonal changes in androgen receptor sensitivity occur in rodents. Consequently, it is not possible to override the wintertime reduction in aggressiveness merely by injecting testosterone. This seasonal shift in responsiveness to androgens has not been demonstrated in voles, but has been investigated in another seasonal breeder, the golden hamster. Injections of testosterone in reproductively regressed male golden hamsters do not elevate the number of aggressive encounters to the level exhibited by hamsters in breeding condition. Presumably, the ineffectiveness of testosterone in stimulating aggressiveness reflects a lack of androgen receptors in the brain regions responsible for organizing aggressive behavior during the non-breeding season. As with mating behavior, very high blood androgen concentrations are required to stimulate aggressive behavior immediately after the hamsters regrow their reproductive systems, as compared with those necessary to sustain aggressiveness in breeding animals (Berndtson and Desjardins, 1974). Desensitization of receptor tissues to steroid hormones is common after a prolonged absence of the hormone (Morin and Zucker, 1978; Powers et al., 1989), and this may be the mechanism by which seasonal changes in the sensitivity of central nervous system tissue are mediated (see Chapter 10). This last statement is somewhat speculative, however. Seasonal changes in receptors are only one of several factors, including changes in metabolizing enzymes, that may mediate seasonal changes in tissue sensitivity.

### Testosterone and the Energetic Costs of Aggression: Lizards

Elevated testosterone concentrations and aggression cause a decrease in survivorship in a number of species. A number of different factors, including injury, energetic costs, exposure to predators, or engaging in more "risky" behaviors, may mediate this effect. In male spiny lizards (*Sceloporus jarrovi*), seasonal changes in testosterone concentrations are tightly correlated with seasonal changes in the intensity of aggression, especially territorial aggression (Moore and Marler, 1987). During the autumnal breeding season, when territorial aggression is most fierce, testosterone concentrations are high; conversely, during the winter, when little territoriality is observed, testosterone concentrations are at their lowest. Interestingly, testosterone is highest during the summer, not during the fall breeding season, in these lizards. Artificial elevation of blood testosterone concentrations by implantation of Silastic capsules during the winter increased aggression above normal summer levels, but not to the level observed during the fall breeding season peak (Moore and Marler, 1987). Males who are implanted with testosterone-filled capsules spend too much time engaged in territorial defense, aggressive displays, and so on to forage adequately. Male lizards treated with testosterone did not survive as long as males implanted with empty capsules, and this decrease in survivorship probably reflects elevated energetic costs associated with aggressive behavior (Marler and Moore, 1988, 1991). Thus, males behaving aggressively during the winter incur a significant cost even in the face of potential reproductive benefits. These costs include the energy expended in increased territorial aggression and displays, as well as longer daily activity levels, which could have exposed the males to greater predation risks (Marler and Moore, 1989; Marler et al., 1995). When oxygen consumption was measured directly, testosterone treatment did not increase resting, or basal, metabolic rates. The approximately 30% increase in metabolism evoked by testosterone treatment appears to reflect primarily the energetic costs of territorial defense (Marler et al., 1995). Food supplements were able to compensate for the testosterone-induced costs of aggressive behavior (Marler and Moore, 1991).

### Do Seasonal Hormone Changes in Primates Correlate with Aggression?

Seasonal breeding is also observed among many primate species. Intermale aggression may increase during the breeding season for some species, including lemurs (*Lemur catta*) (Jolly, 1966) and rhesus monkeys (*Macaca mulatta*) (Michael and Zumpe, 1978, 1993). The frequency of aggressive acts may or may not increase during the breeding season in squirrel monkeys (*Saimiri sciureus*) (Baldwin, 1968; Mendoza et al., 1978). Correlations between periods of high androgen production and aggression are interesting, but do not demonstrate conclusively that elevated androgen concentrations cause aggression in primates. The results of several studies that addressed the relation between decreases in blood plasma concentrations of androgens and receptor sensitivity to androgens have suggested that these correlations probably do represent causation, despite some notable exceptions. Evidence in support of and in conflict with the dominant view that androgens mediate aggressive behavior among primates will be reviewed later in this chapter.

Human males also show seasonal variation in blood testosterone concentrations (Dabbs, 1990; Smals et al., 1976). These seasonal changes have not been shown to cause aggressive behavior; however, this presumption has not been directly tested, despite an abundance of positive correlations. For example, peak incidences of violent urban crime in North America are associated with high ambient temperatures and peak androgen concentrations in some populations (for example, Smals et al., 1976), but such correlations probably reflect factors other than hormone concentrations. For example, as Joan Didion writes in *Slouching towards Bethlehem*, "In Switzerland the suicide rate goes up during the *foehn* [a strong, hot, dry wind], and in the courts of some Swiss cantons the wind is considered a mitigating circumstance for crime" (218–219).

## Increases in Aggression at Puberty

There are countless reports of increased aggression in males undergoing puberty. During puberty, the testes grow larger, and under the influence of LH from the anterior pituitary, the Leydig cells secrete increasing amounts of androgens into the circulatory system. Plasma concentrations of androgens increase at the time of puberty and are associated with the elevation in aggressiveness. Intermale aggression in house mice, as well as isolation-induced aggression, is first observed at the time of puberty (Brain and Nowell, 1969; Levy and King, 1953).

As noted in Chapter 1, male livestock have been castrated prior to puberty since antiquity to make them more docile and manageable. Prepubertal castration is more effective in reducing overall aggression in mice than castration in adulthood (Uhrich, 1938). This observation is not borne out, however, in all species. For example, prepubertal castration of dogs does not necessarily diminish their adult levels of aggression (LeBoeuf, 1970), and prepubertal castration does not preclude male primates from attaining a high social status. For instance, Narses (480–574 A.D.) was a famous Byzantine general and statesman who originally was a eunuch slave in Armenia. He had a reputation for ruthlessness and played an important role in suppressing the Nika riots. Narses served under the emperor Justinian I, who sent him to Italy in 538 A.D. to fight against the Goths. Eventually, Narses rose to become the exarch of Italy.

Although these are interesting exceptions, it is generally true that aggressiveness increases at puberty. The following sections review some specific examples of associations between hormone levels and aggressive behavior that coincide with puberty.

### Is it Adaptive for Rodents to Be Aggressive at Puberty?

In one study, a group of peripubertal male prairie voles (*M. ochrogaster*) was implanted with slow-release capsules of testosterone, while another group received empty capsules. The testosterone-treated males exhibited a higher adult level of aggression in pairwise encounters than the control animals (Gaines et al., 1985). How might such an increase in aggression at puberty be adaptive? Males of many rodent species, including voles, disperse at the time of puberty. Dispersal is a very dangerous time for animals; mortality rates are extremely high during this time. Leaving home exposes the individual to many new threats, including predators and competing males. Dispersing males often find themselves encroaching on other males' territories as they learn to fend for themselves and try to find food, establish territories, and mate with females. Thus, dispersing males have evolved to be aggressive, which presumably increases their odds of survival and success in reproductive competition (Smale et al., 1997).

High blood concentrations of androgens are necessary to elicit dispersal in some mammalian species, but not in peripubertal male Belding's ground squirrels (*Spermophilus beldingii*) (Holekamp and Sherman, 1989; Smale et al., 1997). Male ground squirrels castrated at puberty exhibit dispersal behavior at the same rate and intensity as gonadally intact males (see below). Interestingly, by the time these juvenile ground squirrels disperse, the mating season is over and adult males are no longer maintaining territories with the same intensity as they did at the onset of the breeding season.

### The Timing of Puberty: Birds

In many avian species, reproductive and aggressive behaviors in males are closely linked. Many visual and vocal displays are used to attract females and repel other males simultaneously (Wingfield et al., 1994). Increasing vernal day lengths trigger reproductive maturation in many birds by stimulating gonadal growth and testosterone production (see Chapter 10). Peak concentrations of plasma testosterone correspond to peak levels of intermale territorial aggression in the late spring. At the end of the nesting period, the testes regress in response to the chronic long day lengths. Because long day lengths no longer stimulate the reproductive system, the birds are said to be refractory to photoperiod (day length), or photorefractory. Exposure to short days is then required to break photorefractoriness and allow the birds to respond to the stimulatory effect of long days the following spring.

Note that the photoperiodic control of gonadal function is fundamentally different in birds and rodents. Rodents are reproductively "on" unless exposed to short days, which turns them "off." Eventually, the reproductive systems of rodents break free of the inhibitory effects of chronic short days and regain their function. In other words, they turn "on" despite the short day lengths. The physiological mechanisms underlying this so-called "spontaneous" reproductive development are unknown.

The onset of puberty in most avian species is dependent on photoperiod. However, there is substantial variation in the timing of puberty; for example, some birds breed during their first year, other species breed when they are 1 year old, and other species breed after 2 or more years of age (Follett, 1991). This variation in the timing of puberty corresponds with variation among bird species in the timing of first territorial defense and mating. The majority of nontropical avian species hatch in the late spring and reach adult body size several weeks after hatching, but do not breed until the following spring. This is a reasonable strategy from an adaptive, functional perspective because young males probably could not secure sufficiently suitable territories to induce a female to breed. From a physiological perspective, one might ask why long days do not stimulate the birds to undergo puberty in their first summer. There is increasing evidence that birds that normally breed at 1 year of age hatch in a photorefractory state (Follett, 1991). That is, these birds must experience short days in order to break photorefractoriness and be stimulated by long days. Thus, unless housed under artificial lighting conditions, these birds cannot undergo puberty until spring, when they first experience long days after a period of short days. As you may know, some birds, such as quails and chickens, undergo puberty when less than 1 year of age (Follett, 1991). These birds are not photorefractory at hatching and can be stimulated by long days to undergo reproductive development during their first year.

When circulating testosterone concentrations increase, aggressive interactions among birds increase in frequency, especially during the establishment of territories or social dominance hierarchies (see below; Wingfield et al., 1987). Androgens are important in stimulating territorial behaviors, including singing. Experimental implants of testosterone capsules at the onset of territory establishment increased territory size or intermale aggression in several avian species, including the sharp-tailed grouse (*Tympanuchus phasianellus*) (Trobec and Oring, 1972), red-winged blackbird (*Agelaius phoenecius*) (Searcy and Wingfield, 1980), pied flycatcher (*Ficedula hypoleuca*) (Silverin, 1980), and white-crowned sparrow (*Zonotrichia leucophrys*) (M. C. Moore, 1984). Testosterone provided after territories or social dominance hierarchies were already established, however, usually did not increase territory size or social status (see below; reviewed in Wingfield et al., 1990, but see Cawthorn et al., 1998).

### *Hormones and Dispersal Strategies: Primates*

In contrast to many animals, the pubertal increase in blood concentrations of testosterone among primates is not always associated with elevated aggression. The onset of puberty in captive rhesus monkeys does not result in any discernible increase in aggressive behavior (Rose et al., 1978). Agonistic encounters between young captive male owl monkeys (*Aotus trivirgatus*) and their parents did not change in frequency at puberty, despite large increases in their plasma testosterone concentrations (Figure 8.10).

As in many avian and mammalian species, puberty is associated with dispersal among many primate species (Carpenter, 1940; Charles-Dominique, 1977; Fossey, 1974). Male rhesus monkeys become targets of increasing aggressive outbursts by adult males as they approach puberty at 3 or 4 years of age. This chronic harassment appears to force the peripubertal males to leave the natal troop and attempt to join a new one. Essentially two strategies exist for joining a new

**8.10   Aggressive behavior and puberty.**  (a) Peripubertal androgen levels in three owl monkeys. The shaded horizontal bars indicate the timing of puberty in each monkey. (b,c) The frequency of aggressive encounters with parents did not increase despite large elevations in blood testosterone concentrations during puberty. Source: Dixson, 1980.

troop: the newcomer may burst right into the group and seize membership status, or hang around the periphery and try to sneak into the group. Either strategy has costs, often fatal for the newcomer. Attempts to join a new troop immediately are usually met with strong resistance by the resident males, and a great deal of aggression is aimed at the intruder. Peripheral animals are also in danger because they may starve to death or succumb to a number of parasitic or stress-related illnesses.

Interestingly, several behavioral and hormonal factors predict which strategy an individual male will attempt in joining a new troop (Virgin and Sapolsky, 1997). Young males that are sons of high-ranking females often have "out-going, risk-taking" personalities (Suomi, 1991). These males venture farther from their mothers and engage in more rough-and-tumble play than do orphans or sons of low-ranking mothers. The sons of high-ranking females exhibit low vagal tone (a measure of autonomic reactivity; these individuals show a steady cardiac output and respiratory rate) and low plasma cortisol concentrations. In contrast, males that are not sons of high-ranking females have high vagal tone (heart rate, respiratory rate, and blood pressure are very reactive) and high blood concentrations of cortisol, suggesting that these males experience more stress in their lives. (In the laboratory, males with high vagal tone and high cortisol concentrations are also more likely to abuse alcohol than males with low vagal tone and low cortisol concentrations: Higley et al., 1991; Suomi, 1991.) In seminatural conditions, males with low vagal tone and low cortisol concentrations are more likely to employ the strategy of immediately establishing membership in a troop. In contrast, males with high vagal tone and high cortisol concentrations are more likely to try to sneak into the troop after establishing familiarity from the periphery (Bolig et al., 1992).

In a study of male olive baboons (*Papio anubis*) living freely in stable hierarchies in Africa, subordinate males displayed elevated basal glucocorticoid concentrations, and showed a blunted glucocorticoid response and rapid suppression of testosterone concentrations during stress (Virgin and Sapolsky, 1997). These endocrine characteristics were initially interpreted as reflecting the chronic stress of their social position. However, long-term fieldwork revealed that these endocrine characters do not mark all subordinate individuals. Rather, endocrine profiles differed among subordinate males as a function of their individual "styles of social behavior." One subset of subordinate male baboons was identified that had significantly high rates of copulations, a behavior usually shown only by high-ranking males. Such behavior predicted the onset of a transition to dominance, as this subset of subordinate males was significantly more likely than other subordinates to move to the dominant half of the hierarchy over the subsequent 3 years (Virgin and Sapolsky, 1997). A second subset of subordinate males were the most likely to initiate fights and to displace aggression onto an uninvolved third party after losing a fight. Males in this second cohort generally had elevated testosterone and lower basal glucocorticoid concentrations compared with the remaining subordinate cohort. Taken together, these results suggest that variables other than rank alone may be associated with distinctive endocrine profiles, and that even in the face of a social stressor (such as social subordination), particular behavioral styles may attenuate the endocrine indices of stress (Virgin and Sapolsky, 1997; see Chapter 11).

# Sex Differences in Social Behavior

Males are generally more aggressive than females. Certainly, human males are much more aggressive than females. Many more men than women are convicted of violent crimes in North America. The sex differences in human aggressiveness appear very early. At every age throughout the school years, many more boys than girls initiate physical assaults. Almost everyone will acknowledge the existence of this sex difference, but assigning a cause to behavioral sex differences in humans always elicits much debate (see Chapter 4). It is possible that boys are more aggressive than girls because androgens promote aggressive behavior and boys have higher blood concentrations of androgens than girls. It is possible that boys and girls differ in their aggressiveness because the brains of boys are exposed to androgens prenatally and the "wiring" of their brains is thus organized in a way that facilitates the expression of aggression. It is also possible that boys are encouraged and girls are discouraged by family, peers, or others from acting in an aggressive manner. These three hypotheses are not mutually exclusive, but it is extremely difficult to discriminate among them to account for sex differences in human aggressiveness.

What kinds of studies would be necessary to assess these hypotheses? It is usually difficult to separate out the influences of environment and physiology on the development of behavior in humans (see Chapter 4). For example, boys and girls differ in their rough-and-tumble play at a very young age, which suggests an early physiological influence on aggression. However, parents interact with their male and female offspring differently; they usually play more roughly with male infants than with females, which suggests that the sex difference in aggressiveness is partially learned (Smith and Lloyd, 1978). This difference in parental interaction style is evident by the first week of life. Because of these complexities in the factors influencing human behavior, the study of hormonal effects on sex-differentiated behavior has been pursued in nonhuman animals, for which environmental influences can be held relatively constant. Animal models for which sexual differentiation occurs postnatally are often used so that this process can be easily manipulated experimentally.

## *The Organization and Activation of Aggression: Mice*

With the appropriate animal model, we can address the questions posed above: Is the sex difference in aggression due to higher adult blood concentrations of androgens in males than in females, or are males more aggressive than females because their brains are organized differently by perinatal hormones? Are males usually more aggressive than females because of an interaction of early and current blood androgen concentrations? As with humans, these possibilities are difficult to assess in red deer or Harris's sparrows, but relatively simple to examine in house mice, for which sexual differentiation of the brain occurs postnatally. If male mice are castrated prior to their sixth day of life, then treated with testosterone propionate in adulthood, they exhibit low levels of aggression. Similarly, females ovariectomized prior to day 6 of age but given androgens in adulthood do not express male-like levels of aggression. Treatment of perinatally gonadectomized males or females with testosterone prior to day 6 of age and also in adulthood results in a level of aggression similar to that observed in typical male mice (Edwards, 1969, 1970) (Table 8.2). Thus, in mice, the proclivity for males to act

**Table 8.2**
**Effects of castration and androgen treatments on aggressive behavior in house mice**

| Treatment | | Aggressive behavior in adulthood |
| Before 6 days of age | In adulthood | |
| --- | --- | --- |
| *Males* | | |
| None | None | +++ |
| Castration | None | 0 |
| Castration | Androgen | + |
| Castration + androgen | Androgen | +++ |
| *Females* | | |
| None | None | 0 |
| Castration | None | 0 |
| Castration | Androgen | 0 |
| Castration + androgen | Androgen | +++ |

+++ = normal male levels of aggressive behavior; + = reduced levels;
0 = no aggressive behavior.

more aggressively than females is organized perinatally by androgens, but also requires the presence of androgens after puberty in order to be fully expressed. In other words, aggression in male mice is both organized and activated by androgens. Testosterone exposure in adulthood without prior organization of the brain by steroid hormones does not evoke typical male levels of aggression. The hormonal control of aggressive behavior in house mice is thus similar to the hormonal mediation of heterosexual male mating behavior in other rodent species (see Chapter 3). Aggressive behavior is both organized and activated by androgens in many rodent species, including rats, hamsters, and voles.

The world is much more complex than we often anticipate, however. Even when experimenters use a highly inbred animal model in constant laboratory conditions, it may be discovered that what appeared to be constant conditions in fact contain many variables. Some of these hidden variables may profoundly affect the endocrine–behavior relationships under study. This problem arose in studies of aggression in house mice. In mice, as in other rodent species, fetuses are packed in the uterus like peas in a pod (Clark et al., 1992) (see Figure 3.25), and may thus be influenced by hormones produced by their developing siblings. A female mouse may be situated between two brothers (2M = 2 males), between a sister and brother (1M), or between two sisters (0M). In general, 2M females are more aggressive than their 0M sisters. Presumably, androgens produced by their brothers affect these females' nervous systems (see Chapter 3). This example should remind you that many subtle endocrine influences on behavior are possible.

### Hormones and Dispersal: Ground Squirrels

Male Belding's ground squirrels leave home when they are about 50 days old. Dispersal is a gradual process taking 4–5 weeks to accomplish (Figure 8.11). It is also a robust sexually dimorphic trait: virtually all males disperse, whereas few

(<10%) females leave their natal region (Holekamp and Sherman, 1989). This sex difference in dispersal is common among mammals. A sex difference in dispersal also exists among avian species, but is reversed; that is, female birds are far more likely to disperse from the natal nesting area than males.

As described previously, peripubertal castration does not affect dispersal in male ground squirrels. If the activational effects of androgens are unimportant in sustaining this behavioral sex difference, then it is reasonable to suppose that it is mediated by early organizational hormonal events. In one test of this hypothesis, pregnant ground squirrels were trapped and caged at an outdoor camp near their home burrows (Holekamp, 1986). Their female offspring were injected with testosterone propionate dissolved in sesame seed oil, or with the oil vehicle alone, several days after birth. Immediately after the injections the families were returned to their home burrows, where the mothers successfully reared their offspring. Twelve of the androgen-treated females were re-trapped at 60 days of age or older. Seventy-five percent of them had dispersed from the mother's home bur-

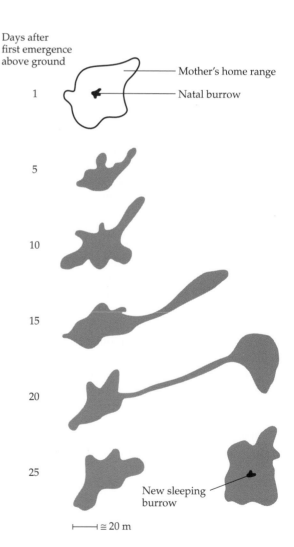

**8.11   Dispersal in male ground squirrels.** Although dispersal sounds like a sudden event, in ground squirrels it requires nearly a month to complete. At about 4 weeks of age, a young male emerges from his natal burrow, and his aboveground activity is limited to an area very close to the mouth of the burrow. After about 15 days above ground, the young male travels throughout his mother's home range, and also ventures well beyond it. Despite spending many hours away each day, he always returns at night until about 7–8 weeks of age (about 25 days above ground), when he establishes a new sleeping burrow and completes the dispersal process. When mapped, the dispersal process is visually reminiscent of an amoeba splitting during reproduction. After Holekamp and Sherman, 1989.

Days after first emergence above ground

1    Mother's home range / Natal burrow

5

10

15

20

25    New sleeping burrow

⊢———⊣ ≅ 20 m

row to a new nest site, following dispersal routes and traveling distances that were comparable to those of males. Approximately 70% of their male siblings had dispersed by this age. Only 8% of the oil-treated females left the natal area by 60 days of age. These results suggest an important role for early organizational effects of androgens on a complex behavior, namely, dispersal (Smale et al., 1997).

### Hormones and Dominance Status: Canines

Hormonal mediation of sexual differentiation occurs both prenatally and postnatally in dogs (see Chapter 3). Female puppies can be masculinized in two steps, by treating their pregnant mothers with testosterone propionate during gestation and then injecting the newborn puppies with testosterone immediately after birth. Such dogs have highly masculinized external genitalia (Figure 8.12) and exhibit male-like behavior. The social signals provided by these masculinized females elicit social confusion among beagles living in small, stable groups, just as the visually disparate signals of dyed Harris's sparrows do. The social confusion results because the behavior of a masculinized female is somehow suspect, or she does not emit the appropriate odors or other sensory signals, or possibly some other feature about her is incongruent with her perceived status.

The dominance hierarchy of a small group of beagles is relatively easy to determine with the right experimental tool. The right tool in this case is a large bone, preferably an oxtail bone, which is simply thrown into the middle of the dogs' pen when all the dogs are present and attending to the "bone provider," namely, the experimenter. During the normal course of events, the highest-ranking dog in a stable group gets the bone, usually with a minimum of conflict, growling threats, or any other hostile gestures. To discover which dog is the second in command, one simply removes the number one dog from the enclosure and repeats the bone competition test. In this way, and in pairwise tests between all of the dogs, the dominance hierarchy of a group can be determined (Beach et al., 1972). A variation of this technique, using chicken feed, was first used in classic studies on the pecking order of domestic fowl (Schjelderup-Ebbe, 1922).

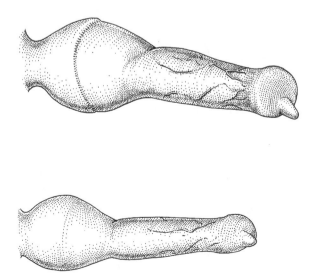

**8.12  Perinatal exposure to androgens masculinizes female beagles.** (Top) The penis of a normal male beagle. (Bottom) The pseudopenis of a female beagle exposed in utero and immediately after birth to androgens. If the penile (or pseudopenile) shaft is retracted, both males and masculinized females display comparable erections. Female dogs exposed to early androgen treatment also display very aggressive behavior and cause social disruption and confusion within small, stable groups. After Beach, 1984.

Both dogs and chickens have relatively linear dominance hierarchies; that is, the highest-ranking individual, A, supplants all others, whereas the second-highest-ranking animal, B, supplants all others except A, and so on down the line. In some species, especially among primates, dominance status may be inherited and thereby relatively fixed over extended periods of time. In other cases, social organization may be quite plastic as low-ranking individuals continually test and overthrow the status quo. Other species do not have linear pecking orders. Dominance hierarchies among more complex animal societies, especially those of primates, may be circular; for example, A is dominant over B, who is dominant over C, who is dominant over A. Other dominance systems involve complex and dynamic cooperative coalitions; for example, A supplants B only with the aid of C (Bernstein, 1981). In general, dominance hierarchies represent a social adaptation that arose over evolutionary time owing to two factors: (1) not all individuals are equal in securing resources, and (2) it is a waste of time and energy to continually reestablish this inequality among group members (Wilson, 1975).

In one study of beagle social organization, the dominance hierarchies were separately determined for a group of five male beagles, a group of five female beagles, and a group of five masculinized female beagles injected with testosterone in adulthood (Beach et al., 1972). Dogs from the different groups were then paired, and their status was determined by which dog won two-dog bone competitions over several consecutive days of testing. In general, normal females, regardless of their rank within their own dominance hierarchy, gave way to males; however, the bottom one or two male dogs often lost to the top one or two female dogs. Female beagles that had not been exposed to testosterone also yielded to the masculinized females. Possession of the bone in virtually all of these interactions was determined without any overt aggressive behavior: if a female got the bone first, she would drop it when the male or masculinized female approached her. These social interactions became more interesting when males and masculinized females were paired in the bone competition. A masculinized female would not yield to a male if she obtained the bone first. The male behaved as if he expected the female to give up the prized bone; he would growl menacingly at her and eventually attack her when she refused to give up the bone. If the male obtained the bone first, the masculinized female would attack him and continue to harry him until he relinquished the bone or counterattacked. The social signals providing information about the masculinized females' status, or their understanding of canine social rules, whatever they may be, were somehow affected by the early hormonal treatment.

The inclination toward high levels of aggression in dogs, as in house mice, requires both early organizational exposure to androgens and activation in adulthood by these steroid hormones (see Chapter 3). Aggressive behavior in males of these species is thus organized and activated by androgens. Early androgen exposure alone elevates the incidence of aggressive behaviors in perinatally castrated males and females above the level observed in normal females, but does not increase aggression to the levels of normal males.

### Flank Marking: Hamsters

Individuals of many mammalian species use chemosensory information to communicate social information (Doty, 1986; Johnston, 1985). One way to distribute chemosensory signals is to engage in scent marking. One type of scent-marking behavior commonly observed among mammals is called "flank marking." Flank marking involves rubbing their sides on a vertical substrate. Males of other mammalian species engage in chin-marking behaviors to the same effect. Syrian hamsters (*Mesocricetus auratus*) engage in flank marking, a behavior that conveys information about dominance (Ferris et al., 1987) or mate choice (Huck et al., 1985). Unlike most other mammals, in which males scent-mark more often than females, female Syrian hamsters flank-mark more often than male conspecifics (Hennessey et al., 1994).

Arginine vasopressin (AVP) plays a critical role in the expression of flank marking (Albers et al., 1992; Ferris, 1992). Microinjections of AVP into the MPOA–anterior hypothalamus, lateral septal nucleus, bed nucleus of the stria terminalis, or periaqueductal gray (PAG) evoke increased flank marking in hamsters (Albers et al., 1986; Bamshad and Albers, 1996). Microinjections of an antagonist for AVP into the MPOA–anterior hypothalamic regions result in a dramatic decline of flank-marking behavior (Albers et al., 1992; Ferris et al., 1993). Castration reduces the amount of flank marking in AVP-treated hamsters, and both testosterone and estradiol treatment rapidly restore flank marking in male and female hamsters, respectively (Huhman and Albers, 1993).

## Sex Differences in Play Behavior: Primates

Although work with altricial rodents has provided remarkable insights into the process of sexual differentiation of behavior, the data generated with these rodents have some fundamental limitations in their application to understanding the process of sexual differentiation of human behavior. People undergo sexual differentiation in utero, not postpartum. Consequently, the organization of sexual differentiation in rodents, in which the hormonal effects occur postnatally, may differ fundamentally from the process in humans. Also, masculinization in rodents depends on aromatization of androgens to estrogens. The aromatization of androgens does not appear to be important in the development and expression of masculine behaviors in primates (reviewed in Resko and Roselli, 1997; Balthazart and Ball, 1998). Although work with nonhuman primates is difficult and expensive, such work is more likely to provide insights into the sexual differentiation of humans than are studies of rodents.

Several fascinating studies that explored the role of gonadal steroid hormones in primate aggressive behavior have been reported. As is the case in humans, males of many nonhuman primate species are more aggressive than female conspecifics. This sex difference in behavior manifests itself early in development during the expression of play behavior. As noted previously, males engage in more rough-and-tumble play, more chasing, and more threatening behavior, and initiate play more often than females (see Chapter 3). The increased proclivity for aggression, either real or in the context of play behavior, in male as compared with female rhesus monkeys appears to require only prenatal exposure to androgens. Castrated male rhesus monkeys, for example, do not differ from intact males in the amount of threatening behavior, rough-and-tumble play, chasing, and play initiation they display (Goy and Phoenix, 1971). Many rodent species, in contrast, require androgens for both early organization and later activation of aggressive behavior. As described in Chapter 3, treatment of pregnant female rhesus monkeys with testosterone propionate produces pseudohermaphroditic female offspring. These androgen-treated females display threatening behavior, initiate play activities, and engage in rough-and-tumble play at frequencies intermediate between those of normal males and normal females (Goy, 1966, 1978; Phoenix, 1974; Phoenix et al., 1968). Thus, the expression of sex differences in play behavior requires the organizational effects of androgens, but not the activational effects.

The role of early androgen exposure in the mediation of sex differences in human aggressiveness has also been examined in "experiments of nature." As described in Chapter 3, girls who were exposed to high concentrations of androgens in utero because their adrenal glands malfunctioned were reported to engage in more rough-and-tumble play than their sisters who did not suffer from congenital adrenal hyperplasia (CAH) (Reinisch, 1974). Although these reports are interesting, observations of this type are less reliable in distinguishing cause–effect relationships than controlled experiments in which researchers are uninformed about the treatment condition of any individual. Recall that because the mothers of the girls were aware of their daughters' medical condition, it is possible that their ratings of the girls' behavior may have been inadvertently biased (see Chapter 3).

### Sex Role Reversals

In some species, females are more aggressive than males. It is interesting to examine these species' behaviors, because studying them may shed light on behaviors among species with more typical sex roles. This section describes some species with reversed sex roles.

**SANDPIPERS.**    Some female sandpipers of the genera *Phalaropus* and *Actitus* exhibit brightly colored plumage in contrast to the dull-colored males of their species (Tinbergen, 1935). Females compete among themselves for access to males, which are the predominant incubators, and are extremely aggressive toward other females (see Box 3.1). These reversals of the typical sex roles are not, however, accompanied by a reversal in the normal male:female ratio of blood androgen and estrogen concentrations. Androgen concentrations are six- to eightfold higher in pre-incubating male than in female Wilson's phalaropes (*Phalaropus tricolor*) (Fivizzani et al., 1986) and spotted sandpipers (*Actitis macularia*) (Rissman and Wingfield, 1984).

Although androgen concentrations are lower in female than in male sandpipers at most times, androgens may still mediate aggressiveness among females. Before pair formation, female testosterone concentrations are quite low and are comparable to values reported for females of other avian species. Females sampled after pairing, however, displayed a temporary sevenfold elevation in blood testosterone concentrations (Fivizzani and Oring, 1986). Thus, female sandpiper territoriality and aggressiveness are not dependent upon male-typical blood androgen concentrations, but may reflect increased sensitivity of brain structures to steroid hormones (Fivizzani and Oring, 1986). There is no sex difference in aromatase, 5α-reductase, or 5β-reductase enzyme activity in the brain, pituitary, or skin of the Wilson's phalarope, suggesting that neural sex steroid hormone receptors or changes in neural circuitry may underlie the sex role reversals observed in this species (Schlinger et al., 1989).

**GOLDEN HAMSTERS.**    Adult female golden hamsters are usually more aggressive than males (Payne and Swanson, 1972). Aggression in these females can be moderated by social influences, particularly housing conditions. For example, ovariectomized females housed individually are more aggressive than intact

Table 8.3
**Effects of housing condition on aggressive behavior in Syrian hamsters**

| Endocrine status | Aggressive behavior | |
| --- | --- | --- |
| | Housed individually | Group-housed |
| *Females* | | |
| Ovariectomized | ↑ | ↓↓ |
| Ovariectomized + estradiol and progesterone | ↑ | ↑↑ |
| *Males* | | |
| Castrated | ↓ | ↓ |
| Castrated + testosterone | ↑ | ↑ |

↑ = increase; ↑↑ = substantial increase; ↓ = decrease; ↓↓ = substantial decrease

females when they are brought into an arena with another hamster; however, group-housed ovariectomized hamsters fight less than individually housed ovariectomized animals (Table 8.3). Treatment of ovariectomized females with estradiol and progesterone causes increased aggression in group-housed animals as compared with intact animals. Housing condition does not significantly affect the aggressive behavior of intact hamsters. As in most other species, castration of male hamsters reduces agonistic encounters, and testosterone replacement therapy ameliorates this reduction. It is interesting to note that male mice and rats have smaller adrenal glands than their female conspecifics, but that the reverse is true of golden hamsters (Chester-Jones, 1955).

Photoperiod can also interact with gonadal steroid hormones to affect female hamster aggressive behavior. There was no difference in aggressiveness between ovariectomized females that were housed under short-day and long-day lighting conditions (Badura and Nunez, 1989; Elliott and Nunez, 1992). However, when treated with estradiol and progesterone, short-day hamsters were more aggressive than long-day females, especially when tested against males intruding into the females' home cage (Elliott and Nunez, 1992; Karp and Powers, 1993).

**SPOTTED HYENAS.**    As described in Chapter 3, spotted hyenas (*Crocuta crocuta*) are remarkable in the similarity of the external genitalia of the two sexes (Kruuk, 1972). As is the case for beagles, there is a rigid dominance hierarchy within each sex (Frank, 1983), but in sharp contrast to beagles, female hyenas dominate males in most behavioral interactions. Do hormones regulate social interactions in this species? If so, are blood androgen concentrations higher in females than in males? These questions are unresolved; conflicting reports exist regarding blood androgen concentrations in this species. One study reported no difference in blood androgen concentrations between male and female spotted hyenas (Racey and Skinner, 1979), but the results of another study indicated the usual sex difference in blood androgen concentrations, with males possessing higher concentrations than females. Individual social status was a much better predictor of blood androgen level than sex; resident animals in general, and the top-ranking individuals of both sexes in particular, exhibited high blood serum androgen concentrations (Table 8.4; Frank et al., 1985; Yalcinkaya et al., 1993).

Table 8.4
**Serum androgen concentrations in Kenyan spotted hyenas**

| Status | Androgen concentration (ng/ml ± SEM) |
|---|---|
| *Males vs. females* | |
| Adult males | 1.93 ± 0.4 |
| Prepubertal males | 0.25 ± 0.1 |
| Parous females | 0.35 ± 0.1 |
| Prepubertal females | 0.18 ± 0.2 |
| *Residents vs. transients* | |
| Residents | 3.15 ± 0.6 |
| Transients | 0.81 ± 0.2 |

*Source:* Frank et al., 1985.

## Individual Differences in Aggression

We all learn early in life that there are large individual differences in the expression of aggressive behavior. Some individuals resort to aggressive tactics with very little provocation, while others virtually never behave aggressively. You may have discovered this variation in preschool when you met your first bully, or you may have learned about it on your paper route when some dogs greeted you happily with wagging tails, whereas other dogs' raison d'être seemed to be to gnaw off your leg. What accounts for these differences in aggressiveness? Are individual differences in aggressive behavior explicable on the basis of blood plasma testosterone concentrations? In other words, are some animals more aggressive because they have higher blood concentrations of androgens, or do these aggressive animals have higher androgen concentrations because they are more aggressive?

Individual differences in aggressive behavior do not correlate with blood testosterone concentrations in mice (Barkley and Goldman, 1977; McKinney and Desjardins, 1973), although they do in rats (Schuurman, 1980). One experimental test of this question first rated male mice as aggressive or not aggressive. All the animals were then castrated, and they all became equally passive. The castrated mice were all provided with equal doses of testosterone and tested for aggressiveness again. Males that were previously aggressive became aggressive with testosterone replacement therapy, and previously nonaggressive males remained docile after testosterone treatment. This study indicates that high circulating concentrations of testosterone are necessary, but not sufficient, for stimulating aggressive behavior. These individual differences in aggressive behavior were probably due to differences in receptor sensitivity or in the ability of androgens to alter the perception of an aggression-evoking stimulus.

There are certainly strain differences among house mice in the extent to which aggressive behaviors are expressed and in the extent to which these aggressive behaviors are mediated by androgens. One systematic study in a Swiss strain of albino mice investigated the effects of castration on predatory, shock-induced, maternal, and isolation-induced aggression. Isolation-induced aggression was generally reduced after castration; post-gonadectomy treatment with testosterone, 5α-dihydrotestosterone (DHT), or estradiol restored this form of aggression (reviewed in Haug et al., 1986). In sharp contrast, castration increased intruding aggression toward lactating females, and treatment with testosterone, DHT, or estradiol reversed the elevated rate of aggressive responses in this situation (Brain et al., 1983). These results strongly imply that steroid hormones do not merely "trigger" aggression, but act to affect the animal's perception of and response to aggression-provoking stimuli (Haug et al., 1986).

In another series of experiments (Whalen and Johnson, 1987), male mice were pitted against either lactating females or males from which the olfactory bulbs had been removed (reviewed by Johnson and Whalen, 1988). Bulbectomized males elicited, but did not initiate, aggressive behavior. Gonadally intact males and castrated males treated with testosterone attacked the bulbectomized males, but did not attack lactating females. Untreated castrated males tended to display tremendous individual differences in aggressiveness, with some attacking either type of opponent, others attacking only one type of opponent, and others failing to attack any opponent. Because castration was associated with large individual variation in aggressive responding, and because androgen treatment reduced that variation, Johnson and Whalen (1988) have proposed that testicular steroid hormones act to induce "behavioral homogenization": in other words, androgens reduce variability in male house mouse aggressiveness. This is an intriguing hypothesis to account for the disparate aggressive responses of males to different aggression-provoking stimuli, although further experiments are necessary to evaluate it fully.

Dominance in more complex social organizations may not be related to blood concentrations of testosterone, especially in stable groups. For example, dominant dogs or squirrel monkeys can be castrated without affecting their position in the hierarchy (Dixson, 1980). Also, treatment of low-ranking individuals with androgens does not change their status in these species.

# Social Experience Feeds Back to Influence Hormone Concentrations

Hormones obviously affect behavior, but it should be emphasized that behavior can feed back and affect hormone concentrations. Tests of male mice in paired aggressive encounters revealed that their androgen levels were suppressed if they lost the fight (Lloyd, 1971). This hormonal suppression lasted for many days after the defeat. Similarly, rhesus monkeys that were defeated by a higher-ranking male had profoundly reduced testosterone concentrations for weeks after the defeat. In contrast, winning males' circulating testosterone concentrations quadrupled within 24 hours of the victory (Bernstein et al., 1974).

## The Challenge Hypothesis: Birds

The influence of social experience on avian hormone concentrations has been studied in a number of different species (Wingfield et al., 1997). In one elegant field study, male red-winged blackbirds were trapped in two different situations. In one condition, a live decoy male was placed in a spring-loaded net trap located near the center of another male's territory. A tape recorder repeatedly broadcast a specific male "advertising" song to ensure an aggressive response from the resident male. As you might imagine, the presence of a male intruder apparently singing with great abandon was certain to elicit a rapid behavioral response from the resident male. First, the resident male increased his rate of singing behavior. Second, he emitted the species-specific wingspread display, showing off his bright red epaulets (Figure 8.13). Because the tape continued to play and the intruder remained in place, the resident male approached and finally attacked the decoy, activating the net trap. A blood sample was immediately obtained. Other territorial males were trapped while foraging, without the use of a decoy. Blood testosterone concentrations were more variable in the birds caught during an escalating aggressive episode than in the foraging males, suggesting that the frequency of pulsatile androgen discharges in the aggressively behaving birds was increasing. There were no significant differences in blood concentrations of corticoids (Harding and Follett, 1979). This study demonstrated that behavior or environmental stimuli can affect hormone concentrations.

It is difficult to discern whether aggressive behavior per se or simply the perception of aggression-provoking stimuli is critical in mediating hormonal responses. Another study on a different avian species begins to address this issue (Wingfield and Wada, 1989). Like red-winged blackbirds, male song sparrows (*Zonotrichia melodia*) exhibit endocrine changes in response to territorial disputes. Again, territorial intrusions were simulated by placing live, caged conspecifics in the center of a male's territory and broadcasting a tape of the conspecific song over a loudspeaker. Responding resident males were caught either 1–4 minutes, 5–10 minutes, or 10–60 minutes after the onset of aggression-provoking stimuli. Control birds were trapped while they were foraging and were not actively engaged in territorial disputes. Blood samples were obtained from all birds and

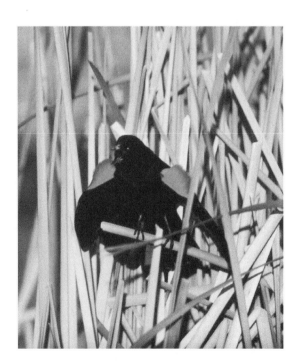

**8.13   Male red-winged blackbird in the wing-spread display.** This behavior shows off the bird's bright red epaulets, and is an aggressive territorial signal to conspecific male intruders.

later assayed for testosterone and LH concentrations. Neither LH nor testosterone concentrations differed between foraging birds and birds involved in territorial disputes sampled 1–10 minutes after the onset of the agonistic interaction. Both testosterone and LH concentrations, however, increased in aggressively behaving birds sampled 10–60 minutes after the agonistic encounter began (Figure 8.14). The initial pulse of testosterone in response to an intruder appeared to be independent from LH regulation, but persistently elevated testosterone concentrations appeared to be mediated by LH in the usual manner (see Chapter 3). Laboratory tests confirmed these field observations.

Additional laboratory studies examined the nature of the stimuli eliciting this behavioral–endocrine response in more detail (Wingfield and Wada, 1989). Simulated territorial intrusion by a heterospecific, a house sparrow (*Passer domesticus*), did not elicit any behavioral or hormonal response in resident song spar-

(a)

(b)

Control    1–4    5–10    10+
Minutes after "invasion"

**8.14   Effects of an intruder on resident song sparrows' hormone concentrations.** After a simulated "invasion" of a male song sparrow's territory, plasma testosterone concentrations begin to rise (a). Note that the rise in testosterone levels 5–10 minutes after the detection of the intruder is not accompanied by a corresponding rise in LH (b), but that the sustained elevation in testosterone seen after 10 minutes appears to be mediated by LH. Source: Wingfield and Wada, 1989.

rows. Further experiments dissected different sensory modalities in order to ascertain the contributions of various sensory inputs in affecting the endocrine system. Tactile cues did not influence hormone concentrations during aggressive encounters among male song sparrows. Song sparrows behaved similarly in response to a tape-recorded song (auditory channel), a voiceless conspecific intruder male (visual channel), or a combination of both stimuli. However, a tape recording alone or a devocalized male alone were less effective in stimulating elevations of LH and testosterone concentrations than a combination of both auditory and visual stimuli (Wingfield and Wada, 1989). These data indicate that the males behaved similarly in response to various stimuli that simulated a territorial intrusion but that a combination of auditory and visual stimuli was necessary to provoke endocrine changes. Had these studies not been designed so well, it might have been concluded that behavior and hormones were not correlated.

A lack of association between hormone concentrations and aggressiveness in birds has been reported in a number of studies. This inconsistency may be explicable on the basis of timing. For example, captive groups of house sparrows were studied over a 2-week period, during which stable social dominance relationships were formed (Hegner and Wingfield, 1987). High-ranking birds were very aggressive during the first week, when the dominance hierarchy was being formed; high-ranking birds had higher blood testosterone, but not DHT or corticosterone, concentrations than low-ranking individuals during this time. High-ranking males continued to behave more aggressively than low-ranking males during the second week of the study, but their testosterone concentrations no longer differed from those of the low-ranking individuals. These results suggest that social rank (attained via agonistic interactions) and blood testosterone concentrations are correlated when social status is being established (Hegner and Wingfield, 1987) or is being actively challenged (for example, Harding and Follett, 1979; Wingfield and Wada, 1989). This may also be true of primates (see below). Hormonal mediation of social status may wane after the initial relationships are formed and stabilized, and that status may then be maintained by nonendocrine factors. Thus, analyses of plasma hormone concentrations after dominance relationships have been established overlook the importance of hormones in mediating agonistic encounters during the formation of these relationships.

Field observations support these laboratory findings. A caged intruder will elicit ferocious fighting and huge surges in testosterone secretion during the early part of the breeding season, when territorial boundaries are being established. An intruder may still elicit aggressive behavior later in the season, when territorial boundaries are more stable, but it is less intense and less sustained, and may not cause an increase in androgen production.

Taken together, these observations of birds have led to the formation of the so-called challenge hypothesis to explain the role of androgens in aggressive behavior. Basically, the challenge hypothesis suggests that androgens are elevated and associated with aggressive behavior only when intermale competition is high; that is, androgen concentrations are elevated in a male by a challenge from another male (Wingfield, 1988; Wingfield et al., 1987). In another example, laboratory tests of aggression in long-term competition between paired Japanese quail showed that testosterone concentrations were elevated in winners during the first 3 days after pairing, but by the 5th day, plasma concentrations of testosterone were indistinguishable between winners and losers (Ramenofsky, 1984).

Generation of the challenge hypothesis has come mainly from comparative studies of avian aggressiveness and hormone concentrations in field-trapped birds (Wingfield et al., 1997). If blood concentrations of androgens and LH are measured in wild male house sparrows, a seasonal change in these two hormones is observed in the population, with high concentrations from about March until late July (Wingfield et al., 1987). In house sparrows, however, as in many other species of birds, a clear relationship between hormone concentrations and aggressive behavior has been difficult to uncover because different birds in the population are engaged in different reproductive activities at any one time. House sparrows breed multiple times throughout the season, and they do not synchronize their reproductive efforts. When blood samples are linked to the stage of the breeding cycle, a clear pattern emerges, showing that LH and testosterone concentrations are elevated during the sexual stage and diminished during the parental stage (Figure 8.15).

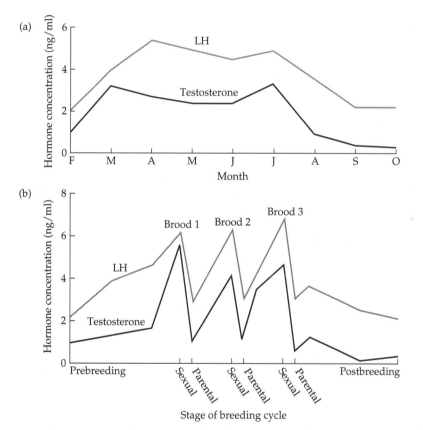

**8.15   Seasonal changes in blood LH and testosterone concentrations in house sparrows.**
(a) When testosterone and LH concentrations from populations of free-living birds are plotted against a yearly calendar, a smooth population-wide seasonal pattern emerges, with a clear elevation in concentrations of these hormones from about March until late July. (b) When blood samples are linked to stages of the breeding cycle, a different pattern emerges: both hormones increase during the sexual stage of the breeding cycle and diminish prior to and during the parental stage of the breeding cycle. Thus, it might be expected that males are more aggressive when they are establishing territories and beginning a breeding effort than at other times. Source: Wingfield et al., 1987.

Figure 8.16 compares blood concentrations of testosterone for several avian species. Two peaks of testosterone are observed among song sparrows; the first corresponds to the establishment of the territory and the second corresponds to the mating period, during which the male guards his sexually receptive mate from other males. Male European blackbirds (*Turdus merula*), like male song sparrows, show no change in blood testosterone concentrations during the second mating episode of the season (Wingfield et al., 1987); this lack of androgen secretion has been hypothesized to reflect that little competition exists for nest sites in these species at this time. Other species, such as European starlings (*Sturnus vulgaris*) and house sparrows, nest in holes, which are scarce, and are extremely competitive; males of these hole-nesting species exhibit an increase in testosterone secretion during each egg-laying period. In contrast, the western gull, like many colonial species, is long-lived, and there is often a skewed sex ratio with excess females; thus, there is little intermale competition. These birds may form pair bonds that last 20 years. There is little seasonal change in the blood plasma testosterone concentrations of male western gulls.

The challenge hypothesis suggests something fundamental about how androgens mediate aggressive behavior, and may account for much of the variation in the relationship between aggression and circulating androgen concentrations found in many species. Additional species will have to be examined to test the challenge hypothesis fully (e.g., Cardwell et al., 1996; Thompson and Moore, 1992).

### Hormones, Competition, and Violent Behavior: Humans

Social status and agonistic behavior may feed back to affect hormone concentrations in humans as well. The testosterone concentrations of male primates fluctuate as their social status changes; blood concentrations of testosterone tend to increase when dominance is achieved or defended, and decrease after defeat (Dixson, 1980). Several studies suggest that a similar effect exists among human males.

Participation in competitive sports is one way in which aggressive behavior is ritualized among humans. In one study, male graduate students participated in doubles tennis matches (Mazur and Lamb, 1980). The team winning the best of five sets split a $200 prize. Blood samples were obtained an hour prior to the match and within an hour of its conclusion. The majority of players whose teams had won decisively displayed post-game elevations in blood testosterone concentrations relative to the losers. Winners of close matches, in which the outcome was not assured until the end, did not differ from losers in their post-game plasma testosterone concentrations.

Male graduate students also participated in another study in which they had the opportunity to win money, but not through any effort on their own part. These individuals were paired, then each member of the pair was given a 50% chance of winning a $100 prize based on a lottery drawing; obviously the men had no influence on the outcome of this contest. A blood sample was obtained immediately prior to the lottery drawing and at four hourly intervals after the recipient of the prize had been determined. The act of becoming a "winner" did not affect blood testosterone concentrations in this situation; blood testosterone concentrations did not differ between winners and losers (Mazur and Lamb, 1980). These results suggest that blood androgen concentrations are more likely to be affected by winning a contest if its outcome is due to the man's own effort.

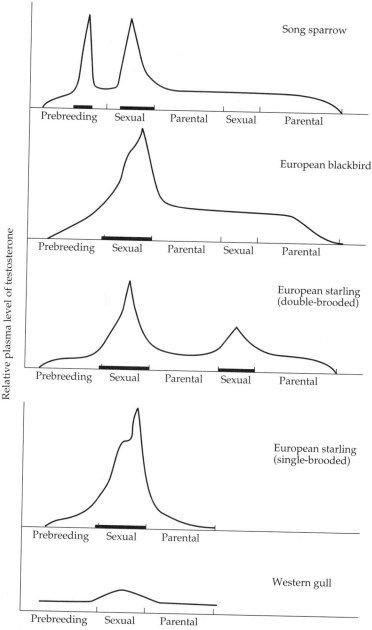

**8.16 Blood testosterone concentrations in birds may reflect competition.** The black bars correspond to periods when male–male aggressive interactions are frequent. During the song sparrow's breeding season, there are two peaks of testosterone; the first peak coincides with territory establishment and the second corresponds with the time of mating, when the male guards the female from other males. However, the second clutch of song sparrows and European blackbirds is not associated with a change in blood testosterone concentrations. Other species, such as the European starling, nest in holes, which are relatively scarce. Consequently, there is much competition over these nest sites, and blood testosterone concentrations increase during each egg-laying period. Colonial species, such as the western gull, display little male–male competition, and there is little change in androgen concentrations during the breeding season. Source: Wingfield et al., 1987.

Consistent with this hypothesis are the intriguing results of a study in which the testosterone concentrations of new recipients of the M.D. degree were evaluated (Mazur and Lamb, 1980). Blood samples were obtained for several days before and after the graduation ceremony. The samples revealed an elevation of blood androgen concentrations 1 to 2 days after graduation. Whether this increase in steroid hormone concentrations reflected the graduates' change in social status or the disappearance of a stress-induced decline in gonadal function requires clarification. Certainly, the stress of intense physical competition can reduce androgen concentrations—even among winners. For example, blood concentrations of testosterone were reduced in both winners and losers of a 26-hour ice hockey cup tournament (Tegelman et al., 1988). In general, mood elevation was related to increased blood androgen concentrations in all of these studies.

The relationship among mood, competitive outcome, and androgen and cortisol concentrations was examined in college varsity tennis players. Saliva samples were obtained before and after six tennis matches, and saliva concentrations of steroid hormones, which reflect blood concentrations of steroid hormones, were measured (Booth et al., 1989). The players' mood was evaluated prior to play as well as after the match. Most players experienced a pre-match anticipatory increase in testosterone. Testosterone was further elevated in winners, especially those winners who reported positive moods, as compared with losers. Performance carried over to the next match in the sense that winners displayed higher and losers displayed lower pre-match testosterone concentrations as compared with their hormone concentrations prior to the previous match. Winning or losing a match did not affect levels of cortisol, a hormone released during stress. Perhaps not surprisingly, top-seeded individuals had lower cortisol concentrations than low-ranking players; cortisol gradually decreased in all players as the season progressed.

Even the vicarious experience of winning or losing can affect testosterone concentrations among fans at sporting events. In one study, self-identified Brazilian and Italian fans provided pre- and post-match saliva samples before and after watching their national team compete in the final match of the World Cup soccer tournament. Mean testosterone concentrations increased among fans of the winning team and decreased significantly among fans of the losing team (Bernhardt et al., 1998). Thus, the performance of sports fans' favorite teams has the capacity to affect more than just civic pride; the testosterone concentrations of the fans can be affected as well. Indeed, female spousal abuse increases in the Washington, D.C., area after the Redskins win football games (White et al., 1992). It is possible that increased testosterone levels, evoked by the vicarious experience of winning, could trigger some men to cross the line into violence.

Studies like those just described that link hormones and behavior directly in humans are valuable because they are comparable to animal studies. However, the vast majority of research on hormones and social behavior in humans has relied on methods quite different from those used for nonhumans. This is not to diminish the value of these other types of correlational studies, but to alert you that conclusions about hormone–behavior interactions in humans are often derived from data that are fundamentally different from the data generated from nonhumans.

Most studies of hormones and human aggression have been based upon three sources of data; namely, hostility questionnaires, interviews, and criminal records. A blood sample may be analyzed and compared with test scores for aggressive tendencies or feelings. These procedures are very different from those used in research on nonhuman animals because the aggressive act is separated in time (by years in many prison studies) from the endocrine variables. Consequently, many contradictions have arisen about the role of hormones in human aggression.

In general, studies that have used psychological rating scales to quantify levels of aggressiveness or hostility have reported no relationship between blood or saliva androgen concentrations and aggressiveness (Doering et al., 1975; Monti et al., 1977; Persky et al., 1977). However, relationships between blood testosterone concentrations and behavior have been reported among aggressive, violent, and antisocial individuals, especially those incarcerated in prison (Ehrenkranz et al., 1974; Kreuz and Rose, 1972). Prison inmates exhibiting high circulating concentrations of testosterone, usually defined as the top 5% or 10% of the normal distribution, had committed violent crimes (Dabbs et al., 1987, 1989; Ehrenkranz et al., 1974), were more unruly in prison, and were judged more harshly by their parole boards (Dabbs et al., 1987, 1989). High testosterone concentrations have also been associated with male juvenile delinquency (Olweus, 1983). Although some studies of criminal populations show no association between plasma testosterone and violent behavior (for example, Matthews, 1979), the consensus is that violence among prison inmates and blood androgen concentrations are positively correlated. A similar relationship was observed among female prison inmates (Dabbs and Hargrove, 1997) (Figure 8.17).

Two related hypotheses have been proposed to explain the association between high androgen levels and human antisocial behavior as observed in delinquent or criminal populations: first, that androgens directly mediate the antisocial activities, and second, that androgens promote a constellation of traits, including social dominance, competitiveness, and thrill-seeking, that may be expressed either as antisocial or as prosocial behavior depending upon the individual's resources and background. For example, the same constellation of traits might be expressed as assaultive behavior in a gang fight among high-testosterone individuals living in an economically depressed neighborhood or as team-spirited competitive behavior among high-testosterone individuals on a college football team. To distinguish between these two possibilities, a large sample of 4462 United States military veterans was examined beginning in 1985. Psychological and medical evaluations and exhaustive laboratory tests, including measurements of blood androgen concentrations, were performed on these men. Analyses of their psychological profiles and saliva concentrations of testosterone indicated that androgens directly mediate antisocial behavior in human males, although socioeconomic status has a small moderating effect (Dabbs and Morris, 1990).

Taken together, these studies suggest that androgens can affect human male aggressiveness and dominance. Some intriguing observations support this contention, albeit in a somewhat indirect manner. Satisfaction with family functioning at midlife, defined as 39–50 years of age in one study, is associated with nonaggressive tendencies among men. Certain psychological factors were related to

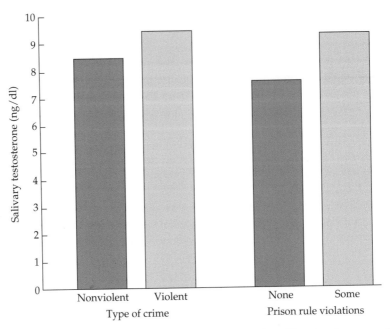

**8.17    Relationship of testosterone concentrations in the saliva of female prisoners and behavior.** High salivary testosterone concentrations are linked to violent crimes and to elevated prison rule violations. Source: Dabbs and Hargrove, 1997.

men's satisfaction with family life at midlife, including androgynous characteristics, marital satisfaction, parent–offspring communication, and emotional expressiveness. Multiple regression analysis revealed that adoption of androgynous behaviors—behaviors that are both masculine and feminine—was linked to low blood concentrations of testosterone. Similarly, marital satisfaction and the quality of the father–child relationship were negatively correlated with testosterone concentrations. In other words, low testosterone concentrations were associated with high marital and family satisfaction. According to this study's authors, dominance, independence, aggressiveness, and competitiveness may not be valuable male traits for maintaining stable family environments (Julian and McKenry, 1989). A similar finding was reported in a study of testosterone concentrations in men with different occupations (Dabbs et al., 1990). The only statistically significant difference was between NFL football players and ministers (Figure 8.18).

Few studies have addressed the role of androgens in aggressive behavior in women; no consistent correlation between androgen concentrations and aggressive behavior has been reported for women (Dabbs et al., 1989; Persky et al., 1982; Dabbs and Hargrove, 1997). However, subtle effects of androgens may influence aggression in women. Saliva testosterone concentrations did not differ between female prison inmates and female college students. But further analyses discovered that testosterone concentrations were highest in women prisoners convicted of unprovoked violent crimes and lowest in women convicted of "defensive" violent crimes, such as killing abusive husbands (Dabbs et al., 1989).

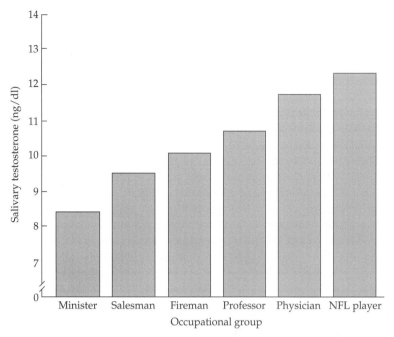

**8.18    Salivary testosterone concentrations among men in six different occupations.** Source: Dabbs et al., 1990.

Other data suggest that androgen concentrations in women, although much lower than those in men, may influence or be influenced by social status. For example, blood testosterone concentrations of female undergraduate students and professional, managerial, and technical workers are higher than those of clerical workers and housewives (Purifoy and Koopmans, 1979). As is the case in males, saliva testosterone concentrations are higher in female attorneys than in female teachers and nurses (Schindler, 1979).

## Physiological Mechanisms Mediating Hormonal Effects on Social Behavior

Where in the brain do androgens act to mediate aggression? Implants of androgen pellets into the preoptic area of the anterior hypothalamus stimulate aggressive behavior in castrated male ring doves (Barfield, 1971) and quail (Watson and Adkins-Regan, 1989). Androgen implants in, or electrical stimulation of, the striatum region also induces aggression in birds (reviewed in Crews and Silver, 1985). There have been many studies employing lesioning or electrical stimulation techniques that have provided evidence that the hypothalamus and several components of the limbic system, including the hippocampus, septum, and amygdala, are involved in avian aggressive behavior. These same general brain regions are also involved in the regulation of aggressive behavior in mammals.

Bilateral implants of testosterone propionate into the septum, but not into the preoptic area, the medial reticular formation (a structure that extends from the medullar brain stem to the midbrain, critical in arousal), or the amygdala, evoked aggressive behavior in castrated white mice (Owens et al., 1974). Lesions of the nucleus accumbens lessen testosterone-dependent aggression in male rats (Figure 8.19; Albert et al., 1990). Androgens also stimulate the hypothalamic tracts to promote aggressive behavior in primates (reviewed in Dixson, 1980). Recent studies have implicated nitric oxide (NO) as a mediator of male aggression (Box 8.1).

Several lines of research have established that reduced brain serotonin concentrations result in increased aggression (reviewed in Albert and Walsh, 1984; Olivier et al., 1995; Olivier and Mos, 1992). For example, a drug that causes 5-HT depletion leads to increased aggression in a variety of species in several different social situations (reviewed in Vergnes et al., 1986). Shock-induced aggression in mice and rats is considered to be defensive aggression, as it results in defensive postures. Mouse-killing behavior in rats is considered offensive aggression. Both mice and rats show offensive and defensive aggression depending on their status as the intruder or resident, respectively, in a home cage (Barr et al., 1975; Nikulina, 1991; Olivier and Mos, 1992). Depletion of 5-HT increases both offensive and defensive aggression (Vergnes et al., 1986). Again, brain 5-HT depletion increases behavioral responsiveness to sensory and painful stimuli (e.g., Lorens, 1978; Telner et al., 1979). Aggressive behavior in response to a wide variety of stimuli can be suppressed by 5-HT or any treatment that elevates 5-HT (Ieni and Thurmond, 1985).

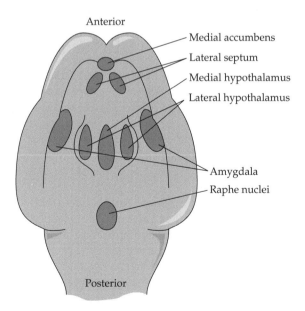

**8.19    Components of the rat brain involved in aggression.** This schematic cross section shows the major components known to be involved in defensive, predatory, and social aggression: the medial accumbens, lateral septum, medial hypothalamus, lateral hypothalamus, amygdala, and raphe nuclei. After Albert and Walsh, 1984.

Box 8.1
# Nitric Oxide and Aggression

Nitric oxide (NO), first identified as an endogenous regulator of blood vessel tone, may also serve as a neurotransmitter (Nelson et al., 1997). NO is an endogenous gas that has several biochemical properties of a free radical. It is very labile, with a half-life of less than 5 seconds; consequently, many studies have manipulated NO indirectly by affecting the synthetic enzyme, nitric oxide synthase (NOS), that transforms arginine into NO and citrulline. Studies that have used this approach have determined that NO plays several critical physiological roles. Three distinct isoforms of NOS have been discovered: (1) a form found in the endothelial tissue of blood vessels (eNOS), (2) an inducible form found in macrophages (iNOS), and (3) a form found in neural tissue (nNOS). Suppression of NO formation, either by the elimination of arginine or by the use of N-methyl-arginine, a potent NOS inhibitor, affects all three isoforms of NOS. The neural isoform, nNOS, is localized at high densities within emotion-regulating brain regions.

In order to examine the specific behavioral role of NO in neurons, mutant mice were created with the *nNOS* gene knocked out (nNOS–/–). Informal observation of these nNOS–/– mice suggested unusual levels of aggressiveness among the male cagemates. When behavioral tests of aggression were conducted using an intruder–resident model, a test of territorial aggression, male nNOS–/– residents engaged in 3–4 times more aggressive encounters than wild-type (WT) mice (see figure at right). Nearly 90% of the aggressive encounters were initiated by the nNOS–/– animals. Similar results were obtained in dyadic or group encounters in neutral arenas. In all test situations, male nNOS–/– mice rarely displayed submissive behaviors.

As noted in Chapter 1, behavioral studies of mice with targeted deletions of specific genes are subject to the criticism that the gene product is missing not only during the testing period, but also throughout development, when critical ontogenetic processes, including activation of compensatory mechanisms, may be affected. To address this criticism, WT mice were treated with 7-nitroindazole (7-NI) (50 mg/kg ip), which specifically inhibits nNOS formation in vivo (Demas et al., 1997). Mice treated with 7-NI displayed substantially increased aggressive behavior in two different tests of aggressiveness as compared with control animals (Demas et al., 1997). The drug treatment did not affect nonspecific locomotor activities. Importantly, NOS activity in the brain was reduced more than 90% in the 7-NI-treated mice. Similarly, immunohistochemical staining for citrulline, a co-product of NO production, revealed a dramatic reduction in citrulline (and, presumably, NO, which cannot be measured directly in cells) in the 7-NI-treated animals (Demas et al., 1997; see figure on the next page). Taken together, these findings suggest that NO formation was virtually eliminated in these experimental animals. Because 7-NI treatment in WT mice caused aggression to be elevated to the levels displayed by nNOS–/– mice, it appears that nNOS is an important mediator of aggression.

As we have seen, plasma androgen concentrations can affect the display of aggressive behavior. There were no differences between nNOS–/– and WT mice in blood testosterone

Photograph courtesy of Jay Van Rensselaer.

Box 8.1 *continued*

concentrations either before or after agonistic encounters. However, recent data on castrated nNOS–/– males suggest that testosterone is necessary to promote increased aggression in these mutants (Kriegsfeld et al., 1997). Castrated nNOS–/– mice displayed low levels of aggression that were equivalent to those observed among castrated WT males. Androgen replacement therapy restored the elevated levels of aggression in nNOS–/– mice. Importantly, inappropriate aggressiveness was never observed among female nNOS–/– mice in these test situations; however, when aggressive behavior was examined in female nNOS–/– mice in the context of maternal aggression, during which WT females are highly aggressive toward intruders, nNOS–/– dams were very docile (Gammie and Nelson, 1999)! No sensori-

motor deficits were found among the mutant mice to account for the changes in aggressive behavior. Taken together, these results suggest that NO from neurons is important in the mediation of aggression in male mice.

From Demas et al., 1997.

Early studies of the inhibitory effects of 5-HT on aggressive behavior used nonselective 5-HT agonists and antagonists (reviewed in Bell and Hobson, 1994; Muehlenkamp et al., 1995). More recently, radioimmunoassay studies have differentiated 5-HT receptors into several subtypes: $5\text{-HT}_{1A,1B, 1D\alpha, 1Db, 1E, 1F}$, $5\text{-HT}_{2A, 2B, 2C}$, $5\text{-HT}_3$, $5\text{-HT}_4$, and $5\text{-HT}_5$ (Bell and Hobson, 1994). Some of these effects could be due to the anti-anxiety (or anxiolytic) actions inherent with the activation of some of these receptor subtypes. However, recent studies have indicated that male-typical offensive aggression is reduced, in the absence of anxiolytic actions, by mixed $5\text{-HT}_{1A}$ and $5\text{-HT}_{1B}$ agonists (Cologer-Clifford et al., 1996).

## Conclusions

How do hormones affect social behavior? Hormones affect social behavior at the level of input systems; for example, androgens affect the perception of aggression-promoting stimuli associated with intermale agonistic interactions (Johnson and Whalen, 1988; Wingfield et al., 1990). Behavior can feed back, as in the case of territorial encounters between house sparrows, to affect hormonal and subsequent behavioral responses to intruders. Androgens, as well as peptide hormones, affect the central processing of stimuli associated with aggressive responding (Johnson and Whalen, 1988; Lincoln et al., 1972; Panksepp et al., 1980b). Steroid hormones also affect social behavior by influencing the effectors involved in aggressive behavior. In the case of red deer, androgens influence social interactions by acting upon the antlers. Hormones, particularly endogenous opioids, may also provide reward properties to social contact or other social interactions.

# Summary

• Social behavior involves interactions between individuals in which one or more of the animals benefits from the interaction. Affiliation refers to behaviors that bring animals together. Aggression is overt behavior with the intention of inflicting damage on another individual. Agonistic behavior is observed when the interests of two individuals are in conflict.

• Affiliative behaviors are affected by glucocorticoids, vasopressin, and oxytocin, hormones that also influence parental behaviors. These hormones appear to function in affiliation by affecting the neurotransmitters dopamine and serotonin. Opioids also mediate affiliative behavior, especially in the context of social grooming or social contact.

• Androgens have been linked to aggressive behavior by three kinds of circumstantial evidence: Seasonal changes in blood androgen concentrations and aggressiveness covary. Aggression is correlated with the onset of puberty, when androgen concentrations rise. Aggression is more common among males than females of most vertebrate species.

• Seasonal changes in hormone concentrations and morphological signals affect aggressiveness in red deer and Harris's sparrows. The interaction between behavior, hormones, and self-perception of one's place in the social hierarchy is complex and subtle for some species. Among rodents, dramatic seasonal changes in social organization occur in response to blood concentrations of androgens.

• The onset of puberty heralds the initial display of aggression in males of many species. Pubertal aggression is linked to dispersal in many avian and mammalian species. Dispersing individuals must be aggressive at this time in order to compete within new social contexts.

• Males are generally more aggressive than females. In rodent species, the sex difference in aggressiveness is organized perinatally and also requires activational actions of androgens in adulthood for expression. The sex difference in aggressiveness among primate species appears to be organized prenatally and does not require androgen stimulation later in life for expression.

• Females of some species are more aggressive than males. Female sandpipers do not usually have higher blood concentrations of androgens than males; however, females show large elevations in blood concentrations of androgens after pairing, suggesting that testosterone may play a role in their aggressive behaviors. Female hyenas are also more aggressive than males; androgen concentrations in adults do not account fully for the behavioral sex reversal.

• There are great individual differences in aggressiveness. In some species, such as mice, aggressive behaviors do not correlate with blood testosterone concentrations, but in other species, such as rats, the degree of aggressiveness and blood concentrations of testosterone are related.

• Social experience feeds back to influence androgen concentrations. Winning an agonistic encounter produces a sustained elevation in blood androgen concentrations in rodents and primates. In contrast, losing results in a chronic reduction of blood androgen concentrations.

• The act of fighting an intruder can elevate blood concentrations of testosterone in many species of birds. Obtaining blood samples during an aggressive encounter increases the likelihood that androgen concentrations will correlate positively with aggressive behavior, especially during the breeding season. The challenge hypothesis suggests that androgens mediate aggressive encounters only during the establishment of territories, or whenever males are highly competitive. Aggression at other times does not elicit the same kind of endocrine response and probably is not mediated by androgens.

• Social experience in competitive sports can feed back and affect human androgen concentrations. Elevation in social status is also associated with high blood androgen concentrations among humans.

• Assessments of human aggression are typically different from studies of aggression in nonhuman animals because the aggressive act is generally removed in time from the blood hormone assessment. Typically, aggression in humans is quantified on the basis of questionnaires or interviews. Nonetheless, prison inmates who have been convicted of violent crimes tend to have high concentrations of androgens.

## Questions for Discussion

1. Suppose that you have obtained blood samples from matadors and bulls immediately after a number of bullfights. You notice that the blood androgen concentration is elevated in the matador whenever he decisively defeats the bull, but that the bull's androgen concentrations are elevated if it gored the matador. Is "winning" the critical factor in determining blood androgen concentrations? What other endocrine events might account for the data?

2. Design an experiment to test the proposition that professional football players are more aggressive than spectators because they have elevated thyroid hormone concentrations. Remember that hormones affect behavior and that behavior can feed back to affect blood hormone concentrations.

3. Johnson and Whalen (1988) propose that androgens cause a behavioral "homogenization" by reducing the variation in response. How might this work? Why is it that some castrated animals retain aggressive behaviors, whereas other conspecifics become docile after castration?

4. How might hormones affect the perception of a threat? How might hormones affect mood in such a way that stimuli become irritating? Design a test of your notions.

# Suggested Readings

Carter, C. S., Lederhendler, I. I., and Kirkpatrick, B. 1997b. *Integrative Neurobiology of Affiliation.* Vol. 807. New York Academy of Sciences: New York.

Dixson, A. F. 1980. Androgens and aggressive behavior in primates: A review. *Aggressive Behavior,* 6: 37–67.

Ferris, C. F. 1992. Role of vasopressin in aggressive and dominant/subordinate behaviors. *Annals of the New York Academy of Sciences,* 652: 212–226.

Insel, T. R., and Winslow, J. T. 1998. Serotonin and neuropeptides in affiliative behaviors. *Biological Psychiatry,* 44: 207–219.

Johnson, F., and Whalen, R. E. 1988. Testicular hormones reduce individual differences in the aggressive behavior of male mice: A theory of hormone action. *Neuroscience and Biobehavioral Reviews,* 12: 93–99.

Svare, B. 1983. *Hormones and Aggressive Behavior.* Plenum, New York.

Wingfield, J. C., Whaling, C. S., and Marler, P. 1994. Communication in vertebrate aggression and reproduction: The role of hormones. In E. Knobil and J. D. Neill (eds.), *The Physiology of Reproduction,* Vol. 2, pp. 1647–1677. Raven Press, New York.

# 9

# Homeostasis and Behavior

I n 1859, 12 pairs of European rabbits (*Oryctolagus cuniculus*) were released from a ranch in Victoria, the southeasternmost state in Australia, in order to provide a ready source of game for hunting. The rabbit population grew exponentially because the animals had no natural predators in Australia. By 1865, one hunting drive successfully killed over 20,000 rabbits. But the rabbits kept multiplying, and by 1900 they presented a serious problem for Australia, where the production of wool is an important economic activity. In addition to being very prolific, rabbits are extremely efficient foragers. Within 40 years after the initial twelve pairs were released, hundreds of millions of their descendants had spread throughout Australia and had destroyed valuable pastures and rangelands required for grazing sheep. The invading rabbits also destroyed many unique habitats, which led to the extinction of several native marsupial species. After

failed attempts by the government to reduce the number of rabbits by using poisons, predators, and other pest control procedures, the myxoma virus (which produces myxomatosis, a disease fatal to rabits), was introduced in 1950. A
myxomatosis epidemic broke out and killed over 99.9% of the rabbits. Only a few
myxomatosis-resistant animals survived. However, these initially rare myxomatosis-resistant animals repopulated the continent once again. In some areas,
only 2 years were necessary to restore the decimated populations. Recently,
Australian government scientists were testing a new rabbit virus, called rabbit
calicivirus (RCD), on nearby Wardang Island to make certain it would work properly. However, before testing was complete, the virus invaded Australia and New
Zealand. In some cases, rabbit mortality has been very high, but in other cases,
only about half of the rabbits in a population have succumbed to RCD. A new
concern in areas of Australia where RCD has drastically reduced the number of
rabbits is that introduced foxes and feral cats will start killing native Australian
species for food. An emergency program to kill foxes and feral cats has recently
been instigated to reduce the damage from this new ecological imbalance. The
"experts" hope that in the long run, everything will balance out, but there is a reasonably high chance that the RCD-resistant rabbits will soon repopulate Australia
and New Zealand.

In their colonization of Australia, the European rabbits were confronted with
a wide variety of environmental conditions. The rapid spread of the animals
throughout the Australian continent required them to adapt to markedly diverse
habitats, including tropical forests, harsh deserts, fertile plains, and barren sea-
coasts. Besides undergoing the obvious climatic and reproductive adaptations,
these pioneering rabbits also had to cope with vastly different levels of nutrient
availability: for example, the prevalence of water and sodium differed widely
across habitats and across seasons. Because physiological systems operate best
within a very narrow range of conditions, rabbits living in different areas were
forced to make very different biological adjustments depending on the habitat they
encountered. For example, maintaining a certain level of sodium chloride, the salt
that is common in your diet, is critical for sustaining life. Sodium chloride is scarce
in some Australian habitats, and rabbits that colonized these areas were successful only to the extent that they coped with the sodium shortages. Rabbits that settled in sodium-rich habitats survived only if they could rid their bodies of excess
sodium.

Individuals are motivated to maintain an optimal level of water, sodium, and
other nutrients in the body. Claude Bernard, the 19th-century French physiologist (Figure 9.1), was the first to describe the ability of animals to maintain a relatively constant internal environment, or *milieu intérieur*. For instance, humans
maintain an optimal body temperature between 36° and 38°C; there are also optimal blood concentrations of sugars, proteins, sodium, potassium, and many other
blood constituents, as well as an optimal blood pH. In 1929, Walter B. Cannon
termed the process by which the body maintains this relatively constant internal
milieu **homeostasis** (from the Greek, "standing the same").

Many homeostatic systems are completely physiological processes; however, many maintenance systems—thirst, for example—also have one or more behavioral components. In yet other cases, physiological mechanisms normally
maintain homeostasis, but behavioral processes may be activated when the nor-

**9.1    Claude Bernard (1813–1878),** a French physiologist who developed the concept of homeostasis.

mal physiological regulatory systems are unable to restore equilibrium. If both adrenal glands are removed from a rat, for example, it will usually perish within a week. However, if salt water is made available, the adrenalectomized rat will drink it, and will survive as well as intact rats in the laboratory (Richter, 1936). Under normal conditions, when the adrenal glands are present, physiological homeostatic systems maintain sodium balance through the action of aldosterone; this steroid hormone, secreted from the adrenals, acts on the kidneys to conserve sodium (Denton, 1982). Without the adrenals, the animal cannot retain enough sodium to sustain its life; however, it can compensate for the missing physiological sodium conservation mechanism by ingesting increased amounts of sodium. Prior to adrenalectomy, a rat, just like you, will avoid drinking seawater (about a 3.5–7% sodium solution), but after adrenalectomy, a rat will avidly drink a saturated salt water solution. When physiological homeostatic systems fail, behavioral maintenance of homeostatic processes is often engaged to sustain life.

Many anecdotal reports describe children, apparently suffering from some sort of nutritional deficiency, who consume seemingly bizarre items to maintain their health. For instance, a child suffering from a calcium deficiency might eat chalk or wallpaper paste in an attempt to ameliorate the calcium shortage. In the recent past, concerned parents admitted such children to the relatively sterile environment of the hospital, where they tragically died because they were no longer able to maintain homeostasis behaviorally (see, for example, Wilkins and Richter, 1940). Even in situations in which the physiological homeostatic systems are undeveloped, homeostasis can be maintained by behavior (recall the behavioral thermoregulation of rat pups described in Chapter 7).

Many homeostatic systems, such as fluid and energy balance, normally require both physiological and behavioral mechanisms to orchestrate a relatively constant internal condition in the face of varying external conditions. Although the physiological mechanisms that mediate homeostatic processes are presented here as isolated events for ease of explanation, it should be remembered that any physiological challenge is met with overlapping, redundant physiological responses. Concurrent physiological and behavioral responses are often mediated or signaled by changes in the release of multiple hormones acting in concert or in opposition. Individual hormones may have multiple physiological and behavioral effects.

This chapter will describe the hormonal and behavioral regulation of several homeostatic systems. Chapters 3–7 have emphasized the parsimonious relationship in which the hormones that mediate physiological reproductive processes have been co-opted during evolution to regulate mating and parental behaviors. Similarly, the hormones associated with physiological homeostatic mechanisms also appear to mediate behaviors critical for homeostatic maintenance. Different species use different hormonal signals to solve similar problems or challenges to their homeostatic processes. In other cases, different species rely on the same hormone to mediate very different solutions to similar problems. For example, female rats and hamsters have evolved two very different ways of coping with the energetic challenges of pregnancy. Rats increase their food intake and gain body fat during pregnancy, while hamsters do not change their food intake appreciably; rather, they utilize most of their established fat stores to meet the energetic demands of pregnancy. The same hormone, progesterone, elicits opposite, but similarly adaptive, responses in these two rodent species.

In this chapter, the conceptual bases of homeostasis will be presented. Then, the interaction among hormones, behavior, and sodium and water balance will be described as a model physiological homeostatic system. The effects of hormones and behavior on energy balance, eating, and body mass maintenance will also be discussed. Finally, the endocrine–behavior interactions controlling specific hungers will be described.

## Basic Concepts in Homeostasis

The archetypal homeostatic device is a thermostatically controlled heating and cooling system. The system in your home is probably controlled by a thermostat (Figure 9.2). A reduction in ambient temperature below the setting on the thermostat (21°C, for example) will activate the furnace, which in turn raises the temperature of the area controlled by the thermostat. When the ambient temperature increases to the "set" temperature, the thermostat shuts off the furnace (an example of negative feedback). If the ambient temperature rises above the set temperature, the cooling system is activated, shutting down if the area becomes too cool. The thermostat acts to keep the room temperature within a relatively narrow range, called the **set point.** The deviation in room temperature from the set point must be one or two degrees before the furnace or air conditioner is activated or turned off; otherwise, the system would be continuously engaging and turning off with only minor changes in temperature.

Similarly, rabbits, humans, and most other mammals maintain an internal body temperature of 37°C, but temperatures in a range between 35° and 38°C are not life-threatening. However, a rapid elevation or reduction in body temperature of just 5°C would seriously endanger the individual. Mammals make physiological, morphological, and behavioral adjustments to maintain body temperature within this relatively narrow range. In common with a thermostat, the optimal set point

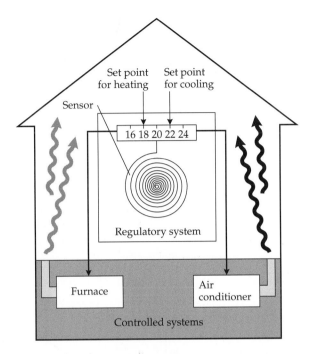

**9.2   The thermostat is a common homeostatic device.** A thermostat has a means to assign a set point and a detector mechanism to determine deviations from the set point and activate corrective measures. In this example, when the temperature decreases sufficiently from the set point, a signal is sent to activate the heating system; conversely, when the temperature increases sufficiently, the cooling system is engaged. Most physiological regulatory systems operate by similar negative feedback control loops.

of an animal can be changed depending on prevailing conditions. As you will learn in Chapter 10, there is a daily program that reduces body temperature significantly during an animal's inactive period, presumably by changing the set point.

When we are ill, our body temperature set point usually changes as well. We often develop a fever, which is an adaptive response, because higher temperatures inactivate or kill the microbial invaders producing the illness. Iguanas provide a good example of this phenomenon. Lizards are poikilothermic, or unable to maintain their body temperature physiologically. A terrarium can be set up in such a way that there is a warm end and a cool end with a relatively smooth temperature gradient in between (Figure 9.3). When healthy lizards were placed in such a terrarium, they settled along the temperature gradient so that their body temperature was 37°C (Kluger, 1978). If the reptiles were infected with bacteria, they *chose* to be feverish; infected lizards positioned themselves in the terrarium so that their body temperatures were elevated a few degrees. In other words, there was a behaviorally mediated change in the set point as a result of the infection. Again, the behavioral generation of a fever has important adaptive consequences. When the infected lizards were prevented from elevating their temperatures, their chances of surviving the infection were reduced (Kluger, 1986). This elegant interplay between physiology and behavior enhances survival.

(a)

Heat source

Terrarium

42°  40°  38°  36°  34°  32°  30°  28°

Temperature gradient (°C)

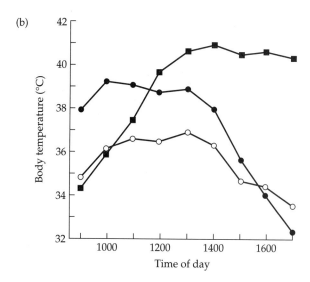

(b)

**9.3  Behavioral thermoregulation in iguanas.**
(a) If an iguana is placed in a terrarium with a
heat source at one end that produces a temperature gradient, it will tend to settle at that
place along the temperature gradient where it
can maintain a body temperature of about
37°C. (b) The behaviorally selected body temperatures of seven green iguanas placed in
such a terrarium over the course of day 1
(open circles); on day 2, after each lizard
received an injection of dead bacteria at 0900
h (solid squares); and on day 3 (solid circles).
Note that the lizards' body temperatures were
raised about 3 hours after the injection and
that the rise persisted until about 1500 h on
day 3. (c) The percentage of iguanas injected
with live bacteria and maintained at temperatures ranging from 34° to 42°C that survived
the treatment; note that the number of animals
surviving is highest at the highest ambient
temperatures. Source: Kluger, 1978.

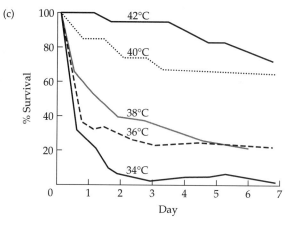

(c)

The thermostat analogy helps us to understand the basic concepts behind homeostasis, but there are several aspects of the control of food and water balance, discussed later in the chapter, that cannot be described adequately by the thermostat analogy. For example, feed-forward mechanisms, anticipation, and learning that occurs with ingestion may modify the basic thermostatic model.

What properties are needed for any system to maintain homeostasis? First, there has to be a *reference value* for the regulated variable (the set point). Second, there must be some sort of *detection mechanism* to detect any deviation from the reference value. Third, the homeostatic system must be able to *mobilize* the organism to make changes that will return the variable to the normal range when deviation occurs. Finally, the detection mechanism must be able to *recognize* when the desired change occurs and shut down the mobilization process through a negative feedback mechanism. Homeostasis requires work, and work requires energy; thus, homeostasis requires energy.

# Fluid Balance

Unicellular creatures living in the ocean rely upon seawater to provide them with the nutrients, oxygen, water, and basic electrolytes (e.g., $Na^+$, $Cl^-$, or $K^+$) necessary to sustain their life processes. These simple animals are at the mercy of the composition and temperature of the seawater; small deviations in water salinity, for instance, may be fatal. To some extent, the evolution of more complex multicellular organisms has required the compartmentalization of "seawater" within the body in the form of extracellular fluid. Essentially, we all carry within us a remnant of the seas in which unicellular organisms evolved—albeit a markedly diluted remnant—to bathe our cells. Homeostatic mechanisms have evolved among multicellular organisms to maintain the composition and temperature of this extracellular fluid at a relatively constant level. The processes regulating intake and excretion of water and sodium, the two main components of extracellular fluid, are closely linked in order to maintain them at ideal levels within relatively narrow ranges. The ability to maintain this relatively constant internal environment despite variable external conditions has allowed the radiation of animals into virtually every niche on the planet. The maintenance of a relatively constant internal environment liberated animals from the sea, or, as Claude Bernard stated, allowed *la vie en liberté,* the free life (Bernard, 1856).

Animals are watery creatures. By weight, mammals are approximately two-thirds water. The proportion of body water varies widely among individuals; in humans, body water content ranges from about 45% to 70% (Rolls and Rolls, 1982). The cells of animals require water for virtually all metabolic processes. Additionally, water serves as a solvent for sodium, chloride, and potassium ions, as well as sugars, amino acids, proteins, vitamins, and many other solutes, and is therefore essential for the smooth functioning of the nervous system and for other physiological processes. Because water participates in so many processes, and because it is continuously lost through perspiration, respiration, urination, and defecation, it must be replaced periodically. Unlike minerals or energy, very little extra water is stored in the body. When water use exceeds water intake, the body conserves water, mainly by reducing the amount of water excreted from the kidneys. Eventually, physiological water conservation can no longer compensate for water use and incidental water loss, and the individual searches for water and drinks. Animals appear to coordinate physiology and behavior so as to maintain body water concentration at some ideal range or set point.

The regulation of sodium intake and of water intake are closely linked to each other (Stricker and Verbalis, 1990b). Part of the reason for this is the way in which the kidney uses sodium to conserve water (Box 9.1). But sodium is also important in the movement of water between the two major compartments in the body; namely, the extracellular and the intracellular compartments. Approximately two-thirds of the total body fluid content is located in the intracellular compartment. The extracellular compartment comprises two separate but interacting parts: (1) the interstitial (between the cells) fluid and (2) the blood plasma. Of the one-third of the total body fluid content located in the extracellular compartment, about 7% is in the blood plasma and 26% is in the interstitial fluid (Figure 9.4). The distinction between the intracellular and extracellular compartments is not merely one of location. The fluids in the two compartments are fundamentally different in composition. Most of the body's sodium and chloride ions are located in the extracellular compartment, whereas most of the potassium ions are located in the intracellular compartment. The differences in fluid composition result from the properties of the cell membranes and blood vessel walls.

Mechanisms exist to balance both the intracellular and extracellular fluid levels. After mammals ingest water, most of it leaves the large intestine and eventually flows into one of the body's fluid compartments, which are separated by membranes. The blood vessel (capillary) walls act as a barrier between the plasma and the interstitial fluid, and permit the flow of all constituents of the plasma except protein into the interstitial fluid. Cell membranes are the barriers between the extracellular and the intracellular fluid compartments. A number of physiological mechanisms are engaged to maintain the extracellular–intracellular differences in sodium and potassium concentrations.

In order to understand the dynamics between sodium and water, and how they affect the behavioral manifestations of thirst, it is necessary to review the concepts of osmolality, osmoregulation, and the regulation of blood plasma volume. Water can pass freely through semipermeable biological membranes, but many solutes, chemical substances dissolved in the solvent (water), cannot. When one compartment has a greater concentration of solutes than the other, the solvent will

**9.4  Body fluid is maintained in separate, but interacting, compartments.** Approximately 33% of the total body fluid content is located outside of the cells, about 7% in the blood plasma and 26% in the remaining interstitial fluid. The other two-thirds of the total body fluid content is located inside the cells.

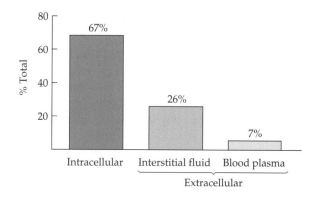

## Box 9.1
# Vertebrate Renal Function

The kidneys are remarkable organs. The human kidneys filter about 30 liters of blood each hour. About 1% of this filtrate is removed as waste and sent to the bladder for elimination. The rest of the blood plasma is reabsorbed in the kidney and returned to the circulation. The kidneys contribute to maintaining fluid balance by either conserving water or eliminating excess water, depending on the body's needs.

The functional unit of the kidney, the nephron, is where the reabsorption of water occurs (see figure). There are about a million nephrons in each human kidney. As the filtrate passes into the nephron at high pressure, it enters a long, convoluted tubule that comprises several sections, each with a specific function: the proximal tubule; the loop of Henle, with its descending and ascending limbs; the distal tubule; and the collecting duct. Water flows passively out of the descending limb into the surrounding tissue, and sodium ions enter because there is a high concentration of sodi-

um in the surrounding regions. The sodium concentration of the filtrate is greatest at the bottom of the loop of Henle; in humans the concentration is about 2%. As the filtrate moves out of the loop into the ascending limb, the sodium is actively pumped out. The ascending limb is impervious to water, so water cannot passively follow the sodium into the surrounding tissue. The filtrate is thus extremely dilute as it leaves the ascending limb of the loop of Henle. As it enters the distal tubule it flows into the surrounding tissue and then into the capillaries by osmosis. The waste filtrate flows into the collecting duct, and eventually moves to the bladder to be voided.

Vasopressin, or antidiuretic hormone (ADH), conserves water by acting on the distal tubules to increase their permeability to water and hence return more water to the circulation. Without ADH, the distal tubules become less permeable, resulting in diuresis, an increase in the amount of water eliminated in the urine.

tend to distribute itself so that the solute concentration on both sides of the membrane is equalized (Figure 9.5). In other words, water moves across the biological membrane to the compartment that has the higher concentration of solutes. The movement of water across a semipermeable membrane into a more concentrated solution is called **osmosis.** The concentration of solutes in a solution is its **osmolality,** and the control of this osmotic concentration is called **osmoregulation.**

Table salt—sodium chloride—is an example of a solute that cannot pass easily through biological membranes. (Although chloride can move in and out of cells, it tends to stay outside cells because it has a negative charge and is attracted to the positively charged sodium ions dissolved in the interstitial fluid.) In most cases, the body's extracellular fluid contains about 8.5 g of sodium chloride per liter, or stated differently, a 0.85% concentration of sodium chloride; this concentration is called physiological, isotonic, normal, or 0.9% saline. If an isotonic saline solution is injected into an animal, it has no effect, because it does not change the concentration of sodium chloride in the animal's interstitial fluid. However, an injection of hypertonic saline, a solution in which the concentration of sodium chloride exceeds 0.9%, will increase the sodium chloride concentration in the interstitial fluid. The resulting increase in interstitial osmolality draws water out of the cells, thus inducing cellular dehydration, a potent stimulus for thirst (Figure 9.6). This type of thirst is called **osmotic thirst,** and is an experience that is well known to anyone who has consumed salty foods. Consumption of sugary foods also causes osmotic thirst because the excess glucose molecules in the interstitial space also pull water out of cells and induce cellular dehydration.

Vasopressin acts to conserve water as blood moves through the kidneys (see Box 9.1). If more water is consumed than needed, plasma osmolality is decreased. Reduced plasma osmolality inhibits thirst and suppresses the release of vasopressin from the posterior pituitary. Inhibition of vasopressin release causes diuresis in the kidney: water is lost from the blood plasma and sent to the bladder for elimination.

In addition to the osmoregulatory mechanisms that regulate intracellular and interstitial fluid balance, a second important fluid regulatory system maintains

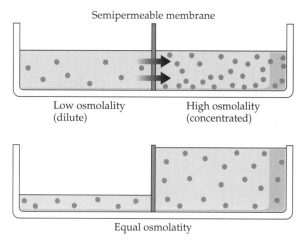

**9.5  Osmosis.** The differences in composition of the different fluid compartments of the body are the result of properties of the cell membranes and blood vessel walls. If compartments containing a dilute and a concentrated solution are separated by a membrane that allows only water to pass through, water will flow into the concentrated compartment until the osmotic pressure between the compartments becomes equal.

Semipermeable membrane

Low osmolality
(dilute)

High osmolality
(concentrated)

Equal osmolatity

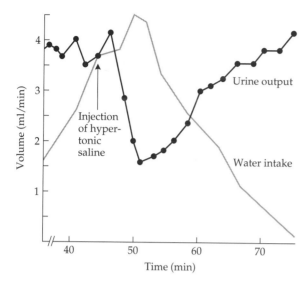

**9.6 Osmotic thirst.** An injection of hypertonic saline, a solution of saline in which the concentration of sodium chloride exceeds 0.9%, will increase the sodium chloride concentration in the interstitial fluid. The resulting increase in plasma osmolality draws water out of the cells, thus inducing cellular dehydration and osmotic thirst, and resulting in increased water intake. Source: Stricker and Verbalis, 1990b.

blood plasma volume. Reduction of blood volume produces a potent stimulus for thirst. This type of thirst is called **hypovolemic thirst,** and it is manifested in the extreme by individuals experiencing hemorrhage; excessive perspiration, diarrhea, or heavy menstrual bleeding can also trigger volemic thirst (Stricker et al., 1987). Volemic and osmotic thirst differ in several important respects. During **hypovolemia,** or low blood volume, water, salts, and other solutes are lost without necessarily pulling water out of the cells. Quenching osmotic thirst merely requires the ingestion of water, but alleviating hypovolemic thirst requires replacement of water, sodium, and other solutes (Figure 9.7).

There are two major ways to induce hypovolemic thirst experimentally. Inflicting a controlled hemorrhage has been the traditional method of causing hypovolemic thirst in animals; however, only acute behavioral changes can be studied with this method. In order to study gradual, long-term changes in behavior, another technique was developed that has been very useful in the study of hormonal effects on thirst and drinking behavior (Stricker, 1968). In this technique, polyethylene glycol (PEG) is injected under the skin of animals. Because PEG is a relatively large colloidal molecule, it cannot cross the blood capillary membranes, and thus remains in the interstitial fluid. The colloidal particles cause an "equiosmotic" sequestration of fluid; that is, both water and solutes are removed from the body fluids, reducing blood plasma volume without significant changes in blood solute content or induction of severe hypotension. The degree of hypovolemia is directly related to the amount of colloidal material injected. When subcutaneous injections of PEG are given to rats, individuals begin drinking 1 or 2 hours later, when their plasma deficits approach 5%, and they continue to drink in short bouts for several hours thereafter (Stricker and Verbalis, 1988).

Hypovolemia compromises kidney function. The reduced blood volume and resulting low blood pressure prevents the kidneys from extracting water effectively. Consequently, hypovolemic rats consume water, but cannot completely correct their blood plasma volume because the ingested water enters all of their

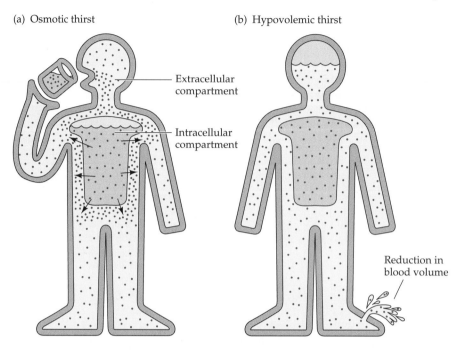

(a) Osmotic thirst          (b) Hypovolemic thirst

Extracellular compartment

Intracellular compartment

Reduction in blood volume

**9.7    Two types of thirst result from different osmotic conditions.**    Osmotic thirst is caused by cellular dehydration—which can occur after ingesting a salty snack or drink—when increased interstitial osmolality occurs and draws water out of the intracellular compartment. Water quenches osmotic thirst. Hypovolemic thirst is caused by the loss of fluids and solutes—such as after hemorrhage. Replacement of both water and solutes is necessary to quench hypovolemic thirst.

fluid compartments. The resulting combination of body fluid dilution and reduced water removal by the kidneys results in reduced blood plasma osmolality, a potent stimulus to stop drinking. Consequently, the rats stop drinking before attaining normal fluid balance. A hypovolemic individual requires salt to restore body fluid osmolality to normal levels. If given access to salt water or salty food, a hypovolemic rat will ingest the proper combination of water and salt to restore blood volume and osmolality to normal levels. Similarly, athletes often ingest salty beverages such as Gatorade after heavy perspiration when they are experiencing hypovolemic thirst. During the normal course of events—that is, during minor dehydration—the experience of thirst is a psychological manifestation of both osmotic and blood volume changes.

 **Thirst** is defined here as a motivation to seek and ingest water (Stricker and Verbalis, 1988; Fitzsimons, 1998). Because thirst is a psychological hypothetical construct, we cannot measure it directly, but can infer it from behavior. In nonhuman animals, the degree of thirst can be operationally determined by the amount of effort an individual expends to drink. Individuals will work harder and endure greater noxious stimuli to obtain water as the length of water deprivation increases. Investigations of human thirst allow the added dimension of verbal reports; people can be asked to rate and describe their thirst (Figure 9.8). In humans, sev-

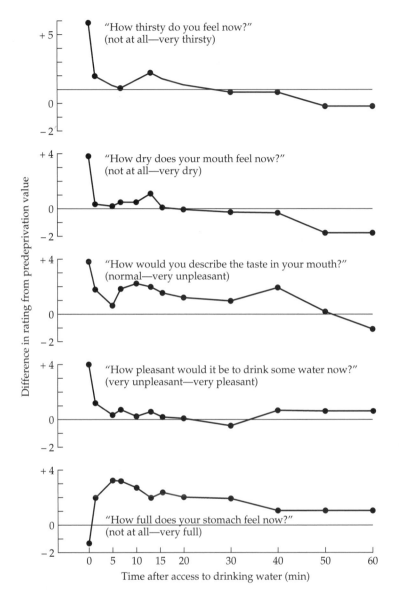

**9.8    Rating of thirst after water deprivation.** A rating scale can be used by human subjects to provide a measure of thirst and other sensations associated with fluid intake. Subjects were deprived of water for 24 hours, then asked to rate their thirst after access to drinking water, and their ratings were compared to their ratings on the same measures before they were deprived of water. Within 5 minutes of drinking, their thirst sensations were ameliorated, and the subjects reported that their stomachs felt full. Source: Rolls and Rolls, 1982.

eral parameters of thirst can be identified and described. For example, water-deprived humans rate the taste of water as more pleasant than do people who are not water-deprived (Rolls and Rolls, 1982).

### Endocrine Regulation of Fluid Balance and Thirst

Vasopressin (ADH) acts on the renal tubules to retain water (see Box 9.1). Occasionally, a genetic error occurs in humans or rats so that ADH is not produced. Individuals lacking ADH suffer from diabetes insipidus (*diabetes*, "run through"; *insipidus*, "weak"), a condition that forces them to ingest copious amounts of water because they are almost constantly urinating. Essentially, all of the extracellular fluid is lost each day and must be replaced. Rats with this mutation, known as Brattleboro rats, urinate 200 ml/day and must drink about that amount daily to maintain their fluid balance. If these rats are injected with ADH, their water intake and urine output drop to the normal levels of about 20 and 15 ml/day, respectively (Figure 9.9).

Two types of stimuli associated with the need to balance body fluids normally evoke the release of ADH from the posterior pituitary. One of these stimuli is the intracellular dehydration of cerebral osmoreceptors. Although virtually all cells in the body shrink in size as water moves into the interstitial space during osmotic dehydration, only these particular cells in the brain signal this condition to the paraventricular (PVN) and supraoptic nuclei (SON) of the hypothalamus, where vasopressin is made. These osmoreceptors are generally located in several brain structures located near the third ventricle, including the lateral preoptic area of the hypothalamus, the subfornical organ, and the organum vasculosum of the lamina terminalis (OVLT) as well as in the area postrema (Figure 9.10). Two different messages are sent from these cerebral osmoreceptors in response to different levels of dehydration. A signal to release ADH from the posterior pituitary occurs in response to mild cellular dehydration. If dehydration persists after maximal reclamation of water has been achieved in the kidneys, then a second signal from the brain osmoreceptors stimulates drinking behavior. This dual control allows physiological water-saving systems to be engaged prior to behavioral responses and thus frees individuals from the need to drink frequently. ADH does not inhibit drinking behavior directly; rather, it causes the kidneys to retain water,

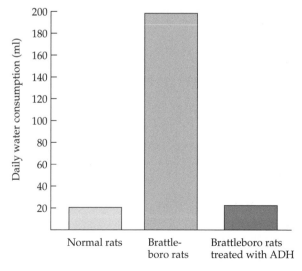

**9.9  Vasopressin (ADH) mediates water consumption.** Normal rats drink about 20 ml of water per day, but rats of the Brattleboro strain, which congenitally lack ADH, drink nearly 10 times as much water and also excrete about 10 times the volume of urine of normal rats. After ADH treatment, Brattleboro rats display normal levels of water consumption and urinary output.

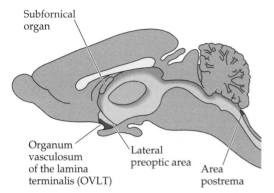

Subfornical organ

Organum vasculosum of the lamina terminalis (OVLT)

Lateral preoptic area

Area postrema

**9.10   Brain structures involved in the mediation of thirst and water intake.** Cerebral osmoreceptor cells respond to dehydration and shrinkage by signaling the paraventricular and supraoptic nuclei to synthesize vasopressin. These osmoreceptors are found in the circumventricular organs seen in this schematic drawing of a mid-sagittal section of the rat brain: the subfornical organ, the area postrema, the organum vasculosum of the lamina terminalis (OVLT), and the lateral preoptic area of the hypothalamus.

which decreases blood plasma osmolality. Reduced plasma osmolality, in turn, inhibits drinking.

Another stimulus that triggers the release of vasopressin is a reduction of blood plasma volume. A loss of blood volume is detected by stretch receptors, called baroreceptors, in the walls of the cardiac blood vessels. These receptors signal the PVN and SON to release vasopressin, which acts as a vasoconstrictor to increase blood pressure (Gauer and Henry, 1963). Hence, the same hormone has two distinct, but related, functions that work in concert when blood pressure drops, and possesses two common names: *antidiuretic hormone,* referring to its effect on the kidneys (and which explains the abbreviation ADH), and *vasopressin,* referring to its effect on the blood vessels. The cardiac baroreceptors also signal the brain directly via the vagus nerve* to stimulate thirst. A diagram of the regulation of fluid intake behavior is depicted in Figure 9.11.

Hypovolemia also stimulates the formation of another potent vasoconstrictor, **angiotensin.** Angiotensin is a hormone that comes from an unusual source: the blood. Because angiotensin is not produced in any endocrine gland, it is often considered a *parahormone.* In any case, a drop in blood pressure during hypovolemia stimulates the brain to signal the kidneys to make an enzyme called renin; the kidneys can also make renin in response to low blood pressure without any neural input. Renin converts a blood-borne substance called angiotensinogen into the various forms of angiotensin, including angiotensin II, the form involved in this response (Figure 9.12). The role of angiotensin in drinking behavior is controversial. In rats, systemic injections of angiotensin (Fitzsimons and Simons, 1969), or injections directly into the subfornical organ (Simpson et al., 1978), increase drinking behavior. However, the doses of angiotensin required to elicit drinking are much higher than the levels of this hormone produced naturally in response to hypovolemia (Stricker, 1978). Furthermore, removal of the kidneys, the source of renin, does not interfere with drinking behavior in response to hypovolemia in rats (Fitzsimons, 1961).

Despite the controversy surrounding the role of angiotensin in regulating thirst, it is well known that this parahormone also stimulates the release of aldosterone from the zona glomerulosa of the adrenal gland. As we saw above, aldosterone is another hormone critical for maintaining fluid balance. Aldosterone

*The vagus (Latin for "wandering") nerve is one of the cranial nerves that make up part of the peripheral nervous system (PNS). It extends far from the head and innervates the heart, lungs, digestive tract, and liver, carrying information between these organs and the CNS.

**9.11    Schematic model of fluid regulation** showing the major organs and regulatory systems involved in maintaining fluid balance in mammals. Source: Rosenzweig et al., 1999.

promotes the retention of sodium in the kidney by stimulating the sodium pump in the ascending limb of the loop of Henle (see Box 9.1). The resulting retention of sodium at high concentrations in the kidneys causes water to be reabsorbed from the blood as it flows through the nephron, and thereby reduces the amount of water sent to the bladder for excretion. Without aldosterone, enormous amounts of water—approximately 30 liters per day in humans—and sodium—about 200 mmol/liter per day—would be lost in the urine.

Pharmacological tools have revealed two distinct types of angiotensin receptors in the brain, type 1 and type 2. Using specific receptor antagonists, it was discovered that only the type 1, and not the type 2, receptors are the primary

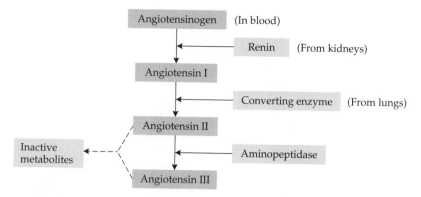

**9.12   Synthesis of angiotensin in humans.** The drop in blood pressure that occurs during hypovolemia initiates the formation of the potent vasoconstrictor angiotensin by stimulating the brain to signal the kidneys to make renin. Renin is an enzyme that converts the blood-borne substance angiotensinogen to three forms of angiotensin: angiotensin I, II, and III. Angiotensin II is the most biologically potent of the angiotensins, but all three exert some effects on water and sodium balance. The kidneys can also make renin in response to low blood pressure without any neural input. After Ganong, 1993.

mediators of angiotensin II-related thirst and sodium intake (Fluharty and Sakai, 1995). Furthermore, intracerebroventricular (icv) administration of angiotensin type 1 receptor antisense oligodeoxynucleotides diminishes drinking behavior in rats (Sakai et al., 1995). Using the antisense technique, it was also discovered that icv administration of mineralocorticoid receptor antisense oligonucleotides reduces sodium appetite in rats (Ma et al., 1997; Sakai et al., 1996) (Figure 9.13). The effects of antisense oligonucleotides that target either the angiotensin or aldosterone receptors demonstrate the role of endogenous angiotensin II and mineralocorticoid in mediating these two types of ingestion, as well as the importance of their actions in the central nervous system.

## Sodium Balance

Humans that consume modern diets and animals maintained on commercial laboratory diets—both of which provide plenty of sodium—have a relatively large reservoir of sodium in the interstitial fluid. This sodium reserve probably serves to buffer the brain from wide fluctuations in sodium availability during large variations in daily sodium intake and loss. When the sodium reservoir is depleted, individuals are motivated to seek and ingest sodium. Sustained sodium deprivation interferes with neural functioning and can rapidly lead to death. The detectors for blood levels of sodium appear to be located in the brain (Andersson et al., 1995; Stricker and Verbalis, 1990b; Weisinger et al, 1982).

Herbivores obtain all of their sodium and much of their water from the plants that they eat. Because there is a wide range of sodium content in plants, herbivores may be exposed to wide variations in sodium availability. Carnivores are not usually under the same sodium pressures as herbivores because the animals that they consume have maintained a relatively consistent sodium level. Es-

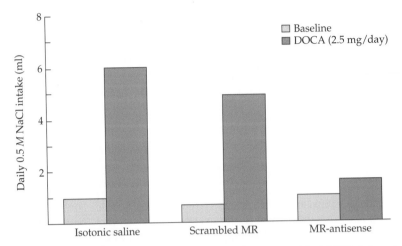

**9.13 Antisense oligonucleotides for mineralocorticoid receptors** block DOCA-induced elevation in saline intake. Deoxycorticosterone acetate (DOCA) (a synthetic mineralocorticoid with about 3% aldosterone activity) causes an increase in salt appetite when injected systemically as shown by the increase in saline ingestion. If the animals are infused with isotonic saline or scrambled mineralocorticoid receptor (MR) mRNA into the amygdala and treated with systemic DOCA, then saline intake is unaffected. If animals are treated with MR-antisense infusion, then saline intake is reduced. After Sakai et al., 1996.

sentially, carnivores have the problem of excreting sodium after a meal because their meals tend to be sodium-rich, whereas herbivores are adapted to retain sodium and excrete potassium after their meals.

Recall that European rabbits in Australia are confronted with environments that vary substantially in sodium availability. These rabbits must cope with these variations in sodium availability in order to survive and reproduce. Rabbits inhabiting the Snowy Mountains in Australia are exposed to an environment that is extremely low in sodium; analyses of the soil and plants in this alpine region revealed a profound lack of sodium (Blair-West et al., 1968). The rain is virtually free of sodium, and the spring snowmelt further reduces sodium availability by leaching it deeper into the ground. In contrast, the food plants of rabbits living in the harsh desert of central Australia are very high in sodium content. Similarly, rabbits inhabiting ocean coastal regions in Victoria are exposed to relatively high levels of sodium in plants because of the high concentrations of sodium in the coastal rain. Researchers have observed differences among the rabbits in these three regions in the quantities of water consumed and urine produced, as well as in other physiological parameters (Table 9.1).

The Australian rabbits occupying opposite ends of the sodium availability continuum are faced with a situation analogous to that of freshwater versus saltwater fishes. Saltwater fishes are essentially bags of fresh water surrounded by a concentrated saltwater solution. There is a high osmotic gradient favoring the movement of sodium ions into these fish, but they have evolved mechanisms to keep sodium out and to remove it from their bodies efficiently. Conversely, freshwater fishes are essentially bags of saline surrounded by dilute water, which cre-

Table 9.1
**Comparison of sodium regulatory indices
of rabbits living in three different habitats in Australia**

| Habitat | Na⁺ in urine (mmol/l) | Aldosterone (ng/100 ml) | Adrenal mass (g) | Zona glomerulosa size (as % of total adrenal cortex) |
|---|---|---|---|---|
| Snowy Mountains | 0.53 | 69.0 | 0.12 | 22.6 |
| Coast | 18.00 | 21.0 | 0.11 | 15.6 |
| Desert | 139.00 | 9.0 | 0.13 | 15.3 |

*Source:* Blair-West et al., 1968.

ates an osmotic gradient favoring the movement of sodium out of the fish. Freshwater fishes have evolved effective sodium-retaining mechanisms to combat sodium depletion.

Modern bony fishes are called teleost fishes, and are thought to have evolved in fresh water, then radiated to environments with vastly different degrees of salinity. Some fishes, termed *stenohaline,* have adapted to specific saline environments and cannot tolerate salinities beyond very specific ranges. In contrast, *euryhaline* species can tolerate wide ranges of salinity. Euryhaline fishes in nature may be exclusively saltwater fishes (for example, the starry flounder, *Platichthes stellatus*), exclusively freshwater fishes (for example, the tilapia, *Sarotherodon mossambicus*), or capable of exploiting their tolerance for a wide range of environmental salinities by migrating between salt water and fresh water (for example, Pacific salmon, *Oncorhynchus* sp., or Atlantic eels, *Anguilla* sp.). Those euryhaline fishes, such as salmon and eels, that move between fresh and salt water rely on hormones—most notably, prolactin, cortisol, and thyroid hormone—to adapt to their changing sodium requirements, and their ability to survive these changes involves a complex interaction among reproductive maturity, day length, and hormonal responses. The extent to which changing hormone levels themselves induce migration or are secondary to other maturational factors remains somewhat controversial.

The Australian rabbits are confronted with the same basic problem as fishes; namely, how to survive in habitats with markedly different sodium availabilities. Several physiological adaptations are evident in rabbits living in sodium-poor habitats. Snowy Mountains rabbits excrete very little sodium in their urine, although there is a notable seasonal cycle of average urinary sodium excretion, which is greater in winter than in summer (Table 9.2). Average blood plasma concentrations of aldosterone mirror the seasonal urinary sodium excretion cycle, as does the average proportion of the adrenal gland made up by the zona glomerulosa, which varies nearly 50% in size. What is the reason for these seasonal variations? During spring and summer, the rapid growth of lush plants further reduces sodium concentrations per gram of plant material in the Snowy Mountains region. Herbivores living under these conditions must consume enormous quantities of food to maintain sodium at a level consistent with proper physiological functioning. Pregnancy and lactation increase this demand even further. During the spring and summer, rabbits living in the alpine regions of Australia display an avid salt appetite. When wooden pegs impregnated with various salts are

Table 9.2
**Seasonal changes in sodium regulatory indices
of rabbits inhabiting the Snowy Mountains of Australia**

| Season | $Na^+$ in urine (mmol/l) | Aldosterone (ng/100 ml) | Adrenal mass (g) | Zona glomerulosa size (as % of total adrenal cortex) |
|---|---|---|---|---|
| Spring | 0.59 | 130.0 | 0.18 | 34.4 |
| Summer | 0.53 | 69.0 | 0.12 | 22.6 |
| Autumn | 2.60 | — | 0.14 | 17.3 |
| Winter | 6.40 | 74.0 | 0.14 | 17.8 |

*Source:* Blair-West et al., 1968.

made available to the rabbits, they clearly prefer NaCl and $NaHCO_3$, but they will also ingest $MgCl_2$ and KCl in smaller amounts (Figure 9.14; Myers, 1967). Thus, these animals possess physiological, morphological, and behavioral adaptations to obtain and to conserve sodium.

In contrast to Snowy Mountains rabbits, rabbits living in the desert inhabit a sodium-rich environment, and their physiological challenge is to limit sodium intake and reduce sodium levels in their bodies. These animals excrete consistently high levels of sodium throughout the year, and have concomitant low plasma aldosterone levels (see Table 9.1). The zona glomerulosa makes up only about 15% of the adrenal cortex. Rabbits living in desert or seashore habitats were never observed to ingest salt from salt licks provided by experimenters.

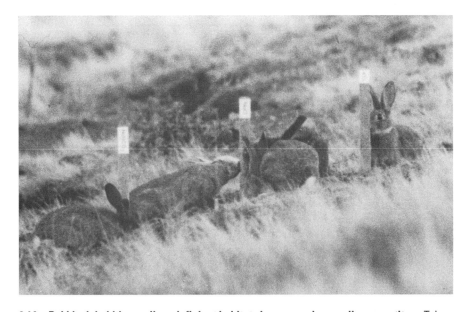

**9.14    Rabbits inhabiting sodium-deficient habitats have voracious sodium appetites.** Telescopic photograph showing rabbits living in sodium-deficient alpine regions of Australia devouring wooden pegs impregnated with sodium. Rabbits in sodium-rich habitats are never observed ingesting sodium-treated pegs.

Regardless of sodium availability in the environment, each rabbit (and every other mammal, including you) must maintain the sodium levels in its body within precise limits. In rabbits and humans, sodium levels are maintained between 135–145 mmol/liter in the blood plasma. Obviously, animals living in sodium-rich habitats must excrete excess sodium to maintain blood sodium levels in the optimal range, whereas animals living in low-sodium environments must avoid losing precious sodium. Australian rabbits provide an example of how physiology, morphology, and behavior are linked to bring about fluid balance and maintain homeostasis.

Although many animals are generalists to some extent, most animals have evolved to inhabit specific environmental niches. Some animals have evolved in habitats that regularly experience sodium shortages, whereas others have evolved where sodium is plentiful. Like rats, golden hamsters (*Mesocricetus auratus*) will perish if subjected to bilateral adrenalectomy. Unlike adrenalectomized rats, however, adrenalectomized hamsters provided with salt water to drink will refuse it and die. Hamsters survive adrenalectomy only if provided with a solution of saline mixed with saccharin. Apparently, the sweet taste of saccharin masks the salty taste of the saline. When provided with a choice between a saccharin solution and a salt water solution, adrenalectomized hamsters will drink the saccharin solution exclusively and invariably perish. Do these facts indicate that hamsters are less intelligent than rats? No. These puzzling results are immediately reasonable in light of the fact that golden hamsters evolved in the desert, where sodium levels are high and water is scarce. They have evolved physiological and behavioral strategies to avoid sodium. It is unlikely that hamsters have ever had a need during their evolution to ingest sodium; consequently, behavioral homeostatic strategies in response to sodium loss from the kidneys are not available to this species. The difference in salt appetite between rats, rabbits, and humans on the one hand and hamsters on the other demonstrates the importance of understanding the evolutionary history of the animals in question when trying to understand the complex web of physiological and behavioral interactions mediating homeostatic processes.

Kangaroo rats (*Dipodomys merriami*) are desert rodents that rarely have access to water in their native habitat and probably never drink it if they do find it. Their water needs are met by chemically liberating water from the seeds they eat. Kangaroo rats have evolved to conserve water very effectively; they rarely urinate, and when they do, the urine is highly concentrated. These small rodents have the longest kidney tubules of any mammal, which accounts for their extreme efficiency in retaining water. Another mammal that has an unusual method of obtaining water is the elephant seal (*Mirounga angustirostris*). During their 4- to 5-month mating season, elephant seals engage in territorial and reproductive behaviors along the shoreline, but do not eat or drink. All the water they need is liberated metabolically by hydrolysis of their substantial fat reserves. Elephant seals, like other marine mammals, have evolved to live in the sea, but their adaptation is limited in that they are no more capable of surviving on seawater than humans. During the nonbreeding season, they get all their water from the fish they consume (LeBoeuf, 1974). Kangaroo rats and elephant seals have adapted to their particular niches over the course of many eons of evolution. The rabbits invading Australia have not been there very long (in evolutionary time), and new mechanisms to balance water and sodium use have yet to evolve; consequently, behavioral adaptations, mediated in part by hormones, are critical for their continued survival.

### How Do Hormones Regulate Drinking Behavior?

The hormones that maintain fluid balance interact with the sensory systems, or input systems, associated with water intake. In a typical study of these interactions, an animal is given a choice between two different drinking bottles (Figure 9.15). For example, a rat may be given a choice between tap water and a normal saline solution. The rat's fluid intake is measured daily, and a preference is calculated. For example, a rat might ingest 8 ml of water and 12 ml of saline during a single 24-hour period. In this case, we would say that saline is preferred over tap water by 67% (8/12). To examine the nature of this preference, the saline could be diluted by half to a 0.45% sodium concentration. If the rat still drinks more of the diluted saline than the tap water, an inference is made that the animal can detect the difference between the two and has a preference. In this manner, a **preference threshold** can be determined by serial dilutions. The preference threshold is the lowest concentration at which preference for the solution over water can be maintained. Obviously, animals will display different preference thresholds for different substances; for example, the preference threshold for sucrose and for sodium solutions is different among most individuals. The **detection threshold** is the concentration at which the animal can tell the difference between solutions. These two parameters are not necessarily identical. Note in Figure 9.15 that the detection threshold for sodium is not different for adrenalectomized and intact animals, although the sodium-deficient animals drink more sodium at low and high concentrations. Adrenal-intact rats can discriminate among different low-sodium concentrations in a test in which they must do so to avoid electric shocks. Presumably, the differences among low sodium solutions make a difference only

**9.15 Adrenalectomy affects saline preference thresholds.** The concentration at which an animal responds differently to different solutions is called the detection threshold. Normal rats (solid line) prefer about a 1% solution of saline over water (the preference threshold), but as the concentration of sodium increases, the rats' preference changes to plain water (the aversion threshold). The shaded line plots the saline preference pattern for adrenalectomized rats, which lack aldosterone. Note that adrenalectomized rats tolerate sodium solutions that normal rats or people would find extremely unpleasant; this change in sodium tolerance helps the adrenalectomized animal maintain behavioral homeostasis.

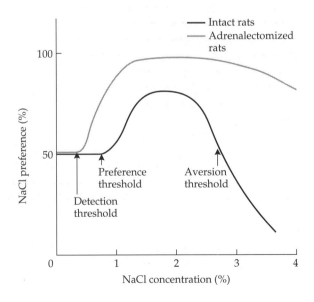

to the adrenalectomized animals. Interestingly, the sensory neurons from the mouth of an adrenalectomized rat reduce their firing rate when sodium is applied to the tongue. Perhaps this is why adrenalectomized rats are able to ingest such high, normally aversive, concentrations of salt.

The hormones associated with fluid balance also mediate behavior by acting on the central processing systems. As described above, during mild cellular dehydration, vasopressin affects central drinking mechanisms indirectly by causing the kidneys to retain water, which results in reduced blood plasma osmolality; reduced plasma osmolality inhibits drinking. After persistent dehydration, vasopressin, aldosterone, and angiotensin II all increase drinking behavior by acting directly or indirectly on the central nervous system. Aldosterone stimulates sodium retention by the kidney and thus maintains osmotic balance, but aldosterone affects drinking behavior only indirectly via its influence on osmotic thirst. Aldosterone may act directly on the CNS to regulate sodium appetite in conjunction with angiotensin. Pharmacological doses of angiotensin elicit drinking behavior, presumably by acting on the subfornical organ in the brain (Simpson et al., 1978; Zigmond et al., 1991). The output systems, the effectors, of water ingestion are essentially unaffected by hormones. Hormones do not appear to increase the efficiency of water intake or otherwise affect the output systems of drinking behavior in any appreciable way.

## Energy Balance

Animals eat to meet the needs of the structural part of the body; that is, to obtain the raw materials to make bone, muscle, and other structures. Animals also eat to obtain energy. All cellular processes require fuel to keep them going. The central nervous system requires substantial energy to function properly. Furthermore, all the vital systems require energy to carry out their functions. Despite this common need for energy, there are fluctuations in the energy requirements of every individual, as the rate of energy utilization varies throughout the day as well as over the seasons. There are also fluctuations in energy acquisition. Eating tends to be episodic, even though the need for energy is more or less continuous (Stricker and Verbalis, 1988). Accordingly, energy acquisition and energy expenditure are never quite balanced. Individuals cannot eat continuously to meet moment-to-moment changes in energy demands; they must occasionally sleep, mate, or hunt for food. Also, food availability is not constant; there are seasonal and daily cycles in food availability. All of this leads to a dynamic relationship between energy acquisition and energy expenditure. When more food is consumed than required, the excess energy is stored in the form of **adipose tissue,** or fat. This stored energy is later tapped when the steady delivery of metabolic fuel from the intestines wanes.

As animals fluctuate between a well-fed and a fasting state, correlated changes occur in the secretion of hormones, neurotransmitters, and neuromodulators. In chronically well-fed animals, blood concentrations of glucose, amino acids, insulin, and leptin are all relatively high; furthermore, body fat stores, lipogenic enzymes, and liver glycogen are also elevated. In contrast, these animals have relatively low blood concentrations of glucagon, glucocorticoids, free fatty acids, lipolytic enzymes, ketone bodies, and hypothalamic concentrations of neuropeptide Y, corticotropin releasing factor, and catecholamines. Among fasting animals, the relative concentrations of all these substances are reversed (Schneider and Wade, in press).

### Metabolism during the Well-Fed State

After a meal, there are two phases of energy utilization and storage: (1) the postprandial phase and (2) the postabsorptive phase. The metabolic interactions that occur in a well-fed individual are outlined in Figure 9.16. The postprandial phase occurs immediately after the ingestion of food. When you eat a meal, a supply of **metabolic fuels**, in the form of simple sugars (e.g., glucose), fatty acids, ketones, and amino acids, enters the bloodstream almost immediately. Unless you are running a marathon immediately after eating, there tends to be an energy surplus after a meal. The excess energy is stored during the postabsorptive phase, and the protein hormone insulin acts to promote such storage. In doing so, insulin lowers the levels of metabolic fuels in the blood.

During the postabsorptive phase, insulin secretion rises while glucagon secretion falls. In the liver, insulin stimulates the conversion of glucose to glycogen, a stored form of sugar. Insulin also facilitates the transport of glucose into muscle

**Well-fed state**

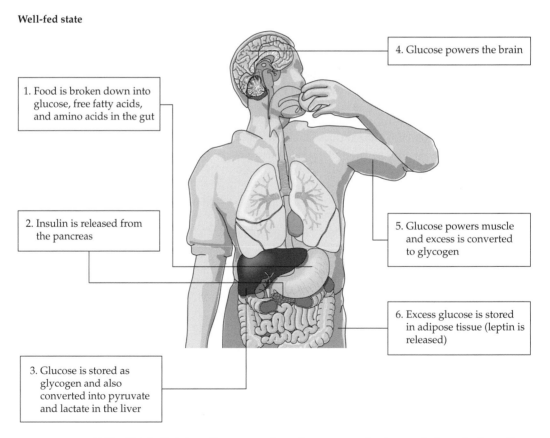

1. Food is broken down into glucose, free fatty acids, and amino acids in the gut

2. Insulin is released from the pancreas

3. Glucose is stored as glycogen and also converted into pyruvate and lactate in the liver

4. Glucose powers the brain

5. Glucose powers muscle and excess is converted to glycogen

6. Excess glucose is stored in adipose tissue (leptin is released)

**9.16   Metabolic interactions among the major components of energy balance in the well-fed state.** After Schneider and Wade, in press.

and fat cells, as well as the transport of amino acids into muscle cells. In peripheral cells, insulin is necessary for glucose oxidation and lipogenesis, processes that result in the storage of fat in adipose tissue. Insulin also prevents the breakdown of glycogen in both muscle and liver cells, as well as the mobilization of fats from adipose tissue. While insulin is the sole hormone responsible for energy storage in vertebrates, many other hormones play a role in energy metabolism. These hormones, which include epinephrine, norepinephrine, glucocorticoids, thyroid hormones, growth hormone, somatomedin, and glucagon, are mainly involved in removing energy from storage.

There are two phases of insulin release: the cephalic phase and the gastrointestinal (GI) phase. During the cephalic phase, a neurally triggered release of insulin from the pancreatic β-cells occurs as a result of the sensory stimuli associated with food intake (Steffens et al., 1990). So even before any new nutrients have arrived in the digestive system, an insulin-induced reduction in blood levels of metabolic fuels may cause an increase in hunger. You have probably experienced the cephalic phase of insulin release when the sights or smells of a favorite meal caused you to feel noticeably more hungry. The primary storage of excess nutrients taken in during a meal occurs in the GI phase, when insulin is released in response to the absorption of nutrients from the gut.

Problems with getting energy into storage are common. Again, insulin is the major actor in this physiological drama, and many metabolic difficulties occur if there are any problems with insulin release. Diabetes mellitus (*diabetes*, "run through"; *mellitus*, "sweet") is a syndrome resulting from insufficient insulin secretion. Individuals with this condition cannot move the surplus energy of a meal into storage; in other words, diabetics cannot make fat. Consequently, extremely high levels of glucose remain in the blood, a condition that is commonly known as high blood sugar. Some of this excess glucose is excreted in the urine, giving the urine of diabetics a characteristic sweetness. The brain does not require insulin to utilize glucose, and can function normally in the absence of insulin. The liver essentially burns no glucose, but rather burns fats. The liver also utilizes fructose and alcohol as energy sources, but few of us can live on honey and beer (at least, not for long). Diabetic individuals become hyperphagic—that is, they eat a lot—because the rest of their cells are being starved. (This observation suggests that the detectors mediating hunger are not located *exclusively* in the brain, as you will see below.) Despite their enormous increase in food intake, diabetics still cannot store fat without insulin. Most cells can use fatty acids to produce energy, although brain cells cannot. Thus, diabetic animals fed a very high fat diet stop being hyperphagic because the energy requirements of their non-neural tissues can be met in this way (Friedman, 1978; Tepper and Friedman, 1991).

In contrast to diabetes mellitus, a condition exists in which individuals produce too much insulin, called hyperinsulinemia (Friedman, 1990). Hyperinsulinemia results in low blood sugar; the most common behavioral symptoms include mental confusion, dizziness, weakness, and hunger. Hyperinsulinemia also usually leads to marked obesity because individuals with this condition feel hungry and eat frequently. Do these hyperinsulinemic individuals have high levels of insulin *because* they are obese and somewhat insulin-resistant (see below), or are they obese because they have high levels of insulin? There is no straightforward answer to this question in humans, and the issue remains unresolved.

Certainly there is evidence that some people may be overly responsive to the cephalic phase of insulin release and become obese because they actually experience greater "hunger" at mealtime than individuals with normal cephalic insulin responsiveness. Their appetite is huge, and they eat larger and longer meals than individuals with a normal cephalic insulin response. There also may be hyperresponsiveness to the GI phase of insulin release in some obese patients.

### Metabolism during the Fasting State

Eventually, the influx of energy from the gut no longer exceeds the body's energy usage requirements. The body must then shift from putting energy into storage to getting it out of storage. This shift in the energy balance occurs, for example, after strenuous exercise or after a prolonged fast. Most of us are confronted with this situation every morning when we awaken and need to break the nighttime fast, or breakfast. Energy reserves are mobilized from storage to meet your energy needs as you become active, even prior to eating your first food of the day.

There are several physiological methods of getting energy out of storage and into the bloodstream during a fast. The metabolic interactions that occur in an

**Fasting state**

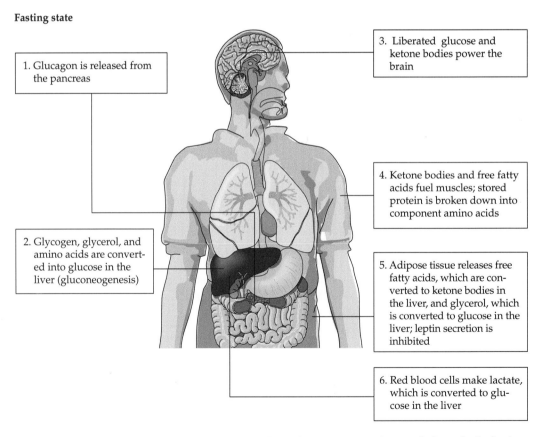

1. Glucagon is released from the pancreas

2. Glycogen, glycerol, and amino acids are converted into glucose in the liver (gluconeogenesis)

3. Liberated glucose and ketone bodies power the brain

4. Ketone bodies and free fatty acids fuel muscles; stored protein is broken down into component amino acids

5. Adipose tissue releases free fatty acids, which are converted to ketone bodies in the liver, and glycerol, which is converted to glucose in the liver; leptin secretion is inhibited

6. Red blood cells make lactate, which is converted to glucose in the liver

**9.17   Metabolic interactions among the major components of energy balance in the fasting state.** After Schneider and Wade, in press.

individual in a fasted state are shown in Figure 9.17. The first method is **lipoly-sis**, or the breakdown of adipose tissue into fatty acids; these free fatty acids are readily used for energy. Second, **glycogenolysis**, the breakdown of stored glycogen in the liver, provides a rapid supply of glucose in the blood. Under extreme conditions, such as during strenuous exercise, glycogen may break down in the muscles for utilization as energy. Normally, the peptide hormone glucagon, released from the α-cells of the endocrine pancreas, is the most important day-to-day stimulator of energy release (Steffens et al., 1990). Glucagon induces both lipolysis and glycogenolysis.

Stored energy in the body can also be released via the sympathetic nervous system. The sympathetic system generally acts as an emergency system, although input to all organs can shift to favor the sympathetic or parasympathetic system in day-to-day regulation as well. Sympathetic nerves that innervate the fat cells can induce lipolysis (Steffens et al., 1990). The liver is also innervated with sympathetic nerves that may signal it to release stored glycogen (Sawchenko and Friedman, 1979). Another backup system that is used during fasting is a process called **gluconeogenesis,** the production of glucose from amino acids. Gluconeogenesis takes place entirely in the liver. Gluconeogenesis results in the production of ketone bodies, a side reaction of making sugar from amino acids; ketone production also results from the incomplete oxidation of free fatty acids (Friedman, 1990). Prolonged fasting, during which muscles are used for energy, produces toxic levels of ketone bodies, a condition called ketosis; the most serious effect of ketosis is the resulting change in blood pH, which has a deleterious effect on neural function. Diabetics with uncontrolled blood sugar levels can also enter ketosis when insufficient insulin is provided and may suffer serious consequences if blood pH fluctuations are prolonged.

Basically, the metabolic system is designed to provide sufficient levels of energy to the brain. As we have seen, the brain must receive a constant supply of glucose via the blood; it cannot utilize fatty acids. During long-term food deprivation, the rest of the body is literally starved to feed the brain. Glucagon release, gluconeogenesis, and sympathetic stimulation of fat breakdown are the most common mechanisms for raising blood sugar levels without eating, but there are additional methods of elevating blood glucose levels during emergencies to keep a relatively constant level of energy supplied to the brain. After prolonged fasting or very demanding exercise, growth hormone can trigger lipolysis in the fat cells. Furthermore, corticosterone or cortisol released during vigorous exercise can induce gluconeogenesis. During stress, epinephrine from the adrenal medulla acts to stimulate glycogenolysis in the liver. Because the brain receives a relatively constant supply of glucose, you might guess that the detectors for changes in blood sugar levels might not be found in the brain, but rather in the periphery, where blood glucose changes are more pronounced. Logical as this assumption may be, it is not completely true. Most metabolic fuel detectors are located in the brain and liver, although fuel detectors are also located in muscle and fat cells.

Problems with the mobilization of fat stores or the monitoring of blood glucose levels may be involved in obesity (Friedman, 1990). The obese person or animal may not be able to mobilize normally the fat stores already present, so these individuals must eat frequently to meet their normal energy demands, and thus continue to deposit more and more fat. Many hormones are involved in maintaining energy balance, and presumably, some of these hormones affect the behavioral systems that are important in maintaining energetic homeostasis. However, the precise role that hormones play in mediating food intake and body mass has not been completely identified. Our inability to link hormones to ingestive behaviors is partially due to a lack of consensus regarding the stimuli eliciting hunger.

In summary, the fasting state is characterized by elevated concentrations of particular hormones (glucagon and glucocorticoids), neuropeptides (neuropeptide Y and corticotropin-releasing hormone), and metabolic substrates (free fatty acids and ketone bodies). Eating results in a reversal of all of these parameters. All of these changes in metabolic fuels, hormones, and neuropeptides are correlated with one another. Which aspect(s) of these changes serves as a signal to the neural mechanisms that control food intake? Do one or all of these factors elicit hunger or control ingestion? Controversy over this question remains, in part because of the complexity of the interactions among these factors. Concentrations of circulating metabolic fuels and fuel oxidation affect both hormone and neuropeptide secretion. Both hormones and neuropeptides affect fuel oxidation. These complex metabolic and endocrine interactions make the determination of the signals controlling food intake difficult.

One way to make sense of all this complexity is to organize the signals into two categories: primary sensory signals and secondary mediators or modulators. Primary sensory signals are those biochemical changes inside the cell that result when metabolic fuels are metabolized to generate cellular energy. For example, changes in glucose metabolism might serve to generate the primary sensory stimulus that controls insulin secretion. Some investigators believe that these primary sensory stimuli also control neuropeptide secretion, and may also control food intake. Secondary modulators are the hormones and neuropeptides that affect food intake. Secondary modulators are usually considered to be "downstream" from the primary sensory stimuli. The secretion of hormones and neuropeptides is controlled by the primary sensory stimuli. Hormones and neuropeptides may have *direct* effects on mechanisms that control food intake, or they may have *indirect* effects on food intake via effects on energy metabolism.

### Control of Food Intake

It was believed for over two decades that mammalian feeding was regulated in a simple way, with two separate centers in the brain controlling hunger and satiety, respectively (Figure 9.18). A "hunger center" that facilitated eating was hypothesized to reside in the lateral hypothalamus because bilateral destruction of this brain region led to nearly complete anorexia (loss of appetite) and subsequent aphagia (absence of eating behavior) in cats and rats (Anand and Brobeck, 1951). Similarly, a "satiety center" that inhibited feeding was hypothesized to be located in the ventromedial hypothalamus (VMH) because lesions of this brain area resulted in hyperphagia and enormous, rapid weight gain (Hetherington and Ranson, 1940). This dual-center theory of the control of feeding was very pervasive in shaping the research and theoretical framework in which experimental outcomes were interpreted. The lateral hypothalamus and the VMH became the key components of putative regulatory systems involving blood glucose (the "glucostat" hypothesis) and triglyceride (the "lipostat" hypothesis) levels (Stricker, 1984).

Further research has displaced the dual-center theory of feeding regulation. Bilateral lesions of the lateral hypothalamus were shown to interfere with all moti-

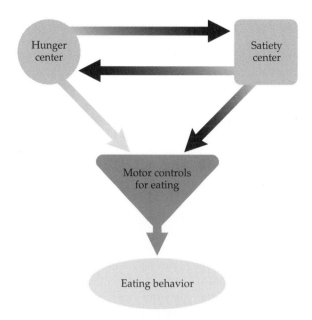

**9.18   The dual-center model of the regulation of feeding.** Until recently, it was believed that mammalian feeding was regulated by mutual inhibitory relationships between a "hunger center" in the lateral hypothalamus and a "satiety center" in the ventromedial hypothalamus, but further research has displaced this notion. The light arrowhead in the figure symbolizes facilitation; the dark arrowheads symbolize inhibition. After Rosenzweig and Leiman, 1989.

vated behaviors, not just feeding (Marshall et al., 1971). Lesions made anywhere along the dopaminergic tracts that pass through the lateral hypothalamus from the midbrain to the striatum while sparing the hypothalamic tissue produce behavioral deficits similar to those resulting from lesions of the lateral hypothalamus (Stricker et al., 1979). Other evidence suggests that the VMH is not a center for satiety, but part of a circuit that regulates feeding via the autonomic nervous system and its effects on energy metabolism, as well as mediating many other types of motivated behaviors. Lesions of the VMH suppress sympathetic nervous system activities while increasing parasympathetic nervous activities, resulting in increased storage of fat while inhibiting lipolysis. This excessive storage of energy as fat leaves a shortage of energy to maintain the animal's daily processes. Consequently, VMH-lesioned animals develop voracious appetites not because a satiety center was damaged, but in order to maintain a steady delivery of metabolic fuel from the intestines. Eventually, as the animals become obese, the fat cells become insulin-resistant—that is, they no longer respond to insulin by taking up more glucose. Thus, food intake and body weight stabilize at this new elevated level, at what is called a new set point. It is now believed that "animals with VMH lesions do not become fat because they eat too much, as was supposed, but instead they overeat because they are becoming obese" (Friedman, 1990; Stricker, 1984; see also Friedman and Stricker, 1976).

As the dual-center control model has proved inadequate to explain feeding behavior, investigators have come to believe that the neuroendocrine system that controls food intake does so via indirect effects on energy partitioning. This idea is known as the metabolic hypothesis. Glucose, free fatty acids, and ketone bodies are metabolic fuels that can be used in chemical reactions (oxidation) to make usable energy for cellular processes. Food intake is responsive to changes in the oxidation of metabolic fuels. In order to study the metabolic signals that control ingestive behaviors, pharmacological agents have been given to animals to block oxidation of specific metabolic fuels. For example, 2-deoxy-D-glucose (2DG) or 5-thio-glucose (5TG) treatment blocks glucose oxidation, whereas methyl palmoxirate (MP) or mercaptoacetate (MA) treatment blocks free fatty acid oxidation. Treatment of satiated rats, dogs, cats, monkeys, and humans with these metabolic inhibitors causes rapid increases in food intake (Friedman and Tordoff, 1986; Ritter and Taylor, 1990; Ritter et al., 1992).

Historically, research on food intake focused on the hypothalamus (e.g., the VMH) and preoptic area. However, brain regions in the posterior, or caudal, parts of the brain are also able to act independently of the hypothalamus to control food consumption. The mechanisms that underlie feeding have been studied in animals that have undergone a surgical procedure to isolate the hypothalamus from the rest of the brain; these animals are termed *decerebrate* animals (Grill and Kaplan, 1990). Decerebrate rats display the ingestive motor program that underlies eating behavior. These studies have demonstrated that even in the absence of information from the hypothalamus, decerebrate rats increase their food intake in response to 2DG and MP, as well as in response to treatment with other peptides that generally stimulate eating (orexinics) (Grill and Kaplan, 1990; Kaplan et al., 1993, 1998; Grill et al., 1997, 1998). These results show that the hypothalamus is not required for the control of feeding, and that metabolic and endocrine signals can act on the brain to control feeding.

Recent data support the idea that areas in the caudal brain stem participate in the control of food intake (Grill et al., 1998). Treatment with metabolic inhibitors that affect food intake increases the activity of neurons in the area postrema and the nucleus of the solitary tract in the brain stem, as well as in forebrain regions such as the PVN of the hypothalamus (Ritter et al., 1992; Horn and Friedman, 1998). 2DG-induced increases in food intake are significantly attenuated in rats that receive varying amounts of damage to the area postrema and the medial nucleus of the solitary tract (Bird et al., 1983; Contreras et al., 1982; Hyde and Miselis, 1983; Ritter and Taylor, 1990). Infusions of 5TG into the fourth ventricle (in the brain stem), but not into the third ventricle (in the hypothalamic area), caused rats to increase their food consumption. Based on these findings, it has been hypothesized that detectors of glucose availability that control food intake may reside in the caudal brain stem.

However, there are also detectors of metabolic fuel availability and oxidation in peripheral tissues outside of the brain. Their presence was demonstrated by showing that metabolic inhibitors could increase food intake in animals in which the abdominal vagus nerve had been cut. Cutting the vagus nerve severs the connection between the brain and the internal organs. MA-induced, but not 2DG-induced, increases in food intake were abolished in vagotomized animals (Langhans and Scharrer, 1987; Ritter and Taylor, 1989; 1990).

Feeding is an extraordinarily complex process that involves several intrinsic inputs, including the amount of fat stored in the body, the levels of glycogen stored in the liver, the biochemical qualities of the food being digested, neural and endocrine signals from the gut, and even the perceived pleasantness of the food (Morley et al., 1985a). Extrinsic factors, such as food availability and, particularly among humans, psychological and cultural influences, also regulate food intake. All of these intrinsic and extrinsic factors are integrated in the CNS to mediate eating behavior. The difficulty of inducing hunger experimentally stands in sharp contrast to the ease with which thirst can be induced, and has prompted the hypothesis that no single stimulus or set of stimuli exist for hunger (Stricker, 1984). **Hunger,** a strong motivation to seek out and ingest food, can thus be broadly considered the psychological state experienced by individuals as satiety from a previous meal wanes.

There are certainly neural signals of satiety. In the blowfly (*Phormia regina*), feeding stops when sufficient food is ingested to overfill the crop sac. The overflow distends the foregut, which activates neural stretch receptors that signal the brain to stop feeding. Cutting the recurrent nerve between the foregut and the brain results in blowflies that continue to eat until they literally burst (Dethier, 1976). Satiety is thus mediated via a simple negative feedback loop (Figure 9.19). Similarly, neural signals of stomach distension in humans (Cannon, 1929; Thompson, 1980), other primates (Moran and McHugh, 1979, 1982), rats (Davis and Campbell, 1973), and dogs (Janowitz and Grossman, 1949) appear to inhibit feeding. The rate of gastric (stomach) emptying may also affect feeding behavior. A slow rate of gastric emptying would inhibit feeding for a longer time than a fast gastric contraction. In humans, a high-fat or high-protein meal leaves the stomach more slowly than a high-carbohydrate meal. Consequently, you actually *may* become hungry sooner after eating carbohydrate-rich Chinese food than after a rich, high-fat meal because of the faster rate of gastric emptying.

More to the point of this chapter, there are endocrine signals that stop eating behavior. To demonstrate this point, an extra stomach and intestines can be transplanted into a rat. In the absence of neural connections, infusion of a liquid diet into the extra stomach results in a corresponding reduction in feeding behavior, even when the original stomach is empty. This observation suggests that some blood-borne product, possibly a hormone, is secreted in response to gastric dis-

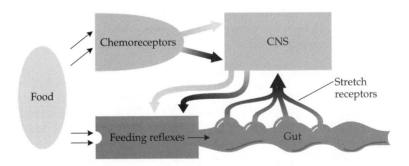

**9.19   Neural control of feeding in the blowfly.**   Satiety in the blowfly is mediated via a simple negative feedback loop. When sufficient food is ingested to overfill the blowfly's crop sac, the overflow distends the foregut and activates neural stretch receptors that signal the brain to stop feeding. If the recurrent nerve between the foregut and the brain is severed, blowflies will continue to eat until they literally burst. After Rosenzweig and Leiman, 1989.

**9.20    Feeding in _Pleurobranchea_** is tightly regulated by hormones. Normally, this sea slug will eat anything less than about one-third of its size. However, _Pleurobranchea_ avoids eating its own eggs because the peptide hormone that stimulates egg laying in this species also inhibits ingestive behavior.

tension by food (Koopmans, 1983). Filling the extra stomach with water does not reduce food intake. Further evidence of a blood-borne factor mediating stomach distension signals was obtained from hungry rats that ate much less after receiving blood transfusions from rats that had recently been fed (Davis et al., 1969). People who have had their stomachs surgically removed still report experiencing the sensation of hunger, but they usually reduce their caloric intake nonetheless (Mills and Stunkard, 1976).

Possibly the most salient example of the endocrine regulation of satiety is provided by a mollusk of the genus _Pleurobranchea_ (Figure 9.20). This sea slug is a voracious cannibal that appears to live by one simple rule: Eat it. Anything less than about one-third its size that wanders too close to a _Pleurobranchea_ is devoured. Those of us who yearn for more simple lives can admire the straightforward rules by which this creature conducts itself, but simple lives can also become complicated. _Pleurobranchea_ eggs are small and are therefore, by definition, food. Obviously, any species that incorporates its offspring into its menu has a problem. However, the peptide hormone that stimulates egg laying in this species also stops eating behavior (Mpitos and Davis, 1973). Treatment with the egg-laying hormone stops feeding behavior within 15 minutes and shortly thereafter causes oviposition (egg laying).

### Peptide Hormones and Food Intake

Simple yet elegant regulatory systems such as that found in _Pleurobranchea_ are uncommon among vertebrates. Instead, there are several complex levels of endocrine mechanisms, usually involving peptide hormones, controlling satiety in vertebrates.

**CHOLECYSTOKININ.**    Cholecystokinin (CCK) is considered to be the hormonal factor most likely to invoke satiety. CCK is a gastrointestinal peptide hormone that is released during feeding to aid with digestion; it was named for its ability to promote the contraction of gallbladder muscle. Administration of CCK to hungry rats, mice, golden hamsters, chickens, rabbits, sheep, cats, dogs, or humans decreases their food intake (Morley et al., 1985b). CCK does not suppress water intake in thirsty animals, indicating that its satiating effect is specific to food intake. When CCK is released during a meal, it binds to peripheral receptors that signal the brain, via the vagus nerve, to stop eating behavior. The effects of CCK on ingestive behaviors can be blocked by cutting the abdominal section of the vagus nerve (Bloom and Polak, 1981). Blood concentrations of CCK diminish only slightly as a meal is digested, suggesting that blood-borne CCK does not mediate satiety; however, CCK concentrations around the vagus nerve vary considerably during the course of a meal, suggesting that local release of CCK mediates satiety via the vagus nerve. It has been proposed that as satiety signals stop, hunger is experienced again. Although this model is an extreme oversimplification of the endocrine control of vertebrate feeding, it suggests that the feedback principles displayed in the blowfly and *Pleurobranchea* could theoretically form the basis of satiety in vertebrates as well.

The exact nature of the inhibitory effects of CCK on feeding and the physiological role of CCK in normal satiety remain controversial. The satiety observed after CCK treatment has sometimes been attributed to the aversive or toxic effects of this compound: in other words, individuals stop eating after CCK treatment because it makes them sick. The aversive effects of CCK have been difficult to sort out. In order to determine whether CCK is aversive in humans, one can simply ask them. In some studies, CCK administration to people at concentrations sufficient to suppress eating behavior caused mild to moderate nausea (Morley et al., 1985b). Nausea, abdominal bloating, cramping, and other symptoms of gastrointestinal distress were reported when CCK was given at doses higher than necessary to suppress food intake. In another study, however, CCK was reported to suppress hunger without nausea or other aversive effects (Stacher et al., 1978). People fasted overnight and were given either saline or one of several different doses of CCK the following morning. They were then seated in a dining room, and a large meal was prepared: "A piece of bread and butter was prepared in the subjects' presence. Fresh, good-smelling chives were cut and put on the bread. Following this, butter was melted in a pan, and bacon and two beaten eggs were added and fried. The aroma and sounds of the food being prepared was aimed to stimulate the subjects' appetite, and in fact, stimulated at least the experimenters' appetite to a rather large degree" (Stacher et al., 1978, 327). Subjects were asked to rate their hunger throughout the preparation of the meal. Those who were injected with saline reported the most "voracious" appetites as the meal was being prepared. There was a dose-dependent relationship between CCK and reported intensity of hunger; higher doses of CCK were associated with lower levels of reported hunger. Note, however, that CCK was not paired with food intake in this study.

In the absence of language, it is even more difficult to ascertain whether CCK inhibits feeding via a true satiating mechanism or through secondary aversive effects. We can simply ask people if CCK makes them feel queasy, or observe them to see if they vomit after CCK treatment, to discover whether CCK causes nausea. But we cannot ask a rat if it is nauseated, and because rats do not vomit, it is difficult to discover whether something is aversive to them. However, learned aversions can be readily established by pairing flavors, such as saccharin, with substances known to produce illness, such as lithium chloride, and presenting the mixture to a rat. Upon subsequent presentations of the saccharin-flavored substance, the animal avoids it, demonstrating that it has learned that the sweet taste predicted the illness induced by lithium chloride. This learned aversion paradigm has been employed to explore the aversive effects of CCK. In some studies, CCK paired with saccharin did not cause rats to develop an aversion to saccharin (Gibbs et al., 1973). Other studies, however, have reported an aversive reaction to CCK in rats (Deutsch, 1982). Further studies are required to understand the precise role of CCK in suppressing food intake. Recent studies, however, have shown that CCK antagonists increase the size of meals consumed after food deprivation, suggesting a physiological role for CCK in normal satiety (Moran et al., 1992).

**BOMBESIN.**    Another peptide that may mediate feeding behavior is bombesin, a small protein consisting of 40 amino acids and distributed throughout the mammalian gastrointestinal and nervous systems (M. Brown et al., 1978), so named because it was originally isolated from the skin of the European frog (*Bombina bombina*) (Anastasi et al., 1971). Experimental injections of bombesin reduce food intake in rats (Gibbs et al., 1979). The mechanism by which this peripheral bombesin treatment affects feeding is unknown; in contrast to CCK, cutting of the vagus nerve does not interfere with the satiating effects of bombesin (Smith et al., 1981a). The satiating effects of bombesin and CCK are additive, further suggesting that they have different mechanisms of action (Stein and Woods, 1981). Intracerebroventricular infusions of bombesin also reduce food intake in rats, indicating a central nervous system mechanism of action (Morley et al., 1985a). Although bombesin inhibits feeding, the extent to which it is important in the normal regulation of feeding remains to be determined (Hostetler et al., 1989).

**NEUROPEPTIDE Y.**    Neuropeptide Y (NPY) is a potent activator of food intake in rats (Levine and Morley, 1984). NPY appears to increase motivation to eat (Flood and Morley, 1991; Woods et al., 1998). Intracerebroventricular  injections of NPY, or injections directly into the paraventricular nucleus of the hypothalamus (PVN), evoke marked food and water consumption in rats, both during the day (when nocturnal animals rarely eat or drink) and at night (Kalra et al., 1991; Levine and Morley, 1984; Stanley and Leibowitz, 1985). NPY is distributed throughout the nervous system; in the brain, it is found in neuron terminals in several regions of the hypothalamus, including the PVN and arcuate nucleus, as well as in the nucleus accumbens, the septum, and the medial amygdala. Cell bodies containing NPY are found in the hypothalamus, hippocampus, caudate–putamen, and throughout the cerebral cortex (Gray and Morley, 1986).

Norepinephrine treatment also stimulates feeding. NPY treatment is neither synergistic nor additive when co-administered with norepinephrine (Morley et al., 1987). Peripherally administered bombesin or centrally administered corticotropin-releasing hormone attenuates NPY-induced food intake. CCK does not inhibit NPY-induced food consumption, and does not affect glucose concentrations in the blood (Morley et al., 1987; Erickson et al., 1997). However, infusion of leptin into the cerebral ventricles inhibits NPY-induced feeding in rats (Yokosuka et al., 1998; McMinn et al., 1998). There seems to be a regulatory "loop" between NPY, which induces food intake, and leptin, which reduces food intake (Rohner-Jeanrenaud et al., 1996).

**CORTICOTROPIN-RELEASING HORMONE.**    Corticotropin-releasing hormone (CRH) acutely reduces food intake and body mass after icv administration (Arase et al.,

1988; Hotta et al., 1991; Rivest et al., 1989). Another regulatory loop appears to exist between NPY, CRH, and the sympathetic nervous system. Discharges of sympathetic nerves to intrascapular brown adipose tissue increased after icv injections of CRH and decreased after icv injections of NPY (Egawa et al., 1990). These results suggest that these two hormones (neuromodulators) have opposite effects on sympathetic activity (Heinrichs et al., 1992). The sympathetic nervous system could communicate between fat depots and the brain; specific endocrine signals could influence the motivation to eat or stop eating, depending on energy stores, energy availability, and energy expenditures.

Endogenous opioids may also mediate food intake (Morley et al., 1983). Treatment of rats (Holtzman, 1975) and other species, including humans (Thompson et al., 1982), with the opioid antagonist naloxone reduces food intake. Apparently, naloxone reduces the hedonic value of food, making its consumption less "rewarding" (Morley et al., 1985a). Ingested sugars and oils are particularly salient cues for the release of endorphins and appear to provide calming and pain-reducing influences (Shide and Blass, 1989). Perhaps this is why we are more likely to reach for a candy bar than broccoli when we are stressed. Several additional peptide hormones also influence feeding, including somatostatin, glucagon, pancreatic polypeptide, motilin, neurotensin, thyrotropin-releasing hormone, and gastrin-releasing peptide.

**INSULIN.**    Recently, increased attention has focused on the role of insulin in the mediation of feeding behavior. There is an obvious association between insulin release and meal termination; hunger ensues when insulin levels drop at the end of the postabsorptive phase (Strubbe et al., 1977). Treatment of rats with streptozotocin, a drug that selectively destroys the pancreatic β-cells and induces diabetes, also causes long-term hyperphagia, demonstrating that lack of insulin can interfere with satiety. Presumably, insulin does not induce satiety directly, but rather by its facilitation of the use and storage of ingested carbohydrates (Stricker, 1984) and via feedback mechanisms involving other hormones as well as the autonomic nervous system (Steffens et al., 1990). It is also possible that the oxidation of metabolic fuels itself generates some kind of signal that controls food intake; thus, the storage and mobilization of fat may indirectly affect food intake by changing the rate of oxidation of metabolic fuels. When neither fatty acids nor glucose are available in the blood for oxidation, as monitored primarily by the liver, then feeding might be induced (Friedman, 1990). It has also been proposed that insulin signals the central nervous system about peripheral levels of metabolic fuels via the cerebrospinal fluid (CSF) (Woods and Porte, 1983). Insulin levels increase in the CSF of baboons immediately after a meal or an intravenous glucose injection (Woods et al., 1981), and icv infusions of insulin reduce food intake and body mass in baboons (Woods et al., 1979).

Several researchers have suggested that tonic levels of central insulin (i.e., insulin in the brain) serve as an important signal to keep body mass and food intake within a healthy range. Thus, obesity might arise from impaired sensitivity to the central insulin signal (Schwartz et al., 1992; Woods et al., 1996). The evidence for this idea is that plasma insulin concentrations are often correlated with body fat content, and infusion of insulin directly into the cerebral ventricles of the brain decreases food intake and causes animals to maintain their body mass at lower levels than before insulin treatment (Chavez et al., 1996).

As noted previously in this chapter, it is difficult to determine whether insulin has direct effects on the mechanisms that control food intake or whether it changes food intake through indirect effects on metabolic fuel availability and oxidation. One way that this issue has been addressed is by dissociating the direct and indirect effects of insulin by measuring food intake in diabetic rats fed different diets (Friedman, 1978; Tepper and Friedman, 1991; Friedman et al., 1985). Diabetic rats, of course, have reduced plasma insulin concentrations, and they eat more food than nondiabetic rats. Untreated diabetic rats also eat more food than diabetic rats treated with insulin (considered alone, these data support the notion that insulin acts in the brain to decrease food intake). However, untreated diabetic rats ate more food than normal rats when fed a low-fat, high-carbohydrate diet, but not when fed a high-fat, low-carbohydrate diet. Thus, insulin concentrations were the critical determinant of food intake. The different levels of food intake can be explained by the differences in metabolic fuel availability in the diets fed to the diabetic rats. Insulin is the hormone that is necessary for peripheral glucose uptake, and therefore, insulin is necessary for the utilization of carbohydrate fuels. The diabetic rats could readily oxidize fats, but not carbohydrates. Consequently, the diabetic rats on the low-fat, high-carbohydrate diet may have been stimulated to overeat by their inability to oxidize the type of fuels that they were ingesting. In contrast, the diabetic rats on a high-fat, low-carbohydrate diet were better able to oxidize the fuels that they were ingesting, and thus did not overeat (Friedman, 1978; Friedman et al., 1985). It is true that when pharmacological doses of insulin are given, metabolic changes in both the body and the brain occur. However, if antibodies to insulin are put into the brain, animals eat more with no effects on metabolism (McGowan et al., 1990). These results imply direct, rather than indirect, effects of insulin.

**THE ROLE OF THE LIVER.**    The liver may generate a signal for satiety. This organ is ideally situated to monitor changes in the concentrations of insulin and metabolic fuels (Granneman and Friedman, 1980). It certainly is important in the mediation of insulin-induced feeding, as elegantly demonstrated by Stricker and his colleagues (Stricker et al., 1977). To understand their experiment fully, the use of metabolic fuels by the brain and liver will be briefly reviewed.

Two metabolic fuels can be used by the brain: glucose and ketone bodies. As described above, the brain primarily uses glucose, and insulin is not required to get energy into nerve cells. During prolonged starvation, the brain can function using ketone bodies as fuel. Fructose, like glucose, is a carbohydrate, but unlike glucose, it cannot easily cross the blood–brain barrier; consequently, fructose cannot be used as a fuel for the brain. The liver, on the other hand, can readily utilize fructose as a metabolic fuel, but it is unable to oxidize ketones and use them for energy. Stricker and his co-workers exploited this disparity in fuel use between the brain and the liver to find out which organ mediated insulin-induced feeding. Rats were infused either with (1) saline, (2) fructose, to "feed" the liver but not the brain, or (3) β-hydroxybuterate, a ketone, to "feed" the brain but not the liver (Figure 9.21; Friedman, 1990; Stricker et al., 1977). All of the rats were also treated with insulin. Insulin treatment of the control animals produced the expected reduction in blood levels of glucose and induced feeding behavior. Infusion of rats with β-hydroxybuterate did not affect insulin-induced feeding. However, infusions of fructose inhibited the onset of insulin-induced feeding, demonstrating

(a)

(b)

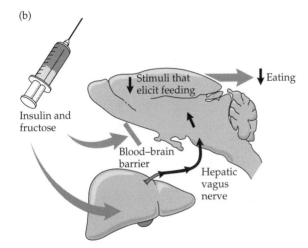

**9.21    The role of the liver in insulin-induced feeding** was determined by injecting animals with insulin to lower blood glucose levels and induce feeding, and then injecting them with either ketone bodies, which can be used as fuel by the brain but not the liver, or fructose, which can be used by the liver but not the brain. Only fructose inhibited insulin-induced feeding, indicating that the liver will block insulin-induced feeding even if fuel levels in the brain are low. After Stricker et al., 1977.

that a "fed" liver, even in the presence of a "starved" brain, was sufficient to block insulin-induced feeding. These results indicate that the liver plays a role in mediating insulin-induced feeding, probably by monitoring its energy stores (glycogen) and communicating this information to the central nervous system via the hepatic branch of the vagus nerve (Friedman and Granneman, 1983; Sawchenko and Friedman, 1979; Steffens et al., 1990; Stricker et al., 1977).

**LEPTIN.**    Leptin, also referred to as the OB protein, is secreted predominantly by white adipose (fat) tissue cells (Zhang et al., 1994) (see Chapter 2). A strain of mice exists that has a mutation in the *OB* gene that results in deficient OB protein. Mice that are homozygous for the *OB* mutation (i.e., *ob/ob*) overeat and become obese. However, when *ob/ob* mice are injected with high doses of leptin, their food intake decreases and their body weights return to normal (Campfield et al., 1995; Halaas et al., 1995; Pelleymounter et al., 1995; Weigle et al., 1995). Individuals of another obese strain of mice, so-called *db/db* mice, produce normal amounts of leptin, but they possess a mutation in the gene that codes for the leptin receptor. Leptin treatment does not ameliorate the obesity of *db/db* mice because of the lack of a functional leptin receptor.

Since the discovery of the role of leptin in food intake and body mass in 1995, there has been great interest in this hormone. Initially, it was hypothesized that leptin concentrations reflect long-term body fat stores. It was thought that when body fat levels, and thus leptin concentrations, reached a particular threshold, food intake would be curtailed. Conversely, when body fat levels, and hence leptin concentrations, fell below a certain minimum, food intake would increase. However, in a number of conditions, such as fasting or exposure to low temperatures, leptin concentrations fall far more rapidly than body fat levels. These results cast doubt on the notion that leptin is a long-term indicator of body fat content (Kolaczynski et al., 1996; Boden et al., 1996; Ahren et al., 1997; Schneider and Wade, in press).

It was also suggested in the mid-1990s that human obesity might arise from insufficiencies in either leptin or its receptor. However, only a very small fraction of human obesity can be explained by mutations in the leptin gene or in the gene that encodes the leptin receptor (Strobel et al., 1998). Effects of leptin treatment on food intake and body mass have been demonstrated only with doses that result in leptin concentrations well above the normal, physiological range. Leptin has significant effects on fuel oxidation and energy expenditure. Thus, as with insulin, it will be difficult to determine whether leptin has direct effects on the mechanisms that control food intake or indirect effects on food intake via its effects on energy metabolism. More research is necessary to determine the functional importance of the natural fluctuations of leptin concentrations. The mechanisms that underlie the effects of leptin on food intake and body mass, and the role of leptin in human obesity, remain unknown.

### Gonadal Steroid Hormones, Food Intake, and Body Mass

As we have seen, the control of feeding, especially in humans, is a highly complex regulatory process involving both the endocrine and nervous systems. To complicate the mediation of food intake even further, gonadal steroid hormones also influence eating and subsequent body mass.

**ESTROGENS AND PROGESTINS.**    After ovariectomy, a female rat increases her food intake and relatively quickly elevates her body mass about 20–25% as compared with a gonadally intact female. The hyperphagia eventually wanes, and her food intake stabilizes to maintain this new elevated body mass. Most of the increased body weight is the result of increased fat deposition (adiposity) (Leshner and Collier, 1973). Locomotor activity, as measured on a running wheel, is permanently suppressed by ovariectomy (Wang, 1923). In other words, ovariectomy leads to a fat rat. Ovariectomy also promotes obesity in other species, including cats, voles, and mice. Ovariectomy does not elevate food intake or body weight in other mammalian species; for example, golden hamsters do not change body mass appreciably after ovariectomy. Bilateral ovariectomy in humans may or may not affect food intake and subsequent body mass.

Estrogens generally have catabolic effects, in contrast to androgens, which, as you know, are generally anabolic (see Chapter 2). Treatment of ovariectomized rats with estradiol benzoate reverses the increase in body mass by inducing a mild, transient hypophagia and prolonged elevation in activity (Mook et al., 1972).

In contrast to the effect of estradiol, treatment of ovariectomized rats with progesterone does not prevent the increase in body mass; progesterone, in the absence of an ovary or estrogen, does not affect food intake, locomotor activity, body fat content, or body mass (Wade and Gray, 1979). In other words, ovariectomized female rats injected with only progesterone are as fat as untreated ovariectomized females. Treatment of an ovariectomized rat with both estradiol and progesterone also fails to prevent the increase in body mass. When gonadally intact females are given progesterone in relatively high doses (for example, 5 mg/day), they experience a weight gain resembling the weight gain observed after ovariectomy (Hervey and Hervey, 1967). Thus, it is reasonable to assume that progesterone blocks the catabolic effects of estradiol on food intake, adiposity, locomotor activity, and body mass. The effects of ovariectomy and progesterone treatment are virtually identical, but nonadditive; that is, both treatments cause the same physiological and behavioral outcomes; namely, a transient rise in food intake with a subsequent elevation in body mass due largely to increased

Ovariectomy

Ovariectomy
+
estradiol

Ovariectomy
+
progesterone

Progesterone
(intact rat)

Ovariectomy
+
estradiol and
progesterone

**9.22    Effects of ovariectomy and progesterone treatment on body mass.** Ovariectomized rats increase their food intake and increase their body mass by 20–25%. Treatment with estradiol reverses these effects, but if estradiol is paired with progesterone, or if progesterone alone is administered, body mass is not reduced. Gonadally intact rats given progesterone increase their body mass in a manner similar to that seen in ovariectomized rats.

adiposity (Figure 9.22). Estradiol replacement therapy, in contrast, temporarily limits food consumption and suppresses adiposity.

If ovarian steroid hormones have these dynamic effects on food intake and body mass, then predictable changes in eating and body weight should accompany estrous cycles, pregnancy, and pseudopregnancy (Wade, 1986). Furthermore, females undergoing seasonal reproductive cycles should also display seasonal fluctuations in food intake and body mass. Homeostatic energy balance does appear to oscillate throughout the estrous cycle. Recall from Chapter 6 that rat estrogen concentrations are highest during vaginal proestrus; eating and body mass are reduced immediately after proestrus (Wang, 1924). The low blood plasma estrogen levels during diestrus are associated with elevated food intake and body mass (Brobeck et al., 1947). Seasonally acyclic golden hamsters increase their body mass when days are short and blood levels of gonadal sex steroid hormones are low (Bartness and Wade, 1985); when the days grow longer and estrous cycles resume, hamsters often display fluctuations in body mass and locomotor activity, and perhaps food intake, similar to those of rats.

Correlations between ovarian steroid hormones and food intake have also been reported for primates. Food intake is higher during the luteal phase, when progesterone levels are high, than at other times during the menstrual cycle in both nonhuman primates (Czaja and Goy, 1975) and women (Dalvit, 1981). These changes in food intake are attributable to the fluctuations in blood levels of sex steroid hormones; ovariectomized rhesus monkeys show cyclic changes in food intake when injected with estradiol and progesterone in a pattern that mimics the hormonal profile of a normal menstrual cycle (Czaja and Goy, 1975). In women, food intake generally, and carbohydrate intake specifically, is higher during the 10-day period prior to menstruation (the luteal phase) than during the 10-day period immediately following the onset of menstrual bleeding (the follicular phase) (Dalvit-McPhillips, 1983; Wurtman and Wurtman, 1989). Carbohydrate metabolism may increase during the luteal phase, thus triggering an increase in physiological energy needs and subsequent elevated intake of this energy source (Pliner and Fleming, 1983; Wurtman and Wurtman, 1989).

As described in Chapter 6, blood plasma progesterone concentrations gradually increase throughout pregnancy; progesterone is also elevated during pseudopregnancy in rats. Food intake, fat storage, and overall body mass increase during both pregnancy and pseudopregnancy (Slonaker, 1924). Ewes entering their first estrous cycle of the breeding season do not display reproductive behavior; this first estrous cycle of the season is called a "silent heat." However, plasma levels of progesterone are high during the luteal phase of the silent heat, and food intake and body mass escalate accordingly during this time (Sadlier, 1969).

How might ovarian steroid hormones affect food intake and subsequent body mass? The most parsimonious possibility is that ovarian hormones affect the brain sites that control food intake and voluntary exercise. Changes in these behaviors would then lead to adiposity and increased body mass. Alternatively, there might be effects on body mass independent from food intake and exercise. One way to distinguish between these two possibilities is to "yoke" the amount of food available to one animal to the food intake of another. In this paradigm, the yoked animal receives the same amount of food per day as is consumed by a counterpart, usually a littermate. Ovariectomized rats still gain weight when they are fed exactly the same amount that a gonadally intact sister eats. In other words, ovariectomized rats appear almost *destined* to gain weight, even when provided with only sufficient calories to maintain a normal body mass in a gonadally intact animal. The same result is obtained in ovariectomized rats yoked to ovariectomized females treated with estradiol. In both cases, the ovariectomized rats are less active than intact or estrogen-treated females, and thus gain body mass. Another way to examine the direct effects of hormones on body mass is to place hormone implants directly into the central nervous system. Implants of estradiol benzoate into the paraventricular nuclei of the hypothalamus or VMH of ovariectomized rats reduce food intake and body weight in a manner similar to systemic injections of estradiol (Butera and Beikirch, 1989; Wade and Zucker, 1970). Estrogen implants elsewhere in the diencephalon do not reliably affect food intake or body weight.

Adipose tissue metabolism is directly affected by steroid hormones. Alteration of the size of the fat deposits is the main effect of sex steroid hormones upon body mass. Adipose tissue contains receptors for both estrogens and progestins (Gray and Wade, 1979; Wade and Gray, 1978). Estradiol and progesterone affect lipoprotein lipase (LPL), an enzyme found in fat cells that mediates the uptake of triglycerides (fatty acids) from the bloodstream by the fat cells, as well as other coordinated changes in fat metabolism. LPL activity is high when fats are being stored; for example, after a meal. LPL activity is decreased by estradiol, but increased by progesterone. Consequently, fat cells cannot store triglycerides when exposed only to estradiol, but concurrent exposure to progesterone enhances fat storage by increasing the amount of triglycerides sequestered from the blood. Why is the body mass effect of progesterone dependent on estradiol? Recall from Chapter 2 that estrogens turn on genes that code for, among other things, progestin receptors in the uterus and elsewhere. Normally, there are receptors for both estradiol and progesterone in the adipose tissue cytosol. After ovariectomy, progesterone receptors disappear from the fat cells. Within 6–12 hours of an estradiol injection, progesterone receptors again proliferate throughout the cytosol (Gray and Wade, 1979). In this case, the progesterone receptors in the fat cells are dependent upon an *anabolic* effect of estrogens.

Clearly, ovarian steroid hormones can significantly affect food intake and body mass, as demonstrated by ovariectomy and hormone replacement studies. Does this effect of steroid hormones play any functional role in the regulation of food intake and body mass, and in the maintenance of energy balance? The answer is probably yes. Pregnancy causes a great increase in food intake in many mammalian species. Pregnancy, and especially lactation, are very energy-demanding activities. The resting metabolic rate of a pregnant mammal more than triples as compared with the nonpregnant animal (Bronson, 1989). A large increase in food intake is required to maintain the fetuses. Fat deposition, and thus body mass, increases during pregnancy in most mammalian species, probably as a hedge against the coming energetic demands. New mother rats, for example, weigh more just after parturition than they did before becoming pregnant. If a pregnant female cannot find sufficient food, or lacks sufficient energy stores, the pregnancy is often aborted. Similarly, a lactating female with insufficient metabolic fuels may kill and eat some or all of her offspring to balance litter size with available metabolic energy supplies (Schneider and Wade, 1989b). Even estrous cycles are suspended if insufficient metabolic fuels are available to the female (Schneider and Wade, 1989a).

There are interesting exceptions to the statement that pregnancy elevates food intake and increases body mass. For example, golden hamsters do not increase their food intake during pregnancy; rather, they draw upon their body fat reserves for energy (Wade et al., 1986). In golden hamsters and Siberian hamsters (*Phodopus sungorus sungorus*), progesterone appears to act in a manner opposite from its actions in rats; that is, progesterone causes a mobilization of fat and substantial decreases in body fat stores in pregnant hamsters (Schneider and Wade, 1987).

Fat deposition increases throughout the first two trimesters of pregnancy in humans. This makes sense when you consider the estrogen and progesterone levels found in the body during pregnancy. But why does fat accumulation virtually stop at the end of the second trimester? The answer to this question is another hormone: prolactin. High blood plasma levels of prolactin inhibit fat production. Prolactin has essentially the same effect as estradiol on fat cells; namely, it reduces LPL activity—except in mammary tissues. Consequently, fat continues to be deposited in the mammary glands through the end of pregnancy.

**ANDROGENS.**   Among vertebrates, males of many species are larger in size and eat more food than females. Much of this difference in size is organized perinatally by androgens, but the activational effects of anabolic steroids also are important in maintaining this sexual dimorphism. In most mammalian species, androgens promote elevated body mass and energy consumption (Wade, 1976). Males generally have more muscle mass than females, and the relatively higher concentrations of circulating androgens in males maintain this sex difference in body mass directly.

Castration decreases food intake and limits weight gain, including muscle mass gain, in rats (Mitchell and Keesey, 1974). The effects of castration on food consumption and body weight can be reversed by low-dose (50–200 µg/day) testosterone replacement therapy (Gentry and Wade, 1976). Bilateral implants of testosterone propionate into the VMH limit food intake in castrated male rats; this action of testosterone presumably reflects the effects of estrogen in this brain region after aromatization of the testosterone. Bilateral implants of dihydrotestosterone, an androgen that cannot be aromatized to an estrogen, into the VMH do not affect food intake (Nunez et al., 1980). These results suggest that androgens have both a central (CNS-induced change in food intake) and a peripheral (muscle mass) mechanism of action on food intake and body mass in male rats.

As is the case in many aspects of behavioral endocrinology, many of the general principles of androgen action have been generated from data obtained from rats. But many species-specific responses to these hormones have been reported that may require future modifications of the current general principles. For instance, a typical male meadow vole (*Microtus pennsylvanicus*) also eats less food and loses body mass after castration (Dark and Zucker, 1984), but individual voles vary markedly and predictably in their response to castration. Adult male meadow voles of identical age vary in body mass from about 35 to over 60 grams; all of the variation is due to differences in body fat stores. Voles heavier than 47 g lost mass after castration, whereas voles lighter than 47 g gained weight after castration. Males weighing about 47 g at the time of castration did not display substantial body mass changes. Testosterone replacement reversed the effects of castration in the appropriate direction for the heavy and light males. The individual differences in body fat content did not reflect differences in blood plasma levels of testosterone, but rather appeared to reflect differences in target tissue sensitivity to androgens (Dark et al., 1987b).

As described in Chapter 6, female garter snakes (*Thamnophis sirtalis parietalis*) are about three times heavier than male conspecifics. The difference in body size is apparent by 3 weeks of age, a time when plasma levels of androgens are high. Androgens appear to *inhibit* growth in male garter snakes. The sex difference in body size can be abolished by castration at any age; that is, castrated male snakes grow as large as females. Treatment with testosterone prevents the female-like body size in castrated males (Crews et al., 1985).

### Seasonal Body Mass Cycles

Several species of rodents undergo seasonal shifts in body mass. Many of us are familiar with sciurid rodents such as squirrels, chipmunks, woodchucks, and marmots that undergo autumnal fattening prior to entering hibernation. As they hibernate, their fat stores are slowly oxidized to provide the energy they need to survive the winter. As will be described further in Chapter 10, these annual cycles of body mass are controlled by an endogenous circannual biological clock and persist for years, even when the animals are housed in laboratories under constant environmental conditions (Figure 9.23) (Barnes and York, 1990; Heller and Poulson, 1970; Mrosovsky, 1985).

Muroid rodents such as deer mice, hamsters, voles, and lemmings also undergo seasonal changes in body mass, primarily by altering the amount of body fat stored. The seasonal cycles of body mass fluctuation in these animals are regulated, for the most part, by day length, or photoperiod. The onset of short days triggers an increase in body fat stores in golden hamsters. Food intake in this species, however, does not change in response to short day lengths, which suggests a direct effect of photoperiod on metabolic pathways. But this is not entirely true either, because the increase in body mass is somewhat independent of seasonal gonadal regression and the subsequent reductions in blood plasma concentrations of sex steroid hormones. As you will learn in Chapter 10, day length is often encoded by melatonin secreted from the pineal gland; removal of the pineal gland therefore blocks reproductive regression in response to short photoperiods because animals cannot discern day length without the pineal melatonin rhythm. However, pinealectomy does not affect short day–induced fattening in golden hamsters (Bartness and Wade, 1984). The mechanism of action of this pineal-independent transducer of day length on body weight is unknown.

Other muroid species adopt an alternative strategy for winter survival. Instead of gaining weight, these animals *lose* body mass in anticipation of winter. A reduction in body mass results in an elevated surface-to-volume ratio, which permits increased heat loss to the environment and a consequent reduction in body fat, resulting in reduced insulation and energy reserves. However, these results of decreased body mass are apparently compensated for by the fact that a small individual has to ingest far fewer calories to maintain itself than a large individual. The resulting reduction in foraging time and concomitant exposure to unfavorable climatic conditions presumably enhances survival. Thus, meadow voles

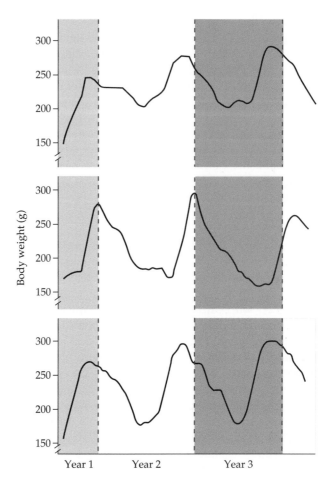

**9.23    Annual body mass changes for three ground squirrels** housed in a laboratory under constant conditions show approximately one-year (circannual) fluctuations in weight gain and loss. These fluctuations correspond to seasonal body mass cycles that occur in nature. After Zucker, 1988.

and other species respond to short days with a *decrease* in food intake and a subsequent reduction in body mass, although the decrease in body mass *precedes* the reduction in food intake in Siberian hamsters (Bartness and Wade, 1985; Dark and Zucker, 1986; Dark et al., 1983). Part of the weight loss can be attributed to reductions in circulating blood plasma levels of gonadal steroid hormones, but most of the effect appears to be due to the direct influence of day length, mediated by melatonin, on metabolic pathways (Bartness and Wade, 1985).

### *Inhibition of Reproduction to Maintain Energy Balance*

When food is abundant and the energetic demands of thermoregulation and foraging are minimal, there is plenty of energy available for the cellular processes necessary for day-to-day survival, as well as for growth and reproductive activities. However, when food is scarce or energetic demands are high, the activities that are necessary for survival take precedence. Thus, mammals have mechanisms to inhibit reproduction when they fall into negative energy balance (Bronson, 1999). Most people reading this book are aware that women who diet or engage in excessive exercise have problems with fertility. Reports of menstrual irregularities, amenorrhea (cessation of menstrual cycles), and diminished sexual desire and sexual activity, as well as infertility, are common among fashion models, women with the eating disorder anorexia nervosa, and athletes or dancers who do not increase their food intake to compensate for their excessive energy expenditure (Schneider and Wade, in press). The fact that reproductive inhibition occurs among females of all mammalian species and is entirely reversible upon refeeding or relaxation of the energy demands should inform us that this is not a pathology or disease, but a biological adaptation for conserving energy in environments in which energy availability may fluctuate (see Chapter 10).

An individual that finds itself hungry in a low-temperature environment must conserve energy, and must also find and eat food. Not surprisingly, the inhibition of reproduction in the service of energy balance is controlled by mechanisms that overlap with those that control food intake. Most of the peptide hormones, neuropeptides, and metabolic inhibitors that increase food intake also inhibit reproduction, and many of the same brain regions are involved in both processes (Schneider and Wade, in press). For example, in Syrian hamsters, estrous cycles can be interrupted by a 48-hour fast. Fat, but not lean, hamsters are protected from this fasting-induced anestrus. It was suggested that the fat hamsters were protected by their ability to use fatty acids as fuels by metabolizing lipids from their fat cells. To test this idea, very fat hamsters were either fasted or fed as much food as they wanted (ad libitum). Half of each group was treated with MP, an inhibitor of free fatty acid oxidation. Fat, fasted hamsters showed normal estrous cycles, but fat, fasted hamsters treated with MP did not. MP treatment had no effect on estrous cycles in hamsters fed ad libitum. Thus, the mechanisms that interrupt estrous cycles are sensitive to signals generated by the oxidation of metabolic fuels (Schneider and Wade, 1989a). Similarly, pulsatile LH secretion is affected by fasting, insulin, and metabolic inhibitors in rats, sheep, and monkeys (reviewed in Schneider and Wade, in press).

Leptin, insulin, neuropeptide Y, corticotropin-releasing hormone, CCK, galanin, nitric oxide synthase, and a variety of other substances are involved in the metabolic control of reproduction. As with the search for the signals that control food intake, the search for the signals that inhibit reproduction is complicated by the fact that hormones might have both direct and indirect influences on reproductive function. As discussed previously, leptin can increase free fatty acid oxidation and can prevent the storage of fat fuels in the form of triglycerides. Does leptin affect reproduction directly through its effects on brain mechanisms that control estrous cycles, or indirectly via its known effects on free fatty acid oxidation? To find out, Syrian hamsters were fasted and treated systemically with either leptin or leptin plus MP. Fasting-induced anestrus was prevented by treatment with high doses of leptin. However, leptin did not prevent fasting-induced anestrus in hamsters pretreated with MP (Schneider et al., 1998). These results suggest that exogenous leptin may affect reproduction via indirect effects on fuel oxidation. It is important to note that there are currently no data to demonstrate that fluctuations in leptin concentrations within normal, healthy physiological

ranges affect human reproduction. Regardless of whether leptin affects reproduction directly or indirectly (or both), the importance of normal daily fluctuations in leptin concentrations will have to be considered in relation to circadian
variation in secretion, as well as variation in the spacing of meals. There are some
data that suggest a threshold effect of leptin on normal pubertal development
(Cheung et al., 1997).

### Specific Hungers

What do we eat? In humans, much of what is consumed is culturally determined:
in other words, we learn what to eat. Many nonhuman animals also learn to eat
foods that improve their health and to avoid foods that make them ill. For example, rats provided with a diet lacking thiamine (vitamin $B_1$) do not seek out foods
rich in thiamine, but rather sample many foods, and over the course of several
days begin to prefer foods containing thiamine. Humans are no better at detecting thiamine deficiencies than rats. In the 19th century, thousands of Asians died
from beriberi, a degenerative disease of the nervous system resulting from thiamine deficiency. The cause of this outbreak of beriberi was the fashion of polishing rice before cooking. The hulls that were removed from the rice contained
the thiamine. Once the practice of rice polishing was discontinued, beriberi
became rare again. Because humans are unable to recognize thiamine in food,
this vitamin has become a common food additive.

In contrast to these learned preferences, some physiological requirements
seem to elicit specific, unlearned hungers. For example, hungers for sodium and
potassium appear to be innate (Milner and Zucker, 1965; Richter et al., 1938). However, even these hard-wired specific hungers can be modified by hormones. Most
animals, even without prior experience, prefer sucrose-laced water over plain
water. This preference is mediated by taste, because preferences also exist for non-
nutritive substances such as saccharin or Nutrasweet over plain water. An argument can be made that the intrinsic preference for sweet tastes is adaptive because
it would increase intake of valuable energy resources. However, the yearning for
chocolate is not necessarily hard-wired at birth, but is an acquired taste.

Female mammals, including rats, mice, hamsters, monkeys, and human infants, consume greater quantities of sweet solutions than their male counterparts
(Wade, 1976; Zucker et al., 1972). This sex difference is hormonally mediated; sex
differences in taste preferences appear to be organized perinatally by androgens
and also activated by sex steroid hormones in adulthood. Generally, estrogens
stimulate sweet solution preferences; ovariectomy reduces the preference for sweet
substances to the level of males (Wade, 1976). Castrated males show sweet solution preferences only slightly greater than gonadally intact males (Zucker, 1969).

Certainly, the taste for sodium and, to a lesser degree, potassium is innate in
many species. Young animals that are sodium- or potassium-deprived seek out
and prefer diets that contain these nutrients; these preferences are immediate and
do not require feedback in terms of improvement of health, as in the case of thiamine. Several vertebrate species, including humans, show early and pervasive
preferences for a slightly salty solution over plain water (Richter, 1936). One patient, a young boy of 3 or 4, was hospitalized because he was undergoing precocious puberty and experiencing development of the secondary sex characters. He
refused the bland hospital diet and died after a week in the hospital. An autopsy
revealed that his adrenal glands were abnormal: the cells of the zona reticularis,

which produce sex steroids, had invaded the zona glomerulosa, which normally produces aldosterone, the major sodium regulator. The parents reported that their son had consumed extremely salty foods and refused most foods that were not very salty at home. In fact, "salt" was one of the first words that he learned to say (Wilkins and Richter, 1940). Thus, failure of the adrenal glands to produce sufficient aldosterone can promote a powerful specific hunger for sodium.

### Conclusions

As already described, many hormonal and neural signals act in concert to balance energy intake and energy expenditure. It appears that hormones affect feeding behavior primarily by affecting the sensory systems related to feeding. CCK has been found to reduce neural activity in the brain regions where sensory information from the taste buds is received (Morin et al., 1983). Similarly, estradiol enhances the neural firing rates of afferent fibers from the tongue. Hormones also probably increase the sensory capabilities of animals hunting for food.

Hormones also have direct effects on the central processing mechanisms controlling food intake. CCK infusions into the brain appear to stop feeding in rats. The hormone's mode of action, and how it would normally cross the blood–brain barrier, are unknown. CCK acts in the periphery by interacting with the vagus nerve (Weatherford et al., 1993). Insulin also exerts direct effects on the central nervous system to stop feeding (Woods and Porte, 1983). Although insulin and leptin are too large to cross the blood–brain barrier, brain capillaries contain receptors for insulin and leptin that enable these hormones to be transported through the capillary walls into the brain interstitial fluid biologically intact (Schwartz et al., 1992). Other peptides have also been proposed to act centrally to mediate food intake (see Morley et al., 1985a for review). Hormones have not been shown to increase the efficiency of effectors of food intake; that is, hormones do not increase chewing frequency or increase efficacy of the muscles involved in feeding.

Although we know a lot about the endocrine mediation of feeding, particularly in rats, there are many different feeding strategies that probably have very different types of controlling mechanisms. For example, some snakes consume a large prey item and then do not eat again for many days as they digest their meal. Similarly, many cats will hunt prey and eat some of it, then leave the remains, or carry them to a resting spot. What cues tell snakes and cats that they are fed? What cues indicate hunger? The endocrine mediation of these signals may very well differ in many respects from that in rats and primates, or it may be identical. Many species go for weeks or even months without eating. Sometimes these fasting individuals are inactive, such as hibernating squirrels, but in other cases, the animals are engaged in other activities, as elephant seals are during the breeding season. The endocrine control of metabolism in these long-term fasting animals and the signals that stop them from feeding require further study. All in all, the study of hormones and homeostasis provides a unique opportunity to investigate the complex interactions among physiology, morphology, and behavior.

## Summary

• Individuals are motivated to maintain specific endogenous levels of water, sodium, and other nutrients. The process by which animals maintain a fairly stable internal environment is called homeostasis.

• Most homeostatic systems operate like a thermostatically controlled heating and cooling system. To maintain homeostasis, a system requires a detection mechanism to note any deviation from a set point. The homeostatic system must also be able to mobilize the organism to make changes to return it to the normal range. Finally, the system must have some way to recognize when the desired change occurs and feed back to stop the mobilization process.

• In multicellular organisms, water and sodium levels are maintained within a narrow range by physiological and behavioral systems. Most water is located inside the cells; the water outside the cells is located both in blood vessels and in the interstitial fluid. Sodium is important in the movement of water between the extracellular and intracellular fluid compartments.

• Movement of fluid out of cells causes cellular dehydration, a potent stimulus for osmotic thirst. Consumption of salty or sugary foods induces osmotic thirst. Cellular dehydration of osmoreceptors in the brain causes ADH secretion from the posterior pituitary, which promotes water conservation by the kidneys. Drinking water alleviates osmotic thirst.

• Volemic thirst is caused by reduced blood volume (hypovolemia). Quenching volemic thirst requires ingestion of water, sodium, and other solutes.

• Hypovolemia stimulates the production of angiotensin II, a potent vasoconstrictor. Angiotensin II may also increase drinking behavior.

• Angiotensin II triggers the release of aldosterone from the adrenals; aldosterone promotes sodium retention and subsequent water conservation by the kidneys. Aldosterone affects drinking behavior indirectly by its influence on osmotic thirst.

• The need for metabolic fuels is continuous, but food intake is episodic; consequently, energy intake and expenditure are never quite balanced. After a meal, there is a surplus of energy that must be stored for later use. Insulin is the only hormone that promotes energy uptake by cells.

• Although insulin is critical for energy storage, many other hormones, including epinephrine, norepinephrine, glucocorticoids, thyroid hormones, growth hormone, somatomedin, and glucagon, are involved in getting energy out of storage.

• The stimuli eliciting feeding are numerous and include physiological signals from fat stores, levels of glycogen stores, and the nature and quality of the food, as well as neural and hormonal signals from the gut.

• Cholecystokinin is released during ingestion and appears to provide an endocrine signal of satiety, acting to inhibit feeding via the vagus nerve.

• Endogenous opioids may alter the hedonic value of food. Treatment with opioid antagonists reduces food intake.

• Several other peptide hormones, including corticotropin-releasing hormone, leptin, neuropeptide Y, bombesin, glucagon, and somatostatin, influence food intake. Neuropeptide Y is a potent inducer of food intake. Most other peptide hormones reduce food intake.

• Insulin may signal the central nervous system about peripheral levels of metabolic fuels via the cerebrospinal fluid. Intracerebroventricular infusions of insulin reduce food intake.

• Gonadal steroid hormones also act to affect food intake and body mass. Generally, estrogens reduce food intake and body mass, as well as increasing voluntary exercise. Progesterone blocks these effects of estrogen. Androgens generally increase food intake and body mass.

• Some small mammalian species undergo seasonal changes in body mass. Individuals of some species elevate body fat levels to increase their chances of winter survival. An alternative strategy is to reduce body mass prior to winter so that less food must be consumed to survive.

• Many species must learn what foods to consume, but some physiological requirements elicit unlearned specific hungers. Specific hungers for sodium and potassium appear to be common in terrestrial vertebrates. Hormones mediate some specific hungers.

## Questions for Discussion

1. In what ways is a thermostat a good analogy, and in what ways is it a poor analogy, for the control of food intake and body mass?

2. Discuss the concept of "set point." In what ways is this concept limited in considering the annual changes in the body mass of squirrels or bears that gain weight prior to entering hibernation?

3. What are the advantages and disadvantages of "hard-wired" taste preferences? What are the advantages and disadvantages of hormonal mediation of taste preferences?

4. How are hormones that have central processing effects on feeding behavior different from or similar to neurotransmitters? Are the distinctions between hormones and neurotransmitters applicable when discussing chemical mediation of behavior in the brain?

5. Why are homeostatic processes controlling body fluid levels important? How would one go about studying the evolution of body fluid regulatory mechanisms?

## Suggested Readings

Bartness, T. J., and Wade, G. N. 1985. Photoperiodic control of seasonal body weight cycles in hamsters. *Neuroscience and Biobehavioral Reviews*, 9: 599–612.

Fitzsimons, J. T. 1998. Angiotensin, thirst, and sodium appetite. *Physiological Reviews*, 78: 583–686.

Fluharty, S. J., and Sakai, R. R. 1995. Behavioral and cellular analysis of adrenal steroid and angiotensin interactions mediating salt appetite. *Progress in Psychobiology and Physiological Psychology*, 16: 177–212.

Hirschberg, A. L. 1998. Hormonal regulation of appetite and food intake. *Annals of Medicine*, 30: 7–20.

Schneider, J. E., and Wade, G. N. In press. Reproductive inhibition in service of energy balance. In K. Wallen and J. E. Schneider (eds.), *Reproduction in Context*. MIT Press, Cambridge, MA.

Stricker, E. M., and Verbalis, J. G. 1991. Caloric and noncaloric controls of food intake. *Brain Research Bulletin*, 27: 299–303.

Stricker, E. M., and Verbalis, J. G. 1988. Hormones and behavior: The biology of thirst and sodium appetite. *American Scientist*, 76: 261–267.

Woods, S. C., Seeley, R. J., Porte, D. Jr., and Schwartz, M. W. 1998. Signals that regulate food intake and energy homeostasis. *Science*, 280: 1378–1383.

# 10

# Biological Rhythms

**W**hen I was about 10 years old, I had a pet hamster. I do not recall his name, but vaguely recall an elaborate funeral upon his demise. What I remember best about this pet was that he had an exercise wheel inside his cage. Every night as I was trying to fall asleep, the hamster would begin to run in his wheel. Because the wheel made a squeaky noise with each revolution, it was very difficult to fall asleep. I tried oiling the wheel, but the nightly squeak continued. Finally, in desperation late one night, I put the hamster and his cage in my closet. As I was closing the closet door, I began to feel guilty, so I switched on the closet light for him. To my amazement, the hamster stopped running, at least until I fell asleep. I switched off the light the following morning. Over the course of the next several days, the hamster began to confine his wheel-running behavior to the period after the light was switched off each morning. Inadvertently, I had created a reverse light–dark cycle for my hamster. He now confined his running behavior to the daytime hours, when he was in my dark closet and I was in school. When I got home from school, I would play with the creature; before retiring, I would turn on the closet light and return the hamster to his cage, where he would curl into a ball and sleep through the night.

As you probably know, some animals (for example, chipmunks, ground squirrels, and chickens) are **diurnal**, or active during the day, and some animals (for example, hamsters, raccoons, and owls) are **nocturnal**, or active at night. Other animals are **crepuscular** (for example, white-tailed deer), or primarily active during dawn and dusk. Animals have evolved to restrict many of their behaviors, including feeding, drinking, mating, and locomotor activities, to specific temporal niches in response to a complex web of selective forces. This temporal variation in behavior presumably reflects temporal variation in underlying physiology. As we will discover, virtually all physiological processes vary over time. Specific to our interests here, endocrine secretion varies markedly over the course of minutes, over the course of a day, and over the course of a year (Figure 10.1). Because of this temporal variation in endocrine function, it should not be particularly surprising to you that behavior, especially behavior that is mediated by hormones, exhibits pronounced temporal variation. Much of this temporal variation is regulated by biological clocks.

The scientific study of biological clocks and their associated rhythms is called **chronobiology** or **biochronometry**. Although biological rhythms have been informally recognized by biologists for many years, the formal study of biological timekeeping began about 40 years ago. One reason that chronobiology took so long to develop as a scientific discipline was that it had to counteract the dogma of homeostasis in biological sciences and medicine. In Chapter 9 we learned that homeostatic processes work to maintain physiological parameters within specific ranges. Biologists and physicians often considered large fluctuations to be pathological, and many resisted the idea of the programmed changes in physiology and behavior that we now understand to underlie homeostatic processes. Many of the specific homeostatic ranges discussed in Chapter 9 are not static, but in fact change over time. To take these changes into account, the thermostat analogy that we used in that chapter may be updated to an automatic thermostat that can be programmed to limit heating or cooling to times when people are likely to be home. This temporal variation increases the efficiency of the home heating system. Similarly, biological clocks increase biological efficiency and thus increase fitness. This chapter will describe such temporal variations generally, and will focus specifically upon the interaction among hormones, biological rhythms, and behavior.

Chronobiology has borrowed terms and concepts extensively from engineering disciplines to describe biological clocks and their associated rhythms. A **rhythm** is a recurrent event that is characterized by its period, frequency, amplitude, and phase (Figure 10.2; Aschoff, 1981). The **period** is the length of time required to complete one cycle of the rhythm in question; for instance, the amount of time required to go from peak to peak or trough to trough. **Frequency** is computed as the number of completed cycles per unit of time (for example, 2 cycles per day). **Amplitude** is the amount of change above and below the average value;

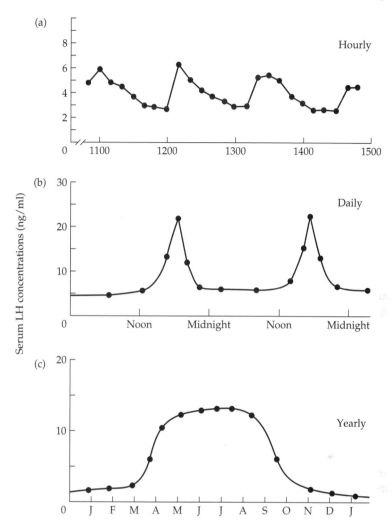

**10.1    Endocrine function shows rhythmic variation over time.** If LH concentrations in hamsters are observed over several different temporal scales, rhythmic release patterns emerge. (a) Assessments every 10 minutes reveal that LH is released in pulses that recur every 30–90 minutes. (b) Samples obtained every 6 hours will not detect 30–90-minute pulses, but reveal a daily rhythm of LH release. These daily surges consist of programmed increases in the 30–90 minute pulse frequency and pulse amplitude that result in elevated blood concentrations of LH. (c) Blood samples obtained once a month from hamsters housed in simulated winter conditions do not detect daily pulses, but an annual pattern of LH secretion emerges, showing that blood LH concentrations are generally higher during the breeding season in spring and summer than during autumn and winter.

that is, the distance of the peak or nadir from the average. The **phase** represents a point on the rhythm relative to some objective time point during the cycle. For example, under normal conditions, the phase of onset of the activity portion of a hamster's activity–rest cycle corresponds closely with the onset of dark. Phase relations among various biological rhythms can also be described; for instance,

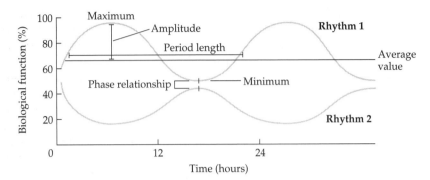

**10.2    Components of biological rhythms.** Rhythms can be analyzed in terms of amplitude, frequency, and period length. The relationship of one rhythm to another is expressed in terms of phase relationships.

the onset of the low body temperature phase of the daily body temperature cycle tightly corresponds with the onset of the sleep portion of the hamster sleep–wake cycle.

## Exogenous versus Endogenous Control of Biological Clocks

Some behavioral rhythms have been recognized since ancient times, but they have generally been attributed to **exogenous** (outside the organism) factors. For example, the activity–rest rhythms exhibited by many species, including my pet hamster, were believed to be caused by daily signals arising from the environment. Thus, one simplistic explanation of how the daily light–dark cycle might drive the activity–rest rhythm of hamsters might be that the light of day is too intense for their eyes, so they rest during the daylight hours and become active after dark. Although exogenous factors may serve a permissive role for biological rhythms, we now know that **endogenous** (inside the organism) timing mechanisms mediate many of the observed rhythms in physiology and behavior.

How is it established whether a rhythm is the result of exogenous factors or an endogenous clock? One type of evidence is provided by isolation experiments. The persistence of a biological rhythm in the absence of environmental cues provides compelling evidence that the rhythm in question is generated within the animal, and not driven by the environment. If a biological rhythm disappears under constant conditions, then it is reasonable to suggest that some cyclic cue in the environment drives the biological rhythm. This logic was first applied to the study of biological rhythms in 1729, when the French astronomer Jean Jacques d'Ortous de Mairan found that the tension–relaxation pattern of a heliotropic plant—a plant with leaves that open during the day and close at night—persisted even when the plant was maintained in the total darkness of a cellar for several days (Figure 10.3; De Mairan, 1729). Augustin de Candolle, a French botanist, expanded on de Mairan's initial observation. Mimosa (*Mimosa pudica*) leaf movements also continued in constant dark conditions, but like most other internally

**10.3   De Mairan's experiment.** Heliotropic plants isolated from sunlight continued to open and close in synchrony with the day–night cycle, suggesting that the rhythm has an endogenous, rather than an exogenous, source. De Mairan's report is the first recorded observation that biological rhythms can persist in the absence of environmental cues.

generated biological rhythms, these free-running rhythms displayed slight to moderate deviations from 24 hours in period length (de Candolle, 1832).

Examples of this sort were reported sporadically over the course of the next 200 years. Although such demonstrations were consistent with the existence of endogenously driven biological clocks, the scientific community largely maintained that these reported rhythms merely reflected rhythms in the environment. From the 1930s through the 1960s, biologists gradually began to accept the existence of endogenous biological clocks, although some scientists continued to argue that the persistent biological rhythms observed when all apparent environmental cues were absent could be explained away as reflecting subtle geophysical forces that simply had yet to be discovered (for example, Brown, 1972). However, recent evidence has convinced virtually everyone that clocks driving behavior and physiology are inside the organism and not driven by the environment. Several types of evidence support this conclusion, all of which will be more fully explored later in the chapter:

1. Animals maintained in constant conditions aboard a spacecraft orbiting far above the earth, presumably far away from subtle geophysical cues, display biological rhythms with periods similar to those observed on earth.

2. Animals maintained in adjacent, but individual, cages in the absence of environmental cues display biological rhythms with slightly different periods, suggesting that they are not being driven by the same subtle geophysical cues.

3. The period (and phase) of the biological rhythms of one individual can be transferred to another individual by means of tissue transplants.

# Types of Biological Clocks and Rhythms

All animals, and virtually all plants (that is, all eukaryotic and some prokaryotic organisms), studied to date possess endogenous biological clocks that mediate biological rhythms. The periods of biological rhythms range from the 1-millisecond cycle of neuronal firing to longer cycles such as the 16-day estrous cycles of guinea pigs, the 1-year cycle of ground squirrel hibernation, the 10-year cycle of the thickening of fur in the arctic lynx, or the 100-year cycle of the flowering of certain species of bamboo (Figure 10.4).

The periods of some biological rhythms, including most central nervous system, cardiovascular, and respiratory rhythms, vary widely within the same individual; for example, the period of heartbeats decreases (that is, the frequency increases) during exercise because heart rhythms are dependent on activity levels. The periods of other endogenous cycles, such as the ovarian cycle, are largely constant for the same individual, but there may be great interindividual or species variation. However, there are four types of biological rhythms that are typically coupled with environmental cues, and the periods of these rhythms do not vary much under natural conditions. These relatively constant biological rhythms mimic the periods of the geophysical cycles of night and day (**circadian**), the tides (**circatidal**), the phases of the moon (**circalunar**), and the seasons of the year (**circannual**) (Table 10.1; Palmer, 1976). These rhythms persist when animals are isolated from the respective environmental cues, but in that case they only approximate the periods of the environmental cues to which they are normally coupled, as we will see below. Thus, the terms for many biological rhythms use the prefix *circa*, from the Latin word meaning "about" (for example, *circa*, "about"; *dies*, "day"; *circadian*, "about a day") (Halberg, 1959). Although conducting an experiment that isolates animals from environmental cues is necessary to determine the extent of endogenous generation of any biological rhythm, it should be noted that the environment often exerts permissive effects on endogenously driven biological rhythms. For instance, chronic food restriction or maintenance in constant bright lights dampens the expression of estrous cycles in laboratory strains of rats.

An important experimental technique used in the study of biological rhythms involves keeping a log of physical activity over time. Basically, the monitoring of activity cycles is adapted to the species under investigation. Often small mammals are placed in a cage equipped with a running wheel, similar to the one in my pet hamster's cage, connected to a counting device that automatically produces a continuous record of activity (Figure 10.5). The locomotor activities of

**Table 10.1**
**Comparison of biological rhythm types**

| Rhythm type | Environmental cycle | Period length Entrained | Period length Free-running |
|---|---|---|---|
| Circadian | Revolution of earth | 24 hours | 22–26 hours |
| Circatidal | Tides | 12.4 hours | 11–14 hours |
| Circalunar | Phases of moon | 29.5 days | 26–32 days |
| Circannual | Seasons of the year | 365.25 days | 330–400 days |

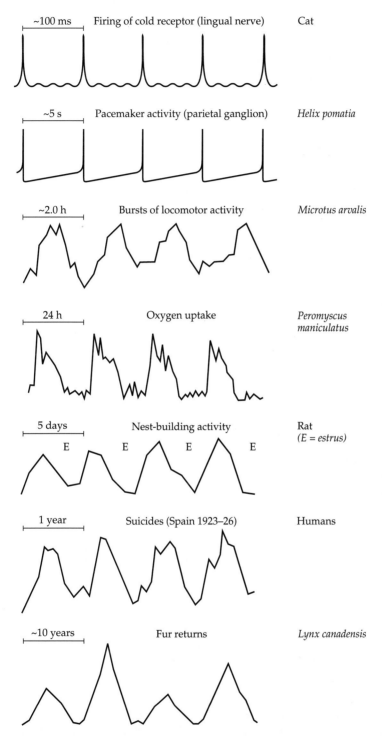

**10.4 The diversity of biological rhythms.** The period lengths of biological rhythms range from milliseconds, such as certain rhythms of neuronal firing (top), to many years (bottom). The longest known period, the time that elapses between flowerings of certain bamboo species, lasts 100 years. Source: Aschoff, 1981.

small birds are often determined by monitoring perch-hopping activities around the clock. Humans can be equipped with electronic monitoring devices that transmit the movements of an individual to a central monitoring station.

**10.5    The collection of behavioral biological rhythm data.** (a) A common method of measuring rhythms in locomotor activity is a wheel-running apparatus that activates a pen with each revolution of the wheel. Sustained wheel-running activity appears as a solid dark bar across the time line for each day (b). The activity record is read like sheet music, with each line representing 24 hours. The period of the daily biological rhythm can be measured from the onset of activity on one day to the onset of activity on the next. The frequency of activity can be measured by counting the number of wheel revolutions each night (c). The amplitude is the distance between the peak and the trough of the number of wheel revolutions. Phase could be measured as the amount of time between the onset of running and the onset of darkness.

Animals display species-specific times of locomotor activity onset that are often linked to the timing of food intake, water consumption, and reproductive behavior. In the case of the hamster—an experimental animal commonly used in studies of biological rhythms—locomotor activity begins right after lights are turned off each day. If lights are turned off at 8:00 P.M. each evening, hamsters begin to run in their wheels at about 8:05–8:15 P.M. each evening. More than 99% of the wheel-running activity is confined to the dark portion of the daily light–dark cycle. Hamsters also confine the majority of their eating, drinking, food hoarding, and sexual behaviors to the dark portion of the daily light–dark cycle. If the environmental light–dark cycles are phase-shifted (e.g., lights are turned off 4 hours later, as in Figure 10.6), then hamsters adapt their activity rhythms to the new regimen in about four or five cycles. The circadian rhythms of other physiological processes, such as adrenocortical hormone release, body temperature, and blood plasma volume, may require longer to adapt to the new time. This process of adaptation to rapid phase shifts in environmental time cues results in what we commonly call "jet lag" when humans travel through different time zones (Box 10.1).

Light serves as a potent environmental time cue, or **zeitgeber** (from the German, meaning "time giver"), for hamsters as well as for most other species (Pittendrigh and Daan, 1976). Temperature is an important zeitgeber for some

**10.6   Wheel-running behavior of a hamster.** When housed in a 12:12 dark–light cycle (lights off for 12 hours, then on for 12 hours), a hamster will confine its wheel running to the dark part of the cycle (top). If the onset of darkness is shifted ahead by 4 hours (arrow), the hamster will adjust to the new cycle. If the dark–light cycle is suspended entirely, and the hamster is housed in constant dim illumination, it no longer expresses a 24-hour cycle of activity, but free-runs with a period greater than 24 hours; this free-running cycle represents the endogenous circadian rhythm of the individual. From Zucker, 1980.

---

## Box 10.1
# Jet Lag

The temporal niche to which humans have been exposed during the past million or so years has remained quite stable (Moore-Ede et al., 1982); it has been estimated that the time required for the earth to rotate once on its axis has slowed by only about 20 seconds during the last million years (Rosenberg and Runcorn, 1975). In contrast, the technological changes of the past century have had staggering and unprecedented effects on our temporal environment. The invention of electric lights has permitted round-the-clock shift work, and powerful security lights keep some environments brightly illuminated 24 hours a day. The development of jet travel has led to abrupt phase shifts not previously encountered by east–west travelers (most jet travel occurs on east–west, rather than north–south, routes because many commercial centers in Asia, Europe, and North America are at similar latitudes).

Jet lag, the physiological and behavioral responses to jet travel across time zones,

involves phase shifts in all the zeitgebers at once. Symptoms include sleep disruption; disruption of digestive processes; impaired psychological processes, including attention, perception, and motivation; and a general feeling of malaise (Office of Technology Assessment, 1991). Most studies indicate that these symptoms are less pronounced when travelers phase-delay (travel west) than phase-advance (travel east). For example, one study discovered that resynchronization of psychomotor performance rhythms took longer for people on eastbound flights than for people on westbound flights, although eastbound travelers could hasten adaptation to local time by being outdoors (Klein and Wegmann, 1974; Moore-Ede et al., 1982). In general, the severity of jet lag symptoms also correlates with the number of time zones crossed. One study showed that physiological adaptation to westbound travel (phase-delay) took less time than adaptation to eastbound travel (phase-advance) for travelers who

---

poikilothermic animals, and possibly a secondary zeitgeber for birds and mammals, but light is the primary zeitgeber among homeothermic animals. If a hamster is placed in constant dim light so that there is no daily zeitgeber, the onset time of its locomotor activity begins to drift (see Figure 10.6). Without the daily light–dark cycle providing a daily reset, the endogenous clock of the hamster can only approximate 24-hour cycles. If a hamster usually begins to run in its wheel at 8:10 P.M., then in the absence of light–dark cycles, it may begin its wheel-running behavior 15 minutes later each day, with wheel-running activity onset at 8:25, 8:40, 8:55, and so on for subsequent days. Other hamsters may begin their wheel-running activities 10 minutes earlier each day. Biological rhythms such as these that are not synchronized with environmental cues are said to be **free-running**. Each individual will display its own free-running period. After a few weeks of constant lighting conditions, it is possible to observe different individuals housed in the same room running in their wheels at different times throughout the day. Thus, the free-running periods of biological clocks are precise, but are not exactly 24 hours. The observation that different hamsters display an array of different free-running periods when housed in the same room suggests that they are *not* synchronized by each other's behavior, and that subtle geophysical cues are *not* providing any temporal information.

crossed four or more time zones. Virtually everyone can easily adapt to 1-hour phase shifts and is adversely affected by 12-hour phase shifts, but there are tremendous individual differences in the effects of temporal phase shifts on performance, as well as in the speed of resynchronization following time shifts (see figure). Studies also show that elderly people have more difficulty with the effects of jet lag than younger people do. Appropriately timed melatonin treatment may provide some relief for the symptoms of jet lag (Arendt, 1998). Outdoor exercise has also been reported to ameliorate jet lag symptoms (Shiota et al., 1996).

However, even a 1-hour phase shift can be significant for some individuals. In many industrialized nations, the entire population undergoes a 1-hour phase shift twice a year with the change from standard time to daylight saving time. It usually requires several days for people to make the adjustment to this biennial time shift in their circadian systems (Monk and Aplin, 1980). In the United States, the rate of traffic accidents increases significantly in the week following the time changes (Monk, 1980). Whether this statistic reflects an impairment of attention and psychomotor coordination because of alterations in our circadian systems, or missed appointments because of incorrectly set watches, is open to question.

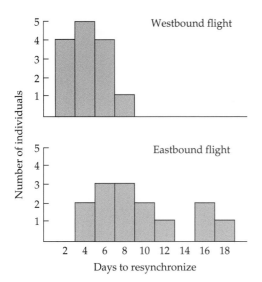

The process of synchronization of endogenous biological rhythms to a periodic cue in the environment—or to a zeitgeber—is called **entrainment**. We will focus on the role of light as a zeitgeber for daily activity rhythms in order to understand the process of entrainment. In order to understand entrainment, a basic understanding of phase-response curves is necessary. **Phase-response curves** are graphic representations of the differential effects that environmental light has on the timing of biological rhythms; these temporal effects depend upon the phase relationship of the light to the circadian organization of the animal in question (Figure 10.7). Exposure to light at different times throughout the day does not result in uniform responses of free-running biological rhythms. If hamsters (or humans) are maintained in constant dark conditions, their biological rhythms begin to free-run, with the period of onset of locomotor activity varying slightly from 24 hours. The circadian period can thus be divided into a "subjective night" and a "subjective day." Because hamsters are nocturnal, the beginning of activity usually coincides with the onset of the creature's subjective night, whereas the rest period begins at the beginning of the animal's subjective day. For diurnal animals, the onset of activity coincides with the beginning of the animal's subjective day, and the rest period begins at the beginning of the animal's subjective night. If free-running hamsters that are housed in continuous darkness are exposed to an

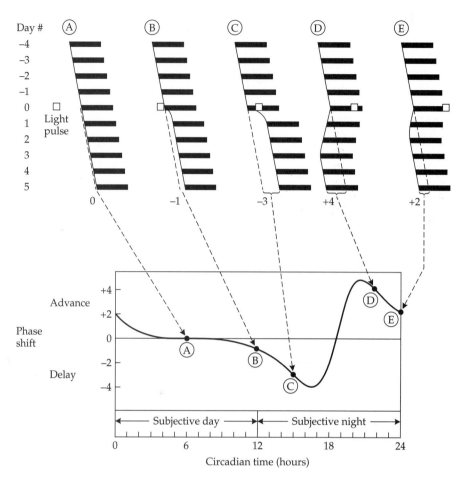

**10.7    Phase-response curve.** A free-running nocturnal individual maintained in constant dark conditions was exposed to a 1-hour light pulse at various times during the subjective day and night. The dark bars at the top of the figure are a schematic record of activity (wheel running), which occurred during the animal's subjective night. (a) When the light pulse was given in the middle of the subjective day, the subsequent activity onset time was unaffected; the middle of the subjective day is thus called the "dead zone." (b) A light pulse at the end of the subjective day phase-delayed activity the next day by about 1 hour. (c) With a light pulse at the start of the subjective night, a substantial phase delay (3 hours) was observed. (d) A light pulse given later during the subjective night caused a substantial advance (4 hours) of activity onset the next day. (e) Finally, a light pulse at the start of the subjective day caused a 2-hour phase advance in activity the following day. The effect of light on endogenous circadian rhythms is involved in entraining them to exactly 24 hours each day. After Moore-Ede et al., 1982.

hour of light at any time throughout the middle of the subjective day, the time of onset of the next bout of locomotor activity is unaffected; that is, for a hamster with a free-running period of 24.25 hours, wheel-running still begins 24.25 hours after the start of the previous bout of activity. However, if the 1-hour pulse of light is given early in the subjective night (or late in the subjective day), then the hamster does not begin its activity 24.25 hours later, but rather delays its activity onset for 1–4 hours, depending on when exactly the pulse of light occurs. If the 1-hour pulse of light is given late in the subjective night (or early in the subjective day), again the hamster does not begin its activity 24.25 hours later, but rather advances its activity onset by 1–4 hours, depending on when exactly the pulse of light occurs. Thus, the largest phase delays can be produced early during subjective night, when a nocturnal animal has just awakened and a diurnal animal has just retired, and the largest phase advances can be produced late during the subjective night; light appears to have little effect on the circadian system during the subjective day of either nocturnal or diurnal animals.

Although phase responses to light are best observed in free-running animals, these effects of light also operate upon animals that are entrained to a light–dark cycle. Light impinges upon the phase-advance and phase-delay portions of an animal's daily cycle of responsiveness to light to reset the biological rhythm to exactly 24 hours—that is, to entrain the rhythm. In an analogous manner, if you owned a wristwatch that gained 15 minutes each day (period = 24.25 hours), you would be the zeitgeber that entrains the watch when you reset it to the correct time each morning. The phase-response curves give clues about what happened to my pet hamster when I created a reverse light–dark cycle. Light, now coincident with the maximal phase-delay portion of the phase-response curve, caused several days of phase delays until a 12-hour shift was attained. The same process occurs when you move across several time zones rapidly (see Box 10.1).

**Ultradian** (shorter than circadian) and **infradian** (longer than circadian) rhythms are biological rhythms that do not correspond to any known geophysical cycles. These names may seem confusing because *ultra* is synonymous with "higher" and *infra* with "lower," but the terms ultradian and infradian refer to the *frequency* of a cycle in relation to a day, rather than to the *period*. If a circadian cycle has a frequency of one event per day, then an ultradian cycle of one event every 2 hours, or every 1/12 day, has a frequency 12 times higher than the circadian cycle. Ultradian cycles are commonly observed; an example is the 90-minute cycle characteristic of REM sleep (Schulz and Lavie, 1985). Ultradian cycles have also been reported for the locomotor activity patterns of other animals, especially newborns (Lavie, 1985). The pulsatile releases of several hormones, including GnRH, LH, testosterone, growth hormone, and corticosterone, are considered ultradian rhythms.

Infradian rhythms, less frequently observed than ultradian rhythms, include biological rhythms longer than a day but shorter than a lunar month. There have been sporadic reports of a 7-day cycle of excretions of urinary ketosteroids and a 21–28-day cycle of excretion of testosterone in human males, but these findings have not been sufficiently replicated. Infradian testosterone rhythms in human males are probably due to exogenous factors, such as pay schedules or exercise patterns, because these types of rhythms are rarely reported for men isolated from social and environmental cues. Generally, infradian rhythms in testicular function are rare among vertebrates. Dormice (*Glis glis*) have been reported to display infradian rhythms of about 60 days in body mass and body fat content (Grimes et al., 1981; Melnyk et al., 1983). The most common types of infradian rhythms are those associated with ovarian cycles; that is, estrous cycles. Hamsters have very brief, 4-day, estrous cycles. Rats, as you may recall, have estrous cycles of 4 or 5 days. Guinea pigs and sheep have estrous cycles of approximately 16 days. Under the right conditions, these cycles are self-sustaining, endogenously generated biological rhythms that do not correspond to any known geophysical cue. Of course, human menstrual cycles roughly correspond to the period of one rotation of the moon around the earth, the lunar month of 29.5 days. However, the length of the human menstrual cycle seems to be only coincidentally similar to the length of the lunar month, rather than reflecting any adaptive link to the lunar cycle (Knobil and Hotchkiss, 1988).

### Examples of Biological Rhythms in Behavior

Examples of the four different types of biological rhythms that occur in nature will be described in this section.

   **CIRCADIAN RHYTHMS.**   Circadian rhythms in many different behaviors have been demonstrated in a very large number of species across animal taxa (Table 10.2). Sexual behavior, learning, parental behavior, aggressive behavior, and other social behaviors show clear circadian cyclicity in occurrence. All of these behaviors have been shown to be affected by hormones, which are often secreted according to a circadian program. These and many of the behaviors listed in Table 10.2 can be modified by experience, but some have to be done correctly during a very precise temporal window. There is a temporal window for emergence from eggs

**Table 10.2**
**Behaviors that display circadian rhythms in birds and mammals**[a]

| Behavior | Birds | Mammals |
|---|---|---|
| Activity | Y | Y |
| Aggression | Y | Y |
| Coprophagy | — | Y |
| Copulation/courtship | Y | Y |
| Drinking | Y | Y |
| Eating | Y | Y |
| Egg laying | Y | — |
| Feeding | Y | Y |
| Food storage | Y | Y |
| Gnawing | — | Y |
| Incubation | Y | — |
| Maternal behavior | Y | Y |
| Nest building | Y | Y |
| Nest departure | Y | N |
| Parental feeding | Y | Y |
| Predation | Y | Y |
| Preening | Y | — |
| Sexual behavior | Y | Y |
| Singing | Y | — |
| Sleep | Y | Y |
| Territorial defense | Y | — |
| Tonic immobility | Y | Y |
| Torpor | N | Y |
| Vocalization | Y | Y |

[a]Dashes in columns indicate behaviors not tested or examined.
*Source:* After Rusak, 1981.

for several species. For example, *Drosophila pseudobscura* larvae mature within their eggs at random times throughout the day, but hatching occurs only in the morning. Thus, there seems to be a biological clock controlling the time at which the larval fruit flies hatch from their eggs (Pittendrigh, 1981). The clock for their developmental activity is set the first time they "see" light in the translucent egg, which is normally at dawn. After developing through the larval to pupal stages, adult flies also emerge from their pupal cases at "lights on" or first morning's light. Why is adult emergence, or eclosion, synchronized in this way? There are significant costs associated with eclosing at the wrong time during the day. The flies need to stretch out and dry their new wings during the early morning, when humidity is high. If the flies are tricked by artificial light into emerging at the wrong time, they suffer a higher mortality rate because their wings may be damaged, and they are also more susceptible to predation. By hatching out in unison, the flies also reduce their individual chances of being consumed by birds or other predators. In other words, synchronous hatching swamps the predators. There is safety in numbers.

Another example of differential mortality rates associated with temporal patterns involves the fledging (nest-leaving) behavior of the guillemot (*Uria lomvia*), a seabird that nests on cliffs in northern Europe (Daan, 1981). The young birds, still somewhat immature and incompletely feathered, leave their nests on the cliffs and glide onto the beach or into the water, where many are eaten by waiting gulls. The peak times for both fledging and predation by gulls are fairly close; however, it is at those times that the highest percentage of the young guillemots survive (Figure 10.8). This is another example of "predator swamping," in this case by fledging in numbers that exceed the carrying capacity (the amount that they can eat) of the

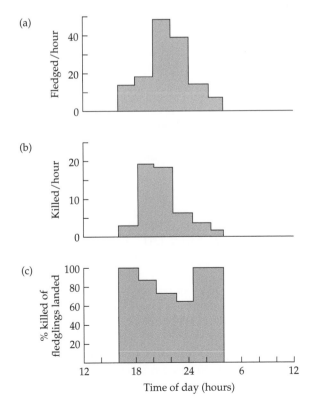

**10.8  Circadian rhythmicity of fledging behavior in guillemots.** Guillemots, seabirds that nest along cliffs near the Arctic Circle, are vulnerable to predation when they first leave the nest, and have evolved to leave at the same time so as to swamp predators and reduce their odds of being eaten. (a) Most guillemot chicks leave the nest by about 2100 (9:00 P.M.). The predators respond to this cycle by feeding during this time (b); however, the best odds of escape for any individual bird also occur during the peak (c), so it is in the best interest of the birds to fledge all at the same time. Source: Daan, 1981.

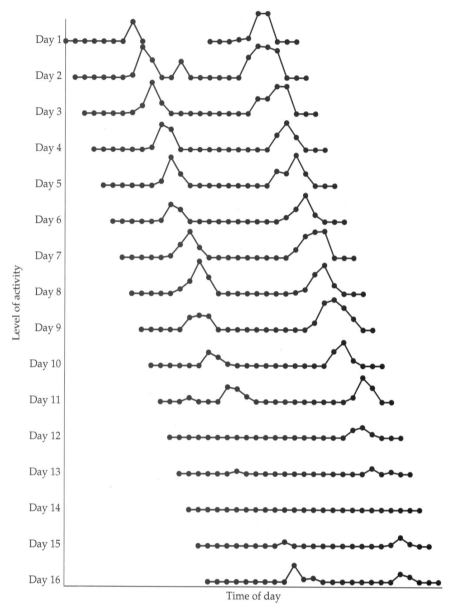

Level of activity

Time of day

**10.9   Circatidal locomotor activity rhythm of fiddler crabs.** Fiddler crabs maintained in
aquaria in constant darkness and constant temperature conditions will become active at approximately the same time as low tide occurs at their capture site, and will maintain this  endogenous biological rhythm for many months. Source: Palmer, 1990.

predators. Young guillemots whose fledging behavior is not synchronized with that
of the others have a high probability of being eaten. Because these birds live above
the Arctic Circle, they must rely on their endogenous biological clocks, which are
synchronized during the early summer when there is still a light–dark cycle, to
make the fledging decision because they are confronted with continuously light
summer days around the time of fledging. Simultaneous hatching in many other

species may also represent a temporal adaptation that has evolved to reduce each individual's odds of becoming a meal.

**CIRCATIDAL RHYTHMS.** An example of an endogenously generated circatidal rhythm can be seen in the locomotor activity pattern of fiddler crabs (*Uca pugnax*) (Palmer, 1990). These crabs are residents of the intertidal zone and can be observed moving along the marsh or beach during low tide, searching for food and mates. The crabs return to their burrows prior to the onset of high tide, when their environment is flooded by the sea. If a fiddler crab is removed to an aquarium, it will retain its cycle of activity, with slight deviations of approximately 2%–3% from the 12.4-hour tidal cycle (Figure 10.9; Palmer, 1990). Its periods of locomotor activity will alternate with quiescence every 12.4 hours and will correspond to the occurrence of low tide in the area where it was collected.

**CIRCALUNAR RHYTHMS.** Lunar cycles of behavior are observed in a limited number of species. Some animals have evolved biological rhythms that permit them to time their behavior within the 29.5-day lunar cycle (Richter, 1968). In general, nocturnal predators increase their activities during the evenings around the time of a full moon, and decrease their activities around the time of a new moon. Prey species show the opposite pattern, avoiding nocturnal activities during evenings with bright moons. Insects may also show this pattern (Figure 10.10a).

(a)

(b)

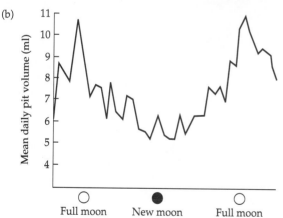

**10.10 A circalunar behavioral rhythm.** (a) The ant lion hunts by building a pit to catch passing ants or other insects. (b) 50 ant lions that were fed a single ant per day and maintained in constant conditions exhibited a circalunar rhythm in the average size of the pits they built; they dug larger pits when there was a full moon and smaller pits when there was a new moon. Source: Youthed and Moran, 1969.

For example, the ant lion (*Myrmeleon obscurus*) hunts by building a pit with steep walls of shifting sands. The ant lion buries itself at the bottom and waits for an ant or other bug to slide into the pit. Its huge pincers pierce the body of its prey, and the ant lion sucks out the body fluids. Perhaps the ant lion could be called the vampire bug because it increases its activities during the full moon. Even in the constant conditions of a laboratory, the ant lion builds a larger pit during full moons than during new moons (Figure 10.10b; Youthed and Moran, 1969).

**CIRCANNUAL RHYTHMS.** Circannual behavioral rhythms include the migratory patterns of birds as well as the hibernation and seasonal changes in body mass observed in several mammalian species. Even when kept in a laboratory for years, birds show 10–12-month cycles of premigratory restlessness, weight gain, and reproductive competence (Gwinner, 1986). Mammals such as ground squirrels also show circannual cycles of weight gain, reproductive competence, and (if the temperature is sufficiently low) hibernation (see below). The functional significance of these annual rhythms usually reflects seasonal changes in energy availability in the environment.

There are also patterns of mixed or hybrid behavioral rhythms. The Pacific palolo worm (*Eunice viridis*) usually spends its time in burrows in the coral off the coast of Fiji and Samoa (Burrows, 1945). But in the months of October, November, and December, on the last day of the last quarter of the moon, at sunrise, a 30-cm

**10.11   Palolo worms display a complex reproductive rhythm.** These epitopes (sea worms) are native to the South Pacific, and move to the ocean surface to exchange sperm and eggs during the months of October, November, and December—but only at sunrise on the last day of the last quarter of the moon. Local residents consider the palolo a delicacy, and make use of their knowledge of its complex reproductive patterns in collecting the worms for eating.

long segment of each worm breaks off and swims to the surface, where it and other worms explode in unison, forming a slurry of eggs and sperm. The local epi-cures are aware of this cycle, which enables them to predict the event in advance and arrive at the coral reefs at dawn on the appropriate days to scoop up hand-fuls of this gastronomic treat. The palolo worms may be consumed raw or roasted, and I have been told that they taste like sushi stuffed with caviar when eaten raw (Figure 10.11). Human knowledge of cyclic behavior, ranging from grunion "runs" on California beaches to the seasonal migrations of caribou in northern Canada, has allowed the exploitation of many animals for food and other resources.

## Usefulness of Biological Clocks

Why have these elaborate timekeeping mechanisms evolved? In other words, what is the adaptive function of biological clocks? As the above examples indi-cate, biological clocks are useful for (1) synchronizing the activities of animals with their environments, including their social environments, thus enabling them to prepare for predictable events (for example, night, winter, or the onset of repro-ductive function in potential mates); and (2) synchronizing the internal physio-logical and biochemical processes of animals in order to promote efficient functioning.

One of the most predictable features of life on earth is the regular pattern of environmental changes associated with the movement of our planet. Life evolved in a cyclic environment. As one chronobiologist wrote, "The rotation of the Earth on its polar axis gives rise to the dominant cycle of day and night; the revolutions of the Earth around the Sun give rise to the unfailing procession of the seasons; and the more complicated movements of the Moon in relation to the Earth and the Sun give rise to the lunar month and to the tidal cycles" (Saunders, 1977). Ex-cept for animals living at the bottom of the oceans or deep within caves, day fol-lows night, and the seasons change. These orderly and predictable changes in the environment have existed since life first began to evolve on this planet, although the timing of these events may have changed over time. The rotation of the earth results in periodic exposure to the radiation of the sun, which causes predictable changes in light and ambient temperatures, as well as associated changes in the relative humidity of the air and in the oxygen levels of aqueous habitats. The bio-logical clocks of animals and plants permit them to start or stop locomotor activi-ties or activate photosynthetic machinery, respectively, in preparation for light (Figure 10.12). All eukaryotic and most prokaryotic organisms tested to date, from unicellular organisms to humans, display circadian rhythms. Of course, circadi-an rhythms have not evolved in organisms that live for less than 24 hours. Similarly, circannual rhythms have evolved only in animals that live for a year or more.

As you know, evolutionary theory describes the morphological adaptation of animals to their environmental niches. Behavioral rhythms can be viewed as adaptations to different temporal, rather than spatial, niches. For example, there are optimal seasons for migration or breeding, and optimal daily times for sleep-ing or feeding. There is a theory that mammals replaced reptiles as the dominant form of life on land because their ability to regulate their internal temperature permitted them to enter the nocturnal niche (Daan, 1981). Presumably, the small, secretive nocturnal proto-mammals were able to exploit the same spatial habitat

**10.12  Linnaeus's "flower clock."**  Linnaeus exploited his knowledge of the activity patterns of heliotropic flowers to design this clock in 1751. He proposed that the clock would operate from 6:00 to 18:00 (6:00 A.M. to 6:00 P.M.), and that the time of day could be determined by noting which flowers were blooming.

used by the reptiles during the day. These early mammals were able to move about at night virtually unmolested because the movements of the cold-blooded reptiles were often constrained to the daylight hours. It is possible that reptilian eggs were devoured by the night-ranging mammals, thus accelerating the reptiles' demise. Although it is fascinating to speculate on these issues, the point to extract from this theory is that adaptations to temporal niches are critical for individual fitness.

The action of biological clocks in synchronizing the bodily functions of an individual has been compared to the role of the conductor in an orchestra. Internal processes may serve to prepare the body for certain activities to occur later; for example, the elevated adrenal secretions coinciding with the morning onset of activity prepare you for increased activity levels and for breaking your nightly fast.

Physiological systems show a wide variety of rhythmic changes. For instance, body temperature, blood plasma levels of potassium, sodium, cortisol, and androgens, and growth hormone and dopamine turnover all show pronounced circadian rhythms (Figure 10.13; Halberg, 1977; Rusak, 1989). Some of these changes may be on the order of 100% to 200% from baseline values. Peak daily cortisol concentrations, for example, which usually occur just prior to or immediately after awakening, coincide with the onset of locomotor activity in the morning. This programmed elevation of cortisol concentrations increases blood pressure and cardiac output prior to the active phase of the day. We know that these increased cortisol concentrations are not driven by the increased activity levels, because the same circadian rhythm is observed in bedridden patients under constant conditions (Aschoff, 1965). In some instances, the production and release of hormones corresponds to the timing of hormone receptor production. Neurotransmitter receptors are manufactured prior to a circadian-programmed increase in neurotransmitter production. Body temperature peaks in mid-afternoon, when people

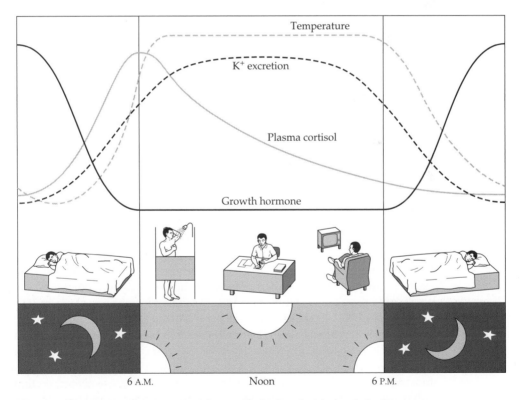

**10.13   Circadian rhythms in human physiology and behavior.** Activity levels, body temperature, urinary potassium excretion, plasma cortisol levels, and growth hormone secretion exhibit circadian rhythms that are closely coupled to the sleep–wake cycle. After Richardson and Martin, 1988.

are most active, but again, muscular activity is not solely responsible for this "heating." If you are inactive in bed under constant conditions, your peak body temperature still maintains a circadian rhythm (Moore-Ede et al., 1982).

# Circadian Clocks

Circadian biological clocks have been the subject of the most study in chronobiology. Several generalizations can be made about circadian biological clocks on a phenomenological level: they are (1) inherited, (2) relatively independent of temperature, (3) relatively independent of chemical influence, (4) entrained (synchronized) only to limited cycle lengths, (5) relatively independent of behavioral feedback, and (6) found at every level of organization within an organism (Pittendrigh, 1981; Pittendrigh and Daan, 1976).

## *Localization of Circadian Clocks*

Where are biological clocks located? Biological clocks are found in both plants and animals, so the nervous system cannot be the fundamental level of organization, although you will soon see that biological clocks in the nervous system play a critical role in the temporal organization of the physiology and behavior of birds and mammals. Because single-celled organisms exhibit circadian rhythms, it is reasonable to suggest that biological clocks are organized at the cellular level (Takahashi, 1991). There are two lines of research attempting to locate the fundamental cellular clock. One approach uses molecular biological techniques to discover the basic features of the clock. The second approach uses classic and molecular genetics to uncover the fundamental properties and location of the clock.

Much has been learned about the mechanisms of the cellular clock through the use of chemicals that promote or block specific cellular functions (Hastings et al., 1991). Typically, a chemical agent is given to an organism that is undergoing regular cycles in constant conditions. For example, providing deuterium oxide (heavy water), which affects cell membrane permeability to ions, to hamsters in constant dark conditions causes them to delay the onset of wheel-running behavior by several hours each night (Richter, 1977; Roberts, 1990). Changes in potassium movement across cell membranes also alter some features of biological clocks; lithium, which can replace potassium in some physiological systems, also can affect biological rhythms (Klemfuss, 1992; Sweeney, 1976). Pharmacological studies such as these have indicated that important components of the biological clock include protein synthesis, membrane structures, calcium, potassium, and other ionic transport mechanisms, and activation of intracellular kinases (Hall and Rosbash, 1987; Takahashi et al., 1993).

The second approach to understanding the mechanisms underlying cellular clocks has been to attempt to identify the genes that control the clock systems, then to identify the actions of those genes (Konopka, 1987; Takahashi, 1993). By studying mutants with unusual free-running circadian rhythms—that is, rhythms with periods substantially greater than or less than 24 hours—and back-crossing these animals with homozygous and heterozygous mates, insights into the locations of the genes that regulate biological clocks can be obtained. Clock mutants have been discovered in the fruit fly (*Drosophila*) and Syrian hamster (Ralph and Menaker, 1988), as well as in other simple plants and animals (Hall and Rosbash,

1987). In the fruit fly, mutants that display no rhythmicity in their behavior, as well as flies that display 19-hour or 28-hour periods, have been discovered. Most of these mutations have been traced to a single gene called *per*, which affects the period of the clock (Box 10.2; Konopka and Benzer, 1971). Whether such genes and their protein products are the ubiquitous mechanisms underlying all biological clocks or are specific to fruit flies requires further investigation. It has been suggested that the mechanisms for biological rhythms may be similar for all organisms in the same way that the cell cycle is shared in common among all organisms (Takahashi et al., 1993).

On a physiological level, circadian oscillators and pacemakers have been discovered in several biological systems. Among vertebrates, the eyes of amphibians, the pineal glands of fishes, reptiles, and birds, and the **suprachiasmatic nuclei (SCN)** of the anterior hypothalamus of mammals contain circadian oscillators (Cahill et al., 1991; Moore and Eichler, 1972; Stephan and Zucker, 1972; Takahashi et al., 1989; Moore, 1997). In most cases, these oscillators and pacemakers were discovered by damaging certain structures and observing that biological rhythms disappeared after their destruction. Several types of evidence suggest that the mammalian SCN contain circadian oscillators: (1) thin slices of SCN tissue continue to display circadian rhythms of electrical activity even when maintained in a culture dish (Shibata and Moore, 1988), and (2) if SCN tissue is transplanted into an SCN-lesioned recipient, the period or the phase of the recipient's rhythm will match that of the donor (Figure 10.14).

The SCN are paired clusters of several thousand neurons located above where the optic nerves cross in the hypothalamus, and below the third ventricle (Figure 10.15). A daily rhythm of glucose utilization in the SCN was first observed in nocturnal rats (Schwartz and Gainer, 1977). Autoradiographic studies in which rats were injected with 2-deoxyglucose revealed that the SCN were metabolically active

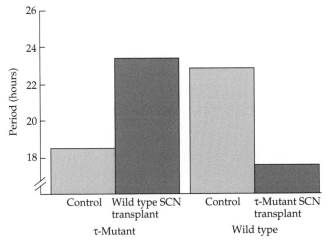

**10.14    Restoration of circadian rhythms with the period of the donor.**    Wild-type (i.e., approximately 24-hour free-running periods) or *tau* mutant (i.e., approximately 20-hour free-running periods) hamsters received SCN lesions, then received SCN transplants from the other genotype. In all cases, the recipient hamsters took on the free-running periods of the SCN donors. After Ralph and Lehmann, 1991.

## Box 10.2
# Molecular Mechanisms of Biological Clocks

Mutant fruit flies whose circadian rhythms show abnormal periodicities have provided important insights into the nature of the cellular biological clock. In a systematic study, fruit flies (*Drosophila melanogaster*) were exposed to a mutagenic compound, then observed for unusual biological rhythms (Konopka and Benzer, 1971). Observations of many mutant flies revealed three general types of mutations that affected biological rhythms: (1) flies with rhythms that had abnormally short periods ($per^s$), (2) flies with rhythms that had abnormally long periods ($per^l$), and arrhythmic flies ($per^0$). These flies differed in the period of their biological rhythms from normal, or wild-type, flies. Through selective mating experiments and the use of so-called visible traits (that is, traits whose genes and chromosomal locations are known), Konopka and Benzer were able to map these different mutations to the same location on the X chromosome. Through the use of what is termed a complementation test, it was discovered that all of the mutations occurred within a single section of the same gene on the X chromosome.

Follow-up studies attempted to isolate the gene, *per,* that was responsible for circadian rhythms in *Drosophila* and to elucidate the mechanism of action of this gene (Hardin et al., 1990; Zwiebel et al., 1991). The *per* gene codes for a protein, PER, that has many branched side chains of sugars (a proteoglycan). The PER protein may act in the cell nucleus to link short-term rhythms into a circadian oscillation (Hardin et al., 1990). Levels of *per* mRNA and the per protein produced in response to the transcription of this gene exhibit a circadian rhythm: there is a 6–8-hour lag between the production of *per* mRNA and the production of the per protein. The various mutant flies showed rhythms in *per* mRNA and per protein synthesis with periods similar to the periods of their other abnormal biological rhythms.

The precise mechanisms of the clock remain unknown. It has been determined that just the 5' end of the *per* gene is sufficient to cause the cycling of *per* mRNA, but is not sufficient to cause cycling in the PER protein product. Thus, the PER protein rhythm does not simply reflect the *per* mRNA rhythm, as might be expected. Administering the wild-type per protein to mutant flies results in normal (that is, wild-type) rhythms of the mutant mRNA in vivo, indicating that the PER protein feeds back to influence *per* gene transcription (Hardin et al., 1990). Other organisms, including humans, possess pieces of genes that resemble the *per* genes in *Drosophila,* and similar molecular mechanisms have been reported for *Neurospora* (a fungus) and mice (Dunlap, 1998).

Another mutant, called *timeless,* exhibits no rhythms in constant darkness. These *timeless* mutants are missing the *TIM* gene, and do not display translocation of the per protein into the nucleus; perhaps the TIM protein is required for nuclear translocation of the per protein.

Another protein that appears critical in both mice and flies (Allada et al., 1998; Gekakis et al., 1998) is called CLOCK. This protein is notable because it contains both a DNA-binding region as well as a site that binds to another protein (Dunlap, 1998). Recently, another *Drosophila* protein was discovered, named CYCLE, that proved to be an important component of the clock mechanism (Rutila et al., 1998). Predictably, flies with mutations for CLOCK or CYCLE did not display any activity by the genes for PER and TIM. It was discovered that CLOCK and CYCLE bind together, then this so-called heterodimer binds to a specific region of DNA, called a promoter, that increases the transcription of the *per* and *tim* genes, but does not appear to affect other gene activities (Rutila et al., 1998; Allada et al., 1998). Furthermore, the PER and TIM proteins also form a complex, which moves into the nucleus to block the special photoreceptors in the eyes and is transduced to the SCN via a special pathway, called the retinohypothalamic tract (RHT), that is distinct from the classic visual system (Figure 10.17; Pickard, 1982; Rusak and Boulos, 1981). An indirect pathway from the intergeniculate leaflet of the thalamus, the geniculohypothalmic tract (GHT), also carries photic information to the SCN (Stopa et al., 1995). Neuropeptide Y appears to be the primary neurochemical signal from the GHT, and may serve to phase-shift the endogenous circadian system (Gillespie et al., 1996; Huhman et al., 1996; 1997; Stopa et al., 1995). A number of neuropeptides have been located in the SCN, including neuropeptide Y, vasopressin, vasoactive intestinal polypeptide, gastrin-releasing peptide, and somatostatin (Duncan, 1998; Hofman et al., 1996; Huhman et al., 1997; Stopa et al., 1995).

Any biological timekeeping system must have an input system (which usually brings light information to the clock), a clock, and an output system, which may be coupled to any number of species-specific physiological and behavioral systems (Takahashi et al., 1993). In some systems, these components may all occur

es may bind to specific receptors within the DNA enhancer region and act to repress or activate gene transcription.

Approximately six different types of binding areas have been located within enhancer regions of DNA, one of which is called the AP-1 complex. The first genes activated when a cell receives a signal are the IEGs, which code for a variety of proteins in the jun family, including jun-B, c-jun, and c-fos. Jun-B and c-fos bind together to form a dimer that binds to the AP-1 receptors in the enhancer regions of other genes to stimulate gene transcription. Thus, activation of IEGs is often the first indication that the genetic machinery within a cell has been activated by an external or hormonal stimulus. In addition to their effects on the enhancer region, IEG proteins can feed back and affect the promoter region, starting or stopping gene transcription.

Light appears to activate IEGs in the SCN of both nocturnal and diurnal animals (Katona et al., 1998). The photomicrographs shown here are in situ hybridization depictions (see Chapter 1) of different magnifications of the SCN from a hamster maintained in constant darkness (top), and from a hamster maintained in darkness and then exposed to a 1-hour pulse of light (bottom). Activation of the c-*fos* gene is seen in the bottom left panel as light areas, and in the bottom right panel as dark spots lying over cells.

**Maintained in darkness**

**After 1-hour light pulse**

Photomicrographs courtesy of Jon Kornhauser.

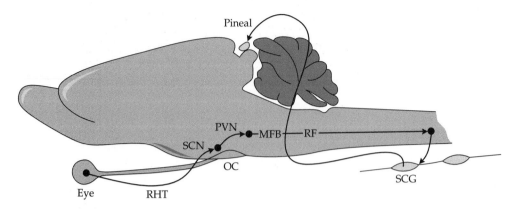

**10.17  Input and output pathways to and from the SCN in mammals.** Environmental light information enters the SCN from the eyes via the retinohypothalamic tract (RHT). One well-characterized output system involves projections from the SCN to the paraventricular nuclei (PVN), from the PVN to the medial forebrain bundle (MFB), and from the MFB to the superior cervical ganglion (SCG). Postganglionic noradrenergic fibers eventually project back into the brain and innervate the pineal gland, where neural information is transduced into a hormonal message. OC = optic chiasm; RF = reticular formation. After Klein et al., 1983.

in the same structure. For example, individual pineal cells from chicks possess a photoreceptor, a clock, and melatonin synthesis capabilities in vitro (Cassone, 1998; Nakahara et al., 1997). Similarly, a photoreceptor is located in the clock cells that are located throughout the head, thorax, and abdominal tissues (including the sensory bristles on the wings and legs) of Drosophila (Plautz et al., 1997). However, it is generally accepted that only the eyes contain photoreceptors that ultimately influence biological rhythms in mammals (Nelson and Zucker, 1981). Thus, the RHT is a critical input path bringing environmental light to the SCN in mammals. Isolated "islands" of brain tissue connected to the SCN continue to exhibit circadian organization (Inouye and Kawamura, 1979). However, a recent study reported that light treatment applied to the popliteal region (the back of the knee) was as effective in entraining biological rhythms of humans as light to the eyes (Campbell and Murphy, 1998). Human volunteers had a fiber-optic device, called a Bill-iblanket (which is typically used to treat premature babies with jaundice) wrapped around their knees; this blanket focused the light of 2400 fiber-optic cables on the skin (Figure 10.18). A relationship was discovered between the timing of the light pulse to the popliteal region and the magnitude and direction of phase shifts (i.e., a phase-response curve; see Figure 10.7). How could lighting the backs of the knees affect the biological clock in the hypothalamus? Perhaps there is some photoreceptor circulating in the blood that conveys light information to the brain. This study might lead to important advances in treating seasonal depression or jet lag. But because these findings have not been replicated, and because there is a long history of laboratory experiments that seem to rule out extraretinal photoreceptors in the entrainment of mammalian circadian rhythms, these findings remain highly controversial. Nighttime melatonin secretion was unaffected by light to the knees in another study (Lockley et al., 1998).

**10.18  Light application to the back of the knee phase-shifts human circadian rhythms.** This device, called a Bil-liblanket, is normally used to treat premature infants with jaundice. The halogen lamp is connected to the 2400 fiber-optic tubes that separate the heat of the light from the skin. In tests of 15 people, light delivered only to the back of the knees was as efficient as light directed to the eyes in phase-shifting body temperature and saliva melatonin daily rhythms. Courtesy of S. Campbell.

Although the eye seems to contain the primary photoreceptor-mediating the effects of light on the mammalian circadian system, the actual photoreceptive units remain elusive. Opsin, the light-sensitive molecule found in the retina, can be ruled out because of the observation that mutant mice with a genetic defect that leads to nearly complete degeneration of the retina continue to show normal entrainment to light shifts (Menaker et al., 1997; Tosini and Menaker, 1998). In some cases, nonphotic cues, such as scheduled handling or injection of saline, can entrain the free-running clocks of adult Syrian hamsters and outbred mice, but not inbred mice (Hastings et al., 1998). Because people who are totally blind (i.e., lack conscious perception of light) usually show entrainment of their biological rhythms, it is likely that humans also possess the capability for nonphotic entrainment of their circadian clocks (e.g., Klerman et al., 1998; Bellastella et al., 1998).

If the SCN are damaged, all circadian rhythms disappear (Figure 10.19). If SCN are transplanted into the brains of arrhythmic, SCN-lesioned hamsters, circadian locomotor activity rhythms are restored (Lehman et al., 1987; Ralph et al., 1990). If *tau* mutant hamsters, which exhibit short (about 20 hours) free-running periods have their SCN destroyed, then receive grafts of fetal SCN tissue from normal hamsters, they develop circadian rhythms that free-run with a period of approximately 24 hours. Similarly, if normal hamsters receive SCN lesions, then receive SCN transplants from *tau* mutant hamsters displaying short free-running periods, the recipient hamsters develop the short free-running rhythms of the donor animal (Ralph and Lehman, 1991; see Figure 10.14). The reappearance of a rhythm in a transplant recipient indicates that the pacemaker cells that generate circadian rhythms exist in the SCN tissue. The phase relationship to the light–dark

**10.19 Disruption of circadian rhythms after SCN damage.** (a) Drinking behavior of a normal hamster in a light–dark cycle (12 h of light and 12 h of dark) displays a 24-hour rhythm (top of panel); in constant dim light, a free-running circadian rhythm of 24.25 hours is displayed. (b) After lesions to both SCN, no temporal organization of the behavior is evident, regardless of lighting conditions. From Zucker, 1980.

cycle can also be transplanted via donor SCN (LeSauter et al., 1997). In some way that is not completely understood, the SCN generate or coordinate overt circadian rhythms within individuals to assure physiological and behavioral temporal synchrony.

Although there have not been any clear demonstrations that the SCN mediate circadian organization in humans, several clinical case studies have reported that anterior hypothalamic damage in the vicinity of the optic chiasm was associated with disturbances in the daily sleep–wake or temperature cycle (reviewed in Cohen and Albers, 1991; Schwartz et al., 1986). In one case study of a 34-year-old female patient, A.H., a tumor was removed from the inferior region of the anterior hypothalamus that included the SCN (Cohen and Albers, 1991). A.H. displayed significant disruptions in her daily body temperature and sleep–wake cycles, as well as impairments in cognitive and behavioral function, after the surgery (Figure 10.20). The disruptions in cognition and behavior appeared to reflect an inability to maintain consistent levels of arousal and/or attention (Cohen

(a) Unscheduled

(b) Scheduled

**10.20   SCN damage disrupts the daily sleep–wake cycle in humans.** (a) The sleep–wake cycle of A.H., a woman whose SCN was damaged during surgery, shows little daily temporal organization in an unscheduled environment (waking periods shown in white; shaded areas represent time asleep). (b) A.H.'s sleep–wake cycle shows daily temporal organization if bedtime, waking time, and meals are scheduled by the nursing staff. Sleep–wake data were obtained every 15 minutes by the nursing staff. From Cohen and Albers, 1991.

and Albers, 1991). Arrhythmic circadian sleep–wake cycles have also been associated with schizophrenia (Wirz-Justice et al., 1997).

What are the SCN output pathways in mammals? Because biological rhythms are so pervasive among physiological and behavioral systems, there are probably hundreds of output pathways leading from the SCN. One well-known pathway is illustrated in Figure 10.17. Light information is transduced into an endocrine message in the pineal gland, which secretes the hormone melatonin (see Figure 2.34). As we shall see below, the length of day (photoperiod) can be measured by the timing of melatonin secretion. Melatonin can phase-shift circadian locomotor activity rhythms in mice (Benloucif and Dubocovich, 1996; Arendt, 1998). Melatonin also affects entrainment in birds (Gwinner et al., 1997) and lizards (Bertolucci and Foa, 1998). Importantly, daily treatment with pharmacological doses of melatonin entrains the locomotor activity rhythms of nocturnal rodents such as rats and mice, but not diurnal chipmunks (Murakami et al., 1997). Despite the diurnal organization of humans, melatonin treatment may be useful in treating jet lag or sleep disorders (Waterhouse et al., 1998; Kripke et al., 1998). However, the safety, toxicology, and teratogenic effects of melatonin have not been determined. Melatonin is sold over the counter in the United States as a nutritional supplement, but is strictly regulated as a neurohormone in Europe (Arendt, 1997; Guardiola-Lemaitre, 1997).

Among mammals, a retinal–SCN axis (with several output pathways, including the pineal gland) appears to underlie the circadian rhythm system. Indeed, this axis appears to exist among all vertebrate species, although there is great diversity among species in the extent to which each component contributes to circadian rhythms. There is greater complexity in the contributions of the component parts of the biological rhythm systems of nonmammalian vertebrates than in mammals. For example, multiple input pathways and multiple oscillators have been discovered in different species of birds (Takahashi, 1991). The input pathways may involve receptors located in the ocular retina, in the pineal gland, or dispersed throughout other brain regions. Extraretinal photoreception can be demonstrated by fitting a bird with opaque contact lenses; the bird will continue to be entrained to the daily light–dark cycle. However, if ink is injected under the scalp of the bird, it begins to free-run, because the light receptors necessary for entrainment are blocked. If the ink is removed, then entrainment is observed again (Groos, 1982) (Figure 10.21).

The central circadian oscillators have been located in several places in birds. The pineal gland is an important circadian clock among many species of passerine (perching) birds (Takahashi et al., 1989; Zimmerman and Menaker, 1979; Gwinner et al., 1997). Several types of evidence suggest that the avian pineal gland contains circadian oscillators: (1) pineal tissue continues to display circadian rhythms of biosynthetic activity even when maintained in a culture dish (Takahashi et al., 1993), and (2) in some species, if pineal gland tissue is transplanted into a pinealectomized recipient, the period or the phase of the donor rhythm is imposed on the recipient (Gwinner et al., 1997). For example, a new circadian phase can be imposed in sparrows by implants of pineal glands from donor birds housed under different light–dark cycles than the recipients (Meijer and Rietveld, 1989). The pineal gland is not required for the expression of circadian rhythms in chickens and Japanese quail. In quail, the eyes control the circadian rhythm of melatonin

*Passer domesticus*

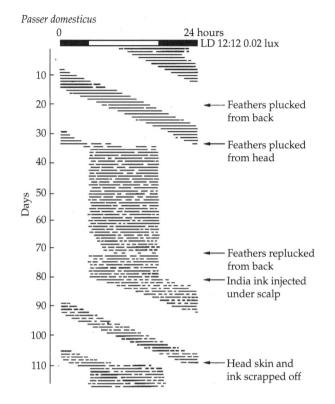

**10.21  Circadian locomotor activity in birds is entrained by non-retinal photoreceptors in the brain.**  If a house sparrow is fitted with opaque contact lenses, the bird will continue to be entrained to the daily light–dark cycle (even under dim illumination) if the feathers on the head are plucked. As the feathers regrow, the bird will begin to free-run. However, if the feathers are plucked again, re-entrainment is attained. If ink is injected under the scalp of the bird, it begins to free-run again because the photoreceptors in the brain necessary for entrainment are blocked. If the ink is removed, entrainment is observed again. From Groos, 1982.

secretion, and also contribute about 30% of the plasma melatonin. If the optic nerves of quail are cut, their activity rhythms are disrupted, but the ocular melatonin secretion rhythms remain intact (Takahashi, 1992). The role of the pineal gland in seasonal breeding is discussed below.

Are there different clocks for rhythms of different lengths, or are longer rhythms simply the result of the multiplication of shorter rhythms? For example, is the 4-day estrous cycle of a hamster the result of a 4-day clock cycling once, or a 1-day clock cycling four times? Another possibility does not involve a clock at all, but rather assumes that estrous cycles simply reflect the cumulative amount of time required to carry out a certain sequence of physiological processes or stages. These hypotheses were evaluated in a study of free-running rhythms in female hamsters. Phase shifts of the circadian rhythm were accompanied by proportionate shifts in the 4-day estrous cycle (for example, if the daily light–dark cycle was changed to 25 hours, then the 4-day estrous cycle changed to 100 hours) (Carmichael et al., 1981; Fitzgerald and Zucker, 1976). If the daily cycle was reduced to 20 hours, then the normally 96-hour estrous cycle was shortened to 80 hours. These findings imply that the circadian rhythm may be, at least partly, the basis of the estrous cycle length. However, it appears that the estrous cycle length is actually a combination of circadian organization and physiological limitations on stage length. Exposing ground squirrels chronically to 22-hour days significantly shortened the circannual rhythm of their reproductive function (Lee et al., 1986). However, in one study comparing normal hamsters (free-running activity periods of about 24 hours) with *tau* mutant hamsters (free-running activity periods of about 20 hours), it was reported that estrus recurred every 96 hours, rather than every 80 hours, in the mutants (Refinetti and Menaker, 1992). This observation indicates that the two rhythms are usually coupled, but that they have distinct underlying mechanisms. Incidentally, gestation required 16 days for both types of hamsters; the timing of gestation did not merely reflect 16 circadian cycles for the *tau* mutant hamsters.

### Circadian Rhythms, Hormones, and Behavior

Hormones may have many effects on daily locomotor activity cycles. As noted previously, hamsters in the laboratory become active 5 to 10 minutes after the lights are turned off. This statement is true of males, but only partially true of females. Female hamsters display an interesting pattern of activity onset that has been termed "scalloping." Every 4th night, coincident with estrus, females show a spontaneous phase advance in their onset of locomotor activity (Figure 10.22). Hamsters are solitary creatures, and it has been speculated that the earlier onset of activity during estrus increases the female's odds of locating a male. The scalloping pattern can be eliminated by ovariectomy. Furthermore, estradiol treatment of free-running, ovariectomized hamsters or rats reduces the period of locomotor activity onset, suggesting a direct effect on the clock itself (Albers, 1981; Morin et al., 1977).

In addition to estradiol, other sex steroid hormones exhibit modulatory effects on biological oscillators. For instance, progesterone lengthens the period of circadian rhythms, possibly by counteracting the effects of estradiol (Takahashi and Menaker, 1980). Sex steroid hormones can also affect daily activity rhythms in males. Castration lengthens and androgen replacement restores the period of free-running locomotor rhythms of male mice (Daan et al., 1975).

Removal of the pituitary gland (hypophysectomy) results in a lengthening of the period of free-running circadian locomotor activity by about 12 minutes per day (Zucker et al., 1980). However, the endocrine sequelae of hypophysectomy are profound. In addition to disruptions in sex steroid hormone production, alterations in many other endocrine functions occur as a result of hypophysectomy. In order to separate the effects of hypophysectomy from other endocrine consequences of this surgery, endocrine manipulations of other systems mediated by the anterior pituitary have been attempted. Investigators have focused on the thyroid gland because of its obvious and direct effects on metabolic processes. Removal of the thyroid gland results in a shortening of the period of free-running circadian locomotor activity in canaries, and thyroid hormone replacement therapy results in a corresponding lengthening (Wahlstrom, 1965). Hypothyroidism induced by the drugs propylthiourea or propylthiouracil has been correlated with lengthened free-running periods of circadian locomotor activity in hamsters (Beasley and Nelson, 1982; Morin et al., 1986). It remains unresolved whether alterations in thyroid hormone secretion per se or exposure to the anti-thyroid drugs accounts for the changes in period length (Morin, 1988). Injections of thyrotropin-releasing hormone (TRH) directly into the SCN phase-advanced wheel running behavior in hamsters (10 and 100 nM doses phase-advanced the behavior 18 and 35 minutes, respectively) (Gary et al., 1996). These hormonal influences on behavioral and physiological cyclic phenomena may eventually provide a key to understanding clock functions directly.

Another example of hormones influencing circadian rhythms is provided by the incubation behavior of pigeons and doves. Recall from Chapter 7 that males and females of these species both incubate the eggs. Each sex, however, incubates during a very specific part of the day: the male sits on the nest for a block of time in the middle of the day, and the female sits on the nest during the remainder of the day. Thus, the primary sex difference in parental behavior among pigeons and doves is in its temporal organization.

In a study of the role of sex steroid hormones in the mediation of this sex difference, gonadally intact ring doves were provided with a nest bowl and eggs and paired in one of the following combinations: (1) male–female, (2) male–male, or (3) female–female. Castrated birds were paired with gonadally intact birds in three additional experimental groups: (1) intact male–castrated male, (2) intact male–castrated male given estrogen and progesterone, and (3) intact female–castrated female given testosterone (Ramos and Silver, 1992). Male–male pairs rarely incubated the eggs; rather, they fought and destroyed the nest. Female–female pairs did incubate, but it was impossible to predict when each member of the pair would be on the nest. Birds paired with castrated partners occasionally incubated, but the castrated birds generally ignored the eggs. However, when castrated birds were injected with sex hormones, they and their same-sex partners incubated the eggs provided. Castrated females injected with testosterone adopted the male-typical time of incubation during the middle of the day, whereas castrated males injected with estrogen and progesterone adopted the female-typical time of incubation (Ramos and Silver, 1992). Additional research is necessary to understand the mechanisms that mediate this sex difference in the timing of incubation and brooding behavior; whether the hormones are affecting the clock itself or the social dominance of the partners requires clarification.

Parental behavior in rabbits is also mediated by daily biological rhythms. In the wild, rabbit pups are delivered in a special nursery den that is usually adjacent to the communal warren. The mother doe returns only once a day to nurse her pups, at intervals that at first seemed to field observers to be irregular—a strategy that could serve to deter predators. During the somewhat frenzied 3–5-minute

**10.22    Estrogen-induced "scalloping" of activity patterns.** Female hamsters kept in chronic dark conditions begin locomotor activity at the expected time on most days, but on the day of estrus, the onset of their running behavior is phase-advanced (arrows) by rising levels of estrogens. From Zucker, 1980.

nursing bout, the pups ingest an enormous quantity of milk, often exceeding a quarter of their body mass (Hudson and Distel, 1989; Zarrow et al., 1965). The female does not interact with her pups during the rest of the day because she is foraging for food. However, the pups *anticipate* their mother's arrival; they emerge from the nesting material prior to the arrival of the doe in order to commence nursing immediately (Hudson and Distel, 1982; Jilge, 1993). What is the basis of this temporal synchrony? Obviously, the ability to anticipate the arrival of the mother indicates that a predictable nursing rhythm exists and that the pups have the ability to measure time.

In the laboratory, rabbits are born during the light portion of the day. Females return to the waiting litter every 23.15 hours, on average, for the first 10 days. The pups manifest anticipatory activity within the first few days of life. What is the zeitgeber for the pups? Remember, they are normally living in a constantly dark burrow, so the light–dark cycle is not available to them as a cue. The zeitgeber for this endogenous biological cycle of anticipatory activity must be the mother herself (Jilge, 1993), but how the mother might actually provide the temporal cue (for example, a nutritional, social, or physiological cue imparted to the infants via her milk), as well as the endocrine correlates of this phenomenon, remains unknown.

What is the zeitgeber synchronizing activity in humans? There are several possible candidates, including light–dark cycles, temperature rhythms, and social influences. Social cues do affect the timing of human circadian rhythms. For example, when a group of people is housed in an underground bunker with no time referents, the entire group may adopt a single free-running rhythm (Coleman, 1986). In some cases, the group members adopt the free-running rhythm of the individual with the most dominant personality (Palmer, 1976). In many other studies, the effects of social cues cannot be untangled from other potential zeitgebers, such as meal times or the timing of the sleep–wake cycle.

The importance of light as an entraining agent for human circadian rhythms has been established for body temperature and the sleep–wake cycle (Czeisler et al., 1980; Dinges, 1984). The role of light in human biological rhythms was emphasized by the discovery that bright light (>2500 lux) suppressed the production of pineal melatonin in humans (Lewy et al., 1980). Melatonin is normally secreted in a circadian fashion, with an extended peak of secretion occurring at night (see Figure 2.34). The duration of this sustained elevation of melatonin varies with the length of the night in a number of mammalian species, including humans (Bartness and Goldman, 1989; Illnerova et al., 1985); this variation provides a means of measuring day length and thus discerning the season of the year, as we will see below (Figure 10.23). Pineal melatonin secretion can be suppressed at night by light, and among many mammalian species, very little light indeed is necessary for this suppression. For example, exposure of hamsters to a very brief (1 msec), dim (0.1 lux—about the illumination provided by a half moon on a clear night) light pulse is sufficient to suppress melatonin production for the entire evening (Milette and Turek, 1986). Thus, exposure to only 1 msec of light per night, strategically placed to occur during the daily melatonin peak, will shorten the length of the nightly bout of melatonin secretion substantially, and affect the animal's perception of seasonal cues.

(a) Long day

(b) Short day

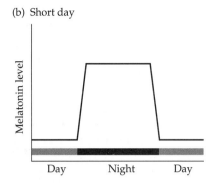

**10.23 Melatonin measures night length.** Melatonin is secreted only at night in both nocturnal and diurnal animals. Hamsters maintained under long-day (i.e., short-night) conditions
display a relatively brief period of melatonin secretion, whereas hamsters maintained under
short-day (i.e., long-night) conditions display an extended period of melatonin secretion.
When the duration of melatonin secretion attains some threshold, a short-day response occurs. After Bartness and Goldman, 1989.

In contrast to hamsters, the melatonin rhythms of humans are unperturbed
by dim light. Over 2500 lux of illumination for about an hour is required to suppress melatonin secretion (Lewy et al., 1980). In one study examining the effects
of very bright light (7000–12,000 lux), typical room lighting (about 500 lux), and
darkness, it was discovered that very bright light presented 3 hours prior to normal awakening was most effective in causing phase shifts in human body temperature (Czeisler et al., 1989). Daytime illumination levels approach 100,000 lux
outdoors, and this is the level of light to which human biological clocks have
evolved to respond (see Chapter 13). For people living at latitudes above 37°N, a
typical December day may include commuting to work in the dark, 8 hours in an
artificially illuminated office, a commute home in the dark, and 5 or 6 hours of
low-level illumination at home. Individuals may not be exposed to 2500 lux of light
for days or weeks at a time, and thus may be functionally considered to be living in
a cave. Under these conditions, the biological clocks of some individuals do not
receive sufficient light to entrain, and begin to free-run. Under conditions that
allow free-running, **internal desynchronization**, the dissociation of rhythms within an individual, may occur (Figure 10.24; Richardson and Martin, 1988). Thus,
rhythms that are normally phase-locked (temporally linked so that all of the cycles
show repeated phase relationships) when entrained may lose this relationship.

Because different rhythms may have different light intensity thresholds for
entrainment, some rhythms may free-run in low-illumination conditions, whereas other rhythms may remain entrained. Desynchronization of these rhythms during the winter may account for a number of sleep, eating, and mood disorders.
One well-known mood disorder, Seasonal Affective Disorder (SAD), which is
associated with dysfunctional biological timekeeping, is described in detail in
Chapter 13. In some cases, treatment with bright lights can ameliorate the affective
symptoms associated with SAD.

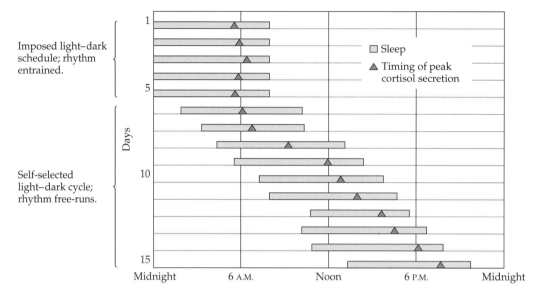

**10.24    Internal desynchronization of circadian rhythms.** Under normal conditions, or under an imposed light–dark cycle, the timing of peak cortisol secretion (triangles) is phase-locked to about 2 hours before awakening. When isolated individuals are allowed to select their own light–dark cycles with a light switch, free-running begins, and the rhythm of cortisol secretion and the sleep–wake cycle change at different rates, so that the peak of cortisol secretion occurs in the middle of the sleep period. Such internal desynchronization is thought to be the underlying cause of jet lag. Source: Richardson and Martin, 1988.

## Circannual and Seasonal Rhythms

The effects of light on daily melatonin production are critical in mammalian **photoperiodism**, the use of day length to time annual cycles. A functional circadian clock is required to measure day lengths, and measurement of day lengths is necessary to make seasonal adjustments in behavior. The duration of melatonin secretion provides mammals this needed information about day length. The duration of the nightly sustained elevation of melatonin secretion varies with the length of the night; in other words, a relatively brief duration of elevated melatonin secretion codes for short nights, or long days, whereas a relatively long duration of elevated melatonin secretion codes for long nights, or short days (Bittman and Karsch, 1984; Carter and Goldman, 1983a). Hamsters experimentally exposed to a brief pulse of light each night, which shortens the duration of melatonin secretion, exhibit a short-night (long-day) hormone profile. They also exhibit physiological, morphological, and behavioral adaptations consistent with long days, such as maintaining complete reproductive function and their "summer" fur coat. Hamsters maintained in short-day light conditions exhibit longer bouts of elevated melatonin secretion, display reproductive regression, and develop a "winter" coat. Although daily melatonin rhythms are observed in birds or reptiles, they do not seem important for these animals.

There appear to be two different types of biological rhythms that account for seasonal behavioral cycles. One reflects an endogenous organization and is commonly observed in animals that undergo seasonal hibernation in burrows and thus do not have access to environmental cues. The second type of seasonal biological rhythm is driven by the environmental day length, but requires an endogenous circadian system to discern day length. There appear to be several instances in which both types of biological clocks interact to permit animals to discern the time of year.

## *Ultimate and Proximate Factors Underlying Seasonality*

Most seasonal changes in behavior reflect strategies to manage an annual energy budget. Many animals and plants are exposed to seasonal fluctuations in the quality of their environments. Individuals generally restrict energetically expensive activities to a specific time of the year. Animals migrate or reduce their general levels of activity when food availability is low. Reproduction, preparation for migration, and other energetically demanding activities have evolved to coincide with abundant local food resources or other environmental conditions that promote survival. Precise timing of behavior is therefore a critical feature of individual reproductive success and subsequent fitness. As noted above, animals have evolved to fill temporal as well as spatial niches.

In some cases, physiological and behavioral changes that occur in direct response to environmental fluctuations have an obvious and immediate adaptive function. For example, reductions in the availability of food or water can lead to inhibition of reproductive function (Bronson, 1989; Nelson, 1987) (see Chapter 9). These types of environmental fluctuations have been termed the ultimate factors underlying seasonality (Baker, 1938). Many animals need to forecast the optimal time to breed so that spermatogenesis, territorial establishment, nest construction, or any other time-consuming preparations for reproduction will be complete at the start of the breeding season. Therefore, seasonally breeding animals frequently detect and respond to environmental cues that accurately signal, well in advance, the arrival or departure of seasons favoring reproductive success. The cues used to predict environmental change may or may not have direct survival value, and can be referred to as proximate factors (Baker, 1938). The most notable example of such a proximate factor is day length, or **photoperiod**, a cue that can serve as a very precise reference for the time of year. Under some circumstances, proximate and ultimate factors may be identical (Negus and Berger, 1987). For example, some individuals may not begin breeding until food cues are detected (Bronson, 1988).

The most salient seasonal rhythm expressed by animals is the seasonal breeding cycle. Many animals, including small, short-lived mammals and birds, mate during the spring and rear their offspring during the summer when food is plentiful; these animals are called long-day breeders. Other animals, such as sheep, deer, and cattle, mate in autumn and have long gestation periods. These large mammals remain pregnant throughout the winter and, in common with small animals, also give birth in the spring, when conditions are most suitable for survival. Animals that mate in autumn are called short-day breeders. Thus, many hormone–behavior interactions associated with the breeding season are mediated by biological clocks. Courtship, copulation, parental care, territorial defense, and aggression all exhibit pronounced seasonal fluctuations in occurrence that are linked directly to seasonal rhythms in reproductive function (Moffatt et al., 1993).

Seasonal changes in behavior are observed even among animals living in the tropics, where the annual cycle of changing day length is not as evident as it is at higher latitudes. Despite relatively constant photoperiodic and temperature conditions, seasonal variation in food availability is common for many tropical species. The irregularly timed onset of rain, or some coincident factor, induces tropical birds such as the red-billed quelea (*Quelea quelea*) to breed in East Africa (Disney et al., 1959); consequently, the onset of breeding in East African quelea varies from year to year (Murton and Westwood, 1980). In West Africa, where the onset of the rainy season is more consistent each year, the quelea display a predictable breeding season (Ward, 1965). In contrast, several species of oceanic seabirds inhabiting equatorial waters experience virtually no detectable seasonal variation in food supplies or other environmental factors. Reproductive activities and molting impose large, conflicting energetic demands on these birds, and so are separated in time (Figure 10.25). However, in this relatively stable environment, breeding and molting may occur at any time of the year, and the frequency of the cycle between these two energetic demands is limited only by the physiological capability of the birds, and varies among species. For example, breeding recurs every 8 months for the bridled tern (*Sterna anaethetus*) (Diamond, 1976), every 9 months for the brown pelican (*Pelecanus occidentalis*) (Harris, 1969) and Audubon's shearwater (*Puffinus lherminieri*) (Snow, 1965), and every 10 months for the swallow-tailed gull (*Creagrus*

**10.25  Annual breeding cycles in birds reflect energy constraints.** North temperate-zone birds may migrate north in the spring, then become reproductively active, establishing territories, courting, and rearing young. After breeding, the birds molt and increase their body fat stores in preparation for the fall migration south. They feed all winter and undergo another molt prior to the next spring migration. Nonmigratory birds must bear the increased energetic costs associated with thermoregulation during the winter. Thus, molting, migration (or winter thermoregulation), and breeding are separated in time in temperate-zone birds so that they can cope with the enormous energetic demands of each activity. Tropical birds may not have the same energetic constraints, so breeding and molting can occur at any time of year, and the frequency of the cycle between these energetic demands is limited only by the physiological capability of the birds.

*fucatus*) of the Galápagos Islands (Snow and Snow, 1967). Thus, mating behavior in some tropical birds is distributed throughout the calendar year.

## Neuroendocrine Mechanisms Underlying Seasonality

There is an extensive literature on the mechanisms regulating seasonal breeding cycles. The principles of seasonality derived from this literature can serve as a basis for the examination of the sparser information base directly related to seasonal changes in behavior. The mechanisms that regulate seasonal reproductive changes may be classified under two categories. One set of mechanisms is directly responsible for timing seasonal rhythms and ensuring that they are synchronized to the annual geophysical cycles. In mammals, the pineal gland and its hormone, melatonin, are involved in mediating the effects of day length on the timing of a wide variety of seasonal changes in physiology and behavior (Goldman and Nelson, 1993). A second set of neuroendocrine mechanisms is directly responsible for regulating changes in the reproductive system. For example, changes in the rate or pattern of pituitary hormone secretion are important for driving changes in reproductive hormones. Seasonal changes in reproductive hormones, especially sex steroid hormones, result in a cascade of seasonal changes in steroid-dependent behaviors. These mechanisms will be referred to as activational mechanisms because they generally involve activational effects of hormones (see Chapter 3; Beach, 1975). In photoperiodic mammals, the various seasonal activational mechanisms are influenced by day length, and thus by pineal melatonin. For some species, including sheep, thyroid hormones play a permissive role in the termination of seasonal reproduction (Thrun et al., 1997).

## Timing Mechanisms

Studies of seasonal rhythms in reproductive physiology have revealed a variety of timing mechanisms. Photoperiodism has been the most widely studied of these mechanisms. For the purposes of this discussion, photoperiodic mammals may be divided into two categories: (1) those that exhibit endogenous circannual cycles that are entrained, or synchronized, by photoperiodic cues; and (2) those that fail to exhibit endogenous circannual cycles in the absence of environmental cues. Deer, an example of the first type, exhibit circannual rhythms of reproductive activity that persist even when the animals are maintained under a constant day length, although these rhythms are not expressed under constant photoperiods of 12 hours or longer. However, changes in day length influence reproductive activity in deer, and natural photoperiodic changes are presumably largely responsible for establishing the seasonal pattern of reproduction (Goss, 1980, 1984; Goss and Rosen, 1973; Plotka et al., 1984). Sheep may also have the capacity to exhibit circannual cycles of reproductive activity in the absence of environmental cues, and these rhythms are clearly responsive to photoperiod under natural environmental conditions (Karsch et al., 1984; Sweeney et al., 1997).

On the other hand, a large number of mammals fall into the second category, and fail to exhibit endogenous cycles when housed under a fixed day length. For example, a variety of relatively short-lived rodent species remain reproductively active so long as they are maintained under long photoperiods. Twelve hours of light per day is the critical photoperiod (i.e., the day length required to maintain reproductive function) for Syrian hamsters; other species, particularly those inhabiting high latitudes, have different critical photoperiods. Although these species require photoperiodic changes for the continuance of seasonal cycles, they still display a prominent element of endogenous seasonal timing. Short day lengths (<12.5 hours of light per day) induce reproductive regression; after several months of exposure to short days, a "spontaneous" activation of the reproductive system occurs. This event seems to be triggered by an endogenous timing mechanism. Many of these species undergo various degrees of torpor in a dark burrow during winter, isolated from environmental cues; this mechanism allows them to prepare for the environmental changes that will take place in the spring (Elliott and Goldman, 1981; Reiter, 1970).

This "spontaneous" activation of reproductive function represents a phenomenon called **photorefractoriness**. In the case of Syrian hamsters, chronic maintenance under short day lengths causes the reproductive system to regress after about 10 weeks. After 20–30 weeks of continuous exposure to short days, the reproductive system is no longer inhibited by the short days, and is now said to be photorefractory. After this time, the hamsters' reproductive systems will become active and remain totally functional, even if the hamsters are kept in total darkness for the rest of their lives. If photorefractory hamsters are switched to long day lengths (>12.5 hours of light per day), after 10 weeks they will be responsive again to the inhibitory effects of short day lengths on reproductive function. In other words, the long days eliminate photorefractoriness. This process is adaptive because it allows preparation of the reproductive system in advance of appropriate breeding conditions.

Perhaps the most striking examples of endogenous timing mechanisms in photoperiodic species are observed in several species of hibernating mammals. Most hibernators undergo gonadal regression before entering hibernation. The gonads shrink, and gamete and sex steroid hormone production stops. Yet when these animals emerge from their hibernacula in early spring, their reproductive systems have been activated, and they are fully capable of breeding. Because the process of spermatogenesis requires several weeks in mammals, reproductive activation in males must begin before emergence from hibernation.

**HIBERNATION IN HAMSTERS.**    Laboratory studies have demonstrated that pituitary gonadotropin secretion and testicular growth begin during the last few weeks of hibernation in Turkish hamsters (*Mesocricetus brandti*). Hibernation is terminated when testosterone levels exceed a certain threshold; this mechanism may serve to coordinate emergence from hibernation with testicular recrudescence (regrowth) (Hall and Goldman, 1980; Hall et al., 1982). The timing of testicular redevelopment in Turkish hamsters is probably accomplished by the same type of seasonal timer that operates in other photoperiodic rodents. Male Turkish hamsters that are exposed to short days in a warm environment do not hibernate, yet these animals exhibit a cycle of testicular regression and subsequent recrudescence very similar in timing to that observed in hibernating males (Darrow and Goldman, 1987). A similar mechanism for temporal coordination of the seasons of hibernation and reproduction appears to exist in European hamsters (*Cricetus cricetus*) (Darrow et al., 1988) and hedgehogs (*Erinacus europaeus*) (Saboureau, 1986).

Males that have just undergone testicular redevelopment produce more androgens and gonadotropins than animals whose reproductive function has been continuously maintained under long day lengths (Berndtson and Desjardins,

1974). This "overshoot" of endocrine activity may have functional behavioral consequences. Recall from Chapter 5 that long-castrated rodents require higher androgen concentrations to maintain mating behavior than do recently castrated or intact animals (Damassa et al., 1977). The brain centers that control reproductive behavior may require sensitization by androgen exposure after prolonged gonadal quiescence in order to respond appropriately (Morin and Zucker, 1978).

**HIBERNATION IN GROUND SQUIRRELS.**    The seasonal organization of reproduction in golden-mantled ground squirrels (*Spermophilus lateralis*) has been the subject of many field and laboratory studies. These squirrels appear to possess an endogenous circannual clock (Berthold, 1837; Gwinner, 1986). When maintained under constant conditions in a laboratory setting, the squirrels display periods of reproductive function every 330–380 days. If the squirrels are exposed to a naturally changing photoperiod, they may entrain their endogenous cycles to exactly 365 days. A typical year in the lives of these squirrels living in northern California would begin with a summer of binge eating and deposition of body fat; body fat levels may double during the weight gain period of the summer. The squirrels then enter a burrow and go into deep torpor. During torpor the body temperature approaches the ambient temperature of the hibernaculum, about 2°–4°C. Contrary to popular belief, the squirrels do not stay in deep hibernation throughout the winter, but arouse every few days. They usually do not eat during this time, and their bodies undergo a programmed utilization of fat stores (although other species may arouse and eat at this time) (Dark et al., 1989). Also, their reproductive systems become activated during hibernation. In males, blood concentrations of androgens rise and eventually become incompatible with torpor, inducing the final arousal in March. Thus, the onset of testicular androgen production in the spring both terminates hibernation and stimulates subsequent mating behavior. When males emerge from their hibernacula, they are fertile, and their high blood concentrations of androgens cause them to defend territories and court females, which emerge a few weeks later. Virtually all females are inseminated during their first day above ground in the spring, despite the fact that they possess very low fat reserves. A litter is born in late spring, and the young squirrels scramble to increase body mass during their first summer.

These seasonal changes in reproductive function, food intake, and body mass also occur in the laboratory when ambient conditions of temperature, day length, and food availability are maintained at constant levels (Zucker et al., 1991). There is a circannual clock in male and female ground squirrels that regulates gonadotropin-releasing factors (primarily GnRH), and ultimately steroid production. In males, the hypothalamic–pituitary axis changes in sensitivity to the negative feedback effects of steroid hormones; during the end of the hibernation period, the negative feedback mechanisms become less sensitive to steroids, and gonadotropins are released that stimulate greater and greater amounts of steroid production (Zucker, 1988a). In female ground squirrels, the feedback system appears to be switched on and off. Ovariectomy at the beginning of the breeding season results in a pronounced elevation of blood plasma levels of LH, indicating that negative feedback mechanisms are operational at this time. If ovariectomy is performed on females at the end of the breeding season, then there is no post-ovariectomy rise in plasma LH; the LH concentrations of ovariectomized squirrels remain basal until the following breeding season (Figure 10.26; Zucker, 1988a).

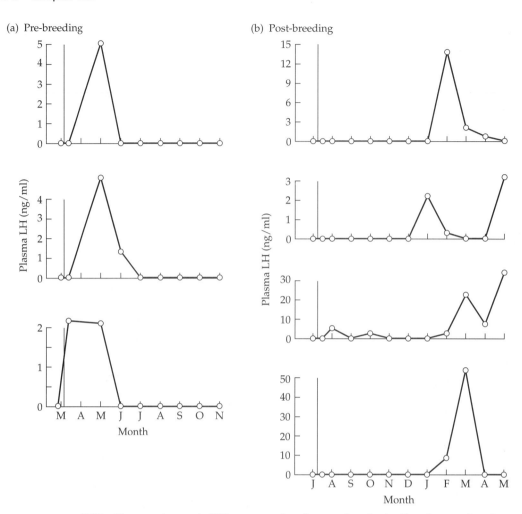

**10.26  Circannual control of LH concentrations in ground squirrels.**  Female ground squirrels show regular annual cycles of breeding in nature and a circannual cycle of reproductive condition under constant conditions in the laboratory. (a) Ovariectomy (vertical line) of 3 female ground squirrels at the beginning of the breeding season leads to the classic castration response of increased LH concentrations because it eliminates negative feedback control. (b) When ovariectomy is performed on 4 different squirrels after the breeding season, no increase in plasma LH concentrations is observed until the next breeding season, suggesting that the steroid negative feedback mechanism is activated only at certain times of the year. Source: Zucker, 1988a.

The annual cycle of body mass changes, with its corresponding changes in food intake, is also programmed by a circannual clock and persists under constant laboratory conditions. It appears that seasonal changes in food intake are secondary to seasonal changes in fat storage and utilization. If the squirrels are limited to levels of food availability comparable to what they were ingesting at the end of the hibernation phase, the animals still manage to gain amounts of body fat comparable to those of squirrels fed ad libitum (without restriction). They accomplish this feat by utilizing other components of the body and reducing activity. Even if the fat is removed by surgical aspiration, the animals make *new* fat cells and are able to catch up to intact control animals in body fat within a year (Dark et al., 1989). Thus, it appears that the circannual clock regulates fat storage and utilization, which causes changes in eating behavior. The exact physiological mechanisms underlying this phenomenon require clarification, but insulin and norepinephrine appear to be involved (Florant et al., 1989).

Thus, a continuum exists for annual cycles, from those that are completely autonomous and in which environmental cues play a limited role as entraining agents, to those that are driven wholly or in part by environmental factors. Ground squirrels are at one end of the continuum, with annual rhythms that are minimally influenced by environmental factors, except that day length *entrains* these rhythms. The annual cycles of Syrian hamsters, at the other end of the continuum, are driven by day length. However, during the winter, an endogenous timer appears to activate reproductive function prior to the mating season, which is coincident with, though not caused by, the long days of spring. Both ground squirrels and hamsters spend part of the year underground in relatively constant environments and require endogenous clocks and temporal processes to time part of their seasonal behavioral cycles.

**BREEDING SEASONS IN BIRDS.** Nonmigrating temperate-zone birds are exposed to an annual cycle of day lengths, and much of their seasonal cycle of behavior is driven by the environmental photoperiod. Like rodents, nontropical birds mate and rear their young during the spring and summer, when days are increasing in length. In contrast to those of rodents, the reproductive systems of temperate-zone birds must be stimulated by long days to function, but it is probably more accurate to state that exposure to short days is necessary to "turn on" their reproductive systems. Breeding for most nontropical avian species is completed by the summer solstice. Some species breed more than once during the breeding season, but most undergo reproductive regression in response to the long days of summer. In other words, the previously stimulatory day lengths act to inhibit reproductive function; the birds are said to be photorefractory because long days no longer stimulate reproduction (Nicholls et al., 1988). In order to break photorefractoriness, the birds must experience a period of short days. After exposure to several weeks of short days, the birds are once again responsive to the stimulatory effects of long days on reproductive function (Nicholls et al., 1988).

## Neural Mechanisms of Endogenous and Exogenous Seasonal Timekeeping

Virtually no information is available regarding the mechanisms of endogenous seasonal timekeeping in either birds or mammals. Attempts have been made to disrupt circannual rhythmicity by lesioning various brain regions. Neither lesions of the paraventricular nuclei (PVN), part of the output pathway from the SCN, nor pinealectomy disrupt circannual cycles of body mass fluctuation in ground squirrels (see Figure 10.17; Dark and Zucker, 1985). Lesions of the SCN disrupt circannual rhythmicity in some individuals; however, most SCN-lesioned squirrels continue to display circannual rhythms, despite the fact that *circadian* rhythms are absent in these animals (Dark et al., 1985). This observation and others in both ground squirrels and birds suggest that circannual rhythms and circadian rhythms may not be regulated by the same neural substrate (Gwinner, 1986).

In contrast to our lack of understanding of the physiological substrate for endogenous seasonal timekeeping, a good deal has been learned about the neuroendocrine basis of photoperiodism in mammals, especially over the past three decades. In virtually all species of mammals that have been carefully examined, pinealectomy severely interferes with most photoperiodic responses (Goldman, 1983). This was first demonstrated in Syrian hamsters, in which removal of the pineal gland prevented the inhibition of reproductive activity that typically occurs following exposure to day lengths of less than 12.5 hours (Hoffman and Reiter, 1965). This observation led to the common belief that the pineal gland exerts an inhibitory effect on the reproductive system (Reiter, 1970).

As we have seen, the pineal hormone, melatonin, has been shown to be the mediator of pineal effects on photoperiodic responses in a wide variety of mammals (Goldman and Nelson, 1993). The rhythm of pineal melatonin secretion is largely regulated by one or more circadian oscillators, probably in the SCN (Darrow and Goldman, 1986; Goldman and Darrow, 1983). In almost all mammals that have been examined, including species (such as the laboratory rat) that are generally considered to be reproductively nonresponsive to changes in day length, the duration of the nocturnal peak of melatonin increases as the photoperiod decreases (Bartness et al., 1993; Darrow and Goldman, 1986; Illnerova et al., 1986; Karsch et al., 1984). In Siberian hamsters (*Phodopus sungorus*) and sheep, daily infusions of melatonin have been administered to pinealectomized animals and reproductive responses have been measured. In both species, responses characteristic of animals exposed to long days (i.e., stimulation of reproduction for hamsters, inhibition for sheep) are elicited by daily melatonin infusions of short duration. Melatonin infusions of longer duration result in short-day responses (Bittman and Karsch, 1984; Carter and Goldman, 1983a,b). In Siberian hamsters, nonreproductive parameters, such as body mass and fat content, are also differentially affected by long-duration and short-duration infusions of melatonin (Bartness and Goldman, 1988a,b). The time of day at which the infusions are given does not appear to be critical in either sheep or hamsters (Bartness and Goldman, 1988b; Carter and Goldman, 1983a; Wayne et al., 1988). Based on these data, it has been proposed that changes in the duration of the elevated phase of the daily melatonin rhythm serve to convey a photoperiodic message to a variety of physiological systems (Bartness et al., 1993; Bittman, 1993; Goldman, 1983; Goldman and Elliott, 1988). Other species, including Syrian hamsters and white-footed mice (*Peromyscus leucopus*), respond to changes in the duration of the phase of elevated melatonin secretion in a manner similar to that reported for Siberian hamsters and sheep (Dowell and Lynch, 1987; Grosse et al., 1993).

In mammals, melatonin binding sites have been located in several brain areas, most notably in the pars tuberalis of the pituitary gland and in the SCN of some species (Bittman, 1993; Weaver et al., 1991). Melatonin may have direct or indirect effects on the release of substances into the hypothalamic–pituitary portal system to regulate LH and FSH release from the anterior pituitary. Hamsters housed under short-day conditions exhibit reduced gene expression for LH mRNA, which may or may not be independent from steroidal activation (Bittman et al., 1992).

Although seasonal changes in the pattern of melatonin secretion similar to those in mammals also occur in birds, birds do not appear to use the melatonin signal to time their reproductive effort (Chakraborty, 1995). Thus, the function of the annual fluctuation in the nocturnal melatonin signal in birds remains uncertain, but it has been implicated in the synchronization of circadian activity rhythms (Gwinner et al., 1997; Heigl and Gwinner, 1995; Menaker, 1968) and seasonal changes in immune function (Bentley et al., 1998). In addition, it may be involved in seasonal changes in the brain areas underlying singing behavior (Bentley et al., 1999). Seasonal neuroplasticity has been documented in several species of songbirds within discrete telencephalic nuclei that are involved in song learning and production (Brenowitz et al., 1991, 1998; Nottebohm, 1981). Increases in the size of these song control nuclei depend largely upon seasonal increases in circulating testosterone and its metabolites (Gulledge and Deviche, 1997; Nottebohm, 1980a; Smith et al., 1995), which are directly related to the annual reproductive cycles of these birds (Dawson, 1983). These seasonal changes  are associated with changes in cell size and cell number in the various song control nuclei (Smith et al., 1997a) (see Chapter 4).

Despite the well-studied role of testosterone in seasonal changes in bird brain morphology, recent studies suggest that there are gonad- and testosterone-independent seasonal changes in the volumes of song control nuclei (Bernard et al., 1997; Smith et al., 1997b).  The annual changes in melatonin secretion may be involved in the regulation of seasonal changes in the structure of the song control system. Presumably, melatonin exerts its effects directly on the neural substrate of the song control nuclei; melatonin binding sites have been found in the song control systems of three songbird species (Gahr and Kosar, 1996; Whitfield-Rucker and Cassone, 1996). In starlings, the high vocal center (HVC), lateral magnocellular nucleus of the anterior neostriatum (lMAN), area X, and nucleus robustus archistriatalis (RA) all contain melatonin binding sites (Gahr and Kosar, 1996; Whitfield-Rucker and Cassone, 1996). Taken together, this evidence suggests that although melatonin does not synchronize the reproductive activity of birds to a specific time of year, it is involved in seasonal modulation of aspects of avian physiology and behavior that have the potential to affect reproductive success.

## Activational Aspects of Timing Mechanisms

Timing mechanisms interact with the neuroendocrine substrates of reproductive function to assure appropriate timing of reproductive activities. In mammals, seasonal changes in reproductive activity are generally associated with changes in pituitary gonadotropin secretion. For example, Syrian hamsters, which are long-day breeders, exhibit decreased circulating concentrations of LH and FSH following exposure to simulated winter day lengths (Figure 10.27; Tamarkin et al., 1976). In sheep, which are short-day breeders, exposure to short days leads to increased LH secretion, manifested as an increase in the frequency of pulsatile LH release (Karsch et al., 1984). These types of changes in pituitary gonadotropin secretion lead to changes in gonadal growth and sex steroid hormone secretion (Berndston and Desjardins, 1974). Thus, the current understanding is that the exogenous factors that mediate seasonal changes in reproductive activity do so primarily via actions on the hypothalamic–pituitary axis. Photoperiod can also alter the ability of steroid hormones to activate sexual behavior.

STEROID-DEPENDENT REGULATION OF REPRODUCTION.    During periods of reproductive activity, one of the important mechanisms regulating pituitary secretion of FSH and LH is the gonadal hormone feedback system (see Chapter 3). In males,

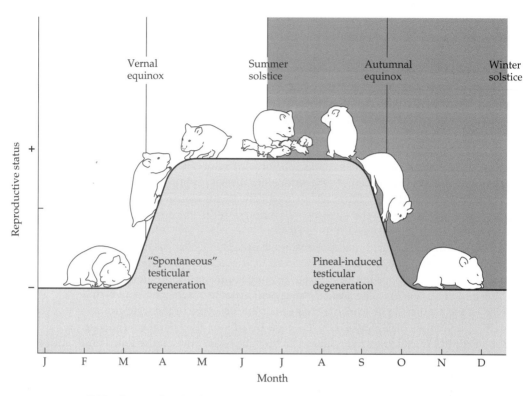

**10.27 Seasonal cycle of reproduction in Syrian hamsters.** During the summer, both male and female hamsters are reproductively competent and engage in breeding activities. When day lengths fall below some critical value in autumn (12.5 hours of light per day in the laboratory), the steroid negative feedback mechanisms of the hypothalamus are enhanced, and become increasingly sensitive to the effects of steroid hormones. Thus, even low concentrations of steroid hormones completely inhibit secretion of GnRH, and consequently LH, which suppresses steroidal secretion in the testes and leads to gonadal regression. Hamsters may spend the winter in torpor in a burrow. In the absence of light, the gonads regrow, and begin to produce steroid hormones and gametes again, in the early spring. Interestingly, the gonads can become functional again when the day length is much less than what is required to maintain the reproductive systems in the fall. After Zucker, 1980.

testicular androgens, especially testosterone, are capable of acting on the hypothalamic–pituitary axis to inhibit the secretion of both gonadotropins. In effect, this feedback system helps to maintain appropriate levels of gonadotropins; that is, the gonadotropins stimulate the biosynthesis and secretion of testicular androgens, and the negative feedback effect of the androgens prevents oversecretion of the gonadotropins. In females, a similar negative feedback system utilizes estrogens and progestins to hold FSH and LH concentrations in check. This system is especially important for regulating the number of ovarian follicles that mature during each ovulatory cycle. As follicles become mature, they produce increasing amounts of estrogen, resulting in decreased levels of gonadotropins and a cessation of recruitment of new follicles (Bast and Greenwald, 1977; Bex and Goldman, 1975). In both sexes, a gonadal peptide hormone, called inhibin or folliculostatin, also serves to inhibit the secretion of FSH (Steinberger and Ward, 1988).

One of the mechanisms that inhibits the secretion of pituitary LH and FSH during seasons of photoperiod-induced reproductive quiescence is an increased sensitivity of the hypothalamic–pituitary axis to the negative feedback effects of gonadal steroid hormones (Ellis and Turek, 1980a; Tamarkin et al., 1976; Turek et al., 1975). Low concentrations of testosterone are more effective in inhibiting post-castration increases in pituitary gonadotropin secretion in male Syrian hamsters (Tamarkin et al., 1976; Turek and Campbell, 1979) and rams (Pelletier and Orta-vant, 1975) when the animals are exposed to nonstimulatory photoperiods. A return to the lower level of sensitivity in response to stimulatory photoperiods is then able to return the animal to a state of reproductive activity via increased pituitary hormone secretion. A similar phenomenon has been implicated in the onset of puberty, when a prepubertal decrease in sensitivity to steroid negative feedback leads to increased secretion of LH and FSH and thus activation of the reproductive system (McCann and Ramirez, 1964; Ramirez and McCann, 1963). The effect of photoperiod on seasonal changes in hypothalamic–pituitary sensitivity is mediated by the pineal hormone, melatonin. Thus, in male Syrian hamsters housed under long-day conditions, administration of melatonin induces an increase in the sensitivity of the hypothalamic–pituitary axis to the negative feedback effects of testosterone (Sisk and Turek, 1982).

**STEROID-INDEPENDENT REGULATION OF REPRODUCTION.** A steroid-independent mechanism has also been implicated in the regulation of seasonal changes in the rate of gonadotropin secretion. Castrated male snowshoe hares (*Lepus americanus*) display seasonal variation in gonadotropin levels despite the absence of negative feedback from gonadal steroids (Davis and Meyer, 1973). Likewise, castration of male Syrian hamsters results in elevated blood concentrations of LH and FSH under both long-day and short-day conditions, although the post-castration gonadotropin levels are higher in animals housed under long-day conditions (Ellis and Turek, 1980b). A steroid-independent effect of photoperiod on gonadotropin secretion is particularly evident in female Syrian hamsters. Under long-day conditions, female hamsters exhibit an approximately eightfold to tenfold increase in baseline serum LH concentrations following ovariectomy, and LH concentrations can be returned to baseline by administration of estrogen (Yellon et al., 1989). After several weeks of exposure to short days, intact female Syrian hamsters become anovulatory, and their serum LH concentrations are very low during most of the day; however, these anovulatory females show large daily pulses of LH during the afternoon (Seegal and Goldman, 1975). This pattern of LH secretion continues following ovariectomy (Bridges and Goldman, 1975) or after combined ovariectomy and adrenalectomy (Bittman and Goldman, 1979). That is, removal of the source of steroid hormones does not result in any detectable increase in the baseline serum LH concentration in short-day female Syrian hamsters, and daily pulses of LH are still apparent in the steroid-deprived animals. These observations suggest that, in female Syrian hamsters, the effect of short days on LH secretion is mediated primarily via a steroid-independent mechanism. Seasonal variations in circulating and pituitary concentrations of gonadotropins have also been observed after ovariectomy in pony mares (Garcia and Ginther, 1976), ground squirrels (Zucker and Licht, 1983), and snowshoe hares (Davis and Meyer, 1973).

**RELATIONSHIP OF BEHAVIOR TO REPRODUCTIVE STATE.** The mechanisms that mediate seasonal changes in reproductive state also affect behavior. A wide variety of behaviors vary in relation to an animal's reproductive state. Some of these, most notably mating behaviors, bear an obvious direct relationship to reproduction. In most vertebrates, mating occurs at about the same time as peak gamete production. Because gametogenesis is a steroid-dependent process in all vertebrates, steroid hormone regulation of mating behavior generally provides temporal coordination between gamete maturation and mating, although exceptions exist (see below). Other behaviors, such as territorial behavior and migration, are less directly related to reproduction, but are frequently associated in an adaptive way with the reproductive process. It is probably because of the need for a close temporal association between fertility and behaviors that are directly or indirectly associated with reproduction that the regulation of many behaviors by the gonadal steroid hormones has evolved. As one would anticipate, the regulation of behavior by reproductive hormones is most evident for those behaviors most closely associated with reproduction; that is, mating behaviors.

The seasonal changes in the display of mating behaviors in many species are regulated primarily by seasonal changes in the amounts of circulating gonadal steroid hormones. In addition, seasonal fluctuations in behavioral *sensitivity* to steroid hormones have also been observed. In castrated male Syrian hamsters, copulatory behavior can be restored by administration of testosterone; however, larger doses of the steroid are required to elicit the behavior in animals exposed to a short-day photoperiod (Campbell et al., 1978; Morin and Zucker, 1978). The various components of masculine sexual responsiveness, including chemosensory behaviors, mounting, intromission, and ejaculation, are not all equally affected by exposure to short days. The effects of short-day exposure on these behaviors in male Syrian hamsters are prevented by pinealectomy (Miernicki et al., 1988). Female Syrian hamsters also exhibit decreased responsiveness to the activational effects of estrogen on lordosis behavior during exposure to short days (Badura et al., 1987). In contrast to males, this decrease in females' behavioral sensitivity to estrogen is not altered either by pinealectomy or by melatonin administration (Badura and Nunez, 1989). It is possible that photoperiod may influence female sexual behavior through a direct neural route. Neural input from the retina to the SCN is probably required for pineal-dependent responses to changes in day length. However, there are also direct retinal projections to the basal forebrain and hypothalamic regions outside the SCN (Pickard and Silverman, 1981; Youngstrom et al., 1987) that concentrate ovarian steroids (Fraile et al., 1987; Morrell and Pfaff, 1978) and may have a role in female sexual behavior.

**DISSOCIATED REPRODUCTIVE PATTERNS.**    Some notable exceptions to the usual association between reproductive hormones and sexual behavior have been reported (Crews, 1984). Some vertebrates exhibit a so-called dissociated reproductive pattern, whereby the production of gametes and mating do not occur at the same time of the annual cycle. In the red-sided garter snake (*Thamnophis sirtalis parietalis*), for example, sperm are produced during the summer and are stored in the male reproductive tract through the 8–9-month period of winter torpor (see Chapter 5). Experiments involving castration and treatment with androgens have revealed that the level of androgens present during the mating phase has no influence on the presence or intensity of mating behavior in these snakes (Crews, 1984). Rather, mating behavior, which persists for about 3 weeks, seems to occur only in snakes that have experienced a period of torpor. The pineal gland may be involved in determining when mating will occur, since removal of the pineal gland prior to entry into winter torpor prevents the display of mating behavior that normally occurs immediately after emergence from hibernation (Crews et al., 1988b; Nelson et al., 1987). A seasonal timing mechanism probably determines the time of mating in this species, and this mechanism may be partially or entirely independent of gonadal hormones. Clearly, for a species that has evolved a dissociated reproductive pattern, it is appropriate for reproductive behavior to be liberated from the influence of sex hormones. In this case, one must suppose that an alternative mechanism is employed to ensure that mating occurs at the proper time.

**AGGRESSIVE BEHAVIOR.**    Perhaps the most general case of seasonal regulation of a behavior by gonadal hormones is exemplified by the male mountain spiny lizard, *Sceloporus jarrovi*, in which a single behavior is largely regulated by testicular androgens during the breeding season in September and October, but is expressed independently of testicular hormones during another phase of the annual cycle. *S. jarrovi* begins to exhibit territorial behavior, expressed as intermale aggression, during the midsummer phase that precedes mating. At this time, castration does not result in a decrease in the level of intermale aggression (Moore and Marler, 1987). During the subsequent mating phase, the level of territorial behavior increases; this increase can be prevented by castration and reinstated by administration of androgens. Castrated mating-phase lizards do not stop showing territorial behavior altogether; rather, aggressiveness declines to a level similar to that exhibited during the earlier, pre-mating phase (Moore, 1987). Yet a third condition occurs in this species subsequent to the mating phase, in which territorial behavior is completely absent and the animals aggregate, tolerating close proximity and even physical contact by members of the same sex. During this phase, administration of androgens fails to stimulate aggressive behavior. It seems that testicular hormones act only to regulate the *intensity* of territorial behavior in *S. jarrovi* and that other, as yet unknown, mechanisms determine the overall annual pattern of territoriality.

There are many reports of seasonal changes in agonistic and territorial behavior among birds and mammals. For example, male starlings (*Sturnus vulgaris*) form rigorously defended territories during the breeding season (Feare, 1984). This territorial behavior is correlated with high circulating levels of androgens. At the end of the breeding season, blood androgen levels diminish, and territorial behaviors stop. The reduction in agonistic behavior allows the formation of so-called winter feeding flocks, which appear to confer advantages in predator avoidance and foraging success (Feare, 1984). Small rodents also display seasonal changes in aggressiveness and territorial behavior. Microtine rodents (lemmings and voles), and probably most rodent species in nontropical regions, form winter aggregations. Animals huddling together in the winter presumably benefit by reducing their energetic requirements. Presumably, the lack of circulating androgens permits the social tolerance necessary for this pattern of behavior to appear (see Chapter 8).

In wood rats (*Neotoma fuscipes*), seasonal changes in aggressive behavior are apparently independent of testicular hormones. The level of intermale aggression increases during the breeding season in this species, but this seasonal increase in aggressiveness is also observed in males that have been castrated postpubertally. Also, the increased aggressiveness continues for some time after the breeding season ends. The independence of aggression from androgen in this species has been hypothesized to have evolved because the greatest threat to reproductive success from conspecific males comes during the breeding season, but the greatest need for nest defense comes later in the year, after the young have been weaned and begin seeking nests of their own (Caldwell et al., 1984).

**DAILY ACTIVITY PATTERNS.**    Field observations of several species of microtine rodents (e.g., *Microtus agrestis, M. oeconomus, M. montanus, Clethrionomys gapperi,* and *C. glareolus*) have indicated a seasonal shift in activity patterns (Erkinaro, 1961; Herman, 1977; Ostermann, 1956; Rowsemitt, 1986). These animals tend to be nocturnal during the summer and diurnal during the winter (Figure 10.28). The adaptive function of this seasonal shift in daily activity patterns probably involves energetic savings. By constraining the majority of its locomotor activity to the daylight hours during the winter, the animal avoids the coldest part of the day; likewise, bouts of activity during summer nights allow the animal to avoid thermal stress or dehydration (Rowsemitt et al., 1982; Rowsemitt, 1986). Predator avoidance may also contribute to the adaptive significance of this seasonal trait.

Testosterone appears to mediate the seasonal shift in activity patterns in montane voles (*M. montanus*). Adult male voles were either castrated or left intact and maintained in long-day or short-day conditions. Testosterone replacement therapy was given to some of the castrated animals via subcutaneously implanted Silastic capsules. Castrated montane voles showed increased diurnal and decreased nocturnal wheel-running activity as compared with intact animals. Castrated voles implanted with testosterone increased their nocturnal activity rel-

**10.28    Photoperiod-mediated shift in activity patterns in montane voles.** Male montane voles maintained under long-day conditions (LD 16:8) change their locomotor activity from a nocturnal to a diurnal pattern if short-day (LD 8:16) conditions are imposed. From Rowsemitt et al., 1982.

ative to voles implanted with empty capsules. There was a great deal of individual variation among the experimental animals. Nevertheless, these results suggest that photoperiod primarily mediates this species' seasonal shift in activity patterns by affecting androgen production; that is, short-day animals tend to be diurnal and long-day animals tend to be nocturnal (Rowsemitt, 1986). Other environmental cues, such as temperature and food quality and quantity, may also affect activity patterns.

Although many subtle effects of steroids on the timing of activity have been reported in other rodent species (Ellis and Turek, 1983; Morin and Cummings, 1981; Morin et al., 1977), assessing the functional significance of these effects on activity rhythms has been difficult. For example, the number of daily revolutions made in a running wheel significantly declines when Syrian hamsters are moved from long days to short days (Ellis and Turek, 1979). This decline in locomotor activity can be mimicked in long-day hamsters by castration, and reversed by testosterone replacement therapy (Ellis and Turek, 1983). Castrated male Syrian hamsters treated with testosterone but maintained under short day lengths do not increase their wheel-running behavior, suggesting that the neural tissues underlying this behavior become insensitive to steroids under short-day conditions (Ellis and Turek, 1983).

**BRAIN SIZE AND LEARNING.**   Seasonal changes in brain weight have been reported for several species of rodents and shrews (e.g., *C. glareolus, C. rutilus, M. oeconomus, M. gregalis, Sorex auraneus,* and *S. minutus*) (Bielak and Pucek, 1960; Pucek, 1965; Yaskin, 1984). Brain weights are greater in summer-captured than in winter-captured animals (Figure 10.29; Yaskin, 1984). The adaptive function of this seasonal variation in brain weight may involve energetic savings. Although the brain constitutes only 2–3% of the total body mass in rodents and insectivores, it uses over 10% of the total energy expended by the animal. It has been suggested that minor reductions in brain mass could result in substantial energetic savings.

A significant part of this seasonal change in brain weight could be attributable to variation in water content; however, several parts of the brain—specifically, the neocortex and the basal portion of the brain (i.e., the corpus striatum)—show seasonal cytoarchitectural changes in rodents and shrews. The relative weight of the forebrain declines during the winter, the relative weight of the hippocampus increases from winter to summer, and the relative weight of the olfactory bulbs, myelencephalon, and cerebellum increases during the winter. A sex difference in brain weight is observed among bank voles (*C. glareolus*) only during the winter months; male brains are heavier than female brains at this time. The absolute and relative weight of the hippocampus is significantly higher in males than in females throughout the year, but the difference is most pronounced during the winter (Yaskin, 1984). Meadow voles (*M. pennsylvanicus*) also show seasonal changes in brain weight. Photoperiod appears to organize the seasonal fluctuation in brain weight in these animals (Dark et al., 1987b); males kept under short-day conditions have smaller brains than long-day males.

Despite the evidence for seasonal changes in brain weight in rodents, there has been relatively little research investigating seasonal changes in learning among mammalian species. In any event, there are a few studies addressing seasonal changes in learning and memory in fishes, reptiles, and birds. It is also known that winter-trapped voles make more errors and require longer to learn mazes than

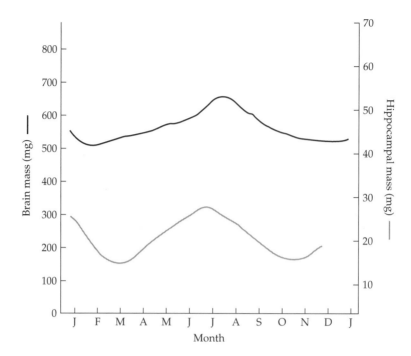

**10.29    Seasonal changes in brain and hippocampal mass** have been reported for several temperate-zone mammalian species, and are shown here for bank voles (*Clethrionomys glareolus*) corrected for changes in body mass. These changes in brain mass may account for seasonal variation in learning and memory, or they may be related to an energy-saving adaptation. Source: Yaskin, 1984.

summer-captured voles (see Chapter 12); the extent to which this seasonal change is mediated by day length requires further study. Among reptiles, seasonal torpor appears to interfere with learning during the winter, but in studies of this phenomenon, it is not clear if learning or memory function is depressed because of cold exposure or if quiescent animals simply cannot make appropriate responses.

As noted above, song learning in birds also fluctuates on a seasonal basis, and the neural tissue underlying song learning changes seasonally. Photoperiod is important in some avian species for the mediation of these changes, including recruitment of new neurons (Nottebohm, 1989); testosterone, or its metabolites, appears to drive the seasonal changes in brain structure and bird song production (Nottebohm, 1981; Bottjer et al., 1986).

There are three types of evidence that support the role of testosterone in mediating the seasonal change in avian singing behavior. First, blood concentrations of testosterone are highest during the onset of the breeding season, and this peak coincides with maximal singing. Second, song production wanes after castration, and steroid replacement therapy (both androgens and estrogens) reinstates singing behavior (for example, Harding et al., 1983, 1988; Heid et al., 1985). Third, several of the song control nuclei (see Chapter 4) concentrate steroid hormones; for example, androgen receptors have been localized with autoradiographic and immunocytochemical techniques in the HVC, RA, lMAN, ICo (nucleus intercollicularis), and nXIIts (Balthazart et al., 1992; Brenowitz and Arnold, 1992), and estrogen receptors have been localized in the HVC and ICo (Brenowitz and Arnold, 1989; Gahr et al., 1987, 1993).

In addition to the seasonal changes in singing behavior, there are substantial seasonal changes in the morphology of several nuclei associated with the control of song. For example, the volume of the HVC and RA increase by 99% and 77%, respectively, among male canaries maintained under spring day lengths (>12 h light/day) relative to birds housed under autumnal conditions (<12 h light/day) (Nottebohm, 1981). Similar results have been reported for several other bird species, including red-winged blackbirds (*Agelaius phoeniceus*) (Kirn et al., 1989), rufous-sided towhees (*Pipilo erythrophthalmus*) (Brenowitz et al., 1991), orange bishop birds (*Euplectes franciscanus*) (Arai et al., 1989), and white-crowned sparrows (*Zonotrichia leucophrys*) (Smith et al., 1991). These seasonal changes in the size of certain brain structures are probably mediated by testosterone or its metabolites.

**MATERNAL BEHAVIOR AND LITTER SEX RATIOS.**   Seasonal fluctuations in the capacity to exhibit maternal behavior have not been examined in detail because it has been widely assumed that seasonally induced reproductive quiescence precludes the display of this behavior during part of the year. However, some environmental factors have been identified as having effects on maternal responses. Several avian species are known to adjust clutch size in response to changes in food availability (Lack, 1954). Syrian hamsters (Huck et al., 1986) and house mice (Marstellar and Lynch, 1987) display increased cannibalism of their young during periods of food restriction. The opportunity to hoard food reduces the incidence of, but does not abolish, cannibalism in Syrian hamsters (Miceli and Malsbury, 1982a). Interestingly, food restriction during development can have effects upon second-generation offspring; litter survival and growth rate are reduced in hamsters born to a dam that had been food-restricted during development. In addition, the sex ratio of litters born to food-restricted female hamsters is skewed in favor of females (Huck et al., 1986). It is unclear whether this bias  reflects a gestational event or an active culling of males via postpartum cannibalism. Montane voles display a similar sex ratio bias toward female offspring when the dam is given 6-methoxybenzoxazolinone (6-MBOA), a plant derivative that is made by young grasses when grazing voles inure the plants during the onset of the breeding season in this species (Berger et al., 1987). Ingestion of 6-MBOA appears to induce the birth of more females during the early portions of the breeding season.

The mechanisms of seasonal changes in maternal behavior may involve photoperiodic changes that modulate behavior through the endocrine system. Increased prolactin levels during pregnancy are required for the induction of the full maternal behavioral repertoire in rats (see Chapter 7; Loundes and Bridges, 1986). In hamsters, decreased prolactin levels induced by the administration of ergocornine or bromocriptine have been related to decreased maternal aggression toward male intruders, increased aggression toward pups, disruption of pup retrieval behavior, and an increased incidence of maternal cannibalism of pups (Wise and Pryor, 1977). Hamsters and several other species experience seasonal changes in circulating concentrations of prolactin that are largely under photoperiodic control (Blank and Desjardins, 1985; Goldman et al., 1981; Martinet et al., 1982; Smale et al., 1988; Worthy et al., 1985). It is not known whether day length also influences prolactin secretion during pregnancy or lactation. However, it has been reported that, while pinealectomized hamsters maintained under a natural photoperiod were able to bear litters during the winter, they displayed a high degree of cannibalism (Reiter, 1973/74). It is possible that the females in this study failed to secrete sufficient prolactin to support maternal behavior, because pinealectomy only partially prevents the effects of short-day exposure on prolactin production in female hamsters (Blask et al., 1986).

**SEASONAL CYCLES OF HUMAN REPRODUCTION.**    Seasonal rhythms in the rates of human conception, mortality, and suicide have been reported (Aschoff, 1981; Becker, 1981). In each case, it is generally necessary to sample a large population to obtain statistically significant data because the fluctuations from season to season are relatively small. Thus, these rhythms are quantitatively different from most of those discussed for other animals, which are far more obvious. Because the human data are derived from populations exposed to both natural and artificial environmental changes, it is clearly impossible to know the underlying causation of these rhythms.

It is interesting to consider the absence of major seasonal fluctuations in human reproductive activity in relation to the selective forces that presumably led to the evolution of reproductive seasonality in other species. Human reproduction is characterized by a relatively long gestation period and an extremely prolonged period of intensive parental care. These energy-demanding processes cannot be compressed into one portion of one year, as is typical for most seasonal species. There may be little selective advantage to beginning this lengthy process at any particular time of year.

With that stated, recent studies have reported a seasonal rhythm in human conceptions. These studies analyzed birth records from many countries from both the Northern and Southern Hemispheres covering over 3000 years of monthly data. At high latitudes, where changes in day length are most pronounced, the most conceptions (computed by back-dating birth records by 9 months) occur at about the time of the vernal equinox (Roenneberg and Aschoff, 1990a). The pattern of human conceptions is reversed 6 months in the Southern Hemisphere as compared with the Northern Hemisphere (Roenneberg and Aschoff, 1990b). Temperature has a moderating effect; conception rates are higher than the annual average between 5° and 20°C and lower than the annual average at extreme temperatures. The influence of photoperiod on conception rates is more pronounced prior to 1930. The authors of the studies conclude that industrialization shielded humans from changes in photoperiod and temperature after that time through artificial lighting and temperature regulation (Roenneberg and Aschoff, 1990b). However, these studies can only be speculative in their conclusions because they are based on correlational data. There are many uncontrolled variables that could provide alternative explanations. However, the possibility of photoperiodic effects on human physiology and behavior remains (e.g., Reiter, 1998; Wehr, 1998).

There are no reports of the existence of endogenous circannual cycles in humans. Collecting such data would be problematic, because the studies necessary to test for the presence of circannual rhythms would require the isolation of individuals under constant environmental conditions for periods of more than a year. Clearly, there are major gaps in our knowledge because there are virtually no data that bear directly on the questions of whether humans are either photoperiodic or circannual. Nevertheless, the growing body of data on seasonal mammals may be useful in pointing the way to obtaining such information for humans. Future research into human seasonality might benefit from a consideration of its potential for contributing to human fitness. For example, seasonal changes in human immune function might be mediated by photoperiod, as they are in other mammalian species (Nelson and Demas, 1995).

## Conclusions

An understanding of the rhythmic nature of behavior is important for behavioral scientists for two reasons. First, an awareness of the daily and annual variation in many behaviors may minimize any unintended influences of time of day or seasonality on experimental results. Care should be exercised in obtaining experimental animals, in maintaining appropriate lighting conditions, and in the timing of data collection. Second, seasonal and daily changes in many phenomena of interest to psychologists and biologists have been documented. Reliable daily and seasonal variation in learning and memory function, perception, communication, developmental rates, social behavior, parental behavior, and mating behavior has been reported for many species. Few data on the mechanisms underlying these seasonal changes in behavior are available. We do know that many hormone–behavior interactions appear to be linked to reproductive cycles, but virtually no data exist on the mechanisms underlying seasonal phenomena not linked to reproduction.

There is a lack of basic information about human seasonality. For example, it is not known if humans are photoperiodic or if they possess endogenous annual cycles. The possibility of seasonal variation in human developmental rates, learning, or perceptual abilities has not been well studied. The extent to which behaviors such as aggression in humans are seasonal, and if so, to what extent these seasonal fluctuations in behavior reflect seasonal changes in human hormone concentrations, also remains unknown. Studies on nonhuman mammals should be useful in obtaining information about the functions and mechanisms of seasonal cycles of behavior. In summary, biological clocks can no longer be ignored in describing normal behavior, treating abnormal conditions, or designing experiments.

## Summary

• Endocrine function varies over a wide range of temporal scales. Many of these temporal changes are the result of biological rhythms generated by endogenous biological clocks. The study of biological clocks and their associated rhythms is called chronobiology or biochronometry. Many homeostatic processes show temporal fluctuations over the course of hours, days, months, or years.

• Some biological rhythms vary in period length, but four general classes of biological rhythms are normally synchronized to the geophysical cycles of day and night (circadian), the tides (circatidal), phases of the moon (circalunar), and the seasons of the year (circannual). These rhythms persist in the absence of the geophysical cues to which they are normally synchronized (entrained) with a period that approximates that of the geophysical cycle. Ultradian (shorter than circadian) and infradian (longer than circadian) rhythms are also observed to persist in constant conditions, but do not correspond to any known geophysical cue.

• Biological rhythms have evolved to synchronize the activities of individuals with changes in their environment, allowing preparation for predictable events, and to synchronize the internal physiological and biochemical processes of individuals to permit efficient function.

• Biological clocks have several formal properties. Biological clocks are inherited, relatively independent of temperature, relatively independent of chemical influence, entrainable only to limited cycle lengths, relatively independent of behavioral feedback, and found at every level of organization within an individual plant or animal.

• Biological clocks are found in single cells. Within multicellular organisms, the various clocks in the body appear to be linked in a hierarchical organization that allows temporal coordination. The master clock appears to be in the suprachiasmatic nuclei of the hypothalamus in mammals and in the pineal gland in some species of birds.

• Hormones can affect daily locomotor activity cycles. Estrogens accelerate clock function, and progesterone lengthens the period of activity cycles. Removal of the pituitary gland and castration also lengthens free-running (nonentrained) activity rhythms.

• Daily rhythms of parental care in ring doves, and possibly rabbits, are mediated by endocrine feedback to biological clock function. Ring doves take care of their young in sex-specific shifts. Adult treatment of castrated ring doves with sex steroid hormones can result in the sex-specific temporal organization of parental care.

• Light is important for entraining biological rhythms to geophysical cycles in virtually all species examined, including humans. Light affects the rhythm of melatonin secretion. Melatonin is produced by the pineal gland during the dark phase of the day, resulting in a sustained elevation in blood levels of this hormone. Long nights (short days) are coded by relatively long periods of sustained elevated melatonin levels. Short nights (long days) are coded by relatively short periods of sustained elevated melatonin levels. Animals use this nightly pulse length of melatonin to assess the time of year.

• Many annual cycles of hormone–behavior interactions have been observed among animals. Most of these seasonal changes in behavior are correlated with seasonal changes in reproductive function. Thus, steroid-dependent behaviors wane when animals become reproductively quiescent and recur during the breeding season, when reproductive hormones are again secreted.

• Some annual cycles are the result of endogenous circannual clocks, whereas others are the result of environmental input; day length may be the most widely used cue in the regulation of seasonal rhythms. Seasonal rhythms in mating behavior, parental behavior, territoriality, aggression, and learning have been reported for a variety of species. Seasonal cycles in human conception have also been recently documented, and these cycles appear to be affected by photoperiod and temperature.

# Questions for Discussion

1. Compare and contrast the concepts of "homeostasis" and "biological rhythms." Are their functions complementary or antagonistic?

2. Why is it important to have an understanding of biological clocks and rhythms in designing or interpreting behavioral endocrinology experiments?

3. Some have noted that males and females of the same species are quite different animals. Similarly, it can be said that animals examined during the summer are quite different animals than those of the same species that are examined during the winter. Defend or refute this statement.

4. What adaptive advantages do biological clocks confer?

# Suggested Readings

Bronson, F. H., and Heideman, P. D. 1994. Seasonal regulation of reproduction in mammals. In E. Knobil and J. D. Neill (eds.), *The Physiology of Reproduction,* pp. 541–584. Raven Press, New York.

Klein, D. C., Reppert, S. M., and Moore, R. Y. (eds.). 1991. *The Suprachiasmatic Nucleus: The Mind's Clock.* Elsevier, New York.

Kupfer, D. J., Monk, T. H., and Barchas, J. D. (eds.). 1988. *Biological Rhythms and Mental Disorders.* Guilford Press, New York.

Nelson, R. J., Badura, L., and Goldman, B. D. 1990. Mechanisms of seasonal cycles of behavior. *Annual Review of Psychology,* 41: 81–108.

Rosenthal, N. E. 1993. *Winter Blues: Seasonal Affective Disorder.* Guilford Press, New York.

Takahashi, J. S., Kornhauser, J. M., Koumenis, C., and Eskin, A. 1993. Molecular approaches to understanding circadian oscillations. *Annual Review of Physiology,* 55: 729–753.

# 11

# Stress

L ife is challenging. The pressure of survival and reproduction
takes its toll on every individual living on the planet. The "wear
and tear" of life eventually leads to death. All things being
equal, animals that live the longest tend to leave the most offspring.
In the Darwinian "game of life," individuals that leave the most successful offspring win. Although some of the variation in longevity
among individuals of the same species merely reflects good fortune,
a significant part of this variation reflects differences in the ability to
cope with the demands of living.

As we saw in Chapter 9, all living creatures are vessels of dynamic equilibrium, or homeostasis. Any perturbation to homeostasis
requires the animal to expend energy to restore the original steady
state. Among birds and mammals, an individual's total available energy is partitioned among many competing needs, such as growth,

cellular maintenance, immune function, reproduction, and thermogenesis. During environmental energy shortages, nonessential processes such as growth and reproduction are suppressed. If homeostatic perturbations require more energy than is readily available after nonessential systems have been inhibited, then an individual's survival may be compromised. All living organisms currently exist because of evolved adaptations that allow individuals to cope with energetically demanding conditions. These demanding conditions may range from final exam week for a well-fed college undergraduate in the United States to finding a meal on the African veldt for a wild dog. Surprisingly, the same neuroendocrine coping mechanisms are engaged in both of these cases, as well as in many other situations.

To illustrate the kinds of demanding conditions animals must face, let's look at the example of wild dogs more carefully. Despite their common name, African wild dogs (*Lycaon pictus*) are more closely related to jackals than to modern dogs (Figure 11.1). However, African wild dogs do possess several characteristics typical of domesticated dogs, including group hunting and the formation of strong social bonds. They live in packs of about 6–8 adults and several pups. Unlike other canine species, however, wild dog packs typically have only one breeding pair (called the alpha pair) (Creel et al., 1996, 1997). In one study, 82% of the alpha females within a pack bred each year, and produced 76–81% of the offspring; only 6–17% of the subordinate females produced any offspring (Creel et al., 1997). Not surprisingly, subordinate females tend to leave their natal packs and attempt to become the alpha female elsewhere, although some subordinate females stay in their natal packs and attempt to rise through the ranks to alpha status.

**11.1　A group of African wild dogs.** Only the alpha pair of each pack breeds. The other adult members of the pack bring food to the pups and otherwise assist in the breeding efforts of the dominant alpha pair. In contrast to many laboratory animals, the alpha animals have higher corticosterone concentrations than subordinate animals of the pack. Courtesy of Scott Creel.

In general, dispersal is a demanding time for young animals (see Chapter 8). They must move to a new area, where they must learn where they can find food and water. Whatever protection they received from their natal pack on their home territory is lost in the new neighborhood, and the dispersing individuals must establish new social relationships. An invading female wild dog faces many challenges when she leaves her natal pack. In order to become the reproductively successful alpha female in a new pack, a new female must attack and dominate the current alpha female of the pack and also defend against the other subordinate females of the group vying for the top position.

In the life of a female wild dog, as in our lives, there are relatively short-term and long-term stressors. A **stressor** may be broadly defined as any disruption to homeostasis. In the case of wild dogs, females experience the effects of short-term stressors when they attempt to establish themselves as alpha females in a new pack, a process that might involve several skirmishes. Subordinate females also experience the effects of long-term stressors to the extent that they forego reproduction. The long-term stressor is likely to be the need to hunt for food not only for themselves, but for the offspring of the alpha pair as well (Creel et al., 1997). Although dominant wild dogs have elevated corticosterone relative to low-ranked individuals, in other species, subordinate females tend to have higher corticosterone concentrations than dominant females.

There are many sources of stressors. Environmental factors, such as temperature extremes, are often perceived as stressors. Stressors can also be physiological factors, such as food or water deprivation. Importantly, psychosocial factors, such as fighting, social subordination, or lack of control in a given situation, can be salient stressors.

The goal of this chapter is to understand the concept of "stress," the hormonal correlates of stress, and the effects of both short-term and long-term stress on behavior. Behaviors that are often affected by stress, including reproductive, parental, and social behaviors, as well as drug abuse, will be emphasized.

## The Stress Response

When a stressor disrupts physiological homeostasis, an individual typically displays a **stress response**. A stress response is a suite of physiological and behavioral responses that help to reestablish homeostasis. The stress response is relatively nonspecific; that is, many different stressors elicit a similar stress response (Selye, 1950). Two endocrine systems, one involving epinephrine (adrenaline) from the adrenal medulla and the other involving glucocorticoids from the adrenal cortex, constitute the major components of the stress response (Stratakis and Chrousos, 1995). Within seconds of perceiving a stressor, the sympathetic nervous system begins to secrete norepinephrine, and both adrenal medullae begin to secrete epinephrine.

In 1915, Walter Cannon (see Figure 12.2) proposed his "emergency theory" of the adrenal glands, which suggested that the secretion of epinephrine from the adrenal medulla increases following an exposure to virtually any stressor, as a means of adapting to that stress. Many physiological studies conducted throughout the 1920s and 1930s demonstrated the stimulatory effects of epinephrine on the respiratory and cardiovascular systems. Epinephrine is usually the hormone that acts first, because only a doubling from resting values causes profound changes in respiration or cardiac tone (e.g., heart rate and blood pressure), whereas norepinephrine concentrations must increase fivefold to have similar effects (Ganong, 1997). This immediate, nonspecific component of the stress response was termed the **fight or flight response** because the physiological changes in cardiovascular tone, respiration rate, and blood flow to the muscles from the trunk could support either of those behavioral responses (Cannon, 1929). Importantly, the catecholamines (norepinephrine and epinephrine), working through a variety of mechanisms, increase blood glucose levels. The elevated blood glucose fuels the fight or flight response. The catecholamines also increase alertness, and as we will see in Chapter 12, enhance learning and memory.

Modern perspectives on stress are less likely to focus on fight or flight than on a psychological feature of stress; namely, the degree of control over the situation. For example, both epinephrine and norepinephrine concentrations increase in the days prior to a Ph.D. final examination, peak on the day of the exam, then slowly return to basal levels (Figure 11.2) (Frankenhaeuser, 1978). As the date of the examination neared, the students' confidence and perceived control of the situation waned, and a stress response ensued. After passing the exam, the students' confidence and sense of control returned.

Other studies have shown that not just epinephrine and norepinephrine, but an entire suite of hormones known to be involved in the mediation of stress, change over the course of the stress response. The **hypothalamic–pituitary–adrenal axis (HPA axis)** is activated, and CRH, ACTH, and the glucocorticoids are released in response to stressors (Figure 11.3). In one classic study, blood samples were obtained from young military recruits prior to their first parachute jump (Ursin et al., 1978). Basal blood hormone concentrations were determined prior to the jump. Hormone concentrations on the day of the jump, as well as on days of

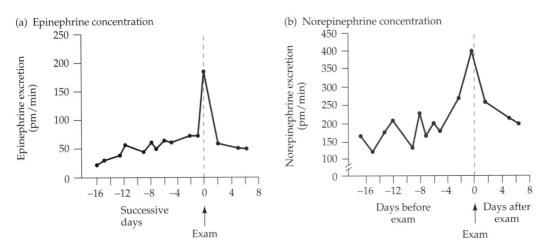

**11.2 Catecholamine concentrations peak on the day of a Ph.D. exam** after showing a consistent elevation in the days prior to the exam. Epinephrine (a) and norepinephrine (b) concentrations both peak on the day of the exam and return to baseline after successfully coping with the stressor (passing the exam). After Frankenhaeuser, 1978.

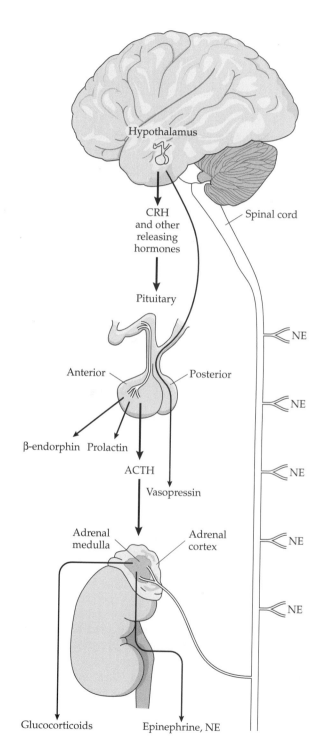

Hypothalamus

CRH
and other
releasing
hormones

Spinal cord

Pituitary

NE

NE

Anterior

Posterior

β-endorphin   Prolactin

ACTH

NE

Vasopressin

Adrenal
medulla

Adrenal
cortex

NE

NE

Glucocorticoids

Epinephrine, NE

**11.3 The hypothelamic–pituitary–adrenal axis releases several hormones in response to stress.** Initially, stress causes the release of epinephrine from the adrenal medulla and norepinephrine (NE) from the sympathetic nervous system. Moments later, the hypothalamus releases CRH and other releasing hormones, which stimulate ACTH and β-endorphin release from the anterior pituitary gland. ACTH stimulates corticosterone secretion from the adrenal cortex. Prolactin is often released from the anterior pituitary during stress as well. Vasopressin is released from the posterior pituitary.

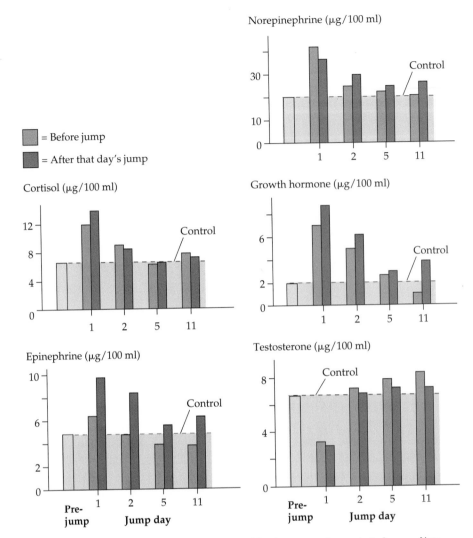

■ = Before jump

■ = After that day's jump

**11.4   Blood hormone concentrations are altered by the stress of parachute jumps.** Note that cortisol, epinephrine, norepinephrine, and growth hormone concentrations were elevated above their own baseline values (pre-jump) and above values for control individuals that were not engaged in parachute jump training (dotted line). Testosterone decreased on the day of the jump, but rebounded the next day to basal concentrations. After Ursin et al., 1978.

subsequent jumps, were also measured (Figure 11.4). Not surprisingly, catecholamine concentrations were high on the day of the jump, although, as the recruits gained confidence, their stress responses were muted. Cortisol and growth hormone concentrations were also elevated on the first jump day, while testosterone concentrations were suppressed on the first jump day (Ursin et al., 1978).

Within minutes of the onset of a stressor, the adrenal cortex begins to secrete glucocorticoids (e.g., corticosterone in most rodents, birds, and reptiles; cortisol in most primates and carnivores) (Stratakis and Chrousos, 1995). Like epineph-

**11.5  Hans Selye** (1907–1982) is considered the founder of modern stress research.

rine, glucocorticoids respond to virtually any stressor. Hans Selye (Figure 11.5) discovered this aspect of nonspecificity when attempting to characterize a new ovarian hormone. In Selye's study, some rats were injected with ovarian extracts that were believed to contain the new hormone, and some other rats were injected with saline as a control procedure (Selye, 1937a, 1950). After several days of injections, it was noted that the rats receiving the ovarian extracts developed peptic ulcers and experienced adrenal hypertrophy and regression of key immune organs (e.g., the spleen and thymus). Unexpectedly, the rats that were injected with physiological saline developed the same symptoms. Because injections of extracts from virtually any tissue evoked the same symptoms, Selye reasoned that the unpleasantness associated with the daily injections, and not a specific ovarian hormone, caused these symptoms (Sapolsky, 1992a). It was soon discovered that stressors, originally termed "nocuous agents" (Selye, 1936), as diverse as frostbite, exposure to formaldehyde, or hemorrhage could also elicit these symptoms (Selye, 1950; but see Kopin, 1995). The common endocrine event underlying these very different stressors was the release of glucocorticoids from the adrenal cortex. Thus, epinephrine and cortisol (or corticosterone) are commonly known as the stress hormones, despite the fact that their major endocrine functions involve metabolism (Selye, 1937b).

### General Adaptation Syndrome

One study was particularly important in forming the basis of Selye's thinking about stress responses (Selye, 1936). Rats were housed in low-temperature conditions for either 2 days, 2 weeks, or 2 months. After 2 days in these conditions, the rats showed hypertrophy of the adrenal cortex, reduced eosinophil (a type of immune cell circulating in the blood) numbers, and atrophy of the thymus, spleen, and lymph nodes. In other words, the rats exhibited a classic stress response. After 2 weeks in the low temperatures, the rats no longer displayed these symptoms, suggesting that they had adapted to the stressor. In other words, the rats had become "cold-adapted" and could tolerate even lower temperatures without exhibiting any further stress responses. After approximately 2 months of exposure to low temperatures, the rats "lost" their "acquired resistance" to the low temperatures and died.

This process of coping with stressors was termed the **general adaptation syndrome (GAS)**. The GAS consists of three stages: (1) the **alarm reaction**, (2) **resistance**, and finally, (3) **exhaustion** (Selye, 1950). The stressor is detected during the alarm reaction stage. Coping with the stressor occurs during the resistance stage. The exhaustion stage is characterized by the termination of the stress response and the onset of stress pathology, which in extreme cases leads to death. Although Selye believed that the exhaustion phase was due to the termination of the stress response, current ideas about stress indicate that the pathological effects of stress result from prolonged activation of the stress response (Sapolsky, 1992b, 1994; Chrousos et al., 1995).

### What Is "Stress"?

Everyone has experienced "stress," and most people can give an example of stress, especially during final examinations week. However, stress has been a notoriously ethereal concept in biology and medicine, and arriving at a consensus for a precise definition has been difficult. "Stress" is yet another type of hypothetical construct or concept. We can easily recognize "stress" in the same way that we can generally recognize "good" and "evil." However, if we try to define the term *stress* precisely, then the concept becomes as slippery as the concepts of good and evil. Consequently, some scientists think the term should be abolished altogether:

> Stress itself is one of those terms that we use to shield us from our ignorances. We would be better off without it. It survives because it is a convenient term to indicate the general topic under discussion. Attempts to provide such a vague concept with a precise physiological definition engender confusion and misunderstanding. (Rushen, 1986)

The concept of stress was borrowed from an engineering term that had a very specific meaning; namely, forces that act against resistance. The term *stress* has often been conflated to include the stressor, the stress response, and the physiological intermediates between the stressor and the stress response (Toates, 1995). Despite the confusing array of uses of the term , however, an impressive scientific literature integrating endocrinology, immunology, psychology, and neuroscience has developed around the concept of stress.

What, then, does it mean to say that an individual is under stress? For the purposes of this chapter, we will use some of the prevailing homeostatic notions of stress to arrive at a working definition. For example, "stress is the recognition by the body of a stressor and therefore, the state of threatened homeostasis; stressors are threats against homeostasis; and adaptive responses are the body's attempt to counteract the stressor and reestablish homeostasis" (Chrousos et al., 1998). Similarly, Robert Sapolsky (1994) defines a stressor as "anything that throws your body out of homeostatic balance–for example, an injury, an illness, subjection to great heat or cold." Considered together, stress is the sum of all nonspecific effects of factors that can act upon the body to increase energy consumption significantly above some resting, or basal, level. In the short term, the stress response is adaptive and helps individuals cope with emergency situations; in the long term, the stress response tends to be maladaptive (Selye, 1936, 1937a; Sapolsky, 1992b, 1994). Both short-term and long-term stress responses can affect hormone–behavior interactions.

# Physiological Effects of the Stress Response

Almost immediately after exposure to a stressor, a physiological stress response with several components begins to unfold: within seconds, the sympathetic nervous system secretes norepinephrine, and the adrenal medulla secretes epinephrine; within minutes, the adrenal cortex begins to secrete glucocorticoids, and several other hormones including prolactin, glucagon, thyroid hormones, and vasopressin are secreted from various endocrine organs. The stress response has many adaptive effects:

- Increased immediate availability of energy

- Increased oxygen intake

- Decreased blood flow to areas not necessary for movement

- Inhibition of digestion, growth, immune function, reproduction, and pain perception

- Enhancement of memory and sensory function

Imagine that a rabbit is being chased by a fox. How does the stress response affect the rabbit in this situation? First, the rabbit needs a quick energy supply in order to sustain the sprint back to its warren. In such an emergency, the need for metabolic fuel is acute, large, and unpredictable (Sapolsky, 1992b, 1994). The immediate release of catecholamines raises respiration and cardiovascular rates within seconds; the body requires increased energy availability to sustain these high rates. The most obvious physiological change that occurs in response to a stressor is an immediate increase in available levels of glucose and oxygen in the blood. Epinephrine increases the delivery of oxygen to the tissues, and raises sympathetic tone (i.e., the activation level of the sympathetic nervous system). Glucocorticoids, which are secreted within minutes, affect metabolic pathways to ensure that adequate energy is available to the individual to cope with the increased need for metabolic fuels. Blood flow is temporarily rerouted to the muscles and away from the digestive system or other processes not critical for coping with the emergency situation. In other words, the rabbit's lunch can be digested later (if there is a "later"). Responses to injuries that might curtail movement (e.g., pain, inflammation) are inhibited by the stress-induced release of endorphins. If a rabbit that suffered scrapes and scratches as it darted into the brambles stopped to nurse its wounds, it would likely become the fox's dinner. Energetically expensive activities such as growth, reproduction, and immune function are also suppressed until after the emergency has passed. After the rabbit is safe in its nest, the stress response subsides, parasympathetic tone increases, and metabolic rate returns to baseline.

Importantly, both the predator and the prey are experiencing similar stress responses during the chase, despite their disparate roles. This is another example of the nonspecificity of the stress response. If the attempts of the fox to obtain food are unsuccessful, it will experience a prolonged stress response, the effects of which we will see below.

Other physiological responses to stressors occur within minutes after perception of the stressor. Corticotropin-releasing hormone (CRH) is released from the hypothalamus into the portal blood system. The CRH travels to the anterior pituitary gland, where it stimulates specific cells to secrete ACTH, which enters the general blood circulation and provokes the adrenal cortex to produce and secrete glucocorticoids.

The stress response often includes an increase in blood concentrations of vasopressin, which acts to increase blood volume and blood pressure and makes the delivery of energy to the large muscles more efficient. Vasopressin is also involved in the release of ACTH from the anterior pituitary (de Kloet et al., 1991). The anterior pituitary gland also secretes prolactin, which functions in the stress response to suppress reproduction temporarily by acting at multiple sites within the hypothalamic–pituitary–gonadal (HPG) axis (Figure 11.6) (Van de Kar et al., 1991). The α-cells of the endocrine pancreas are stimulated to secrete glucagon. As you will recall from Chapter 2, glucagon serves to increase energy availability. The β-cells of the pancreas are inhibited by glucagon from secreting insulin. Endorphins and enkephalins are released to provide relief from pain; these hormones also suppress GnRH, thereby inhibiting reproductive function. Essentially, all of the physiological sequelae in the response to a stressor involve making more energy available for immediate use. Again, all processes that are involved in future survival or reproductive success (e.g., energy storage as fat, production of gametes, growth) are put on hold until a future is certain (Sapolsky, 1994).

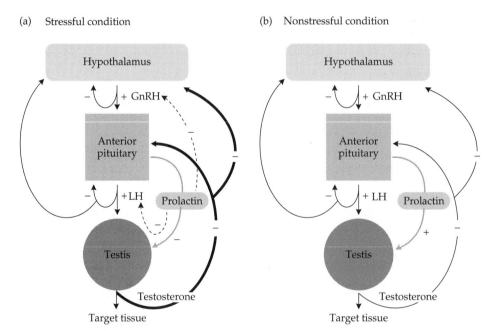

(a) Stressful condition

(b) Nonstressful condition

**11.6 Prolactin inhibits reproductive function** temporarily during stressful conditions (a) by acting at multiple sites within the hypothalamic–pituitary–gonadal (HPG) axis. The Leydig cells become less responsive to LH and produce less testosterone, and the negative feedback mechanisms in the pituitary and hypothalamus are accentuated so that any testosterone produced causes further reductions in GnRH and gonadotropin secretion. Normally, prolactin at low concentrations facilitates testosterone production (b).

# Pathological Effects of the Stress Response

In the short term, the stress response is adaptive, and for the most part, the neuroendocrine mechanisms underlying the stress response are conserved across vertebrate phylogeny. Generally, the stress response serves to help an individual cope with an emergency energetic crisis. Ideally, the stress response is activated by stressful stimuli, then the system is deactivated shortly after the emergency subsides. For example, if a female wild dog were trying to integrate herself into a new pack, she would probably be met by aggressive rebuffs from the females currently in the pack. Whether she decided to stay and fight or to run away, she would experience a short-term stress response that would increase her ability to mobilize and burn energy. If she were accepted into the pack, then a new social hierarchy would be established, fighting would decrease, and the stress response would be terminated. However, if she were driven from the pack, and she had to hunt for food or water alone in an unfamiliar territory, she would probably experience a long-term stress response, especially if her solo hunting success was low. Prolonged stress shifts the useful, adaptive short-term stress response to a pathological condition that can jeopardize health and survival  (Sapolsky, 1992b, 1994).

Stress-related pathologies are a common contributing factor to human disease. Many of us perceive "foxes" (i.e., stressors) all around us—paying the bills, writing textbooks, public speaking, or dealing with our personal relationships may all evoke a full-blown stress response. Our bodies remain engaged for emergency action even though we may remain physically inactive. The consequences of this chronic stress are mainly negative. Some of us may try to alter our perception of stress-evoking situations by ingesting alcohol or other drugs. As you will see below, stress accentuates the effects and the addictive properties of these substances. Some of us may use various psychological coping strategies, such as visualization, to alter our perception of stressors, others will go through life seemingly unaware of stressors, and a few will embrace stressors, actually seeking out various experiences that engage the HPA axis, such as working in a big city trauma center, parachuting, or riding roller coasters.

The pathological effects of chronic stress involve cardiovascular, metabolic, reproductive, digestive, immune, and anabolic processes (Table 11.1) (Sapolsky, 1992a, 1994; Brown, 1994). A high pulse rate and elevated blood pressure are useful for explosive activities such as pursuing or evading prey, but are well-established contributors to the development of atherosclerotic plaques leading to heart disease, embolisms, and strokes. The breakdown of glycogen and lipids to elevate blood glucose concentrations cannot continue indefinitely. With prolonged glucocorticoid secretion, myopathy (i.e., muscle loss) is inevitable, and in severe cases stress can even induce the irreversible loss of muscle cells in the heart. Reproductive function is also inhibited by high glucocorticoid concentrations. This has obvious negative consequences for the reproductive success of animals in the wild that are confronted by demanding environmental conditions. An important consequence of stress for reproductive function in humans is that infertile couples often experience an escalating effect of stress on fertility that interferes with the infertility treatment (Agarwal and Haney, 1994; Greenfield, 1997). In other words, the stress of experiencing infertility, or the stress of the treatments, causes more stress and consequently reinforces the infertility. Prolonged inhibition of diges-

**Table 11.1**
**Pathological effects of long-term stress responses**

| Acute stress response | Pathological state associated with chronic stress |
|---|---|
| Shift from energy storage to energy use | Fatigue, myopathy; steroid diabetes |
| Increased cardiovascular tone | Hypertension |
| Inhibited digestion | Peptic ulcers |
| Inhibited growth | Psychosocial dwarfism |
| Inhibited reproduction | Impotence; anovulation; loss of libido |
| Compromised immune function and inflammatory responses | Impaired disease resistance; cancer |
| Enhanced cognition | Accelerated neural degeneration during aging |
| Enhanced analgesia | |

*Source:* Sapolsky, 1992b

tion during stress can also lead to ulceration and chronic bowel distress syndrome. Peptic ulcers can develop as a result of suppressed immune function that allows the proliferation of bacteria, especially *Helicobacter pylori,* in the stomach and digestive tract that can attack the lining of the stomach or duodenum. In general, chronic immunosuppression, as seen in AIDS patients, compromises long-term survival. Stress adds to AIDS-associated immunosuppression to reduce the chances of survival (Capitanio et al., 1998; Evans et al., 1997). Chronic stress also inhibits growth and repair processes. You might notice that your fingernails are more likely to be flimsy or brittle, or that your hair grows more slowly, during stressful periods in your life. Chronic stress in children, usually as a result of parental deprivation and abuse, can inhibit growth hormone and result in a condition called psychosocial dwarfism, as we will see below.

The pathological long-term effects of chronic stress affect many hormone–behavior interactions. As we have seen, reproductive function is impaired in chronically stressed individuals (Welsh et al., 1999). Recall that only the alpha pair of each pack of African wild dogs breeds. A series of studies was conducted to discover why social subordinates do not breed, even though they are reproductively mature. It was hypothesized that subordinate wild dogs were reproductively suppressed by stress. These studies were conducted with the hope of reversing the recent population declines in this endangered species (Creel et al., 1996). By collecting feces from individual animals whose social status was known, the investigators were able to assay hormone concentrations (measured indirectly by assaying fecal metabolic breakdown products of the hormones of interest) without disturbing the animals (Monfort et al., 1998). In contrast to the investigators' expectations, these studies, as well as studies of African dwarf mongooses (*Helogale parvula*), indicated that the *dominant* animals had high glucocorticoid concentrations (Figure 11.7) (Creel et al., 1996). It is possible that the dominant animals are exposed to the chronic psychological stressor of potentially losing their status. In any event, these results contrasted with the findings of previous laboratory studies that had reported that subordinate rats, mice, and primates were more highly stressed than the dominant members of their social group (Sapolsky, 1992b).

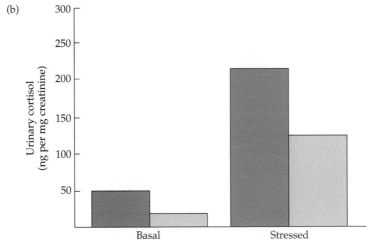

**11.7 Corticosterone concentrations are elevated in dominant wild dogs and mongooses.** In contrast to the findings in most laboratory animals, the alpha individuals (dark bars) in groups of (a) free-living African wild dogs and (b) captive mongooses have higher corticosterone values than subordinate animals (light bars). In other words, the dominant individuals appear to be more stressed than subordinate individuals. After Creel et al., 1997.

## *Perinatal Stress*

The damaging effects of chronic stress are not limited to adult animals. As will be described in this section, fetal animals and newborns are also affected, and these effects of stress can have prolonged consequences.

**PRENATAL STRESS.**    Although we would all do well to try to limit the effects of chronic stress in our lives, sometimes they have already affected us before birth (Herrenkohl, 1986; Takahashi, 1998; Weinstock, 1997). A series of studies have examined the effects of prenatal stress on the physiology and behavior of rat pups. If pregnant dams are placed in clear plastic restraint devices under bright lights for 30–60 minutes each day during days 14–21 of their 21-day gestation, they respond with increased activation of the HPA axis. Importantly, their offspring display permanent changes in their brain morphology, physiology, and behavior. Maternal stress alters blood testosterone concentrations in fetal male rats, shifting the peak to 2 days earlier than that in nonstressed males (Ward and Weisz, 1980; Ward, 1984). When tested as adults, sons of stressed mothers often failed to ejaculate in mating tests (Ward et al., 1994), even though their adulthood concentrations of testosterone and LH were normal (I. L.Ward et al., 1996). The shift in the timing of the testosterone peak blocked the development of the normal sexual dimorphism of the brain, affecting the sexually dimorphic nuclei (SDN) of the medial preoptic area as well as the spinal nucleus of the bulbocavernosus (SNB) and the dorsolateral nucleus (DLN) of the spinal cord (Kerchner and Ward, 1992; Kerchner et al., 1995). The sex difference in the size of the rostral anterior commissure was also found to be altered by prenatal stress (Jones et al., 1997). Furthermore, when exposed to restraint stress as adults, both male and female rats whose mothers had experienced stress during gestation displayed an attenuated prolactin response (Kinsley et al., 1989), suggesting a permanent effect of prenatal stress on the HPA axis. Prenatally stressed female rats did not display any disturbances in normal estrous cycles, sexual behavior, pregnancy, parturition, pup survival, or maternal behavior when tested as adults (Beckhardt and Ward, 1983; but see Herrenkohl, 1986).

Recall that rat dams tend to spend more time licking the anogenital regions of male pups as compared with female pups (Michel and Moore, 1995), and that this sex difference in eliciting maternal attention is mediated by testosterone. If dams are stressed while pregnant, they show no preference in grooming between their male or female offspring (Power and Moore, 1986). Presumably, the prenatal stress affects testosterone secretion so that the male and female offspring do not vary in the critical testosterone-dependent variable that dams normally use to discriminate male from female pups.

Prenatal stress impairs subsequent negative feedback within the HPA axis in adult rats, which often results in elevated basal corticosterone blood concentrations (Henry et al., 1994). Subjecting pregnant rat dams to either stress or exogenous glucocorticoid administration decreases hippocampal type I glucocorticoid receptors in their offspring; this decrease has been hypothesized to account for the impaired negative feedback of the HPA axis in adulthood (Barbazanges et al., 1996). Damage to the hippocampal cells mediating negative feedback results in elevated glucocorticoid levels. Again, the process of prenatal stress is mediated by the HPA axis. If a pregnant female is adrenalectomized prior to stress or corticosterone treatment, the negative feedback mechanisms are not impaired in her adult offspring (Figure 11.8) (Barbazanges et al., 1996). The offspring of stressed rat dams are more likely to self-administer drugs such as cocaine and amphetamines as adults than their unstressed peers (Deminiere et al., 1992; Diaz et al., 1995; see below). These results may have important implications for drug abuse in children of stressed parents.

Prenatally stressed human infants have reduced birth weights, experience developmental delays, and also display attentional deficits, hyperanxiety, impaired social behaviors, and possibly impaired strategies for coping with stressful conditions as adults (Weinstock, 1997). It is possible that the same kind of dys-

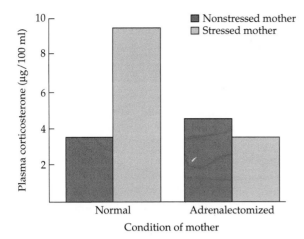

**11.8   Adrenalectomy prevents the elevated stress response in rats stressed in utero.** Corticosterone concentrations are elevated in response to restraint stress in adult rats whose mothers were stressed while pregnant. Adrenalectomy prevented this elevated stress response. After Barbazanges et al., 1996.

regulation of the HPA axis observed in rats exposed to prenatal stress serves as a precursor to the HPA disinhibition observed in many instances of human depression (Weinstock, 1997). Like prenatal stressors, exposure of humans to glucocorticoids in utero has a number of negative consequences, including low birth weight, which in turn is associated with adult cardiovascular and metabolic disorders such as hypertension, insulin resistance, hyperlipidemia, and ischemic heart and brain disease (Nyirenda and Seckl, 1998).

Human studies of prenatal stress, of course, are correlational; it would be unethical to manipulate stress levels in women in order to observe the effects on their babies. However, long-term studies of monkeys can be used to investigate the long-term consequences of prenatal stress for the behavior and reproductive success of adult humans. The effects of prenatal stress on the human HPA axis have been carefully modeled in rhesus monkeys (Clarke et al., 1994). To induce stress experimentally, pregnant rhesus monkeys were exposed to random loud noises throughout mid- to late pregnancy. Their offspring displayed low birth weights, impaired neuromotor development, attention deficits (Schneider, 1992b; Schneider and Coe, 1993), and impaired cognitive function (Schneider, 1992a) as compared with their nonstressed peers. Additionally, enhanced stress responsiveness, higher frequencies of abnormal coping behaviors, and impaired social behaviors were observed in the offspring of female rhesus monkeys that were chronically stressed during pregnancy (Clarke and Schneider, 1993; Clarke et al., 1994).

**NEONATAL STRESS.**   Animal models have also been developed to determine the effects of stress in newborns. Several experimental paradigms have been examined to explain individual differences in coping with stress as adults. According to the leading hypothesis (Levine et al., 1967), early stressful experiences affect reactions to stress later in life. If a rat pup experiences certain types of mild stress, then it appears to be better able to cope with stress later in life. Human handling of pups or brief separation of pups from their mother evokes stress responses in the pups. However, upon the return of the pups to their mother, the rat dam spends extra time licking them. This gentle stimulation appears to reverse the negative effects of the stress on the pups and is responsible for the so-called "stress immunization" effect that allows the pups to cope with stress better as adults (Figure 11.9) (Liu et al., 1997). One way this is hypothesized to occur is by changing the densities of hippocampal glucocorticoid receptors, which are important in the negative feedback regulatory mechanisms of adults (Liu et al., 1997), as we saw above.

A commonly used experimental paradigm for assessing separation stress involves the separation of infants from their mothers at different ages and for differing periods of time (Levine et al., 1991). Typically, rat pups are isolated in novel test arenas and receive a saline injection; this combined treatment of isolation plus injection is considered to be a mild stressor (e.g., Suchecki et al., 1993). If 6-, 9-, or 12-day-old rat pups are isolated from their mother for 24 hours, then baseline ACTH concentrations are elevated. The elevated ACTH concentrations are significantly higher in stressed than in nonstressed animals, and the magnitude of the increase becomes higher as the pups age (Suchecki et al., 1993). Corticosterone concentrations show a similar effect, and the effect of mild stress on corticosterone concentrations persists for at least for 4 days (Rosenfeld et al., 1992). Again, postnatal exposure to mild stressors blunts adult stress responsiveness (Levine et al., 1967; Sapolsky and Meaney, 1986). In contrast, elevated stress responses are observed throughout life in pups exposed to moderate or strong stressors (Rots et al., 1996). For example, severely stressed pups may have long-term decreases in food intake and body mass in response to endogenous pro-inflammatory cytokines such as interleukin-1β (Kent et al., 1997).

**11.9  Stress responses are reduced in offspring that received maternal attention as pups.** Both ACTH (a) and corticosterone (b) concentrations were lower before, during, and after a 20-minute restraint stress in rats (indicated by the shaded area) that had received a high (shaded circles) amount of maternal licking after separation as pups than in those that received a low amount (solid circles). After Liu et al., 1997.

Maternal tactile and feeding cues are sufficient to suppress the elevated concentrations of ACTH and corticosterone resulting from 24 hours of maternal deprivation (van Oers et al., 1998). Interaction with an anesthetized lactating female rat is sufficient to block the enhanced corticosterone stress response associated with isolation (Stanton and Levine, 1990). Thus, it appears that the contact comfort of the mother is sufficient to prevent the stress response to isolation, although her grooming and licking behaviors are also important (Liu et al., 1997). Impairment of HPA function is more marked in female than in male rats exposed to isolation stress (McCormick et al., 1995).

These studies on isolation-induced stress are reminiscent of the famous biopsychological studies conducted on rhesus monkeys by Harry Harlow and colleagues, in which the factors that represent "motherness" were investigated. In these studies, infants were separated from their mothers immediately following birth. In one series of studies, infants were provided with two surrogate mothers. One surrogate, made of a wire frame, had a nipple protruding from its midsection, and gave milk to the infant; the other surrogate mother provided no nutrition, but her wire frame was covered with a soft material to which the infant could cling to derive contact comfort (Figure 11.10). When stressed by an intruder, the infant ran to the so-called "cloth mother" (Harlow and Harlow, 1965; Harlow et al., 1971). Neither of these surrogate mothers provided any social instructions, however. When these isolated infants grew up, they were socially inept and generally fearful (Harlow et al., 1971). Only some reversal of this social impairment was possible (Harlow et al., 1971). Some of the best improvements in social behav-

**11.10 Infant rhesus monkeys cling to cloth "mother" for contact comfort** when stressed by a novel toy. These infants were reared with two surrogate mothers, a wire mother that provided nutrition, and a cloth-covered wire mother that provided no nutrition, but had a soft surface. From Harlow, 1959.

ior in these formerly isolated monkeys were obtained by pairing them with pet dogs (Mason and Kenney, 1974; Mason and Capitanio, 1988).

**PSYCHOSOCIAL DWARFISM.**　Psychosocial dwarfism is a relatively rare syndrome found among human infants that are reared in situations in which they experience little or no physical contact during development, as in orphanages where the staff does not regularly interact with the children (Widdowson, 1951). This syndrome is characterized by lack of growth and development despite adequate nutrition, disruption of normal sleep cycles, a selective disruption of normal patterns of growth hormone secretion, and an absence of tissue responsiveness to exogenous growth hormone (Schanberg and Field, 1987). This last feature of the syndrome distinguishes psychosocial dwarfism from hypopituitary dwarfism, in which treatment with growth hormone restores normal growth. Patients with psychosocial dwarfism, however, usually recover after placement in a hospital or home environment where more social and physical stimulation is available (Figure 11.11). As seen with rhesus monkey infants, young animals, too, require tactile stimulation provided by physical contact with their mother (or some other adult) for normal somatic growth and development.

What are the physiological factors that mediate these stimulatory effects of tactile contact in facilitating growth and development? A series of beautifully constructed studies have addressed this question in rats. When maternal tactile stim-

**11.11 Psychosocial dwarfism** is a rare occurrence seen most frequently in severe cases of child abuse, and is usually reversible after termination of the stressors. This girl was drinking from puddles in the street and eating from garbage cans before admission to the hospital at age 15.3 years (left panel). At admission, her height was in the normal range for 9-year-old children, and she displayed abnormal GH release. Both LH and FSH were nondetectable. After 1 month in the hospital, she grew 2.5 cm, and began to undergo puberty. At age 16 (center panel), she was living in foster care, and displaying significant GH release. Growth continued, and at 16.9 years (right panel) she had grown 27.5 cm. Courtesy of Dr. Claude Migeon.

ulation of rat pups is restricted, either by isolating or anesthetizing the rat dam, the pups' growth is reduced, and at least three biochemical changes occur (Schanberg and Kuhn, 1985). First, levels of the enzyme ornithine decarboxylase (ODC) are sharply reduced immediately after separation from the mother in all tissues examined, including brain, liver, heart, kidney, and spleen (Schanberg and Field, 1987). ODC is the first enzyme required in the synthesis of polyamides, which are involved in the regulation of protein synthesis, and hence in tissue growth and development. ODC concentrations return to normal within 2 hours of the reunification of pups and dam. Placement of the pups with an anesthetized mother, who continued to lactate, provided warmth, and supplied all noninteractive maternal cues, did not prevent the rapid decline in ODC concentrations in the pups.

Clearly, something that the mother rat does stimulates ODC activity. As previously noted, mother rats retrieve their pups and lick them. When isolated pups were stroked with a damp paintbrush in a way that roughly approximated the tongue movements of the dam, the reduction in ODC concentrations was prevented (Table 11.2). Other forms of sensory stimulation, such as tail pinching, were ineffective in preventing the decline in ODC concentrations in isolated pups.

The decrease in ODC concentrations in many different body sites suggests that either a general metabolic or an endocrine signal mediates the effects of tactile stimulation. Blood plasma concentrations of growth hormone (GH), but not of prolactin or thyroid-stimulating hormone, decreased in pups after maternal separation, whereas blood concentrations of corticosterone increased (Schanberg and Kuhn, 1985). GH regulates ODC activity in the brain and other tissues. Stroking with a wet paintbrush also normalized GH concentrations in isolated pups. In an attempt to counteract the diminished concentrations of ODC after separation, isolated and unstroked pups were injected with growth hormone, but it was discovered that the tissues of these pups were unresponsive to the hormone. Stroking with a paintbrush maintained tissue responsiveness to GH.

After GH is secreted from the anterior pituitary gland, it binds, along with several types of somatomedins, to receptors on the surfaces of cells. Cells that bind GH are stimulated to grow and divide. The physiological mechanisms by which tactile stimuli increase GH secretion from the anterior pituitary, and how they induce tissue sensitivity to GH, are not yet known. But research into this fascinating area should provide more answers about how maternal behavior influ-

### Table 11.2
### Effect of stroking on ODC activity and serum GH concentrations in maternally deprived rat pups

|  | ODC serum concentration (% control ± SEM) | | | Serum GH concentration (% control ± SEM) |
| --- | --- | --- | --- | --- |
|  | Brain | Heart | Liver |  |
| Control | 100 ± 13 | 100 ± 6 | 100 ± 13 | 100 ± 20 |
| Deprived[a] | 68 ± 8 | 36 ± 7 | 32 ± 6 | 25 ± 7 |
| Deprived and stroked | 134 ± 15 | 93 ± 15 | 199 ± 41 | 82 ± 17 |

*Source:* Schanberg and Kuhn, 1985.
[a] $p < 0.05$ or better compared to controls for all values.

ences hormone concentrations, growth, and development in the offspring of rats and humans. This research has several practical applications; one important outcome has been the practice of stimulating growth and development in premature infants by increased handling in perinatal intensive care nurseries (Schanberg and Field, 1987). A low-tech improvement in premature infants' health, and a shorter hospital stay, are certainly impressive outcomes of these interesting studies in rats.

Glucocorticoids might also be involved in psychosocial dwarfism; however, cortisol concentrations are usually normal or in the low normal range in affected children. As mentioned above, glucocorticoid concentrations in young rats rise dramatically after maternal separation. In human children, only a doubling of glucocorticoid concentrations is sufficient to arrest growth (Sapolsky, 1994). Glucocorticoids can suppress growth by suppressing GH, inhibiting GH receptor sensitivity, and decreasing protein production and DNA synthesis. Whatever is actually suppressing the growth of afflicted children, the good news is that removing them from the stress-inducing environment allows them to catch up on their growth. In Table 11.3, the effects of emotional factors on growth are obvious in a single boy suffering from psychosocial dwarfism.

### Reproductive Dysfunction

Every individual has limited energy resources, which must support maintenance of the body as well as reproduction. Other energetically expensive activities, including immune function and growth, must also be partitioned out of the total energy budget. Consequently, from an evolutionary perspective, there is a tradeoff among competing energetic requirements, so that growth or immune function may be compromised to support reproduction when energy is somewhat limited (Ots and Horak, 1996). Alternatively, reproduction or immune function may be compromised when energy availability is significantly reduced.

Reproductive suppression in response to stress occurs on several physiological and behavioral levels, and can have potentially severe effects on both humans and nonhuman animals (Welch et al., 1999). Stress is an important contributory factor in human sexual dysfunction and infertility. Stress-induced reproductive impairments may also have a marked economic impact in domestic animals (Moberg, 1991); stress can reduce milk production in cows and egg production in chickens (Welsh et al., 1999). In sum, the scientific study of the effects of stress on reproductive function has important clinical and practical applications.

| | Plasma GH | Growth | Food intake |
|---|---|---|---|
| Event | concentration (ng/ml) | (cm/20 days) | (kg/day) |
| Hospital admission | 5.9 | 0.5 | 1663 |
| 100 days post-admission | 13.0 | 1.7 | 1514 |
| Favorite nurse on vacation | 6.9 | 0.6 | 1504 |
| Favorite nurse returns | 15.0 | 1.5 | 1521 |

**Table 11.3**
**Effects of external events on growth in a child with psychosocial dwarfism**

*Source:* Saenger et al., 1977.

**MALES.**    A variety of stressors have been reported to suppress male reproductive function. Stress inhibits testosterone production, and low testosterone concentrations reduce both sexual motivation and performance (see Chapter 5). The
release of CRH and endogenous opioids can directly suppress the release of GnRH
(Hulse and Coleman, 1983; Jacobs and Lightman, 1980; Rasmussen et al., 1983;
Rivier et al., 1986). CRH-containing neurons in the paraventricular nucleus (PVN)
of the hypothalamus have been classified into two types: (1) vasopressin-positive
and (2) vasopressin-negative neurons. Stress causes certain neurotransmitters to
trigger the release of CRH from both types, and of vasopressin from the vasopressin-positive neurons. CRH travels to the anterior pituitary, where it binds to
specific G protein-associated receptors in the ACTH-releasing cells. Activation of
these CRH receptors stimulates the protein kinase A pathway. CRH and its receptors have also been identified in the testes and ovaries, suggesting that this releasing hormone may also directly inhibit steroid production (Welsh et al., 1999). In
the brain, vasopressin binds to its receptor ($V_{1A}$), which activates the protein
kinase C pathway.

Both CRH and vasopressin can stimulate expression of the genes for pro-opiomelanocortin in the anterior pituitary. Recall from Chapter 2 that POMC can be
processed by various enzymes to yield several peptides, including ACTH and β-
endorphin. There is some evidence that different environmental stressors determine which enzymes are produced in order to cleave specific peptides from the
POMC precursor molecule (DeWied, 1997). POMC-derived peptides may feed
back to inhibit GnRH secretion (Welsh et al., 1999). For example, both endogenous
and exogenous opiates can inhibit GnRH secretion (Figure 11.12) (Cameron, 1997;
DeWied, 1997; Genazzani and Petraglia, 1989; Rivier and Rivest, 1991). Sexual
motivation and performance are impaired in male heroin addicts. More than half
of the female heroin addicts interviewed in one study experienced menstrual
abnormalities while taking heroin or methadone (Santen et al., 1975; Smith et al.,
1982). Detailed endocrine studies revealed impaired gonadotropin secretion in
most of these cases (Santen et al., 1975). Naloxone, an opioid antagonist, reverses
the effects of opioids on reproductive suppression in humans and nonhuman animals (Genazzani and Petraglia, 1989; Gilbeau and Smith, 1985).

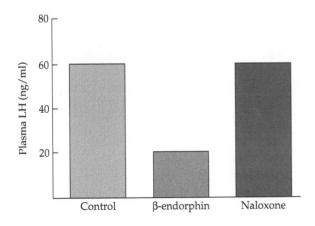

**11.12 Opiates suppress gonadotropin produc-
tion.** Plasma LH concentrations are reduced
after endorphin treatment; the reduction in LH
by endorphin is reversed by treatment with the
opiate antagonist, naloxone. After Kalra et al.,
1990.

ACTH stimulates the production and secretion of glucocorticoids from the zona fasciculata and zona reticularis of the adrenal cortex. Glucocorticoids can inhibit reproduction in several ways. First, glucocorticoids suppress GnRH and LH secretion via negative feedback (Welsh et al., 1999). Glucocorticoids have also been reported to inhibit the formation of proteins necessary for the production of hormone receptors, steroidogenic enzymes, and several intracellular signaling molecules (Rivier and Rivest, 1991). Cortisol inhibits testosterone secretion in men (Cummings et al., 1983) by acting on testicular LH receptors (Bambino and Hseuh, 1981). Glucocorticoids also suppress spermatogenesis somewhat directly. The testosterone-producing Leydig cells have glucocorticoid receptors that appear to be involved in the normal process of cell growth, metabolism, and energy use. However, when glucocorticoid concentrations increase for long periods of time, an enzyme that normally neutralizes glucocorticoids at basal concentrations is overwhelmed, and testosterone production is curtailed (Ge et al., 1997). The resulting low testosterone concentrations may fail to support spermatogenesis, so that sperm counts fall and stressed individuals become infertile (Ge et al., 1997), especially if they are subordinate animals. In contrast, when dominant rats are housed under stressful conditions, their testosterone concentrations increase; it appears that dominant rats have higher levels of the enzyme that counteracts elevated glucocorticoid concentrations to ensure fertility (Monder et al., 1994). Thus, social status appears to affect testicular enzymes that, in turn, mediate androgen production and fertility (Figure 11.13).

A moderate amount of activity or exercise actually stimulates testosterone concentrations (Figure 11.14) (Elias, 1981; Grandi and Celani, 1990). However, as my grandmother used to say, "too much of a good thing is often a bad thing." Excessive exercise can be interpreted by the body as stress; strenuous exercise, such as running a marathon, causes sustained glucocorticoid secretion and leads to low testosterone concentrations in men (Dessypris et al., 1976; MacConnie et al., 1986; Grandi and Celani, 1990; Luger et al., 1987).

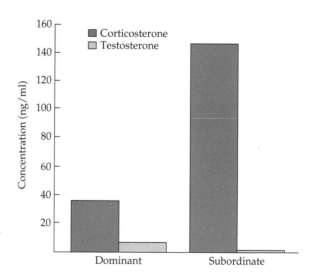

**11.13 Dominant male rats have lower corticosterone and higher testosterone concentrations than subordinate rats.** For this experiment, rats were housed in a special seminatural apparatus that allowed investigators to see their social interactions. After Blanchard et al., 1995.

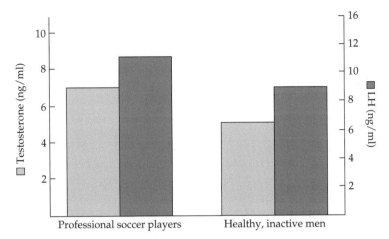

**11.14 Exercise elevates testosterone in men.** Men who engage in vigorous exercise display significantly higher testosterone and LH concentrations as compared to healthy, but inactive, men. However, it remains to be determined if this statistically significant elevation in hormone concentration is behaviorally significant; that is, do increased testosterone values of 1–2 ng/ml in men make a difference in the number of their aggressive encounters, mating partners, or babies sired. After Grandi and Celani, 1990.

As noted earlier in the chapter, prolactin is released during stress. Elevated blood prolactin concentrations can inhibit male reproductive function in a variety of ways, including enhancement of the sensitivity of the negative feedback mechanisms to testosterone (Bartke et al., 1977a,b; McNeilly et al., 1983). Treatment of hyperprolactinemia in men improves their potency in advance of any enhancement of blood testosterone concentrations (Buvat et al., 1985). The net result of all of these interactions is straightforward: chronic stress inhibits circulating testosterone concentrations. The decrease in testosterone suppresses both sexual motivation and performance, and also impairs fertility.

The long-term secretion of epinephrine also interferes with reproductive function. Recall from Chapter 5 that both the sympathetic and parasympathetic nervous systems must act together "in opposition" to generate a penile erection. In order for an erection to be initiated, the parasympathetic nervous system must be activated (Meisel and Sachs, 1994). In some species, such as rats and dogs, activation of the parasympathetic nervous system causes a specific muscle to pull up (contract) the penile bone (os) during sexual excitement. In other species, such as humans, that have hemodynamic penile erections, activation of the parasympathetic nervous system increases blood flow into the penis and blocks blood from draining out via the veins. As the penis fills with blood, it stiffens to permit intravaginal insertion. As copulation proceeds, the rest of the body maintains high sympathetic tone; that is, the sympathetic nervous system increases heart rate, blood pressure, and breathing rate, and moves blood from the periphery to the central trunk. The autonomic input to the genitalia retains its parasympathetic tone until sufficient stimulation occurs, then parasympathetic input suddenly terminates. Simultaneously, the sympathetic inputs to the penis are activated, and ejaculation occurs (Meisel and Sachs, 1994).

During stress, it becomes increasingly difficult to establish parasympathetic activity in the penis because of the stress-induced high sympathetic output (Rous, 1996). In humans, this can result in problems with achieving or maintaining penile erection; that is, stress can cause erectile dysfunction (impotence) (Smith, 1988; Morokoff et al., 1987). If the sympathetic input to the penis is activated too fast, as is also the case during stress, then premature ejaculation results (Smith, 1988). Premature ejaculation would severely affect the reproductive fitness of males of species in which females require sufficient stimulation to induce ovulation or functional corpora luteal formation (see Chapter 6). The consequences of premature ejaculation for human reproductive fitness have not been evaluated. But premature ejaculation can interfere with sexual relations, and represents one of the most common complaints heard by sex therapists. One way for a male to postpone ejaculation is to take a deep breath. Inflating the lungs triggers a salvo of parasympathetic signals that delays the switch from parasympathetic to sympathetic input to the penis (Rous, 1996). Problems with impotence and premature ejaculation are very common during times of stress. Because sexual behavior can proceed with very low concentrations of testosterone in experienced human males, the most common effects of stress on human copulation typically involve epinephrine and sympathetic signals.

**FEMALES.**    As we learned in Chapter 6, successful ovulation and the onset of mating behavior in females typically depend on the precise timing of neuroendocrine events. Stress, however, often disrupts this timing (reviewed in Chrousos et al., 1998). Stress can interrupt estrous cycles in laboratory animals, domesticated animals, and zoo animals and menstrual cycles in women (i.e., amenorrhea) (Welsh et al., 1999; Xiao and Ferin, 1997). Women with functional hypothalamic amenorrhea (no menstrual cycles and no pulsatile release of GnRH from the hypothalamus), but not other types of anovulation, display elevated cortisol concentrations (Berga et al., 1997). Stress can also interrupt pregnancy or lactation if the stressful conditions are sufficiently severe.

As noted in Chapter 9, mammals have mechanisms to inhibit reproduction when they fall into a negative energy balance (Bronson, 1999). Women who diet rigorously or exercise strenuously often have problems with fertility (Figure 11.15) (Arena et al., 1995; Constantini and Warren, 1994). Reports of menstrual irregularities, amenorrhea, and reduced sexual desire and sexual activity, as well as infertility, are common among fashion models, women with the eating disorder anorexia nervosa, and athletes or dancers who do not increase their food intake to compensate for their excessive energy expenditure (Arena etal., 1995; Schneider and Wade, 1999). Reproductive inhibition occurs among females of all mammalian species and is entirely reversible upon refeeding or relaxation of the energy demands (Cameron et al., 1993).

Fasting increases blood glucocorticoid concentrations and is generally considered to be a stressor. Suppression of reproductive function in the service of energy balance is controlled by mechanisms that overlap with those that control food intake. As we saw in Chapter 9, most of the peptide hormones, neuropeptides, and metabolic inhibitors that increase food intake also inhibit reproduction, and many of the same brain regions are involved (Schneider and Wade, 1999). Mechanisms that interrupt estrous cycles are sensitive to signals generated by the

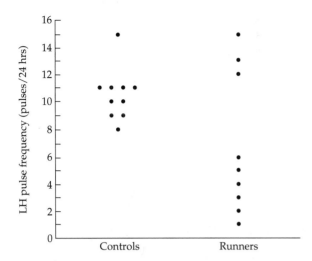

**11.15 Effects of exercise on LH pulse frequency.** LH pulses are less frequent in women who are long-distance runners, which may be related to the reported incidence of amenorrhea among such women. Source: Veldhuis et al., 1985.

oxidation of metabolic fuels. For example, treatment of well-fed female hamsters with 2-deoxyglucose (2-DG), which prevents glucose utilization, suspends estrous cycles (Schneider and Wade, 1989a). Thus, stress appears to interrupt estrous cycles by affecting metabolic pathways. It is likely that stress-evoked interruption of menstrual cycles in humans is mediated by the same pathways.

There are a variety of mechanisms underlying stress-impaired female reproduction. All of the neuroendocrine impairments of GnRH and gonadotropin secretion that were described previously for males also occur in females. One additional mechanism of reproductive impairment in females appears to be a side effect of overactive adrenal cortices. In addition to glucocorticoids, the adrenal glands also secrete androgens in both males and females. Even though the amount of androgen (primarily androstenedione) released by females' adrenals is only about 2–3% of male concentrations, it can interrupt female reproductive processes. Many of these androgens are converted to estrogens in fat cells, and during food shortages, less estrogen is produced in the fat cells. More importantly, increased androgen concentrations wreak havoc with the negative feedback mechanisms of GnRH and the gonadotropins.

**SEX DIFFERENCES.**    Sex differences in the neuroendocrine response to stress have been reported in rats. Female rats usually have higher basal corticosterone concentrations than male rats (Critchlow et al., 1963; Kitay, 1963). In response to stress, female rats generally display higher ACTH and corticosterone concentrations than stressed males do (Handa et al., 1994; Patchev et al., 1995; Viau and Meaney, 1991). These sex differences in stress responses are activated, rather than organized, by hormones; ovariectomy in adulthood eliminates the sex difference in the HPA axis, and estradiol replacement therapy restores the HPA sexual dimorphism (Kitay, 1963). Using 2-DG autoradiography, it was discovered that stressed female rats display higher glucose utilization than stressed males in several brain regions, including the hypothalamic ventromedial nuclei, arcuate nucleus, medial preoptic area, and the hippocampal CA1 layer and dentate gyrus (Figure 11.16) (Brown et al., 1996).

**11.16 Sex differences in glucose utilization under stress.**    Females (top) show greater brain utilization of glucose, seen here as dark areas, than males (bottom) under stress. This difference is seen in all brain regions, but is especially prominent in the CA1 region and dentate gyrus of the hippocampus. From Brown et al., 1996.

## Stress and Social Behavior

Research on the effects of social factors on stress arose from ecological research in the 1950s and 1960s investigating the dramatic population cycles observed in voles (*Microtus* spp.), lemmings (*Lemmus* spp.), and wild mice (*Mus* spp.) (e.g., Bronson, 1967; Calhoun, 1961, 1962; Chitty, 1961; Christian, 1950, 1959; Christian et al., 1965; Clough, 1965; Southwick, 1955a,b; Thiessen and Rodgers, 1961; Wynne-Edwards, 1965). Similar studies of avian species emerged at about the same time (e.g., Kluver and Tinbergen, 1953; Siegel, 1959, 1960). To study population cycles in the laboratory, a few animals are generally put in large (typically 3 × 3 meters) cages, provided with excess food and water, and allowed to breed and raise their young. Because rodents are particularly well adapted for rapid reproduction, the population in these cages soon increases to amazing levels. But at some point, the population crashes. Why? It is not due to a lack of food or water, because these are replenished daily. It is not due to other challenging conditions such as extreme temperatures, inclement weather, or a buildup of predators, which might explain population crashes in the field, because all of these factors are controlled in the lab. The animals that died in these circumstances appeared to have enlarged adrenal glands and showed a variety of problems associated with high circulating glucocorticoid concentrations (Thiessen and Rodgers, 1961). Were the animals stressed because they had inadequate space as populations increased? If rats were housed individually in cages with about 30 cm$^2$ of floor space, they did not exhibit any of the signs of stress. If ten rats were housed together in a cage of about 300 cm$^2$, however, stress responses were evident in the grouped animals, despite the fact that all the animals had the same average amount of floor space. In fact, even if the group-housed rats had 32 times more floor space than the individually housed rats, they still exhibited stress responses (Myers et al., 1971). Clearly, something about the increasing social interactions at higher population densities caused the stress responses in the animals.

A number of studies have indicated that socially dominant animals have relatively low circulating levels of glucocorticoids, whereas subordinate individuals typically display relatively high circulating glucocorticoid concentrations (reviewed in Sapolsky, 1994). These differences are particularly salient during times of social instability. In some cases, as noted with African wild dogs, the dominant individuals tend to have elevated glucocorticoid concentrations compared with subordinate animals (Creel et al., 1996, 1997). Thus, in some cases, it is stressful to be "top dog," and in other cases, being at the bottom of the social ladder is stressful. These differences probably reflect social factors such as the amount of harassment within a social group or the extent to which social positions are out of the control of the participants (e.g., inherited).

Marmosets and tamarins exhibit an interesting reproductive strategy whereby only one female per social group breeds. The other, subordinate adult females are reproductively suppressed by a combination of olfactory, behavioral, and other signals from the dominant female (Kuederling et al., 1995; Saltzman et al., 1996; Abbott et al., 1997). The subordinate females have low circulating estrogen concentrations, but their GnRH levels are indistinguishable from those of dominant females (Abbott et al., 1997). It appears that their anovulation is caused by their inability to generate an LH surge (Abbott et al., 1997). This phenomenon has been termed "social castration."

Intense stress can cause brain damage in many species, including primates. For example, a group of captive vervet monkeys (*Cercopithecus aethiops*) was studied at a primate center in Kenya. In the group-housing enclosures, social hierarchies developed, and the animals at the top of the hierarchy made life miserable for the lower-ranked individuals. The net result of the constant harassment was that many of the monkeys at the bottom of the social hierarchy died at a relatively young age. When these animals were autopsied, it was revealed that their adrenal glands were enlarged, and gastric ulcers were evident. Other signs of chronic stress were apparent upon microscopic examination of the deceased individuals. Neurons in the CA1 region of the hippocampus had atrophied in comparison with the same region in high-ranked individuals (Uno et al., 1989) (Figure 11.17). Atrophy of brain regions has also been observed in rats that have been subjected to intensely stressful conditions (Sapolsky et al., 1985; Sapolsky, 1992b). Furthermore, CAT scan examinations of humans that had been subjected to torture have revealed significant degeneration in some brain regions (Jensen et al., 1982).

**11.17  Neural degeneration associated with stress.** The hippocampal regions between the arrows in a normal monkey (a) and a monkey subjected to stress (b) show large deficits in the number of pyramidal cells present in the stressed monkey compared with the normal monkey. From Uno et al., 1989.

The functional consequences of hippocampal atrophy for learning and memory are discussed in Chapter 12, but one example is useful here. Individuals that experience intensely stressful events (e.g., combat, torture, work camps) often suffer later in life from a constellation of symptoms called post-traumatic stress disorder (PTSD) (Yehuda et al., 1993). Even 50 years after their liberation, individual Holocaust survivors with PTSD displayed low urinary cortisol excretion compared with Holocaust survivors without PTSD (Yehuda et al., 1995). Combat soldiers from the Vietnam War era displayed similar dysregulation in the HPA axis (Yehuda et al., 1995). In cognitive tests, Vietnam veterans with combat-related PTSD displayed significant deficits in short-term memory (Bremner et al., 1993). Whether these deficits in memory reflect underlying hippocampal damage by long-term elevated cortisol secretion remains to be determined, but the possibility certainly exists.

Based on this evidence, it is apparent that chronic, intense stress impairs several physiological and behavioral systems. Additional research is necessary to determine the effects of intermittent, moderate stress—the type of stress experienced by most of us—on physiological and behavioral functions.

## Seasonal Fluctuations in Stress Responses

The experience of being captured generally causes an animal to experience a rapid surge of epinephrine and glucocorticoids. If blood samples are obtained immediately after an animal is captured, reproductive hormone concentrations are also generally much higher than if they are obtained a few hours post-capture (e.g.,

Licht et al., 1983; Mahmoud and Licht, 1997; Mendonca and Licht, 1986; Orchinik et al., 1988; Tyrrell and Cree, 1998). Obtaining multiple blood samples provides a more complete endocrine profile than a single blood sample, which might be obtained at the peak or nadir of a pulse of hormone secretion. Obviously, the interval of time between capture and the blood sample is important when trying to determine hormone concentrations in wild-caught animals. Techniques to assay glucocorticoid by-products in urine or feces have allowed the study of the relationship between social dominance and corticosterone values in unrestrained animals, as in the study of wild dogs and dwarf mongooses described earlier in this chapter. Another variable that is important in assessing hormone–stress–behavior interactions is the time of year. A study of greylag geese (*Anser anser*), for example, revealed that a complex interaction exists among social status, stress, and season of the year (Kotrschal et al., 1998).

Redpolls (*Acanthis flammea*) are birds that live in the challenging arctic conditions of Alaska. Both males and females showed the typical marked elevation in blood corticosterone concentrations when held captive for about 1 hour, indicating that they responded similarly to many other vertebrates (Wingfield et al., 1994). However, the amount of post-capture corticosterone elevation varied across the year (Figure 11.18). Corticosterone elevations were generally blunted during January, and were maximal during June, when the birds were breeding. It appeared that birds with the highest fat stores secreted the lowest amounts of glucocorticoids post-capture (Wingfield et al., 1994). Similar effects have been reported for other birds living at high latitudes, including white-crowned sparrows (*Zonotrichia leucophrys gambelii*), snow buntings (*Plectrophenax nivalis*), and Lapland longspurs (*Calcarius lapponicus*) (Romero et al., 1997, 1998a–d). The seasonal modulation of corticosterone secretion appears to be regulated at multiple sites within the HPA axis; during the winter (or during the energetically expensive, feather-replacing molting process), the system appears relatively insensitive to the effects of exogenous ACTH in stimulating corticosterone production (Romero et al., 1998a–d).

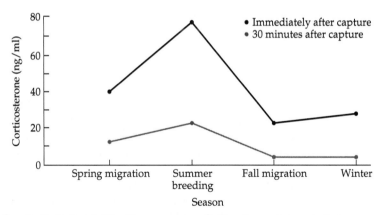

**11.18 Seasonal changes in the stress response.** Corticosterone concentrations were measured in blood samples obtained from white-crowned sparrows immediately or 30 minutes after capture. Note that the stress response was blunted during the fall and winter. After Romero et al., 1997.

Because glucocorticoids are released whenever energy requirements rise significantly above baseline, it is reasonable to expect temporal changes in glucocorticoid levels. As you may recall from Chapter 10, there is a marked circadian rhythm of glucocorticoid secretion. Glucocorticoids are secreted just prior to awakening each day to help increase blood glucose levels prior to increasing energy demands. Similarly, one might predict that glucocorticoids would be secreted during energetically demanding times across the year, such as molting, migration, or winter. Challenging winter conditions such as low ambient temperatures and decreased food availability can directly evoke a stress response in mammals (reviewed in Nelson and Demas, 1996). In the case of Arctic birds, it appears that special adaptations have evolved to blunt corticosterone secretion during the winter, when the birds' fat stores are too low to power a full stress response.

## Psychological Factors in Stress and Coping

Approximately 50% of women incarcerated in prison camps during the Second World War stopped menstruating. Obviously, prison camps are extremely stressful environments. But why were only 50% of the women affected?

In many cases of stress (e.g., capture in a net), the actual stressor is psychological, rather than physical. However, the secretion of epinephrine resulting from capture usually increases heart and lung functioning well above baseline, and both of these activities are energetically expensive; the subsequent glucocorticoid secretion several minutes after capture generates energy to power the heart and other muscles normally involved in the "fight or flight" response. The perception of stressors, the amount of epinephrine released in response to perceived stressors, the number of available receptors for epinephrine and glucocorticoids, the amount of binding proteins available to transport adrenal steroid hormones through the blood, and a host of other factors vary from one individual to another. Consequently, individual differences in stress responses are common, and specific causes for individual differences in stress responsiveness are not easily explained. Individual differences in the perception of and responsiveness to stressors—in other words, psychological differences—appear to account for many of the differences among humans responding to stress (Mason, 1975).

As we discovered earlier in this chapter, early individual experiences can modulate stress responses in adulthood. For instance, how children responded to a cold pressor test (a test of bodily reactions to a hand placed in a tub of iced water for 1 minute) in 1934 predicted their health problems as adults (Wood et al., 1984): Over 70% of the individuals that "over-reacted" to the test as children developed cardiovascular disease as adults, compared with fewer than 20% of the individuals who had displayed little or no reaction to the test 50 years previously (Wood et al., 1984).

One experimenter deprived two monkeys of food to study individual differences in response to stress (Sapolsky, 1992a). Although both individuals were deprived of any nutrition, and both should have showed an equal energy deficit and an equivalent rise in stress hormones, one monkey was fed a non-nutritive, flavored placebo. That monkey did not display elevated glucocorticoid secretion, but the other individual did. It seems that the first monkey did not *perceive* things to be as stressful as the second one (Sapolsky, 1992a).

Most scientists now accept the power of psychological variables to modulate stress physiology (Sapolsky, 1994). What are these variables? Among individuals of vertebrate species, the main psychological factors that modulate stress responses include: (1) control, (2) predictability, and (3) outlets for dealing with frustration.

### Control, Predictability, and Outlets for Frustration

Individuals suffer fewer stress-related pathologies if they can control the situation causing the stress (Gatchel et al., 1989). Controlling a stressful situation is a type of coping behavior. Rats were subjected to intermittent electric shocks in one early study (Weiss, 1968). One rat was able to depress a lever to decrease the rate of shocks. Another rat received a shock whenever the first rat did, but could not control the frequency of the shocks. Subsequently, the second rat showed higher glucocorticoid secretion than the rat that could moderate the shocks (Weiss, 1968). Predictable stress is easier to cope with than random presentation of stressors. In studies comparable to the one just described, predictability reduces the stress responses of individuals. For example, if warning signals are given to rats prior to shocks, those rats have lower glucocorticoid concentrations than rats that receive no warning stimuli (Sapolsky 1992a) (Figure 11.19). The ability to engage in displacement behavior—having an "outlet"—also ameliorates the effects of stress. When rats are shocked, they show relatively low glucocorticoid secretion if they can chew on a piece of wood or attack another rat (Sapolsky, 1992a). It is common knowledge that the effects of stress in humans can be ameliorated by displacement behaviors such as engaging in a hobby or moderate exercise.

Even modest activity can lessen the effects of stress. A study of children moving from kindergarten to primary school noted that many children engage in stereotypic "leg swinging" when confronted by the twin stressors of constraint to a desk and learning complex new cognitive skills (e.g., reading, writing, and arithmetic). Leg swinging appears to induce a shift from sympathetic to parasympathetic nervous system activation. Children engaged in leg swinging display a

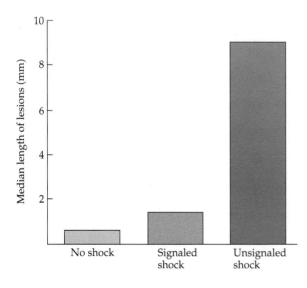

**11.19 Predictability of shock determines pathological stress responses** in rats. This graph depicts the lengths of gastric ulcerations in rats that were given electric shocks, either signaled or unsignaled by a warning bell. Although rats in both conditions heard the same number of warning bells and received the same number of electric shocks, the contingency of the bell and shocks provided a psychological factor that mediated the physical response to stress. After Weiss, 1972.

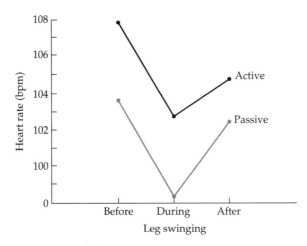

**11.20  Leg-swinging displacement activity reduces heart rate.** Leg swinging by first-grade children engages the parasympathetic system, which reduces heart rate, regardless of whether the children are involved (active) or uninvolved (passive) in learning activities. After Soussignan and Koch, 1985.

small, but consistent, reduction in heart rate during and after this displacement behavior (Figure 11.20) (Soussignan and Koch, 1985).

We began this chapter by discussing individual differences in reproductive fitness, and how survival and reproductive success are intertwined. Individual differences in the perception of stressors appear to be among the most important factors that determine the consequences of long-term stressors. Indeed, individuals who are in extremely stressful situations may avoid post-traumatic stress disorder by adopting an *illusion* of control, such as carrying a "lucky" charm (Gatchel et al., 1989).

## Stress and Drug Abuse

Stress increases the use of psychoactive drugs, including alcohol, cocaine, amphetamines, heroin, and nicotine (Goeders, 1997; DeVries et al., 1998). Cocaine abuse has been the most thoroughly studied in humans and animal models, and will serve here as an example of the effects of stress and hormones on substance abuse. Cocaine is a psychomotor stimulant, and is a very powerful reinforcer, or reward for a particular behavior. Self-administration of cocaine (e.g., individuals learn to bar-press for an I.V. hit of cocaine) can be established in several different species, including humans. If given ad libitum access to cocaine, individuals of several species, including rats, rhesus monkeys, and humans, will eventually self-administer lethal doses (Johanson et al., 1976; Bozarth and Wise, 1985; Dworkin et al., 1987).

The rewarding properties of cocaine, and of other psychomotor stimulants, are mediated by dopamine (Koob, 1992; DiChiara, 1995; Wise, 1996). Specifically, the mesocorticolimbic dopamine system, which originates in the ventral tegmental area and projects primarily to the nucleus accumbens (NAc), has been implicated in the mediation of the rewarding properties of psychomotor drugs (Koob, 1992). In vivo microdialysis has revealed that cocaine administration increases extracellular dopamine levels in several brain regions, including the NAc, medial prefrontal cortex, and striatum (Levy et al., 1994; Carboni et al., 1989; Pettit and Justice, 1991). This increase in dopamine results from the binding of cocaine to the dopamine transporter molecule, which effectively blocks dopamine reuptake by the presynaptic neuron. Blocking reuptake of dopamine usually causes more dopamine to be available in the synapse to interact with the dopamine receptors (Pettit and Justice, 1991; Defts et al., 1990). The increase in synaptic concentrations of dopamine potentiates the rewarding effects of cocaine (Defts et al., 1990). Dopamine-depleting lesions of the NAc reduce cocaine self-administration in rats (Defts et al., 1990). Experimental treatments that elevate dopamine transmission in the NAc facilitate the development of psychostimulant self-administration (Wise and Rompre, 1989). Predictably, mice lacking the gene that encodes the dopamine transporter do not display addictive behaviors associated with cocaine use (Giros et al., 1996). Because of conflicting results, the effects of dopamine agonists and antagonists on cocaine's rewarding properties and on addictive behaviors remain controversial (see Goeders, 1997 for review).

Corticosterone is secreted after administration of several psychoactive drugs, including alcohol, cocaine, amphetamines, heroin, and nicotine (Goeders, 1997; DeVries et al., 1998). Corticosterone increases dopamine transmission in the mesocorticolimbic pathway via several mechanisms (Deutch and Roth, 1990). For example, glucocorticoids increase dopamine release (Koob and Bloom, 1988; Wise and Rompre, 1989), decrease dopamine metabolism (Rothschild et al., 1985), decrease dopamine reuptake at the synapse, and modify the binding of dopamine to postsynaptic receptors (Biron et al., 1992). Predictably, glucocorticoids have reinforcing properties in rats (Piazza et al., 1993) and produce feelings of euphoria in some humans (Hall et al., 1979; Ling et al., 1981).

If the influence of glucocorticoids is removed, either by drugs or by adrenalectomy, then rats neither acquire nor maintain cocaine addiction; it appears that corticosterone blood concentrations must be more than 150 ng/ml before rats will initiate cocaine self-administration (Goeders et al., 1996, 1997). Treatment of rats with corticosterone or exposing them to various types of stressors increases their propensity to self-administer morphine (Shaham and Stewart, 1994), heroin (Bozarth et al., 1989), cocaine (Bozarth et al., 1989; Goeders and Guerin, 1996a), and amphetamines (Maccari et al., 1991; Piazza et al., 1991). Stressful stimuli can reinstate heroin self-administration in rats in which the behavior has been extinguished (Shaham and Stewart, 1995). Stress also initiates craving in recovering heroin or crack cocaine addicts (Childress et al., 1994). Thus, glucocorticoids appear to enhance the reinforcing effects of abused drugs in both humans and nonhuman animals. Treatments for substance abuse might be developed that inhibit the additive effects of glucocorticoids on psychoactive drugs. As these studies show, stress affects both physical and mental well-being, and stress increases substance abuse.

Stress is the "wear and tear" of life. Stress affects us all. How well we cope reflects how well we will age, which diseases we might avoid, and ultimately affects our reproductive function, as well as our reproductive fitness.

## Summary

- All living animals are dynamic systems of equilibria, or homeostasis. Serious disruptions in homeostasis are called stressors. Stressors may be environmental, physiological, and psychosocial.

- Stressors are met by a stress response, which is a suite of physiological and behavioral reactions to reestablish homeostasis. The stress response is nonspecific, and consists of epinephrine release from the adrenal medulla, norepinephrine release from the sympathetic nervous system, and glucocorticoid release from the adrenal cortices. The nonspecific feature of the stress response was also termed the "fight or flight" response by Walter Cannon.

- Hans Selye studied the process of coping with stressors, which he termed the General Adaptation Syndrome (GAS). The GAS consists of three stages: (1) the alarm reaction, (2) resistance, and (3) exhaustion.

- Stress is a difficult concept to define precisely. For the purposes of this chapter, stress is defined as all the nonspecific effects of factors that can act upon the body to increase energy consumption significantly above basal levels. The adaptive features of the stress response include an increase in the immediate availability of energy, an increase in oxygen uptake, a decrease in blood flow to areas not necessary for movement, and inhibition of digestion, growth, immune function, reproductive function, and pain perception, as well as enhancement of memory and perception.

- The pathological features of chronic stress include fatigue, myopathy, hypertension, gastric ulcers, psychosocial dwarfism, impotence, anovulation, loss of libido, compromised immune function, cancer, and potentially accelerated neural degeneration during aging.

- Prenatal stress can demasculinize male reproductive behaviors, but has little effect on female sexual behaviors. Mild stress during infancy can provide "stress immunization" and blunt stress responses later in life. Severe stress during infancy enhances stress responses.

- Psychosocial dwarfism is a rare syndrome found among human children that are raised in very stressful situations. GH is suppressed in these individuals; if they are removed from their stressful environments, they can catch up in their growth.

- Stress impairs male sexual behavior (motivation and performance) by suppressing testosterone. Stress also affects female sexual behavior by interrupting the precise timing of neuroendocrine events necessary for successful ovulation and sexual behavior.

- Crowding evokes dramatic stress responses. The social interactions among individuals vary according to species. In some social groups, it appears that the high-ranked individuals display pronounced stress responses, whereas in other social groups, low-ranked individuals display stress responses. These stress responses vary according to time of day, time of year, and age of the individual.

- Stress enhances and maintains substance abuse. Glucocorticoids function to accentuate the effects of dopamine to increase the rewarding properties of drugs of abuse.

• Individual variation in the stress response reflects variation in many physiological parameters, but also reflects differences in the perception of stressors.

## Questions for Discussion

1.  Discuss Hans Selye's quote, "Life is stress. Stress is life." Is stress truly a necessary component of life?

2.  A common problem with animals in zoos is failure to mate. Ling Ling and her "friend" Hsing Hsing, a pair of giant pandas given to the U.S. National Zoo by the People's Republic of China in 1972, provide a good example. It was hoped that these beautiful and mysterious animals would breed and produce young. Although Ling Ling became pregnant a few times, she never successfully brought a pregnancy to term. She lived for 20 years at the National Zoo. How might stress have impaired her reproduction? How could stress generally affect the breeding of captive animals?

3.  Using thermometers and pH meters, infertile couples often try to maximize the odds that sperm and ova will meet in the oviduct(s). Given the effects of stress on reproductive function, how might you, as a clinician, advise (or treat) a couple undergoing fertility treatment?

4.  Generate several hypotheses to account for individual variation in responsiveness to stress.

5.  Given what you now know about the pathological effects of chronic stress, what sort of pharmacological interventions do you think would help to ameliorate the negative consequences of stress?

## Suggested Readings

Chrousos, G. P., McCarty, R., Pacak, K., Cizza, G., Sternberg, E., Gold, P. W., and Kvetnansky, R. (eds.). 1995. Stress: Basic mechanisms and clinical implications. *Annals of the New York Academy of Sciences*, 771.

Levine, S. 1993. The psychoendocrinology of stress. *Annals of the New York Academy of Sciences*, 697: 61–69.

Meaney, M. J., Diorio, J., Francis, D., Widdowson, J., LaPlante, P., Caldji, C., Sharma, S., Seckl, J. R., and Plotsky, P. M. 1996. Early environmental regulation of forebrain glucocorticoid receptor gene expression: Implications for adrenocortical responses to stress. *Developmental Neuroscience*, 18: 49–72.

Sapolsky, R. M. 1992. *Stress, the Aging Brain, and the Mechanisms of Neuron Death.* MIT Press, Cambridge, MA.

Sapolsky, R. M. 1998. *Why Zebras Don't Get Ulcers: An Updated Guide to Stress, Stress-Related Diseases, and Coping.* W. H. Freeman, New York.

Welsh, T. H., Kemper-Green, C. N., and Livingston, K. N. 1999. Stress and reproduction. In E. Knobil and J. D. Neill (eds.), *Encyclopedia of Reproduction*, 662–674. Academic Press, San Diego.

# 12

# Learning and Memory

**M**any of us maintain vivid memories of frightening events. A colleague of mine recounts a terrifying experience that occurred during a boyhood game of kickball. He ran after a wayward ball, hoping to stop it before it rolled into the street. He made a valiant rescue attempt, but tripped on the curb and sprawled onto the pavement in front of an oncoming car. The driver slammed on the brakes and the car screeched to a halt, centimeters from him. Thirty-five years later, my colleague insists that he can remember every detail of the incident, including the pattern of the front grille of the car. Now an entomologist, he claims that he can even identify, from memory, the genus of dead moths that were stuck to the front of the car. It is difficult to judge the accuracy of such accounts, but memories of stressful events in our lives seem to be particularly salient. In humans, the phenomenon of vivid memories of important, stressful events has been termed "flashbulb memory" (Brown and Kulik, 1977). Flashbulb memory is probably not a separate category of memory function, but rather may represent a class of memories that are more frequently rehearsed or more strongly encoded. Depending on their age, people are likely to have flashbulb memories of what they were doing when they heard about the attack on Pearl Harbor, the assassination of President Kennedy or John Lennon, the suicide of Kurt Cobain, or the explosion of the space shuttle *Challenger*. Positive stressful events such as weddings, births of children, or winning lotteries are also remembered with great clarity (McCloskey et al., 1988). Other memories, however, are more fragile. For example, what you ate for dinner last night should be easily recalled, but you probably cannot remember what you ate for dinner a week ago, unless it made you ill.

Thus, some memories are relatively permanent while others are fleeting, and generally, important events are remembered better than unimportant events. My friend the entomologist cannot remember the front grille of every car that he has ever seen. The grille pattern of most cars is a trivial detail to him, and probably to you as well. Somehow, the brain sorts trivial and important events, and it has been proposed that hormones released during stress or high arousal may act as a physiological "marker" of importance. As animals evolved, memory systems may have co-opted the endocrine signals of physiological stress to signal important events. At an ultimate level of causation, the marking of important events could enhance learning about adaptively significant aspects of the world. Presumably, the entomologist learned about the dangers of running into a street from just one experience, or one "trial." The hormones secreted as he fell into the street and immediately thereafter notified his brain about the importance of the event. He can confidently claim that he learned from his experience because he never again ventured into the street without first checking for traffic.

## Components of Learning and Memory

Many recent studies have demonstrated an important role for the endocrine system in mediating learning and memory. In order to understand these hormonal effects, it is useful to understand several components of learning and memory. **Learning** can be defined as a process that expresses itself as an adaptive change in behavior that results from experience. **Memory**, the encoding, storage, and retrieval of information about past experience, is necessary if learning is to take place.

All animals appear to be capable of changing their behavior as a result of experience. The most generalized and simple type of learning is habituation; more complex types of learning include active avoidance, passive avoidance, and appetitive learning. **Habituation** is usually considered to be a loss of response after repeated exposure to a stimulus. Habituation can be functionally important in all kinds of behavior. When young ground squirrels around my university campus first emerge from their natal burrows in the spring, they seem very fearful. They scurry back home each time someone walks too close or when the shadows of the trees move about on the lawn. Eventually, they habituate to the harmless shadows and the comings and goings of students, and go about their business of collecting food from the trash barrels. Habituation occurs in the central nervous system and is regarded as learning not to respond. The neuronal mechanism of habituation has been studied in simple invertebrate systems and involves a reduction in the amount of neurotransmitter released into the synapse. The phenomenon of habituation can be demonstrated in a few cells living in a glass dish.

Habituation is fundamentally different from fatigue or sensory adaptation. Fatigue is loss of efficiency in the performance of a motor act after numerous, rapid repetitions. For instance, the loss of response that is experienced after performing several chin-ups is due to fatigue in the muscles, and is not usually attributed to forgetting how to do chin-ups. Sensory adaptation occurs at the level of the sensory receptor: in short, sensory receptors that are repeatedly exposed to a stimulus stop sending nerve impulses to the central nervous system. Thus, in sensory adaptation, the messages do not reach the CNS; in habituation, the messages reach the CNS but essentially are ignored. Sensory adaptation is considered a way for the nervous system to protect itself from being overwhelmed by sensory input. For example, the pressure of our clothes on hairs wired to cells that sense mechanical pressure is continuous, but sensory adaptation spares us from being overwhelmed by a neural barrage that offers little new information about the world.

To date, no studies have directly examined the effects of hormones on a simple cellular learning system. The direct effects of hormones on the mechanisms of habituation could be studied by the sequential introduction of several hormones; the effects of each hormone on neurotransmitter release could then be catalogued. Presumably, some hormones might facilitate neurotransmitter release, whereas other hormones might inhibit it. In the absence of an understanding of the mechanisms of hormonal action on the simplest types of learning, understanding more complex types of learning is difficult.

Nonetheless, animal behaviorists have developed several ways to study more complex types of learning in nonhuman animals, and these methods have shown that complex types of learning are affected by hormones. **Active avoidance** describes a situation in which an animal must do something—that is, act—to avoid a noxious situation. For example, a rat is placed in a box that is divided into two parts. A warning bell is sounded, then the rat receives a mild foot-shock. The rat can escape the foot-shock by going to the other compartment. After a few trials, the rat will learn to move to the other compartment when it hears the bell, thus avoiding the shock. Once the rat has learned to leave the compartment every time the bell is sounded, it is removed from the test box—called a shuttle box because the animal shuttles back and forth—and receives no more practice. After a period of time, the rat is returned to the shuttle box, and the strength of the association between the bell and the foot-shock—that is, the degree of learning—is assessed. A rat that leaves the compartment when it hears the bell is said to have a stronger memory than a rat that does not leave. The strength of the memory decreases as the interval between training and testing increases. In general, memory fades with time, and a strong foot-shock is remembered longer than a mild foot-shock.

**Passive avoidance** refers to a slightly different learning situation in which an animal must learn to suppress some behavior that would otherwise be exhibited. For example, rats prefer dark compartments to illuminated ones. A rat may be placed in an illuminated compartment that is adjacent to a dark one. When the rat goes into the dark compartment, which it prefers, it receives a foot-shock, and must travel back into the illuminated part of the shuttle box to escape the shock. The next time it is put into the illuminated compartment, the rat should avoid entering the dark compartment if it remembers its past noxious experience there. In other words, the rat inhibits its inclination to enter the dark compartment of the box and therefore passively avoids the unpleasant stimulus. The length of time that the rat remains in the lighted compartment is an indication of the strength of its memory for the noxious experience. Both active and passive avoidance learning are examples of aversive conditioning, or **aversive learning**.

Another type of learning is called **appetitive learning**. In this situation, an animal learns to perform some task that is rewarded with food, water, or some other pleasant experience. For example, a rat may learn to navigate a maze if it receives a food reward at the end. We learned in Chapter 6 that a female rat or chimpanzee will press a bar to gain access to a male when their estrogen concentrations are high.

A memory system is required in order for adaptive changes in behavior to result from experience. Current situations must be compared with prior events that are in some way encoded in memory. There are many types of memory systems; a nervous system is not necessarily required for a memory system to be present. The immune system of vertebrates, for example, has a memory for microbes and responds vigorously to previously encountered agents. Likewise, calculators and computers have sophisticated memory systems. All memory systems share the ability *to enter information into storage (acquisition and consolidation), to retain information, and to retrieve information from storage*. These three components of memory must operate or learning will not be observed. Hormones could affect any of these components of memory, as well as affecting learning directly. It is rare to measure learning directly; only the results of learning can be measured and quantified. Consequently, statements about the effects of hormones on learning and memory are typically based on their effects on performance, or observed behavior.

In addition to a functional memory system, successful learning involves several psychological components; namely, motivation, attention, and arousal. These components, like learning itself, are hypothetical psychological constructs designed to describe features of behavioral performance. These hypothetical constructs cannot be measured directly; only performance on a test designed to assess one of these constructs can be measured. For example, if your professor gave you an examination to test your learning of behavioral endocrinology, but only asked questions about geography, you would probably complain that the test was not a valid measure of your learning. Sometimes tests cannot discriminate one hypothetical construct from others. For example, if you leave an answer blank on the exam, your professor does not know whether your failure to answer reflects a failure to learn the material, a failure to attend to the material when it was presented in class, or a failure to be sufficiently motivated to answer the question. Probably, your professor will assume that a failure in learning occurred and assign a grade accordingly.

Learning, motivation, arousal, and attention interact and affect one another. In fact, one of the few laws in psychology states that learning is an inverted U-shaped function of arousal (Figure 12.1; Yerkes and Dodson, 1908). That is, learn-

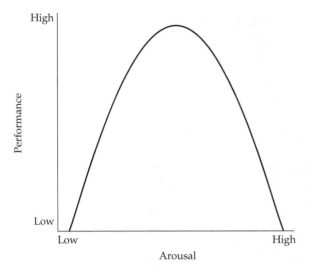

**12.1   Arousal and learning.** Optimal performance on learning tasks occurs at moderate levels of arousal. If arousal is either too low or too high, learning is adversely affected. Because hormones are involved in arousal, they can have effects on learned performance. Source: Yerkes and Dodson, 1908.

ing does not occur in subjects that are too highly aroused (excited, agitated) or insufficiently aroused (asleep). Hormones are involved in arousal, motivation, and probably also in attention and emotion.

## The Effects of Hormones on Learning and Memory

In 1915, Walter Cannon (Figure 12.2) proposed his emergency theory of the adrenal glands, which suggested that following an exposure to stress, the secretion of epinephrine (adrenaline) from the adrenal glands increases as a means of adapting to that stress (see Chapter 11). Many physiological studies conducted throughout the 1920s and 1930s demonstrated the stimulatory effects of epinephrine on the respiratory and cardiovascular systems. Few experimental studies, however, examined the behavioral effects of epinephrine until after the Second World War, when the acute fear "paralysis" that occurred in some soldiers going into combat was thought to be caused by excessive discharge of the adrenal medullary hormones (see Kosman and Gerard, 1955). Animal studies were conducted in order to investigate the effects of noxious stimuli (aversive conditioning) on adrenal secretions. In these studies, the effects of adrenal hormones on learning and memory were discovered, and they laid the groundwork for studies of the effects of many other hormones on learning and memory.

### Epinephrine

More is now known about the role of epinephrine in learning than about the role of any other hormone. Reliable assays and better agonists and antagonists have been available longer for epinephrine than for other hormones. One can measure the amount of epinephrine released during learning and demonstrate that it is released in situations in which learning typically occurs.

In general, epinephrine enhances memory, and the memory-enhancing effects of epinephrine are both dose- and time-dependent. Responses to different concentrations of epinephrine follow an inverted U-shaped curve; that is, low and

**12.2   Walter B. Cannon** first proposed that the adrenal glands secrete epinephrine in response to stress, the so-called emergency theory of adrenal function.

high blood levels of epinephrine impair memory, whereas moderate epinephrine levels enhance memory (Parsons and Gold, 1992). Because epinephrine is released in response to stressful events, a reasonable possibility is that epinephrine potentiates the effects of the noxious stimuli used to train animals in active avoidance tasks. Animals perform better in avoidance situations after receiving a moderate than after a mild foot-shock. If epinephrine potentiates the effects of shock, then (1) epinephrine should be released when the shock occurs, and (2) epinephrine treatment paired with mild foot-shocks should produce learning comparable to that observed in animals experiencing moderate foot-shocks. Both of these effects have been demonstrated. For example, the optimal level of epinephrine for memory enhancement in rats is 1500 picograms/ml of blood serum, and this level is typically found in rats that show optimal performance in avoidance tasks (Figure 12.3; Gold, 1987). If a mild foot-shock produces blood epinephrine levels of 1000 pg/ml, and this shock is paired with an injection that raises epinephrine levels another 500 pg/ml, then the exogenous and endogenous epinephrine sum, and the animal exhibits optimal learning (Gold, 1987).

The best time to administer epinephrine is immediately after training; treatment before training, or when a substantial period of time has elapsed since training, is not effective in enhancing memory (Figure 12.4). These temporal constraints are consistent with the hypothesis that epinephrine influences memory by potentiating the effects of noxious events. My friend the entomologist was extremely stressed as a boy by observing the car bearing down on him. Possibly, his adrenal glands began releasing large quantities of epinephrine immediately after his learning "trial," and the elevated levels of epinephrine enhanced his memory to the extent that he vividly reports the incident 30 years later.

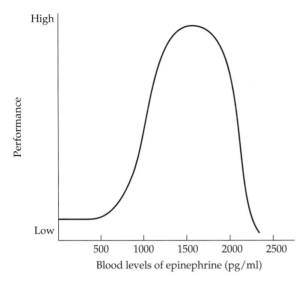

**12.3   Effects of epinephrine on performance.** The effectiveness of doses of epinephrine in enhancing performance on memory tasks follows an inverted U-shaped curve. The optimal dose in rats is about 0.1 mg/kg, which yields a blood level of epinephrine of about 1500 pg/ml. Source: Gold and Van Buskirk, 1975.

How does epinephrine enhance memory? Again, learning and memory involve encoding, storing, and retrieving information. Epinephrine, as well as other hormones, could facilitate any or all of these processes. The precise mechanisms of memory have yet to be elucidated, but neuroscientists certainly agree that the memory for active and passive avoidance tasks resides in the brain. Epinephrine is a molecule that is too large to cross the blood–brain barrier, although it is produced by a very few neurons in the brain as a neurotransmitter (Weil-Malharbe et al., 1959). We are faced with an apparent paradox: How can epinephrine affect learning and memory processes if it cannot get to the neurons in the brain? Obviously, epinephrine must affect some process outside of the brain

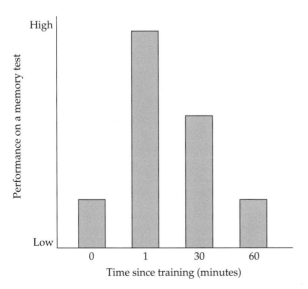

**12.4   The effects of epinephrine on memory are time-dependent.** Injections of epinephrine (1 mg/kg) are most effective in enhancing memory if given 1 minute after training; the beneficial effects of epinephrine diminish 60 minutes after training. After Gold, 1987.

that subsequently influences the brain. There are currently two working hypotheses regarding how epinephrine affects memory: (1) epinephrine affects memory via its effect on blood glucose levels, and (2) epinephrine activates peripheral receptors that directly influence brain function.

**THE GLUCOSE HYPOTHESIS.**    One of the many physiological consequences of epinephrine secretion in a stressed animal is hyperglycemia, an increase in blood glucose levels. In general, glucose enhances memory; the dose–response curve again resembles an inverted U-shape (Figure 12.5; Gold, 1986; Parsons and Gold, 1992). The effects of glucose are time-dependent; injections of glucose delayed by 1 hour after training have no effect on retention and performance. These features are all common to glucose and epinephrine. The doses of glucose and of epinephrine that are most effective in enhancing memory both result in plasma glucose levels comparable to those found naturally in response to optimal training conditions. Glucose injected directly into the brain also enhances memory (Gold, 1987).

Additional evidence that epinephrine produces its effects on memory by raising blood glucose levels is based on negative findings. The memory-enhancing and memory-impairing effects of epinephrine treatment can be blocked by treating animals with adrenergic antagonists—drugs that block peripheral epinephrine receptors—but these blockers have no effect on memory enhancement produced by glucose treatment. These results are consistent with the notion that glucose release is a memory modulation step that occurs subsequent to the release of epinephrine. Because adrenergic antagonists block the receptors by which epineph-

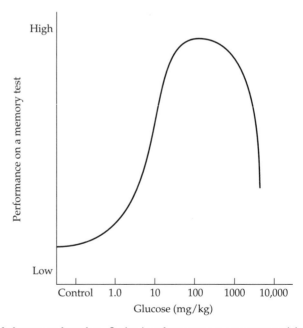

**12.5    Effects of glucose on learning.** Optimal performance on a memory task is attained with a dose of 100 mg/kg of glucose provided within 1 minute of training. Lower or higher doses, or doses provided later after training, do not enhance memory function. Source: Gold, 1987.

rine acts, they prevent the effects of epinephrine, as well as those of treatments that act through epinephrine on memory. But the effects of glucose, which are "downstream" from the peripheral epinephrine receptors, remain intact. The most effective agents that are known to enhance human cognitive performance (i.e., improve learning and memory) share a common feature: they all elevate blood glucose levels (Table 12.1).

How does glucose produce its effects on memory? As we have seen, the brain requires a constant supply of glucose in order to function (see Chapter 11). Elevated blood glucose levels permit more glucose to enter neurons, which in turn stimulates an increase in the release of the neurotransmitter acetylcholine from neurons in the brain. Increases in acetylcholine levels in the brain synapses are characteristic of all known cognitive enhancers (see Table 12.1). Thus, cognitive enhancers must work by increasing glucose, which increases acetylcholine release, or by increasing acetylcholine levels directly. The neurobiological mechanism(s) by which glucose improves memory do appear to involve acetylcholine release. In a study of rats in a simple "T-maze," microdialysis revealed that acetylcholine levels were elevated in glucose-treated rats during memory testing (Ragozzino et al., 1996). The severe memory deficits observed in patients with advanced Alzheimer disease or AIDS are correlated with a marked reduction in neurons that secrete acetylcholine. Obviously, cognitive enhancers that increase the release of acetylcholine or prolong its life have great clinical significance.

The study of impaired learning and memory represents another approach to understanding the effects of hormones. Memory function in old rats diminishes in a fashion similar to the decline observed in normal elderly people. Epinephrine enhances the memory of very old rats; however, treatment of elderly human patients with epinephrine to enhance their memories would not be wise, considering the cardiovascular effects of this stimulating hormone.

Unlike epinephrine, glucose is a relatively safe compound with which to study memory in humans. In a recent study, the effects of glucose on memory were tested in a group of healthy 70-year-old people. Individuals of this age typically have memory impairments even if they do not suffer from dementia or other aspects of Alzheimer disease. These 70-year-olds scored less well on a standard memory test than college students tested at the same time. Following the test of

### Table 12.1
### Agents that enhance cognitive performance

| Substance | Effect |
| --- | --- |
| *Nootropics*[a]*:* Aniracetam, piracetam, pramiracetam, oxiracetam<br>*Others:* Amphetamine, epinephrine, glucose, hypertonic saline, painful stimuli, stress, vasopressin | Elevation of glucose |
| Choline, lecithin, physostigmine, phosphatidylersine | Elevation of synaptic ACh, but not glucose |
| Phlorizin[b] | Inhibition of glucose transport |

[a]Pharmacological cognitive enhancers.
[b]Although phlorizin interferes with brain glucose utilization, it still enhances memory performance by some unknown means.

memory, the elderly subjects were asked to drink a glass of lemonade that had been prepared with either saccharine or glucose. Another memory test was then administered. Those individuals who had received glucose showed improved memory function relative to those who drank lemonade prepared with saccharine. It was noted that the glucose utilization efficiency of an individual predicted memory function among the aged, but not the young, subjects. Elderly people often have problems regulating their blood sugar levels. The normal decline in memory function during aging may thus reflect a diminishing ability to regulate blood levels of glucose. The extra glucose provided in the study probably allowed the brain cells to function better in the elderly subjects (Hall et al., 1989).

Recent studies have confirmed that glucose enhances both memory storage and retrieval in healthy elderly humans (Manning et al., 1998b). Glucose also improves learning and memory in people with Alzheimer disease, as well as in adults with Down Syndrome (Korol and Gold, 1998; Manning et al., 1998a). Although earlier studies on college students failed to discover any effects of glucose on performance, more recent studies have revealed glucose enhancement of learning and memory in this age group when the tasks are challenging (Korol and Gold, 1998). In these challenging memory tests on college students, it was demonstrated that glucose augmented memory for material in a paragraph. Glucose also seemed to improve attentional skills in the students as well. However, neither face and word recognition nor working memory (usually defined as the nonpermanent storage of information that is being processed in a cognitive task) were influenced by glucose treatment (Korol and Gold, 1998).

If unregulated blood glucose levels interfere with learning, then diabetic animals and humans should exhibit learning difficulties. Surprisingly few studies, however, have addressed the relationship between diabetes and learning and memory in humans. Most of the studies on people have shown no strong correlation between learning and memory and insulin-dependent diabetes (Helkala et al., 1995; Crawford et al., 1995; Ryan and Williams, 1993; Wolters et al., 1996) or insulin-independent diabetes (Worrall et al., 1996).

In contrast to the lack of data on humans, several studies have documented the effects of diabetes on the acquisition of passive avoidance tasks in nonhuman animals. Treatment of rodents with streptozotocin destroys the insulin-secreting β-cells of the pancreas, inducing diabetes (see Chapter 9). Streptozotocin-induced diabetic rodents display modest, but consistent, deficits in passive avoidance learning (Leedom et al., 1987). Surprisingly, administration of a drug, phlorizin, that inhibits glucose transport into cells causes significant *enhancement* of memory performance in diabetic rats in comparison to control rats (Hall et al., 1992). The physiological mechanisms underlying these cognition-enhancing effects of phlorizin remain unspecified.

A common test of spatial learning in rats is performed with the Morris water maze, and rats rendered diabetic with streptozotocin also display deficits in spatial learning in this test (Figure 12.6) (Biessels et al., 1996). The "maze" consists of a round tank that is about 1.3 meters in diameter, filled with milky-white water; hidden below the surface of the water is a small platform, which the animal must find and climb onto in order to stay above water (Morris et al., 1982). The rat is released into the water at different points along the edge of the tank. An animal does not have to be food-restricted to learn this task, which has its own built-in

(a) The Morris water maze

(b) Water maze trajectories

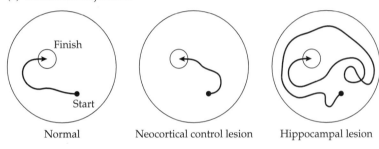

| Normal | Neocortical control lesion | Hippocampal lesion |

**12.6  Spatial memory can be assessed in the Morris water maze.** (a) In the Morris water maze, rats must swim to find a submerged platform. The platform is visible here, but in testing conditions it is hidden below the surface of milky water. The rat requires relational learning because there are usually large extra-maze cues around the tank. (b) Representative swimming paths of rats in the Morris water maze. Rats learn to navigate to the platform from any position in the tank if they are normal or have had their neocortex lesioned. However, if the hippocampus is lesioned, the rat swims aimlessly until it randomly discovers the submerged platform. After Morris et al., 1982.

motivation—the water is at room temperature, and so is unpleasant, and presumably the rat does not want to drown. The rat is initially trained to find the platform while it is visible. After training, the water in the tank is made opaque, and the rat must depend on its memory to recall where the platform is located. The animal uses its spatial memory to locate the platform based on extra-tank visual cues.

Streptozotocin-treated rats were tested in the Morris water maze to determine whether their learning deficits could be prevented or reversed by insulin treatment (Biessels et al., 1998). Three experimental groups were evaluated: (1) rats that received streptozotocin, but no insulin, (2) rats that received streptozotocin, but also received insulin so that diabetes never developed, and (3) rats that received insulin 10 weeks after streptozotocin treatment began (i.e., after the onset of diabetes). Insulin prevented, but did not reverse, the deficits in performance in the Morris water maze in the streptozotocin-treated rats. In the next part of the experiment, in vitro hippocampal long-term potentiation (LTP) was assessed. LTP is a change in the pattern of neuronal firing that has been linked to learning (Teyler and Discenna, 1984). Hippocampal LTP was impaired in the diabetic rats. Insulin treatment that began at the same time as streptozotocin treatment prevented diabetes and prevented the hippocampal impairments in LTP; insulin treatment that began 10 weeks after the onset of diabetes only partially restored LTP (Biessels et al., 1998). Thus, it seems that insulin affects spatial memory in diabetic rats only if provided from the onset of diabetes.

Other studies have demonstrated that memory can also be enhanced by fructose, a sugar that is not metabolized by the nerve cells in the brain; other glucose analogues that are not well metabolized by the brain also improved retention (Messier and White, 1987). These latter studies also indicated that a much higher dose of glucose is optimal for memory enhancement than previously reported (e.g., 2.0 g/kg versus 0.1 g/kg) (Messier and White, 1987). The basis for this discrepancy in effective doses is not apparent. Perhaps at high doses these other sugars act at peripheral sites to activate membrane glucose transport mechanisms; at lower doses, the glucose may affect memory more directly via actions on neural function or processing.

**THE PERIPHERAL-RECEPTOR HYPOTHESIS.**   The second working hypothesis for how epinephrine modulates memory is that it activates peripheral receptors that communicate with the central nervous system (McGaugh, 1989). In order to discover which neural receptors are involved in the memory effects of epinephrine, specific receptor agonists (mimics) and antagonists (blockers) have been employed.

The effects of epinephrine on memory can be blocked by both $\alpha$- and $\beta$-adrenergic antagonists (Sternberg et al., 1985, 1986). In one study, rats were injected with an $\alpha$- or a $\beta$-adrenergic antagonist—phenoxybenzamine or propranolol, respectively—30 minutes before they received either an injection of epinephrine or a foot-shock (which caused endogenous levels of epinephrine to rise). Glucose concentrations did not rise very much after epinephrine or foot-shock treatment in rats pretreated with the $\beta$-blocker, propranolol; however, glucose concentrations increased after epinephrine treatment or foot-shock in rats pretreated with the $\alpha$-blocker, phenoxybenzamine (Manning et al., 1992). The mnemonic (memory-enhancing) effects of clenbuterol, an adrenergic agonist that crosses the blood–brain barrier, can be blocked only by centrally acting $\beta$-adrenergic antagonists (Introini-Collison and Baratti, 1986). These data suggest that epinephrine acts on peripheral adrenergic receptors to initiate its effects on memory (McGaugh, 1989).

The amygdala has been considered for years to be involved in emotions. This almond-shaped part of the limbic forebrain (at the base of the temporal lobe) is also involved in learning and memory, both directly and indirectly via its close association with the hippocampus (Figure 12.7). Electrical stimulation of the amygdala can increase memory retention (McGaugh and Gold, 1976). In a series of elegant experiments, it was demonstrated that memory can be modulated by post-training injections of epinephrine and norepinephrine directly into the amygdala. The increased retention induced by intra-amygdala injections of norepinephrine can be blocked by concurrent administration of $\beta$-adrenergic antagonists

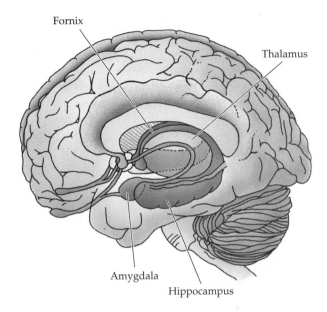

**12.7  The amygdala and associated structures** seen in a "cutaway" lateral view of the human brain.

such as propranolol (Gallagher et al., 1981). The effect is observed only if the nor-epinephrine and adrenergic antagonist are injected on the same side of the brain; in other words, the effect is stereospecific. Like that of epinephrine, this effect of norepinephrine is dose- and time-dependent. The generality of the effects of adrenergic compounds on memory is supported by research on olfactory memory in honeybees. Post-learning injections of norepinephrine into bee brains affect memory; retention is enhanced by moderate doses and impaired by high doses of norepinephrine (Menzel, 1983; Menzel and Michelsen, 1986).

In one fascinating study of humans, individuals read either an emotionally charged story or a similar story that was judged by other people as more emotionally neutral (Cahill et al., 1994). Some individuals were treated with propran-olol, a potent β-adrenergic antagonist, which significantly impaired memory of the emotionally arousing story, but did not affect memory of the neutral story (Cahill et al., 1994). The researchers who conducted this study were able to rule out the possibility that the drug had nonspecific effects on attention or motiva-tion. These results support the hypothesis that highly charged emotional memo-ries require activation of β-adrenergic receptors (Cahill et al., 1994).

The effects of epinephrine, administered either peripherally or centrally, could hypothetically be mediated via increased release rates of adrenocorticotropic hor-mone (ACTH). However, the memory-enhancing effect of post-training epineph-rine administration is not blocked by dexamethasone, an artificial steroid that blocks the release of ACTH. Therefore, it appears that ACTH does not mediate the memory-enhancing effect of epinephrine (McGaugh et al., 1987), although ACTH has its own potent effects on memory (described below).

The two working hypotheses explaining how epinephrine affects memory are not incompatible. Epinephrine elevates blood glucose concentrations, which increases the amount of glucose that enters the neurons. The neurons thus release higher concentrations of acetylcholine into the synapses. Epinephrine also appears to act directly on neurons to enhance their function. These direct, central effects of epinephrine may reflect endocrine activity, or epinephrine could affect memory directly (perhaps after entering the brain through the cerebrospinal fluid, thus circumventing the blood–brain barrier) by acting as a central neurotransmitter. There may be other mechanisms underlying memory enhancement by epinephrine as well.

There is convincing evidence that many peptides previously characterized as hormones also function as neurotransmitters in the central nervous system, including vasopressin, oxytocin, the opiates, and cholecystokinin (CCK). Of course, epinephrine and norepinephrine have been known for some time to function as both hormones and neurotransmitters. When there is evidence for a central site of action, as in the case of epinephrine, ACTH, vasopressin, the opiates, and CCK, one must consider the hypothesis that these chemical messengers exert their effects centrally by acting as neurotransmitters, rather than as hormones. This observation may account for the ability of these compounds, which cannot cross the blood–brain barrier, to act in the brain.

### Adrenocorticotropic Hormone (ACTH)

In 1950, Hans Selye introduced the concept of the general adaptation syndrome as a model for the physiological coping strategies of an animal enduring stress (see Chapter 11). According to this model, stress causes the release of ACTH from the anterior pituitary, which induces the production and release of glucocorticoids by the adrenal cortex. These hormones, along with epinephrine and norepinephrine, presumably prepare an animal to react to threatening stimuli—the so-called "fight or flight" response. In his early work, Selye assumed that the "stress" hormones had a relatively permanent effect upon the central nervous system (i.e., learning), as well as affecting the immediate ability to respond (Selye, 1956). Many prominent learning theorists of the mid-1950s attempted to explain avoidance learning in terms of an anxiety-reduction model. It was hypothesized that an interruption in the "anxiety mechanisms" (i.e., the pituitary–adrenocortical axis) would disrupt the acquisition of an avoidance response.

In one early study, two groups of rats were tested on an active avoidance task. The pituitary gland was surgically removed in one group of rats; the control group received a sham operation. Recall that the pituitary is also called the hypophysis; the removal of this gland, therefore, is often called a hypophysectomy. The control rats acquired the avoidance task much faster than the hypophysectomized animals (Applezweig and Baudry, 1955; Applezweig and Moeller, 1959). Injections of ACTH into the hypophysectomized animals restored their performance to the levels of the control animals. It is important to note that ACTH only *restores* performance in endocrine-deficient animals; ACTH treatment of intact animals does not enhance normal learning and memory performance (Murphy and Miller, 1955). Consequently, this peptide is not a candidate as a cognitive enhancer (see Table 12.1).

In general, a deficit in ACTH leads to slower acquisition and poorer retention of information. Remember, however, that the surgical removal of the pituitary gland is not a minor physiological disruption. Hypophysectomy not only reduces ACTH levels, but affects many other endocrine and regulatory systems as well (see Chapter 2). DeWied (1964) tried to control for these problems by providing hormone "cocktails" to hypophysectomized rats. The addition of growth hormone and thyroid-stimulating hormone had restorative effects; that is, the animals were much healthier. Without the replacement of ACTH, however, the memory deficits were still observed.

Does ACTH act through the CNS or via the adrenal glands to affect memory? The best way to answer this question is to remove the adrenal glands. ACTH appears to act upon the CNS through a nonadrenal route because it enhances acquisition of avoidance tasks even in rats that have been adrenalectomized. Because adrenalectomized animals lack feedback control, their ACTH levels rise. Furthermore, ACTH injections in rats lacking both pituitary and adrenal glands also restore learning. Therefore, the effect of ACTH on memory is independent of its classic endocrine effects (DeWied, 1974).

Not only ACTH, but also small pieces of the ACTH molecule, devoid of any effect on the adrenal glands, affect learning (for example, DeWied, 1974, 1977). The first hint of this possibility was evident in a number of studies in which the administration of α-MSH (melanocyte-stimulating hormone) and β-MSH restored avoidance responses in hypophysectomized rats (Kastin et al., 1975). Recall that ACTH is made from pro-opiomelanocortin (POMC), a giant molecule that is also the precursor of several other hormones, including α-MSH and β-MSH as well as the endorphins and enkephalins. Alpha-MSH and β-MSH share the same sequence of amino acids with ACTH at positions 1–13 (see Figure 2.23). Treatment with smaller ACTH fragments, such as $ACTH_{1-10}$ or $ACTH_{4-10}$, also restored learning (DeWied, 1969, 1974). These fragments do not affect adrenocortical function. However, administration of $ACTH_{11-24}$ or $ACTH_{25-39}$ had no effect on avoidance responding (DeWied, 1974). In another series of studies, amino acids were systematically removed from both ends of the ACTH molecule; each ACTH fragment was then tested in vivo to determine its behavioral "potency" (DeWied, 1974, 1980). Through a long series of studies testing various bits and pieces of the ACTH molecule, it was determined that the behaviorally active portion of the ACTH molecule resides at the amino end of the molecule, $ACTH_{4-8}$. Artificial analogues of the ACTH molecule have also been produced and examined for behavioral effects. ACTH analogues with a D-isomer of phenylalanine at position 7 exhibit behavioral effects that are opposite to those of comparable ACTH analogues with the normal L-isomer of phenylalanine at position 7. The D-isomer analogue facilitates extinction (i.e., decay of active avoidance responding), while the L-isomer form delays extinction (DeWied, 1980). This kind of dissection of a behavioral response using molecular techniques should prove to be a powerful research tool for probing the physiology underlying avoidance responding.

ACTH can also protect against amnesia, the failure to remember. Substances that protect against forgetting are called **antiamnestics**. Three experimental techniques can induce amnesia: exposing animals to $CO_2$ immediately after training, administering a strong electric shock after training, or treatment with protein synthesis inhibitors (Quartermain, 1976). ACTH attenuates the amnestic effects produced by these experimental manipulations. If a rat is trained to leave the dark half of a box when it hears a bell to avoid a mild foot-shock, and is then exposed to $CO_2$ immediately afterward, the rat will display a low level of memory for the task. If another rat is trained on the same task, given an injection of ACTH, and immediately given $CO_2$, its memory is less impaired. It is not known whether ACTH is affecting arousal, attention, encoding, retrieval, or some combination of those factors in this paradigm.

How does ACTH reach the brain to affect memory processes? ACTH consists of 39 amino acids and therefore, like epinephrine, is too large to cross the blood–brain barrier. There are five likely hypotheses explaining how ACTH affects the brain, but few data exist to refute or support any of them.

1. After release from the anterior pituitary, ACTH may flow backward through the portal blood vessel system into the brain (see Figure 2.6). There is only weak evidence for this possibility.

2. ACTH may leak into the cerebrospinal fluid. This route would circumvent the blood–brain barrier, but this hypothesis is based on pure speculation; there are no supportive data.

3. The ACTH may have been in the brain all along. The peptides released by the pituitary, as you will recall, are also produced in the brain itself. Hypophysectomy does not change brain concentrations of ACTH. Recall, however, that hypophysectomy produces learning deficits that can be restored with peripheral ACTH injections.

4. Small ACTH fragments may exist freely in the blood and pass through the blood–brain barrier.

5. Finally, ACTH, like epinephrine, may influence some process outside of the CNS that ultimately affects the neuronal activity of the brain. Although this mechanism may seem reasonable, there are also no data in support of this possibility.

As we have seen, ACTH and its memory-enhancing fragments come from the giant precursor molecule POMC. The precursor molecules of many hormones are cleaved by specific enzymes into two or more pieces. The active form of the hormone is thus liberated from the precursor molecule. It has been hypothesized that different enzyme systems are stimulated by the environment to induce different cleaving patterns of the giant molecule; in this way, various environmental stimuli may produce different hormones. It is also possible that different cleaving enzymes for separating the POMC molecule reside in different cells, and that certain environmental factors induce certain cells to produce their specific enzymes.

ACTH has been administered to humans in several studies. In general, ACTH does not affect the performance of normal volunteers, children with learning disabilities, or elderly experimental subjects on learning tasks. However, $ACTH_{4-10}$ can affect attentional and motivational processes without directly affecting learning in humans (DeWied, 1980).

Another question one could ask is how ACTH (and $\alpha$-MSH) might increase retention. An easy answer is that ACTH might increase arousal. In other words, the firing rates of neurons might increase, or the likelihood of an action potential might be enhanced by the presence of this peptide. The aversiveness or reward properties of a stimulus might thereby be increased. Intraventricular injections of ACTH in rats cause regionally specific changes in cerebral deoxyglucose uptake, an index of brain cell activity (Dunn et al., 1980). ACTH might produce its antiamnestic effect in this way by giving access to weak memory traces. The mechanism by which ACTH, or hormones in general, affect retention is still largely speculative, and the real answers await advances in the neurobiology of learning and memory. Once the biochemical processes of memory are understood, the role of ACTH and other hormones will be more easily described.

## *Vasopressin and Oxytocin*

Vasopressin, as we saw in Chapter 9, promotes water uptake in the kidney tubules and is thus also called antidiuretic hormone (ADH). Brattleboro rats, which have a congenital lack of vasopressin, suffer from diabetes insipidus, a condition that occasionally occurs in humans and is marked by the production of large quantities of dilute urine and concomitant intake of liters of water. In addition to the difficulties that Brattleboro rats have with managing their water economy, these animals also have difficulty learning shuttle-box avoidance skills (DeWied, 1980, 1984). They forget these tasks very quickly. The deficit in their performance appears to be due to memory problems rather than learning dysfunction. Homozygous Brattleboro rats avoid the compartment in which they have been shocked when their retention is tested immediately after the learning trial; however, if a delay occurs between training and testing, they rapidly reenter the compartment in which they have been shocked. Treatment with vasopressin immediately after the learning trial raises the subsequent avoidance behavior of homozygous Brattleboro rats to the level of their heterozygous cousins, which have normal vasopressin levels.

As these experiments demonstrate, vasopressin is an antiamnestic; like ACTH, it blocks forgetting or prolongs memory. Injections of vasopressin can also prolong memory in normal animals. In contrast to an injection of ACTH, which may delay forgetting for 6–8 hours, vasopressin treatment prolongs memory for noxious experiences by days or weeks (DeWied, 1980). The effects of vasopressin on memory are dose- and time-dependent (DeWied, 1984). The memory-enhancing effects of post-training treatment with vasopressin in normal rats require the presence of an intact adrenal gland or prior treatment with epinephrine (McGaugh, 1989).

Injections of vasopressin antagonists directly into the septum (an area of the brain that is rich in neurons in which vasopressin serves as a neurotransmitter) abolish the ability of a male rat to recognize (remember) the odor of a conspecific male that he has previously encountered (Peele and Vincent, 1989). Castration also abolishes this social recognition and reduces the number of vasopressin neurons in the septum. Testosterone replacement therapy reverses these effects of castration. In this case, vasopressin most certainly functions as a neurotransmitter within the septum, but its influence on social behavior is androgen-dependent in rats and mice (Bluthe et al., 1993). Both working memory (discussed later in the chapter; see Figure 12.11) and reference memory (long-term) as assessed in a radial-arm maze (see below) are improved by vasopressin and vasopressin analogues (Dietrich and Allen, 1997a,b). Intranasal treatment with vasopressin slightly improved verbal memory of elderly humans (Perras et al., 1997). Generally, inhibitory avoidance learning was improved by vasopressin and impaired by oxytocin (Boccia et al., 1998).

Oxytocin appears to have a variety of effects on memory function, but the majority of studies have implicated oxytocin as an amnestic peptide. When given intraventricularly, oxytocin enhances forgetting; rats given oxytocin in this manner forgot the noxious experience associated with an active avoidance paradigm (Bohus et al., 1982). However, there are several studies indicating that systemic injections of oxytocin can *enhance* memory (DeWied, 1984), but usually only in constrained situations or under specific conditions (Boccia et al., 1998). Furthermore, it appears that the memory-impairing effects of oxytocin are observed only when it is given intracerebrally (i.e., icv) (Engelmann et al., 1996). When memory for stimuli associated with pups was tested in adult female rats, all of the rats performed this task well as long as the test was performed within 180 minutes (Engelmann et al., 1998). Treatment with icv oxytocin did not affect this task; however, treatment with an oxytocin receptor antagonist, but not an arginine vasopressin receptor antagonist (V1), impaired the development of this type of memory (Engelmann et al., 1998).

Oxytocin promotes smooth muscle contraction and is therefore critical to milk letdown and the uterine contractions of birth. One possible adaptive function of the amnestic properties of oxytocin is the dulling of memories of the pain associated with giving birth, thereby increasing the probability that females will repeat the process (Carter et al., 1992).

Taken together, the effects of oxytocin on learning and memory are inconsistent, sometimes contradictory, and not well understood. The results of one study have suggested that oxytocin may have intrinsic reinforcing properties (Liberzon et al., 1997). If something "positive" occurs in a particular place, an individual will spend more time in that place in the future. For example, if a rat is given an injection of morphine in the right half of its cage, it develops a place preference and spends more time in the right half of the cage. Thus, one can determine whether a substance has positive reinforcing properties by observing whether or not a place preference develops. If rats are injected with oxytocin, a slight place preference develops, suggesting that oxytocin has intrinsic reinforcing properties (Liberzon et al., 1997).

### Endogenous Opiates

Opiates attenuate pain or the emotional response to pain. There is some controversy regarding whether the endogenous opiates, the endorphins and enkephalins, are truly hormones, but they are included here because they seem to fulfill the definition of a hormone as presented in Chapter 2. These substances have clear effects on learning and memory. In general, opioids have amnestic properties in avoidance learning paradigms, but seem to enhance the reward properties of trial-and-error learning situations. Although true amnestics act directly on memory storage, retrieval, or both processes, opioids probably ameliorate the noxiousness of an aversive stimulus so that it is not *perceived* as aversive, thus appearing to act as amnestics.

Opiate receptors may play a part in reinforcement and reward. This suggestion was first prompted by the observation that opiates such as morphine and heroin have reinforcing effects that cause some people to become addicted to the drugs. However, opiate receptors in humans presumably did not evolve to permit people to become drug addicts. Consequently, a search for the endogenous opioids that fit these receptors began, and the functional significance of these natural, internal "pain killers" was sought. The reinforcing effects of opioids were

**12.8    The distribution of opioid receptors,** shown as light areas in these darkfield autoradiograms of horizontal (top) and coronal (bottom) sections of rat brain. There are several opiate receptor types; μ, δ, and κ types are shown here. The locations of these receptors correspond to the locations of brain sites at which electrical stimulation has reinforcing effects. Rats will press a lever repeatedly to cause opiates to be microinjected into these sites, thus activating these receptors. Courtesy of Alfred Mansour and Stanley J. Watson.

found to be caused by the activation of opiate receptors in the brain (McGaugh, 1983). This finding suggests that the release of endogenous opiates may play a role in the reinforcement of behavior.

Neurons that contain opiate receptors are found in several regions of the brain in which electrical stimulation has reinforcing effects, including the hypothalamus, nucleus accumbens, and periaqueductal gray matter (Figure 12.8). Rats will press a lever repeatedly to cause opiates to be injected into their brains, thus activating these receptors. Further, morphine and other opiates increase the rate of responding (bar pressing) for electrical brain stimulation, whereas naloxone, an opiate receptor blocker, decreases the response rate (Schaefer, 1988). One can imagine situations in which other hormones might have reward properties (e.g., rats housed in cold rooms bar-pressing for thyroid hormones); however, there have not been any reports of animals bar-pressing for non-opiate hormones. Rats will also show a place preference in response to systemic injections of morphine; that is, they will prefer the part of a cage where they received morphine injections on previous days (Amalric et al., 1987). This effect is also blocked by injections of naloxone.

Infant rats also experience the positively reinforcing properties of exogenous opioids. In one experiment, 5-day-old rat pups were isolated from their mothers and siblings, placed in the presence of a novel odor (orange extract) for 30 minutes, then injected either with a low dose of morphine (0.5 mg/kg) or with saline. Five days later, these rats were tested to determine their responses to another presentation of the orange odor. Pups were placed in a small cage containing plain bedding chips in one half and bedding chips mixed with orange extract in the other. Testing lasted 10 minutes, and the percentage of time spent in each half of the cage was recorded (Figure 12.9). Rat pups that had experienced morphine injections after exposure to the novel odor of orange spent 73% of their time over the orange-scented bedding. In contrast, control animals (injected with saline) spent only 34% of their time over the orange odor. Pretreatment with naltrexone, another opiate antagonist, before conditioning blocked the positive association between the morphine state and the orange odor (Weller and Blass, 1988).

A similar paradigm has been used to test the effects of other substances on learning and memory. When opiate receptor agonists, including morphine, β-endorphin, and enkephalin, were given to adult rats immediately after training in low doses, their memory was impaired in a dose- and time-dependent manner (McGaugh, 1989). Opiate antagonists ameliorate the memory-impairing effects of opiates and their agonists. Studies have demonstrated that retention is enhanced by post-training administration of opiate antagonists, including naloxone, naltrexone, diprenorphine, levallorphan, nalmenfene, and β-funaltrexamine (McGaugh, 1989). The memory-enhancing effects of these opiate antagonists are also dose- and time-dependent, and have been found in studies using several types of training tasks, including passive avoidance, active avoidance, habituation, and appetitive spatial learning (McGaugh, 1989). Opiate antagonists also block the amnestic effects of electroconvulsive shock therapy (ECT) (Collier et al., 1987), but have had mixed results in human patients with memory disorders (McGaugh, 1989).

The amnestic effects of post-training, peripherally administered met-enkephalin can be blocked by the centrally acting opiate antagonists naloxone and naltrexone, as well as by the peripherally acting antagonist MR 2263 (Zhang et al., 1987). The memory-modulating effects of both central and peripheral injections of met-enkephalin (and peripheral naloxone) are attenuated in adrenal-denervated (or demedullated) animals (Conte et al., 1986). Denervating the adrenals prevents the release of epinephrine and norepinephrine. Of course, removal of the adrenal medulla also eliminates the release of many endogenous enkephalins and endorphins (see Chapter 2). Amnesia can be produced in adrenal-demedullated rats if epinephrine is administered prior to training (Conte et al., 1986). Taken together, these results suggest that peripheral injections of opiates affect memory via epinephrine. Predictably, injections of met-enkephalin elevate blood levels of glucose, probably by stimulating epinephrine secretion. This finding may seem contradictory to the results of previous studies indicating that epinephrine and glucose enhance memory. However, recall that the effects of epinephrine and glucose follow an inverted U-shaped curve; levels too high or low reduce performance on learning and memory tasks. Only moderate levels of epinephrine and glucose enhance learning and memory.

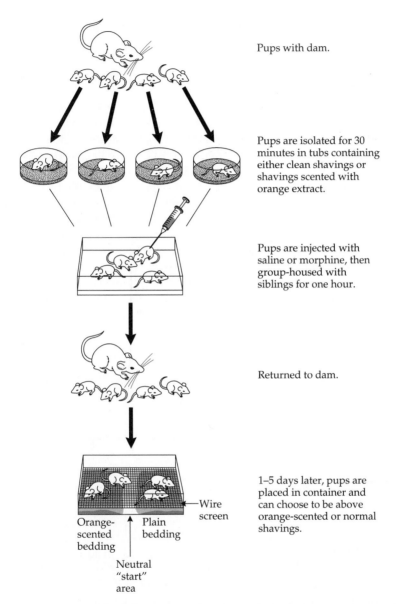

Pups with dam.

Pups are isolated for 30 minutes in tubs containing either clean shavings or shavings scented with orange extract.

Pups are injected with saline or morphine, then group-housed with siblings for one hour.

Returned to dam.

1–5 days later, pups are placed in container and can choose to be above orange-scented or normal shavings.

Wire screen

Orange-scented bedding

Plain bedding

Neutral "start" area

**12.9   Opiates enhance learning in rat pups.**  Pups that were separated from their mothers and isolated for 30 minutes in tubs containing either clean bedding or orange-scented bedding were injected with either saline or morphine, then group-housed with their siblings for 1 hour before being returned to the dam. After 1–5 days, the pups' preference for clean versus orange-scented bedding was measured. Pups that had received morphine injections after exposure to the novel orange scent showed clear preferences for that odor. After Weller and Blass, 1988.

### *Cholecystokinin*

All animals need to find food in order to survive, so it is advantageous for animals to remember where food has been found in the past. Therefore, one might suspect that hormones involved with feeding might modulate memory function. At an ultimate level of explanation, it makes sense that hormones involved in feeding and digestion would be co-opted to enhance memory because the ability to remember the details of successful foraging behavior would have high survival value (Flood et al., 1987).

Cholecystokinin (CCK) is a gastrointestinal hormone that is released during feeding. CCK has been assigned several behavioral functions, including involvement with post-feeding satiety (Smith et al., 1981b). Injection of CCK inhibits feeding by rats via the vagus nerve (Bloom and Polak, 1981; Moran et al., 1992) (see Chapter 9). CCK has also been discovered in brain tissue.

CCK modulates learning and memory. In one recent study (Flood et al., 1987), two groups of hungry mice and one group of mice with free access to food were given a number of trials to learn to avoid an electric shock in one arm of a T-maze (Figure 12.10). The mice with free access to food and the mice in one of the food-restricted groups were given access to food immediately after training. The free-access mice tended to eat very little, but the hungry mice feasted. Mice in the other food-restricted group received food 3 hours after training. During the next week, food was provided freely to all the animals. At the end of the week, all of the mice were tested again in the T-maze. Access to food immediately after training

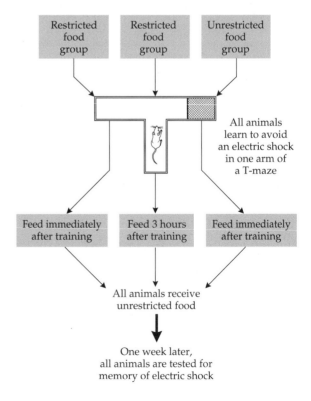

**12.10  CCK enhances memory in mice.** Mice from two food-restricted groups and from a group that had been fed freely learned to avoid an electric shock in one arm of a T-maze. One of the food-restricted groups was fed immediately after training, and one was fed 3 hours after training; the freely fed group was fed immediately. When the animals were tested a week later, the food-restricted mice that were fed immediately after training showed the best retention, probably because the food caused these hungry mice to secrete CCK shortly after training. After Flood et al., 1987.

enhanced memory retention for the aversive experience in the hungry mice, as compared with either the hungry mice for which feeding was delayed by 3 hours or the mice that received food freely. Presumably, the hungry mice that were fed immediately released CCK in response to their meal, which enhanced their memory of the shock. CCK injected intraperitoneally also enhances memory in mice. The memory-enhancing effects of CCK can be blocked by cutting the vagus nerve, which suggests that peripherally administered CCK produces its memory effects by activating ascending vagal fibers (Flood et al., 1987).

CCK also affects learning and memory functions in young rats. Young rats, like many animals, are neophobic; that is, they avoid novel experiences. This aversion can be blunted by pairing a novel odor (orange extract) with injections of CCK in a paradigm similar to that used to test the effects of morphine (see above; Weller and Blass, 1988). In fact, 24 hours after the CCK injections, rat pups preferred an orange-scented test arena, whereas pups injected with saline still avoided the orange scent. An antagonist (L-364,718) that selectively blocks peripheral CCK receptors completely eliminated CCK-induced conditioned odor preferences. These results strongly support the hypothesis that CCK affects learning in rats via a peripheral site of action. CCK "conditioning" follows an interesting developmental course: CCK-induced olfactory preferences were observed in rats that were 5, 11, or 22 days of age, but 28-day-old rats failed to exhibit CCK-conditioned preferences (Weller and Blass, 1990). Perhaps the ontogeny of CCK-supported conditioned preferences reflects natural events that correspond to the weaning process.

## Sex Differences in Learning and Memory

Many recent studies have demonstrated sex differences in learning and memory performance, but determining whether a sex difference in performance truly reflects learning and memory functions, rather than other hypothetical psychological constructs, is difficult. In general, female rats learn active avoidance tasks faster than male conspecifics, but males do better at passive avoidance tasks (Beatty, 1979; Heinsbroek et al., 1988). These results may not reflect sex differences in learning and memory per se, but rather may reflect a sex difference in general activity levels. Because male rats generally are less active in open field situations than females, it may be "easier" for males to perform a passive avoidance task (that is, suppress a behavior) than for females, and "easier" for females to perform an active avoidance task than for males.

One common test of learning in rats uses a radial-arm maze (Figure 12.11). Males use different strategies than females to solve radial-arm mazes, and these strategies can be manipulated by early hormone treatment (Williams et al., 1990). In one study, eight of the twelve runways of a radial-arm maze were always provided with a food treat (baited); four arms were always devoid of treats (unbaited). The solution to the maze involved making only one trip down each of the eight baited arms and avoiding the unbaited arms. This task, therefore, involved long-term, or reference, memory to recall which of the twelve arms were always baited, as well as short-term, or working, memory to recall which of the eight baited arms had already been visited on that particular trial (Olton and Samuelson, 1976; Williams et al., 1990). Male rats and females treated with estrogen prior to day 10 of age learned the task faster than female rats or males castrated on day 1

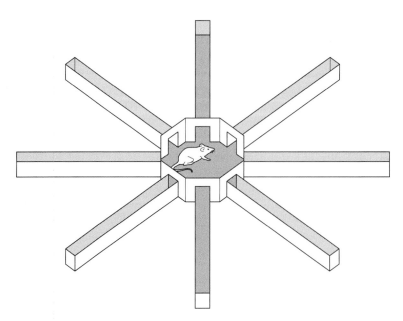

**12.11    The radial-arm maze,** popularized by David Olton, is a common apparatus used in assessments of spatial memory. The maze is open at the top, and may have 8, 12, or even 36 arms; the greater the number of arms, the more difficult the maze. During training, the subject learns that only some of the arms are baited (have a reward) at the end. To solve the maze successfully after training, the subject must make only one trip down each baited arm and avoid exploring the unbaited arms, a task that requires both long-term memory, to recall which of the arms are always baited, and short-term memory, to recall which of the baited arms has been visited during the current trial. After Olton and Samuelson, 1976.

(Williams et al., 1990). After the task was learned, there were no differences in subsequent error rates.

The strategies used by rats to solve the radial-arm maze were probed by manipulating potential cues in the interior of the maze (called landmarks) and orientation cues outside the maze (geometry). Females used both landmarks and geometry to solve the maze, whereas males and masculinized females used only geometry to learn the task. In other words, males and masculinized females learned fewer total cues and could master the task faster than females or feminized males (Williams et al., 1990). This effect is thought to be mediated by hormonal effects on the hippocampus (see Chapter 3).

The higher error rate of female rats in mazes may not represent errors in memory, but rather inappropriate exploratory behaviors, as well as increased levels of general activity that are scored as errors (Beatty, 1979). Males are generally more anxious than females. When rats are placed in an open arena, females show more locomotor activity, rear up and look about less, and defecate less than males (reviewed in Beatty, 1979; Johnston and File, 1991). These sex differences in behavior can be reduced by anxiolytic drug treatment of males or by early endocrine manipulation (Stevens and Goldstein, 1981; Stewart and Cygan, 1980). These animal models of spatial learning indicate that males perform better on spatial learning tasks than females in most cases, and that hormones are likely to mediate the sex difference in performance (Gaulin and FitzGerald, 1989; Williams et al., 1990). Early hormone exposure may influence visuospatial learning among humans as well (see Chapter 4).

These models also show that the effects of sex hormones on learning performance may be indirect, and may be influenced by a variety of extrinsic and intrinsic factors, such as stress. An interaction between sex and the stress of novelty or electric shock has been demonstrated in several recent studies. Males generally perform better than females in the Morris water maze. Prior familiarization with the maze, however, reverses the sex difference in performance of this spatial learning task by increasing the females' performance (Galea et al., 1996). In another recent study, stress impaired learning of a simple associative task (i.e., eye blink) in female, but not male, rats. In fact, stress facilitated the males' performance (Wood and Shors, 1998). These findings underscore the difference between learning and performance.

### Androgens

The effects of androgens on learning and memory have been studied for over 70 years (Tuttle and Dykshorn, 1928). In one of the best early experiments, male rats were castrated at 20, 50, 90, 130, or 170 days of age and later tested for maze-learning ability (Commins, 1932). Castrated and intact animals performed equally well at learning the mazes. An extensive review of these early studies (Stone and Commins, 1936), including the reviewers' own work, in which castration failed to affect performance on a light-discrimination task or on three different mazes, led to the conclusion in 1936 that castration does not affect learning in rats.

Many studies since then have investigated the role of testicular androgens in learning and memory, and the results of these studies generally agree with the early pronouncement that gonadal androgens do not affect learning and memory. This appears to be true of humans as well as nonhuman animals. For example, neither testosterone replacement therapy in hypogonadal men nor testosterone treatment of normal men revealed changes in learning and memory performance (Alexander et al., 1998). In some cases, however, castration has small or subtle effects on learning, especially spatial learning or learning that affects anxiety levels.

As we have seen, female rats generally outperform males in the acquisition of active avoidance tasks, although the effect is small (Haaren et al., 1990). In these strains, neither neonatal nor postpubertal castration affects performance. However, neonatal castration of males treated in utero with the anti-androgen cyproterone acetate raises their performance to levels typical of females, demonstrating that prepubertal organization by sex steroid hormones must be responsible for the difference in performance (Beatty, 1979). Similarly, it has been hypothesized that early organizational effects of androgens account for sexually dimorphic responses to Pavlovian fear conditioning (Anagnostaras et al., 1998).

Studies on seasonally breeding animals have documented a correlation between peak androgen concentrations and peak learning abilities. Goldfish trained in several tasks, including learning to swim with a tethered float, conditioned avoidance tasks, and maze learning, exhibit seasonal changes in learning ability (Agranoff and Davis, 1968; Shashoua, 1973). Maximal learning occurs between January and March, prior to spawning, when the gonads are developing and blood concentrations of steroid hormones are high. Poor learning is observed during the summer, after the spawning season. Photoperiod may regulate this seasonal cycle of learning ability in goldfish.

A sex difference in spatial learning performance has been reported for meadow voles (*Microtus pennsylvanicus*) and deer mice (*Peromyscus maniculatus*) (Galea et al., 1995, 1996). During the breeding season, males of both species outperform females, but the sex difference disappears when the animals are not in breeding condition (Galea et al., 1996). In female voles, there was a significant correlation between plasma estradiol concentrations and retention, whereas there were no performance differences between males with low and high testosterone concentrations (Galea et al., 1995).

As described in Chapter 10, seasonal changes in brain size in several species of rodents are likely to be mediated by seasonal changes in androgen levels. Changes in learning and memory should correspond to these seasonal changes in brain mass, but this proposition essentially remains untested. In North America, over 90% of learning studies are performed on laboratory rats (Burkhardt, 1987), which are not particularly seasonal.

There is a seasonal change in maze-learning ability in voles. Home range size shrinks during the winter in both meadow (*Microtus pennsylvanicus*) and prairie voles (*M. ochrogaster*). In one study, winter-trapped voles were compared with spring-trapped voles on their ability to learn mazes (Gaulin and FitzGerald, 1989). Males captured and tested during the winter made more errors while learning the mazes and required more trials to negotiate the maze without making any errors than animals tested during the spring. These results may reflect seasonal changes in brain size; brain weights are proportionally heavier in spring-trapped than in winter-trapped voles (Gaulin and FitzGerald, 1989; Yaskin, 1984). The difference in maze-learning abilities may also reflect differences in motivation between winter- and summer-captured animals.

Testosterone does seem to have some positive reinforcing properties. A place preference develops in rats that have testosterone injected into the nucleus accumbens (Packard et al., 1997). The rewarding properties of testosterone might help to explain some of the abuse associated with anabolic androgens (see Chapter 13).

### *Estrogens*

Estradiol appears to enhance spatial memory in a reliable, but subtle, manner (Luine, 1994; Daniel et al., 1997). It is important to note, however, that simple statements like this one must be qualified. Estrogenic effects on learning and memory are complex and depend on many factors, including the timing of hormone administration and the gonadal state of the individual being assessed.

Estradiol seems to enhance memory when the task is difficult. In general, estrogens appear to enhance consolidation, and slightly enhance acquisition, of spatial reference memory tasks (Daniel et al., 1997; Luine et al., 1998; Fader et al., 1998) and of two-choice water-escape working memory tasks, a version of the Morris water maze (O'Neil et al., 1996). In contrast, several studies in rats and humans have demonstrated that spatial memory is impaired during the periovulatory portion of the ovarian cycle, when estradiol concentrations are normally high (e.g., Frye, 1995; Galea et al., 1995; Korol et al., 1994; Warren and Juraska, 1997).

In one of the first studies of the effects of estradiol on memory, castrated male rats were deprived of food (reduced to 85% of their baseline body mass to motivate them to find food in a maze), and trained on an eight-arm radial-arm maze. These males were implanted with either empty Silastic capsules or capsules containing estradiol benzoate; males possessing the estradiol capsules had circulating estradiol concentrations of about 90 pg/ml of blood serum (Luine, 1994). Beginning 3 days after capsule implantation, the performance of the males was assessed over twenty trials. There was no difference between estrogen-treated and control rats in performance (Figure 12.12) (Luine, 1994; Luine and Rodriguez, 1994). In the next eight trials, a 1-hour delay between the fourth and fifth arm choice was added. When the task was made more difficult by the 1-hour delay, the males treated with estrogen exhibited a small, but reliable, improvement in performance as compared with the control animals (Luine, 1994). In another study, both low (40 pg/ml) and high (200 pg/ml) doses of estradiol resulted in improved choice accuracy in a twelve-arm radial-arm maze by young and aged female rats (Williams, 1996). In yet another study, estrogen treatment of ovariectomized female rats augmented working memory, but not reference or working-reference memory (Luine et al., 1998). Similarly, estrogen treatment enhanced the performance of ovariectomized female rats during acquisition of an eight-arm radial-arm maze when provided for 30 days then removed prior to training (Figure 12.13) (Daniel et al., 1997). These results suggest that chronic treatment with estradiol is required to produce an effect on memory, and that estradiol may induce changes in neuronal form or function that persist well after the hormone capsule is removed.

The hippocampus mediates spatial memory (Olton et al., 1978). Infusion of a water-soluble form of estradiol directly into the hippocampus enhances the memory of ovariectomized rats for the Morris water maze, but only if given immediately after training (Packard et al., 1996; Packard and Teather, 1997). Estradiol treatment 2 hours post-training did not affect retention (Packard and Teather, 1997). Estradiol receptors are located within the hippocampus, especially in the CA1 region, but also in the CA3 region and dentate gyrus (Loy et al., 1988; Maggi et al., 1989; Gould et al., 1990) (see Figure 12.15). Estrogen treatment and natural-

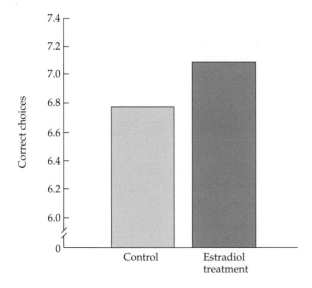

**12.12  Estradiol improves spatial memory.** Male rats were implanted with either an empty Silastic capsule (light bar) or with a capsule containing estradiol (dark bar). The bars represent the average number of correct choices on an eight-arm radial-arm maze after a 1-hour delay between the fourth and fifth visits across several trials. After Luine and Rodriguez, 1994.

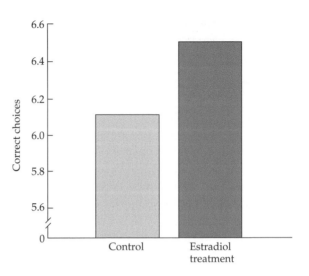

**12.13   Estradiol during training improves spatial memory.** Ovariectomized female rats were implanted with capsules containing either an inert substance (light bar) or estradiol (dark bar) prior to or during training on an eight-arm radial-arm maze. Estradiol-treated females performed better than females that did not receive hormone replacement therapy. Adapted from Daniel et al., 1997.

ly high estrogen concentrations around the time of ovulation are associated with an increase in the density of dendritic spines in the CA1 region (Gould et al., 1990; Woolley et al., 1990a; McEwen et al., 1995; reviewed in Desmond and Levy, 1997) (see Chapter 4). The results of studies that have attempted to correlate hormone-induced changes in hippocampal circuitry with spatial learning performance in rats have been equivocal (Woolley, 1998). However, hippocampal LTP varies across the estrous cycle in association with these changes in connectivity (Warren et al., 1995). Hippocampal LTP is facilitated by estrogen treatment in awake rats (Cordoba-Montoya and Carrer, 1997), and estrogen also affects basal forebrain cholinergic neurons that might be important in passive avoidance, attentional tasks, as well as spatial learning (Gibbs, 1997). Prenatal gonadal steroids also affect hippocampal cell morphology; males have larger CA1 and CA3 pyramidal cell field volumes and cell body sizes than females (Isgor and Sengelaub, 1998).

In one study, estrogen treatment of postmenopausal women was found to enhance verbal memory and maintain the ability to learn new material (Sherwin, 1996, 1997, 1998). In contrast, postmenopausal women participating in a short-term estrogen replacement therapy study with a randomized, double-blind cross-over design showed no significant effects of estrogen (Polo-Kantola et al., 1998). The differences between the results of these studies may reflect differences in the memory tasks assessed. In another study of humans, male-to-female transsexuals receiving estrogen treatment prior to surgical sex reassignment did not differ from women on any tests of learning and memory (Miles et al., 1998). Estrogen administration has been shown to enhance memory and reduce neuronal loss associated with Alzheimer disease in postmenopausal women (Simpkins et al., 1997), and to reduce the damage caused by blood reperfusion (restoration of blood flow) after a cerebral ischemia (stroke) (Hurn et al., 1995).

Taken together, the effects of estrogens on memory seem to be slight and to affect only certain aspects of spatial memory. Recently, it has been hypothesized that the effect of estrogens on memory in females might reflect aspects of maternal behavior, rather than nonspecific effects on learning and memory (Woolley, 1998).

## *Glucocorticoids*

This chapter began by describing how memory was enhanced by stressful events. Acute stress does appear to promote lasting memories. However, chronic stress seems to have the opposite effect. Long-term stress, or chronic treatment with corticosterone, impairs memory (Luine, 1994; Luine et al., 1994; de Quervain et al., 1998). Thus, corticosterone (or cortisol) appears to function as an amnestic in most of the studies reported to date (McLay et al., 1998).

In one study, male rats were stressed by being placed in clear plastic containers for 6 hours per day for 3 weeks. The animals were not completely immobilized, they could move in the restraint device (Luine et al., 1994; Luine, 1994). After 21 days of this stress treatment, the rats were food-restricted, trained, then tested on an eight-arm radial-arm maze. The performance of the restraint-stressed rats was impaired compared with that of rats that were not restrained (Luine et al., 1994). A different strain of rats was used in a follow-up study (Luine, 1994). These rats were restrained for 3 weeks, trained, and tested on an eight-arm radial-arm maze, as before. A blood sample was obtained, and blood concentrations of corticosterone were assayed. Rats with the highest corticosterone concentrations displayed the most errors in performance. Similarly, a study that correlated corticosterone consumption (provided in the rats' drinking water) and maze performance indicated that rats consuming the most corticosterone made the most errors in a radial-arm maze (Luine et al., 1993). Essentially, corticosterone treatment impairs spatial learning in rats in a variety of testing situations (McLay et al., 1998). Treatment with RU38486 (a progestin and glucocorticoid receptor antagonist commonly called RU-486) infused directly into the dorsal hippocampus improved the performance of male rats in the Morris water maze (Oitzl et al., 1998).

The previously described studies on the effects of glucocorticoids on learning and memory were conducted exclusively on acquisition and long-term memory storage. Recently, a study provided evidence that stress and corticosterone also impair memory retrieval (De Quervain et al., 1998). Rats were trained to locate a submerged, hidden platform in a Morris water maze. After the rats were trained, they received a foot-shock (i.e., a mild stressor), either 2 minutes, 30 minutes, or 4 hours prior to testing. During the test, the platform was removed. In this situation, rats with good memories spend more time swimming over the area of the tank where the platform was previously located. Rats with poor memories swim around somewhat randomly, usually along the edge of the tank, suggesting that they do not recall where the escape platform ought to be. Rats shocked 30 minutes prior to memory testing performed poorly compared with rats tested 2 minutes or 4 hours after foot-shock (Figure 12.14) (De Quervain et al., 1998).

Like estradiol, corticosterone causes restructuring of the hippocampus and parts of the so-called hippocampal circuit (Figure 12.15). The hippocampus and related brain structures are rich in glucocorticoid receptors. Treatment of rats with corticosterone or inducing chronic stress decreases the number of pyramidal cells, dendrite length, and number of dendritic branch points in the CA1 and CA3 regions of the hippocampus (Watanabe et al., 1992; Woolley et al., 1990b; Sapolsky et al., 1985). Somewhat paradoxically, very low corticosterone concentrations also cause degeneration in a brain region closely associated with the hippocampus, the dentate gyrus (Sloviter et al., 1989; Conrad and Roy, 1992). After adrenalectomy,

**12.14  Retrieval of spatial learning is impaired by stress.** (a) The amount of time spent in the target quadrant (T) as compared with the opposite quadrant (O) of the water maze. Rats spent less time in the target quadrant 30 minutes after foot-shock, but this impairment was reversed 4 hours after foot-shock. (b) Representative swimming paths of a nonstressed control rat and a stressed rat. Note that while the nonstressed rat had swum in the general area of the platform, the stressed rat appears to have swum across all areas of the maze randomly. After De Quervain et al., 1998.

hippocampal cell numbers decrease by approximately 50% (Gould et al., 1991; Conrad and Roy, 1992; Luine, 1994). Specifically, hippocampal granule neurons decrease in number when corticosterone concentrations are low. Predictably, spatial memory is impaired by adrenalectomy (Gould et al., 1991; Conrad and Roy, 1992). Thus, there seems to be an ideal range of corticosterone concentrations, above or below which hippocampal-dependent spatial learning is impaired.

Humans with altered glucocorticoid concentrations may also display changes in memory. For example, patients with Cushing syndrome, whose adrenal glands produce excessive cortisol, have reduced hippocampal volumes (Starkman et al., 1992). In contrast, patients with Addison disease, whose adrenal glands produce insufficient cortisol, show necrosis of the granule cells in the hippocampus and

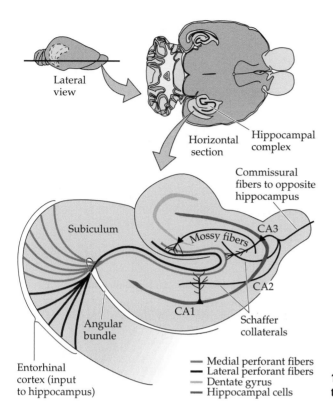

**12.15  Connections and components of the hippocampal circuit.**

display impaired memory (Maehlen and Torvik, 1990). These clinical observations in humans support the hypothesis that glucocorticoids can affect memory. Taken together, the evidence shows that estradiol and corticosterone modulate cellular morphology and function in the hippocampus, and in some cases alter spatial learning and memory (Figure 12.16). Further research is necessary to determine whether these hormones affect other parts of the brain and other types of learning, and to determine the extent to which other hormones affect neuronal morphology and function.

Importantly, adult neurogenesis, a phenomenon known to occur in the hippocampal region of rodents and primates, is responsive to glucocorticoid concentrations in the blood. Glucocorticoids and stress inhibit the production of new hippocampal neurons (Gould et al., 1998). Although any potential association between adult neurogenesis and hippocampal-dependent learning remains undetermined, it is plausible that these new neurons participate in some way. Thus, chronic suppression of neurogenesis by repeated stress might contribute to diminished spatial navigational learning (Gould et al., 1998).

### Other Hormones

Melatonin treatment appears to improve short-term memory in male rats (Argyriou et al., 1998). Treatment with the melatonin  receptor antagonist luzindole blocked the melatonin-induced enhancement of short-term recognition memory.

**Control: Memory normal**

CA1
pyramidal cell

CA3
pyramidal cell

Granule cells

**Repeated stress: Memory impaired**

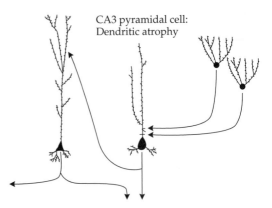

CA3 pyramidal cell:
Dendritic atrophy

**Adrenalectomy: Memory impaired**

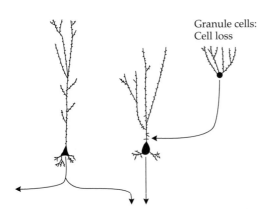

Granule cells:
Cell loss

**Elevated estradiol: Memory enhanced**

CA1 pyramidal cell:
Increased spine density

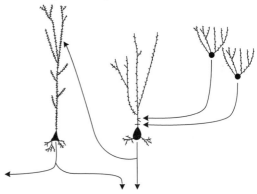

**12.16  Behavioral effects of hormone-induced changes in hippocampal circuitry.** A simple schematic circuit of three hippocampal cell types illustrates structural changes caused by hormones and associated effects on performance in memory tasks. After Luine, 1994.

Transgenic mice that overexpress bovine growth hormone display impaired inhibitory avoidance learning, but not appetitive learning (Meliska et al., 1997).

The effects of hormones on learning and memory are usually subtle and often specific to a given situation or task. The exact mechanisms by which hormones affect learning and memory function await additional advances in the understanding of the neurobiological mechanisms of learning and memory. Hormones may change structures in the brain, the activity of specific neural cells, the uptake or release of neurotransmitters, or act in a coordinated way through all of these mechanisms.

# Summary

- The hormones that are associated with adaptation to stress enhance learning and memory.

- There are two hypotheses regarding how epinephrine affects memory: (1) epinephrine may affect memory via its effect on blood glucose levels, and (2) epinephrine may activate peripheral receptors that directly influence brain function.

- Elevated blood glucose levels facilitate the movement of glucose into neurons. More glucose entering neurons stimulates the release of more acetylcholine into the neuronal synapses.

- Elevated glucose levels may be a common pathway by which several hormones enhance memory. Hormones may increase blood sugar levels directly (e.g., epinephrine) or act through another agent (e.g., vasopressin) to increase blood sugar levels.

- Many peptides previously characterized as hormones also function as neurotransmitters in the CNS, including vasopressin, oxytocin, CCK, and the opiates. Epinephrine and norepinephrine have been known for some time to function in both roles. When there is evidence for a central site of action of hormones on memory, as in the case of epinephrine, ACTH, vasopressin, the opiates, or CCK, one must consider the hypothesis that these chemical messengers exert their effects centrally by acting as neurotransmitters, rather than as hormones.

- The lack of ACTH impairs memory formation, and its presence can also protect against amnesia. A small piece of the ACTH molecule, devoid of endocrine activity, contains the features of the molecule that affect memory. The physiological mechanisms underlying the effects of ACTH on memory are unknown.

- Vasopressin also blocks forgetting and appears to act via its stimulatory effect on epinephrine secretion.

- Oxytocin may act as an amnestic agent; it promotes forgetting. The mechanisms of its action are not known.

- Endogenous opiates seem to have amnestic properties in avoidance learning paradigms, but appear to enhance reward properties in trial-and-error learning tasks.

- CCK enhances memory, but requires an intact vagus nerve to act.

- Sex differences in learning and memory performance are common; however, these differences may be due to sex differences in spatial abilities, exploratory behaviors, or general anxiety levels.

- In rats, androgens do not have major effects on learning and memory. In some species, enhanced learning and memory are reported during the breeding season, when blood concentrations of androgens are high.

- Estrogens appear to enhance spatial learning in animals and other forms of memory in humans.

- Glucocorticoids or chronic stress impair spatial learning and memory. However, if glucocorticoid concentrations are too low, impairments in memory are also observed.

## Questions for Discussion

1. Nearly all of the research on the effects of hormones on learning and memory has been conducted on laboratory rats and mice. Discuss the implications and limitations of this approach to studying learning.

2. In Chapter 10, it was established that hormone levels vary on a circadian basis. It was also documented that performance on a variety of cognitive skills varies as a function of time of day. In most studies on the effects of hormones, learning, and memory, rodents are tested during the experimenters' work day (the rodents' rest period). Discuss the proposition that hormones affect learning and memory by shifting circadian rhythms of performance to different times of day.

3. Glucagon, secreted from the α-cells of the pancreas, acts in opposition to insulin and elevates blood sugar levels. Design a study to test the effects of glucagon on learning and memory. Discuss your predicted outcomes.

4. Opioids often act as reinforcers, or rewards, for behavior and consequently have marked effects on learning and memory. Discuss the possibility of other hormones acting as reinforcers and their potential influences on learning and memory. What are these hormones, and under what conditions would you expect them to exert effects on behavior?

## Suggested Readings

DeWied, D., Diamant, M., and Fodor, M. 1993. Central nervous system effects of the neurohypophyseal hormones and related peptides. *Frontiers in Neuroendocrinology*, 14: 251–302.

Korol, D. L. and Gold, P. E. 1998. Glucose, memory, and aging. *American Journal of Clinical Nutrition*, 67: 764S–771S.

Luine, V. N. 1994. Steroid hormone influences on spatial memory. *Annals of the New York Academy of Sciences*, 743: 201–211.

McGaugh, J. L. 1989. Involvement of hormonal and neuromodulatory systems in the regulation of memory storage. *Annual Review of Neuroscience*, 12: 255–287.

Sherwin, B. B. 1997. Estrogen effects on cognition in menopausal women. *Neurology*, 48: S21–S26.

# 13

# Hormones and Mood

**H**ormones have been implicated throughout this book in the regulation of many diverse behaviors. As we have seen, hormones can affect behavioral thresholds, changing the probability that a given stimulus will elicit a specific response in a particular environmental setting. In addition to overt behaviors, hormones can also affect mood. In some cases, hormones appear to lower the threshold for the appearance of nonadaptive behaviors and feelings in humans. It should be apparent from the previous chapters that individuals display a wide range of responses to the same hormone, and that a substantial range of hormone concentrations occur normally in both humans and nonhuman species. Individuals that occupy either end of the continuum of endocrine responses or hormone levels may display or experience atypical behaviors or moods. Hormonal imbalances caused by pathology, inherited predisposition, or the effects of foods, drugs, or toxins may underlie a number of behavioral disorders or cause psychological distress to individuals. Some of the behavioral pathologies that arise because of hormonal dysfunction have been described in previous chapters.

This chapter will focus on a few select examples of the ways in which hormones can affect mood in humans. The examples that were chosen are those that have been the most consistently studied and in which the relationships between hormones and mood are best established. First, the role of hormones in perimenstrual syndrome will be addressed. Second, correlations between various hormones and depression will be described; the role of sex steroid hormones in postpartum depression, as well as the influence of melatonin on seasonal affective disorder, an unusual, recurrent type of depression, will be presented. Finally, the phenomenon of nearly psychotic aggressive behavior, commonly called "roids rage," in individuals that chronically abuse anabolic steroid hormones will be discussed.

Most of the experimental work presented in the previous chapters was based upon animal research. This chapter, however, focuses on human behaviors and feelings. Animal models are usually inappropriate for elucidating the relationship between hormones and human mood changes. Consequently, most of the studies described in this chapter employ self-reports. Studies that attempt to correlate human mood changes with endocrine events typically involve people reporting their moods, which are then correlated with measurements of hormone concentrations. The effects of endocrine manipulations or natural endocrine fluctuations can then be assessed.

## Perimenstrual Syndrome

**Perimenstrual syndrome (PMS)** is probably the best-known behavioral phenomenon associated with hormones. A large number of clinical studies have shown that the normal changes in steroid hormone concentrations associated with the menstrual cycle are often associated with changes in the behavior and feelings of women (see Figure 6.18). In some instances, the symptoms of PMS appear to be a direct result of these hormonal changes. Other studies suggest that PMS symptoms result from physiological changes that are caused by the endocrine changes. However, still other studies suggest that cognitive factors, including social expectations, influence the occurrence of PMS symptoms in the absence of hormonal correlates. Because some symptoms continue or increase in intensity during menstruation, the term *perimenstrual* is used here instead of the more common term, *premenstrual syndrome*. Use of the word *syndrome* does not imply "abnormal" or "diseased," but rather refers to a cluster of physiological and emotional symptoms that appear to be linked.

### The Social Context of PMS

There is much controversy surrounding PMS. As we shall see, the prevalence and the defining symptoms of PMS, as well as the physical and psychological factors associated with it, remain subjects of debate; in fact, the very existence of the syndrome has been questioned by some researchers. Over the past 25 years, PMS has changed from a relatively unknown medical condition to a well-known social phenomenon. North American men and women use the term "PMS" to communicate a widely shared cultural understanding about the behavior and moods of women. For example, an article about powerful women in Washington, D.C., described one such "scary" woman: "Known as the PMS poster child . . . her prima donna ways are legendary" (*Washingtonian*, April 1992, 67). Most North American adults understand this description to mean that the woman in question is possibly aggressive, certainly assertive, and probably cranky. These traits are often tolerated or even applauded in men. Does the assignment of these character traits to PMS trivialize the accomplishments of powerful women?

PMS must be considered within a social context because it affects only one sex and because its image is not positive. Feminist social scientists have noted that several cultural phenomena have interacted to establish PMS as a biologically based illness that affects only women and to make it a part of the social fabric (Brown-Parlee, 1990, 1991). For example, the increased awareness of PMS in North America has coincided with an increase of feminist ideas in public forums. A discussion of the meaning of feminism is beyond the scope of this book, but one of its central tenets is that equal opportunities for economic and political power should exist for women and men. This demand is reasonable in the North American political system because justice demands equal treatment for individuals who are equal. In theory, women should not have difficulty in making their case for equality. If, however, men and women are not biologically equivalent, then making an argument for equal economic and political opportunities for men and women is more difficult (Young, 1990). Some feminists have argued that the "pathologization" of normal menstruation is an attempt on the part of the male-dominated biomedical community to demonstrate that women and men are unequal in ways that disqualify women from holding positions of economic and political power.

Certainly, the biomedical community is not the objective, culture-free, unbiased fellowship of truth seekers that is often portrayed as its ideal. During the first feminist movement early in the twentieth century, scientific evidence of the reproductive frailties of women provided by the medical community was used to support the view that women should not participate in higher education, vote, or drive automobiles. Others argue that many women actively participated in the "conspiracy" to medicalize PMS, apparently embracing it for the advantages of the "sick" role that accompanies it, especially the exemption from accountability for behaviors and feelings for which they would normally be held responsible. According to this argument, some women diagnosed with PMS have thereby been empowered by physicians to be "out of control" and have received subtle cultural acceptance of aggression and power that they typically may not express. The extreme version of this view is evident when PMS is used to justify violent crimes. In France, for instance, women defending themselves in court can plead a special form of temporary insanity if their crimes were committed during the late luteal phase of their menstrual cycle. In North America, PMS is not acceptable as a legal defense.

The feminist position does not question the reality of PMS, but it does question the existence of biological mechanisms underlying PMS, as well as emphasizing the potential limitations that the acceptance of PMS as a biologically based illness places on women, who are thus assumed to be subject to "raging hormones," "out of control," or "dysfunctional." From a social perspective, the important question is not whether women fluctuate in their moods or even in their level of aggressive behavior, but rather whether their functioning is impaired by these monthly fluctuations. The vast majority of research from the social sciences has not detected any significant impairments of this sort (Ussher, 1989).

## What Is PMS?

A consideration of PMS from a biomedical perspective leads to several problems with the characterization of this phenomenon. Consequently, understanding the relationship between hormones and the mood changes associated with PMS is difficult. The first issue that is often raised in biomedical discussions of PMS is whether PMS is a real phenomenon. Before this issue can be directly addressed, a distinction between illness and disease needs to be made. PMS is not a disease; it is a response to a natural cycle, and there is no known underlying pathology. However, PMS may be considered an illness, since a woman suffering from symptoms associated with menstruation can visit a physician, receive a diagnosis of PMS, get treatment, and report amelioration of the symptoms. This scenario suggests that PMS is real and should be considered an illness. One interesting issue, the significance of which remains unresolved, is the fact that approximately 50% of women that receive placebo treatments for their PMS symptoms report improvements. There are few other illnesses for which this is true. Of course, there is a placebo response for other symptoms not associated with PMS: approximately 30% of both men and women respond to placebos for many symptoms. With PMS, there is reason to believe that the placebo effect wears off after 3 months. However, few clinical investigations of PMS have extended beyond 3 months. As you might expect, correlating hormonal changes with the symptoms of PMS becomes challenging under these circumstances.

If the reality of PMS is accepted, several other problems remain to be addressed. First, estimates of the prevalence of PMS vary widely, despite many cross-cultural studies that have indicated that some women in all societies examined report perimenstrual symptoms. The frequency of perimenstrual symptoms reported in different studies varies between 20% and 90% of North American and European women. A meta-analysis of all published reports yields a prevalence rate of about 45% of all women. Most of these women rate their symptoms as mild; however, some women are debilitated by PMS. The frequency of severe PMS symptoms ranges between 2% and 10% (Logue and Moos, 1986). It is generally accepted that about 3–5% of women experience PMS symptoms to a degree that interferes with their usual functioning. This variation in prevalence rates is due in part to differences in the criteria used to define the syndrome (Endicott et al., 1981). The prevalence estimates reflect the types of symptoms included in each study (for example, psychological versus physiological), as well as the severity of symptoms included (Table 13.1). A corollary of this problem is that all of the PMS data are based on self-reports. In some studies, the self-reports are retrospective; in others, they are prospective or concurrent with the symptoms. In no other area of behavioral endocrinology is the introspective, or self-report, method the primary technique used to generate behavioral data to correlate with hormonal data. Obviously, self-reports of PMS symptoms can be influenced by many factors; for example, simply being asked about the symptoms is likely to increase the per-

**Table 13.1**

**Percentages of women who report perimenstrual symptoms in two tests designed to assess PMS**

| | Test | |
|---|---|---|
| **Symptom** | **Menstrual Distress Questionnaire**[a] | **Premenstrual Assessment Form**[b] |
| Breast pain | 35 | 84 |
| Weight gain | 34 | 83 |
| Swelling | 36 | 77 |
| Backaches | 24 | 74 |
| Sadness | 43 | 76 |
| Anxiety | 30 | 70 |
| Skin blemishes | 34 | 69 |
| Dizziness | 5 | 25 |

[a]Severity ratings from "mild" to "severe"
[b]Severity ratings from "slight" to "extreme"
*Note:* Tests were administered during the perimenstrual period.
*Source:* Logue and Moos, 1986.

ceived severity of the symptoms (Brown-Parlee, 1991). Women are also likely to rate their symptoms as more severe when asked about their perimenstrual period after the fact as compared with during the experience.

A second problem with PMS is that neither the premenstrual nor menstrual periods are well defined. When should symptoms be considered part of PMS? If they appear 3 days prior to menstruation? If they appear 5 days prior to menstruation? If they appear 10 days prior to menstruation? Also, how long after the onset of menses should symptoms be included? Menstruation may continue for 3 days in some cases or 8 days in others. Is a menstrual period of 3 days equivalent to an 8-day period? Because there is no consensus about which data should be included, there is substantial difficulty in comparing PMS studies with one another.

A third problem with PMS is the lack of consensus concerning its symptoms. PMS was originally described in 1931 as "premenstrual tension." Symptoms of this condition included severe psychological tension, weight gain, headaches, and edema (swelling) that occurred 7–10 days prior to the onset of menses (Frank, 1931). Because these symptoms may also occur in postmenopausal women, as well as in men and children, diagnosis of PMS requires the additional criterion of regular recurrence. Thus, symptoms must manifest themselves on a cyclical basis and end with the onset or offset of menstruation. The current diagnostic criteria for the so-called Late Luteal Phase Dysphoric Disorder, as described in the *Diagnostic and Statistical Manual of Mental Disorders*, Fourth Edition (DSM-IV), published by the American Psychiatric Association in 1995, can be found in Box 13.1. Within the past decade, the recognized symptoms of PMS have included anxiety, sadness, irritability, bloating, breast enlargement, dysmenorrhea (painful menstruation in the absence of identified pelvic pathology), increased appetite, fatigue, depression, headache, edema, insomnia, emotional lability, dizziness, confusion, asthma, constipation, thirst, nausea, weight gain, aggression, acne, boils, epilepsy,

## Box 13.1
# Diagnostic Criteria for Late Luteal Phase Dysphoric Disorder

A. In most menstrual cycles during the past year, symptoms in B occurred during the last week of the luteal phase and remitted within a few days after onset of the follicular phase. In menstruating females, these phases correspond to the week before, and a few days after, the onset of menses. (In nonmenstruating females who have had a hysterectomy, the timing of luteal and follicular phases may require measurement of circulating reproductive hormones.)

B. At least five of the following symptoms have been present for most of the time during each symptomatic late luteal phase, at least one of the symptoms being either (1), (2), (3), or (4):

  (1) marked affective lability, e.g., feeling suddenly sad, tearful, irritable, or angry

  (2) persistent and marked anger or irritability

  (3) marked anxiety, tension, feelings of being "keyed up," or "on edge"

  (4) markedly depressed mood, feelings of hopelessness, or self-deprecating thoughts

  (5) decreased interest in usual activities, e.g., work, friends, hobbies

  (6) easy fatigability or marked lack of energy

  (7) subjective sense of difficulty in concentrating

  (8) marked change in appetite, overeating, or specific food cravings

  (9) hypersomnia or insomnia

  (10) other physical symptoms, such as breast tenderness or swelling, headaches, joint or muscle pain, a sensation of "bloating," weight gain

C. The disturbance seriously interferes with work or with usual activities or relationships with others.

D. The disturbance is not merely an exacerbation of the symptoms of another disorder, such as Major Depression, Panic Disorder, Dysthymia, or a Personality Disorder (although it may be superimposed on any of these disorders).

E. Criteria A, B, C, and D are confirmed by prospective daily self-ratings during at least two symptomatic cycles. (The diagnosis may be made provisionally prior to this confirmation.)

*Source:* DSM-IV, 1995.

---

rhinitis, herpes outbreaks, conjunctivitis, fever, reduced sex drive, increased sex drive, moodiness, impaired motor coordination, craving for sweet or salty foods, and backaches (Brooks-Gunn, 1986; Clare, 1985; Reid and Yen; 1981; Sanders et al., 1983; Wurtman and Wurtman, 1989). Obviously, not every symptom is experienced by every woman with PMS, and not all women who experience PMS necessarily have the same symptoms, or experience them with the same severity, from one period to the next. Thus, the enormous variety and range of symptoms, as well as the varying severity of the symptoms and the difficulty of matching groups of experimental subjects so that their respective symptoms are similar, impede research on the physiological correlates of PMS. All of these caveats necessarily constrain causative statements about PMS and the mood effects of hormones.

Many factors influence the severity of PMS symptoms, but these correlates are not well defined. For example, women with long and heavy menstrual bleeding report more perimenstrual symptoms than women with brief and light menstrual flows (Logue and Moos, 1986). Also, age affects PMS symptoms. The severity of PMS symptoms reported by women increases during the late teens and twenties and subsides during the thirties. Women older than 20 who are using oral contraceptives report fewer PMS symptoms than women taking the Pill who are younger than 20 years old.

In terms of psychological influences, recent stressors can greatly enhance the severity of PMS symptoms (Schlotts, 1988). During the 1940s and 1950s many psychoanalytic theories were offered to explain PMS symptoms. These male-oriented psychoanalytic theories focused on women's supposed "disgust" or "shame" surrounding menstruation itself, and the symptoms that preceded menstruation were considered conversion reactions (essentially psychosomatic symptoms) to adapt psychologically to this anxiety. From this psychiatric perspective, many attempts have been made to correlate psychological profiles with PMS. Women with a history of affective illness report more PMS symptoms than women without such a history. Women who score high on psychological scales of neuroticism also are more likely to report PMS symptoms than women who rate low on these psychological scales (Endicott et al., 1981). However, the nature of the interplay between physical and psychological factors in mediating PMS has not been completely elucidated.

Is PMS one syndrome with a single cause, or a number of ailments with differing underlying causes? Generally, physiological symptoms are more prevalent during the menstrual phase than during the premenstrual phase of the cycle, whereas psychological symptoms are reported more frequently during the premenstrual than during the menstrual phase (Logue and Moos, 1986). Abdominal swelling and breast tenderness, however, are prominent premenstrual symptoms. Four major subtypes of PMS have been identified. These subtypes are based on prospective, rather than retrospective, reports; that is, questionnaires that are filled out during the perimenstrual period rather than afterward. Prospective questionnaires based on 19 different symptoms have led to the designation of four major subtypes of PMS (Logue and Moos, 1986): (1) Premenstrual Tension-A (PMT-A) includes anxiety, irritability, mood swings, and nervous tension; (2) PMT-H includes body weight gain, swelling of extremities, and sensations of bloating; (3) PMT-C includes increased frequencies of headaches, craving for sweet foods, increased appetite, pounding heartbeat, fatigue, and dizziness, and (4) PMT-D includes depression, mild amnesia, crying, confusion, and insomnia. PMT-A and PMT-H are the most commonly occurring subtypes, affecting 57% and 56%, respectively, of the approximately half of the women in one study that scored positive for premenstrual tension (Abraham, 1980). Perimenstrual changes characterized by a depressive syndrome (PMT-D) have been linked to mild or subclinical affective disorders (Endicott et al., 1981). If it is true that different symptoms cluster together, then it seems unlikely that a single hormonal factor associated with the menstrual cycle underlies PMS. The possibility that different subtypes of PMS exist, and that women may experience more than one subtype of PMS simultaneously, suggests that several hormonal conditions, sometimes contradictory ones, may be related to PMS.

### Hormonal Correlates of PMS

Because most of the mood changes associated with PMS occur during the late luteal phase, when progesterone concentrations in the blood are peaking and estrogen concentrations are decreasing, the first hormonal hypothesis about PMS proposed that progesterone played a role in the mood changes. However, when all studies are considered together, no consistent differences in progesterone concentrations between women who report PMS symptoms and women who do not suffer from PMS have been found. For instance, women who suffer from PMS have higher progesterone concentrations 10 days prior to menstruation than women who do not report PMS symptoms (O'Brien et al., 1979); however, these differences in progesterone concentrations are not evident 4 days prior to menstruation. Perhaps women who experience higher concentrations of progesterone experience greater "withdrawal" from this steroid hormone or its precursors or metabolites.

How might this work? The major inhibitory neurotransmitter in the brain is GABA (gamma-aminobutyric acid), a simple amino acid that is formed in one step from glutamate. GABA-secreting neurons are found throughout the brain in vertebrates. When GABA interacts with its receptor on the postsynaptic cell, chloride ($Cl^-$) channels are opened, which causes the inside of the postsynaptic neuron to become more negatively charged and less likely to fire an action potential. Neuroscientists have discovered that a class of drugs called the benzodiazepines binds to receptors that are often closely associated with, but different from, the GABA receptors. Activation of the benzodiazepine receptors appears to enhance the inhibitory effects of GABA on the neural firing of the postsynaptic neuron. The benzodiazepines are drugs such as Librium, Valium, and Xanax that have anti-anxiety or calming effects, which are presumably the result of enhancing the inhibitory effects of GABA. These drugs are very effective at therapeutic doses, but have potential for abuse and addiction at high doses. Moderate to severe withdrawal symptoms, both psychological and physiological, are associated with the discontinuation of benzodiazepines. Several steroid hormones, particularly the progestins, have been reported to affect GABA neurons and may interact with benzodiazepine receptors (Bitran and Dowd, 1996; Bitran et al., 1995; Majewska, 1987). "Addiction" to, and withdrawal from, steroid hormones may account for many of the mood-altering effects of these substances—including PMS.

Progesterone has been reported to alleviate some PMS symptoms, but certainly not all of them (Backstrom et al., 1983; Daugherty, 1998; Rubinow et al., 1988; Tiemstra and Patel, 1998; Zweifel and O'Brian, 1997). Progesterone vaginal suppositories administered in a double-blind study failed to affect symptoms in women who reported severe PMS symptoms (Maddocks et al., 1986). Combining progesterone with thyroid hormones, however, has been reported to be very effective in alleviating depressive symptoms of PMS (see below).

Blood estrogen concentrations have also been implicated as a factor affecting PMS. Estrogen affects fluid retention, hyperplasia of mammary tissue, and carbohydrate metabolism. Accumulation of estrogen in the limbic system has been hypothesized to account for the emotional and other CNS manifestations of PMS (Reid and Yen, 1981). However, mean serum levels of estrogens and progesterone do not differ between women with severe and with mild symptoms of PMS (Backstrom et al., 1983), and no data have supported the notion that estrogen treatment ameliorates PMS symptoms, although estrogen therapy is known to elevate mood (Daugherty, 1998; Fink et al., 1996; Halbreich, 1997; Pearlstein et al., 1997; Rubinow et al., 1998).

Again, no physiological abnormalities have been consistently linked with steroid hormone concentrations associated with the menstrual cycle in women diagnosed with PMS (Schmidt et al., 1991; Young and Korszun, 1998), nor have abnormal responses to normal levels of gonadal steroid hormones been reported (Schmidt et al., 1991). These findings are puzzling because virtually all current biomedical treatments for PMS putatively correct some physiological abnormality associated with the luteal phase of the menstrual cycle. The two most common courses of treatment for PMS include (1) providing some hormone that is believed to be suppressed in PMS patients or (2) suppressing endogenous hormone concentrations in the belief that PMS is a manifestation of elevated hormone concentrations (Schmidt et al., 1991).

The failure to identify any specific physiological aspects of the late luteal phase underlying the symptoms of PMS led one research team to suppress the entire luteal phase of the menstrual cycle in the hope of suppressing the symptoms of PMS. Using the progesterone antagonist mifepristone in a double-blind study, they arrested the luteal phase in the subjects, causing an artificial follicular phase to occur. If the symptoms of PMS are caused by the endocrine events associated with the luteal phase, then women who do not experience a luteal phase should not experience symptoms. However, women who were treated with mifepristone and did not experience the luteal phase reported no change either in the timing or the severity of their PMS symptoms (Schmidt et al., 1991). These results suggest, but do not prove, that the endocrine events associated with the luteal phase of the menstrual cycle are not directly responsible for the symptoms of PMS.

What, then, is causing the distress of PMS? There is evidence that preventing sex hormone cycling entirely in women with PMS abolishes the symptoms. Treatment with the GnRH agonist leuprolide, which eliminates menstrual cycles, significantly reduced symptoms in double-blind, crossover studies (Brown et al., 1994; Helvacioglu et al., 1993). It is possible that target tissue sensitivity to steroid hormones changes during the menstrual cycle differently in women with PMS than in women who do not experience PMS symptoms. In a recent study, ten women with PMS were given leuprolide, and their symptoms were ameliorated. If leuprolide was provided with either estradiol or progesterone, however, the nonaffective symptoms were restored (Schmidt et al., 1998). Thus, PMS symptoms do appear to reflect abnormal responses to normal concentrations of steroid hormones.

As implied above, PMS may reflect a pathological state induced by the chronic fluctuations in hormone concentrations associated with long-term menstrual cycles. That is, women may become dependent upon the elevated steroid hormone concentrations present during ovulation and pseudopregnancy (the luteal phase), and the psychological symptoms associated with PMS may reflect withdrawal of these gonadal steroid hormones. Abrupt withdrawal from gonadal steroid hormones may also be responsible for the postpartum depression reported by many women (see below).

Antidepressants that alter serotonin availability at the level of the receptor appear to be useful in treating depression associated with PMS (Yonkers, 1997). Thus, the current medical therapies of choice include GnRH agonists (usually reserved as a treatment of last resort), benzodiazepines (e.g., alprazolam), and selective serotonin reuptake inhibitors (SSRI) (e.g., fluoxetine) (Altshuler et al., 1995; Mortola, 1997).

Menstrual cycles were probably rare until recently in human history. In extant hunting and gathering societies, cultures that probably reflect over 99% of human evolutionary history, postpubertal females are either pregnant or lactating for most of their reproductive lives (Figure 13.1). Puberty occurs at a later age than in Western civilizations, and because of the high risk of death posed by childbirth, relatively few women survive until menopause. Women are reproductively successful only to the extent that they bear babies, and the high rate of infant mortality demands high pregnancy rates. Each pregnancy interrupts at least nine menstrual cycles. Menstruation does not begin immediately after parturition in most cases; lactation also prevents menstruation, so most women experience 2 years of lactational amenorrhea (cessation of menstrual cycles) between pregnancies. Thus, the reproductive life of a typical woman in such societies lasts for less than 20 years, and within those two decades she experiences probably fewer than 10 to 20 menstrual cycles (Dennis, 1992).

Contrast 10 to 20 menstrual cycles with an extreme, but not uncommon, reproductive scenario for a present-day North American female. If a woman begins menstruating at 12 and continues until her first pregnancy at 35 years of age, she will experience nearly 300 uninterrupted menstrual cycles. After the weaning of a single child, this hypothetical woman can expect another 100 menstrual cycles. Thus, PMS may be an unavoidable consequence of Western civilization and the abnormal physiological milieu of chronic, long-term cyclic fluctuations in hor-

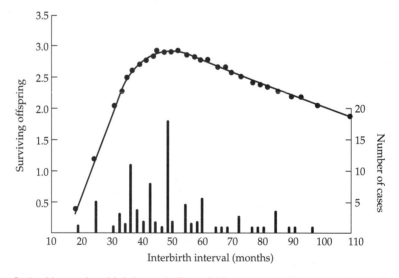

**13.1  Optimal human interbirth interval.**  The solid line, generated by a computer model, represents the number of surviving human babies for various interbirth intervals, based on a calculation that takes offspring survival into account ([reproductive life span/interbirth interval] × probability of offspring survival if born at that interval); the dots represent individual cases upon which the model is based. Thus, the optimal birth spacing is about 50 months. The vertical bars represent actual birth intervals in a hunting–gathering society, the !Kung, which roughly correspond to the computed optimum. After Blurton Jones, 1986.

mone concentrations that accompanies it. This is not to say that widely spaced pregnancies are not a reasonable goal for individuals and for ameliorating the ecological pressures of the increasing human population on this planet, but those incentives do not negate the possibility that these recent (on an evolutionary scale) changes in the physiological conditions to which the nervous systems of women are subjected could cause changes in behavior and mood. From this perspective, it is remarkable that more women do not report fluctuating mood changes associated with repetitive cycles of hormone surges and withdrawals. A similar explanation involving uninterrupted ovarian cycles has been put forward to explain the increase in the incidence of ovarian cancer (Schildkraut et al., 1997).

One way that hormones may affect mood indirectly is via food intake. Recall from Chapter 8 that food intake and body mass increase in rodents and primates after ovulation, when blood plasma estrogen concentrations are low and progesterone concentrations are high (Blaustein and Wade, 1976; Bowen and Grunberg, 1990; Czaja, 1978). Women display a similar pattern of caloric intake and body mass change associated with their menstrual cycles. Consumption of carbohydrates in particular is higher during the luteal phase than during the follicular phase of the human menstrual cycle (Dalvit, 1981; Pliner and Fleming, 1983; Kurzer, 1997). Women crave carbohydrate-rich foods more frequently during the luteal phase than during the follicular phase. These carbohydrate cravings occur more frequently during the luteal phase regardless of the occurrence or severity of PMS symptoms (Cohen et al., 1987), indicating that they are a normal component of the menstrual cycle and do not necessarily represent "symptoms" of PMS (DSM-IV, 1995; cf. Severino and Moline, 1989). One study explored the relationship between carbohydrate cravings and PMS using a computer-assisted vending machine that dispensed snacks that varied in their caloric components. When women were sequestered in a nutrition ward and given access to this machine, those who suffered from PMS increased their average snack intake by approximately 500 more calories per day than women who did not report PMS symptoms, despite equally caloric meals. The snacks chosen by women with PMS symptoms were invariably carbohydrate-rich and rarely contained protein, although protein intake in the two groups was equivalent at mealtimes (Wurtman and Wurtman, 1989). An increased intake of carbohydrates may affect mood by increasing the availability of tryptophan, the precursor of serotonin, to the brain (see below for details of this mechanism).

Other studies have implicated dietary calcium in some PMS symptoms (Thys-Jacobs and Alvir, 1995). Low estrogen concentrations may deplete calcium reserves and affect CNS function. Treatment of PMS with calcium dietary supplements ameliorates many symptoms (Thys-Jacobs and Alvir, 1995; Thys-Jacobs et al., 1998). In one definitive clinical study, 466 women with moderate to severe PMS symptoms were recruited from 12 outpatient clinics across the United States. The women received either calcium (1200 mg elemental calcium/day) or a placebo pill in a randomized, double-blind study. In this large study, calcium treatment reduced four separate symptom factors (negative mood, water retention, food cravings, and pain) by approximately 50% by the third menstrual cycle of treatment (Thys-Jacobs et al., 1998). Placebo treatment caused a 30% reduction in PMS symptoms after three menstrual cycles. Overall, calcium supplementation seems to be a simple, inexpensive, and effective treatment for PMS (Thys-Jacobs et al., 1998).

The roles of calcitonin and parathyroid hormone in PMS symptoms remain unspecified, although a secondary hyperparathyroidism has been reported in women suffering from PMS (e.g., Thys-Jacobs and Alvir, 1995). Blood concentrations of aldosterone also vary during the menstrual cycle. High concentrations of aldosterone during the late luteal phase cause retention of sodium by the kidneys. The retention of sodium leads to water retention and feelings of bloating during the perimenstrual period (Janowsky et al., 1973).

All of these data indicate that many hormones may be involved at several different levels to cause PMS symptoms. Determining the exact constellation of endocrine events responsible for PMS will require further synthetic research on a number of different experimental levels.

### Cognitive Features of PMS

Although negative mood changes are commonly associated with PMS, some women report positive mood changes and increased performance during the perimenstrual phase of their menstrual cycles (Logue and Moos, 1988; Parlee, 1980). Approximately 5–15% of women experience elevated energy levels and an enhanced sense of well-being during the perimenstrual phase. Although many other women report reduced energy and activity levels during the perimenstrual phase of the cycle, some women may not accurately report their activities. In one study, women wore electronic activity monitors and also answered questionnaires. Despite their reports of lethargy during the premenstrual period, the women's actual behavior indicated an increase in activity (Endicott and Halbreich, 1982).

A significant minority of women also report increased performance on particular types of tasks. For example, a battery of cognitive tasks, including tests of reaction time and mental arithmetic skills, was administered every other day to women undergoing normal menstrual cycles. Reaction times and speed of mental calculations improved during the late luteal phase (Wuttke et al., 1975). Similar results have been reported for some women for perceptual motor skills, critical thinking abilities, and intelligence test scores (Cormack and Sheldrake, 1974; Jensen, 1982; Logue and Moos, 1988; Wuttke et al., 1975). Finally, many women report an increase in sexual interest during the perimenstrual phase (Halbreich et al., 1982; Logue and Moos, 1988; Taylor, 1979). A heightened sex drive may represent reduced concern about unwanted pregnancies during the perimenstrual phase. However, women taking oral contraceptives also report an increase in sexual activities premenstrually, as well as during the time of ovulation (Englander-Golden et al., 1980; see Chapter 6).

Obviously, both endocrine and cognitive factors interact to influence PMS. As we have seen, the symptoms of PMS can be affected by social expectations, and these symptoms can be improved by placebo treatments (Koeske, 1980; Parlee, 1982; Ruble, 1977). These facts, along with the lack of consistent endocrine correlates of PMS symptoms, have led some researchers to suggest that these symptoms are "all in the head" of the sufferers. However, the interaction of complex endocrine signals with cognitive factors is not unique to PMS. By analogy, recall that rat maternal behavior can be elicited after many days of exposure to pups, immediately after parturition, or after several days of specifically timed hormonal treatments involving at least three different hormones (see Chapter 7). In the latter case, the endocrine manipulations must still be combined with several days of exposure to pups prior to the onset of maternal behavior. Adults can overcome their fear of pups and begin acting maternally by means of frequent exposure to pups, the endocrine environment of pregnancy, or some combination of hormones and behavior. In other words, there is an interaction between cognitive (reduction in fear) and endocrine factors (the hormones that reduce the processing of fear-inducing chemical stimuli). Further research will have to focus on this interaction, keeping in mind that various subtypes of PMS are probably mediated by different underlying causes. A more holistic, integrative approach to the study of PMS may be required before the physiological, behavioral, and social causes of PMS are understood.

## Hormones and Depression

The symptoms of **depression** include reduced mood (profound sadness); low self-esteem and feelings of worthlessness; general fatigue; feelings of guilt; disturbances (usually reductions) in sleep, sex drive, and food intake; anger; absence of pleasure; and agitated or retarded motor symptoms (DSM-IV, 1995). Agitated motor symptoms include pacing or hand-wringing; retarded motor symptoms include slow body movements or speech. In severe cases, delusions and hallucinations may be present.

Patients exhibiting the symptoms of depression are generally suffering from "clinical" depression. The term **major depression** describes a depressed state characterized by very severe symptoms that last chronically for at least 2 weeks. **Dysthymia** is characterized by less severe symptoms that last much longer, at least 2 years. Both of these types of depressive disorders occur in the absence of other psychological or physical problems, and are considered **primary depression.** **Secondary depression** refers to depression that results from some other physiological or psychological dysfunction. Individuals who are depressed for a transient period of time because of some clearly identifiable stressor or environmental stimulus (for example, grieving the loss of a friend or relative) are generally labeled "normal," "reactive," "neurotic," "exogenous," or "justified" depressives, or are said to be suffering from bereavement reactions (Corsini, 1984). The bouts of depression in these individuals are usually short-lived and exhibit a benign outcome; that is, individuals recover fully on their own without treatment. Another distinction made among types of clinical depression is between **bipolar** and **unipolar** depression. Bipolar depression is depression in the presence of at least one episode of **mania,** or elevated mood, which often involves inordinate feelings of confidence, power, and creative energies. Unipolar depression is depressed affect (mood) in the absence of manic episodes. Many of the studies on depression cited below used experimental groups that included both unipolar and bipolar depressives. Because the physiological mechanisms underlying these two subsets of depression may differ, the clumping of all of these individuals into one experimental group may mask hormonal correlates of depression, even though individuals in both groups often respond to the same antidepressant drugs.

Depression is typically considered to be at one end of a mood continuum with mania at the other end (Figure 13.2). Depressed individuals vary in both the severity and the duration of their symptoms. The prevalence of depressive symptoms is determined by means of psychological tests such as the Hamilton rating scale and

| Depression | Melancholia | Normal | Hypomania | Mania |

**13.2    Continuum of mood from depression to mania.** People may display unusual mood elevation or mood depression in response to environmental conditions. When these mood extremes persist and interfere with normal function, they become clinically significant.

the Zung self-rating scale (Hamilton, 1960). Studies of the endocrine correlates of depression use scores on these tests to measure the effects of hormone treatments. A number of endocrine correlates have been associated with depression.

**THYROID HORMONES.**    The hormones of the hypothalamic–pituitary–thyroid axis have been implicated in depression (see Figure 11.2) (Musselman and Nemeroff, 1996; Sauvage et al., 1998). Administration of thyrotropin-releasing hormone (TRH) stimulates the release of thyroid-stimulating hormone (TSH) from the anterior pituitary gland and subsequent hormone production by the thyroid gland. Administration of TRH to depressed individuals has been attempted in several studies. In one such study, five patients that achieved a certain composite score on psychological tests were considered to be depressed (three were diagnosed as unipolar and two were bipolar) (Kastin et al., 1972a). Depression was reduced in four of these five patients by TRH treatment, as indicated by their improved scores on subsequent rating tests. Amelioration of the depressive symptoms varied in duration from 3 hours to several weeks, and the latency of action of TRH varied from 1 to 72 hours. No improvement of the depressive symptoms was reported when the patients were treated with saline. All of the depressed patients showed a smaller than normal TSH elevation in response to the TRH stimulation, which is unusual in the absence of thyroid dysfunction. Although protein-bound iodine levels, basal metabolic rate, and rate of radioactive iodine uptake—all indicators of thyroid function—are usually within the normal range in depressed patients, the thyroid response to TSH is significantly lower in depressed patients than in nondepressed individuals (Ehrensing et al., 1974; Takahashi et al., 1974), suggesting some subclinical endocrine malfunction.

The depressive symptoms of PMS have also been associated with thyroid function. In one study, the responses of TSH and prolactin concentrations to TRH administration were examined in women who reported PMS symptoms and in women who did not. Previous studies on depressed patients had found both blunted and enhanced TSH secretion in response to TRH. TRH had also been found to stimulate prolactin release in nondepressed women, but did not affect prolactin levels in depressed patients (Roy-Byrne et al., 1987). TRH was given during both the follicular and luteal phases. There were no significant differences in basal or maximal elevations of TSH or prolactin in response to the treatment between women with and without PMS symptoms, and neither TSH nor prolactin values differed between the luteal and follicular phases. However, the women with PMS showed much greater variation in TSH response to TRH treatment than the control women; that is, sometimes TSH levels were augmented, but other times they were reduced (Roy-Byrne et al., 1987). Women without PMS showed stable responses of TSH to TRH. Variable TSH response to TRH could be present in a subgroup of women that suffer depression as part of their PMS symptoms.

In addition to changes in the response of TSH to TRH, recent studies have shown that depressed patients often exhibit (1) a very high level of antibodies against the thyroid gland, (2) high cerebrospinal fluid TRH concentrations, and (3) enhancement of antidepressant efficacy with co-treatment with triiodothyronine (T3) (Musselman and Nemeroff, 1996; Sauvage et al., 1998).

**GROWTH HORMONE AND PROLACTIN.**    Basal growth hormone (GH) concentrations have been reported to be in the normal range in depressed patients. However, impaired GH responses to insulin-induced hypoglycemia in depressed patients have been reported by many investigators (for example, Sachar et al., 1973). Depressed patients also display inadequate GH responses to serotonin stimulation as compared with nondepressed patients. TRH, which does not affect GH concentrations in normal individuals, evokes an abnormal increase in GH in depressed patients (Maeda et al., 1975). Elevated blood plasma prolactin concentrations have also been reported in depressed patients (Sachar et al., 1973; Nicholas et al., 1998). Although the results of correlative studies linking GH and prolactin to depression are somewhat contradictory (for example, TRH increased prolactin concentrations in depressed patients in one study [Maeda et al., 1975] and decreased prolactin concentrations in another [Ehrensing et al., 1974]), they point to a fundamental difference in endocrine function between depressed patients and nondepressed individuals, and suggest differences in the physiological mechanisms underlying their endocrine feedback control systems (Dinan, 1998; Nicolas et al., 1998).

**CORTISOL.**    Excessive cortisol production has been reported in nearly 50% of depressed patients examined (Figure 13.3a) (Carroll, 1980). These increased serum cortisol concentrations do not appear to reflect the stress of coping with depression, because cortisol concentrations are at their highest 3–4 hours after sleep onset, when stress levels should be lowest, and decrease throughout the daylight hours, when stress levels are presumably highest (Carroll, 1980). Because cortisol is normally secreted in a pronounced circadian pattern, with peak concentrations measured in the early morning, this disturbance of the diurnal rhythm of cortisol secretion suggests an abnormal disinhibition of the neural centers regulating the release of adrenocorticotropic hormone (ACTH), the tropic hormone from the anterior pituitary gland that stimulates adrenal output.

Cortisol normally counteracts the hypoglycemic effects of insulin; however, depressed patients do not show this response. High doses of insulin given during the diagnostic insulin tolerance test (ITT) suppress blood glucose levels, but glucose levels cannot be restored by cortisol in depressed patients (Carroll, 1980). The function of the hypothalamic–pituitary–adrenal axis in depressed patients has also been assessed by means of the dexamethasone suppression test (see Figure 13.3b–c). Administration of 1 to 2 milligrams of dexamethasone, an artificial steroid that mimics cortisol, at midnight normally suppresses blood plasma cortisol concentrations for 24 hours via a negative feedback mechanism. Dexamethasone failed to suppress cortisol production in 46% of depressed patients examined (Carroll et al., 1968). In most cases, plasma concentrations of cortisol were suppressed the morning after dexamethasone treatment, but increased shortly thereafter (Carroll et al., 1976). This inappropriate response to dexamethasone indicates a failure of the normal neural inhibiting mechanism for ACTH/cortisol secretion. It seems likely that a complex relation between the serotonergic system and the HPA axis (see

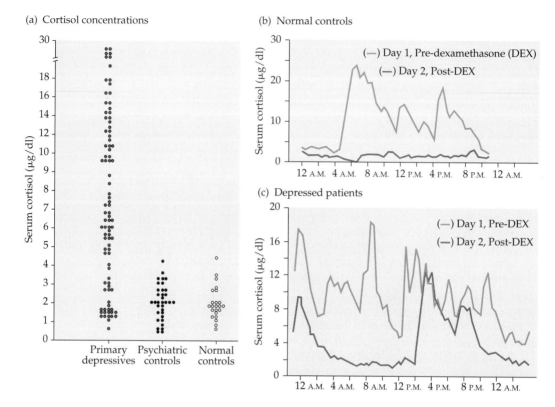

(a) Cortisol concentrations

(b) Normal controls

(c) Depressed patients

**13.3    The HPA axis and depression.** (a) The hypothalmic-pituitary-adrenal (HPA) system. (b) Dexamethasone inhibits the normal circadian pattern of cortisol secretion on day 1 of treatment. (c) Dexamethasone often fails to suppress cortisol concentrations of depressed individuals. (d) The negative feedback features of the HPA axis appear to be impaired in depressed people because blood cortisol concentrations are often higher in depressed than in nondepressed individuals. From Rosenzweig et al., 1999.

Figure 11.3; McAllister-Williams et al., 1998) underlies the hypersecretion of cortisol, the failure to respond normally to dexamethasone by suppressing cortisol production, and the disturbance of the circadian rhythm of cortisol secretion.

Taken together, these findings in depressed patients of (1) high basal cortisol concentrations due to cortisol hypersecretion, (2) the failure to respond normally to dexamethasone by suppressing cortisol production, (3) high cortioctropin-releasing factor (CRF) concentrations in the cerebrospinal fluid, (4) a blunted ACTH response to treatment with endogenous CRF, and (5) the disturbance of the circadian rhythm of cortisol secretion appear to indicate a central disinhibition of the HPA axis during depressive episodes (Heuser, 1998; Mitchell, 1998; Musselman and Nemeroff, 1996; Plotsky et al., 1998). These changes in the HPA axis appear to be state-dependent; that is, these factors normalize with the elevation of mood (Murphy, 1997; Plotsky et al., 1998).

In all of these examples of hormonal changes in depressed patients, it is unclear whether depression causes a change in hormone production or whether changes in hormone production cause depression. When depression is secondary to some endocrine dysfunction, then more definitive statements can be made about the direction of causality. For example, individuals suffering from primary hypothyroidism often present symptoms of depressed affect and intellect. However, patients suffering from primary adrenal disorders show conflicting mood responses to cortisol concentrations. For instance, patients with Cushing disease have adrenals that produce excessive cortisol, and depression is often a symptom of this disorder; however, patients with Addison disease have adrenal glands that produce insufficient cortisol, and depression is a defining symptom of this disease as well. Thus, an inverted U-shaped function exists for the effects of cortisol concentrations on mood (Figure 13.4).

**ESTROGEN.**   Deficits in estrogen have been associated with depression (Fink et al., 1996; Halbreich, 1997; Zweifel and O'Brien, 1997). In one double-blind study, estrogen treatment was given to 40 women who were hospitalized with severe depression. None of the women who received placebo treatment showed changes in their affect; in fact, 47% of those patients deteriorated in their mood. However, over 90% of the depressed women treated with estrogen significantly improved their mood (Klaiber et al., 1979). It should be noted that substantial pharmacological doses (15–20 times the recommended therapeutic doses) of estrogen were administered in this study. Administration of estrogen in physiological doses improves mood in normal women (Sherwin and Gelfand, 1985; Sherwin and Suranyi-Cadotte, 1990), but not in clinically depressed women (Schneider et al., 1977). However, estrogen treatment seems to ameliorate depressed affect in postmenopausal women (Fink et al., 1996; Halbreich, 1997; Pearlstein et al., 1997; Rubinow et al., 1998; Zweifel and O'Brien, 1997). It is possible that estrogen plays a role in postpartum depression (discussed below).

### Postpartum Depression

For most women, the postpartum period is a time of mother–infant bonding. However, a significant minority may suffer from postpartum depression. Like PMS, **postpartum depression** is a well-known outcome of the endocrine changes associated with reproductive function (Deakin, 1988; Hendrick et al., 1998; Llewellyn et al., 1997). Also in common with PMS, there is confusion regarding a

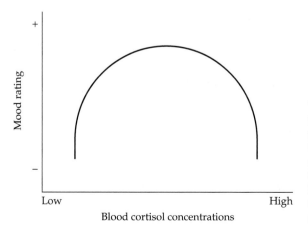

**13.4   Cortisol and mood.** Mood rating in self-reports shows an inverse U-shaped relationship with blood cortisol concentrations, with optimal mood ratings corresponding to moderate blood cortisol concentrations. If blood cortisol concentrations become too high or too low, as in Cushing disease or Addison disease, respectively, then mood ratings typically drop into the depressed category.

precise definition of postpartum depression, as well as uncertainty that it is a unique disorder (Hamilton et al., 1988; Hopkins et al., 1984).

Many women experience mild to severe depression within a few days of giving birth (O'Hara et al., 1991; Susman, 1996). The mildest type of postpartum depression is called either "maternity blues" or "baby blues" and typically lasts only 24–48 hours. A case of maternity blues is usually manifested by periods of crying and sadness; about 50% of women in North America display these symptoms after giving birth. Mild to moderate postpartum depression is experienced by about 15–20% of women; this type of postpartum depression may last 4–8 weeks. Its symptoms include depressed affect, insomnia, crying, irritability, feelings of inadequacy, reduced coping ability, and fatigue. In very rare cases (fewer than 0.01% of women giving birth), women display a temporary, but severe, form of depression called postpartum depressive psychosis (Hopkins et al., 1984).

The exact precursors to postpartum mood disorders have not been specified, but a combination of biological, social, and psychological factors, including a personal or family history of depression, may be involved. Because dramatic changes in blood concentrations of estrogens, progesterone, and prolactin occur at the time of parturition, most studies of the hormonal correlates of postpartum mood changes have investigated the role of these hormones (O'Hara and Zekoski, 1988; Llewellyn et al., 1997). As in the case of PMS, no consistent correlation between mood changes and these hormones has been identified (George and Sandler, 1988; Gitlin and Pasnau, 1989; Kuevi et al., 1983; O'Hara et al., 1991).

Recently, a relationship between opioid peptides, specifically β-endorphin, and postpartum mood changes has been reported (Deakin, 1988; Ferin, 1984; George and Sandler, 1988). Blood plasma concentrations of β-endorphin change during pregnancy: concentrations are relatively constant during the first two trimesters, begin to rise during the end of pregnancy, peak during parturition, and then drop immediately afterward (Newnham et al., 1983, 1984; Smith et al., 1990). Because β-endorphin concentrations plummet within hours of parturition, it has been suggested that maternity blues, and perhaps other more severe postpartum mood disorders, may result from this "withdrawal" of endogenous opiates (Newnham et al., 1984). In support of this hypothesis, women who displayed the highest incidence of depressive symptoms from gestational week 38 through day 2 postpartum, as well as 3 months postpartum, had the greatest decreases in plasma β-endorphin concentrations after parturition (Smith et al., 1990). Increases in anxiety and tension are also associated with the postpartum decline in plasma β-endorphin levels (Brinsmead et al., 1985). Although several correlative studies have established a relationship between opioids and postpartum mood, direct experimental evidence remains lacking.

There are several social changes that occur after the delivery of a baby that may lead to postpartum depression (Nonacs and Cohen, 1998; Hendrick et al., 1998). For instance, hospitalization may affect depressive symptoms in some women; also, the change in status to parent can be a sufficiently significant life event to cause anxiety and depression (Richman et al., 1991). Although a fair amount of descriptive work has been done, only recently have data been collected that seem to indicate that postpartum depression may not reflect only endocrine changes. Women who remain at home with their children are more likely to display depressive symptoms than women who have careers outside the home (Gotlib et al., 1989). Not surprisingly, perhaps, women bringing unwanted pregnancies to term are more likely to become depressed than women with planned pregnancies. Men are nearly as likely as women to suffer postpartum depressive symptoms within 2 months of their child's birth (68% versus 82% respectively) (Richman et al., 1991).

In one study, repeated measurements of women's moods revealed that 25% exhibited increased depressive symptomology during pregnancy. However, only 10% of the women in this study met the diagnostic criteria for depression, and only 7% could be diagnosed as depressed postpartum (Gotlib et al., 1989). These results indicate that mild depression may be common during and immediately after pregnancy, but that debilitating depression is rare. Also, these data suggest that endocrine changes may not necessarily be the primary cause of postpartum depression: a similar incidence of depression was seen in men, and in women both *during* and *after* pregnancy, despite very different hormone concentrations at those times.

### Seasonal Affective Disorder

Seasonal changes in behavior are legion in animals and humans (see Chapter 10). One seasonal rhythm in humans that has received much attention during the past several years is winter depression, or seasonal affective disorder (SAD). SAD is characterized by depressed affect, lethargy, loss of libido, hypersomnia, excessive weight gain, carbohydrate cravings, anxiety, and inability to concentrate or focus attention, occurring during the late autumn or winter (Rosenthal et al., 1988). In the Northern Hemisphere, symptoms usually begin between October and December and go into remission during March. These symptoms do not merely reflect the holiday blues, because individuals suffering from SAD in the Southern Hemisphere display symptoms 6 months out of phase with Northern Hemisphere residents (Terman, 1988). With the onset of summer, SAD patients regain their energy and become active and elated, often to the point of hypomania or mania. Prevalence rates in the population range from 1% to 10%, with higher prevalence rates reported at higher latitudes (Rosenthal, 1993). Women seem to be affected by SAD more often than men (Kasper et al., 1989): the sex ratio of SAD prevalence in one epidemiological study was 3.5 women to 1 man. Over 80% of respondents to newspaper advertisements recruiting experimental subjects with SAD were women (Rosenthal and Wehr, 1987). Among menstruating women suffering from SAD, PMS is common during the fall and winter; often their PMS symptoms are reduced during the summer (Thase, 1989). Three features atypical of depression— hyperphagia, carbohydrate cravings, and hypersomnia—set SAD apart from nonseasonal depression. SAD is frequently diagnosed as "Bipolar II" depression or "Atypical Bipolar Disorder," particularly if hypomania or mania are present (DSM-IV).

Improperly entrained circadian rhythms may be involved in SAD (Lewy et al., 1985, 1988; see Chapter 10). It has been hypothesized that changing the onset of sleep time resets biological clocks, resulting in amelioration of the depression (reviewed in Lewy et al., 1988). In one study, a depressed patient was phase-advanced in her sleep–wake cycle by 6 hours; her depression was temporarily ameliorated by this treatment (Wehr et al., 1979). Four of seven other patients who underwent spontaneous remission from depression also displayed a spontaneous phase advance of their times of awakening (Wehr et al., 1979). Lithium, tricyclic antidepressants, and estrogen, all of which are used to treat depressive illnesses, also affect endogenous timekeeping mechanisms (Wehr et al., 1979). The fact that these pharmacological agents and sleep–wake cycle manipulations are both effective in ameliorating depression suggests that they work via similar mechanisms involving biological clocks.

More recently, bright lights have been used in place of sleep–wake therapy in the treatment of SAD. When patients are exposed to bright light, usually for a few hours in the morning or evening, signs of remission of the SAD symptoms are often apparent within a few days (Figure 13.5a; Rosenthal et al., 1988). Phototherapy, like sleep–wake therapy, may work by phase-advancing biological rhythms. Bright light has been suggested to possess two antidepressant effects: (1) light treatment in the

(a)

(b)

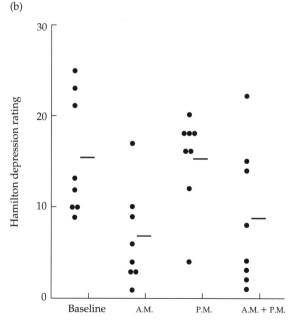

**13.5  Light box therapy may ameliorate seasonal affective disorder (SAD).** (a) Individuals suffering from SAD can sometimes obtain relief using daily light therapy, whereby they sit in front of a light box for 1–2 hours early each morning during the autumn and winter. Light boxes produce bright illumination (>2500 lux), which is thought to help resynchronize biological rhythms. (b) Individual (solid circles) and average (horizontal bars) ratings of mood on the Hamilton rating scale for eight individuals with SAD at baseline and after morning (A.M.), evening (P.M.), or combined (A.M. + P.M.) light treatment. Light treatment that took place during the morning resulted in significantly improved mood (that is, lower depression scores) as compared with baseline mood or evening treatment. Photograph in (a) courtesy of Lightbox Company of New England. Source: Lewy et al., 1987.

morning may ameliorate depression by realignment of inappropriately entrained circadian rhythms, and (2) light may also serve as a general "energizer . . . of mood in a way that may be attributable wholly or in part to a placebo effect" (Lewy et al., 1988). Light treatment at different times during the day results in differing rates of mood improvement (Figure 13.5b; Lewy et al., 1987).

Serotonin may be involved in the symptoms of SAD (Skwerer et al., 1988; Wurtman and Wurtman, 1989). Tryptophan, an amino acid that normally circulates in the blood at low concentrations, is converted to serotonin in the brain, specifically in the raphe nuclei (Cooper et al., 1986). Diet affects this conversion process because carbohydrates stimulate pancreatic β-cells to secrete insulin, which in turn facilitates the uptake of sugars and non-tryptophan amino acids into peripheral cells. This results in a relatively high ratio of tryptophan to other amino acids in the blood, and because tryptophan competes with the other amino acids for access to central nervous system tissue, carbohydrate ingestion results in more tryptophan crossing the blood–brain barrier, and thus higher production of serotonin (Figure 13.6). Serotonin concentrations feed back to regulate the intake of carbohydrates. It is possible, therefore, that patients suffering from SAD have cyclic disruptions in their serotonin–carbohydrate regulating mechanisms (Wurtman and Wurtman, 1989). Serotonin is also involved in normal sleep onset, and faulty sero-

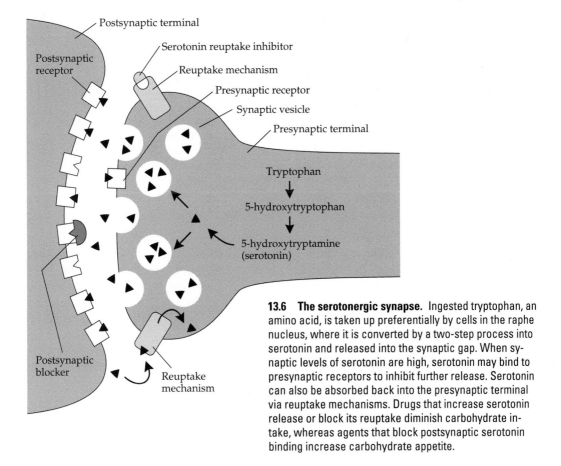

**13.6  The serotonergic synapse.** Ingested tryptophan, an amino acid, is taken up preferentially by cells in the raphe nucleus, where it is converted by a two-step process into serotonin and released into the synaptic gap. When synaptic levels of serotonin are high, serotonin may bind to presynaptic receptors to inhibit further release. Serotonin can also be absorbed back into the presynaptic terminal via reuptake mechanisms. Drugs that increase serotonin release or block its reuptake diminish carbohydrate intake, whereas agents that block postsynaptic serotonin binding increase carbohydrate appetite.

(a)

(b)

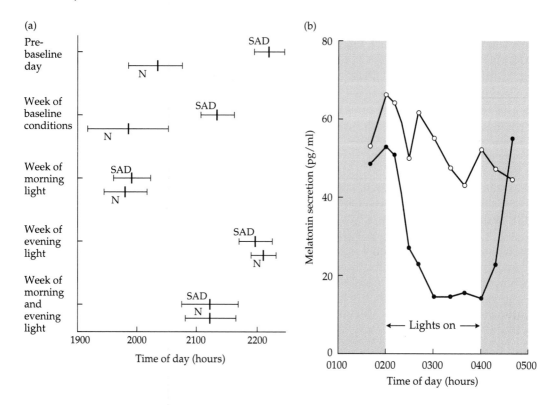

**13.7   Light exposure affects both onset time and level of melatonin secretion.** (a) Average melatonin secretion onset times for normal subjects (N) occurred nearly 2 hours earlier than for SAD patients prior to experimental light treatment (pre-baseline). After a week of bright light treatment, the average melatonin secretion onset times for N and SAD individuals coincided, regardless of the timing of the light treatment. (b) Effects of light pulses on human melatonin secretion. The open circles represent the effects of light pulses of an intensity of 500 lux; this level of illumination is about that found in a typical office or brightly lit room. The solid circles represent light pulses of 2500 lux, which are much more effective in suppressing melatonin secretion. Source: Lewy et al., 1987, 1980.

tonin regulation may also contribute to the hypersomnia reported in SAD patients. If it is true that symptoms of SAD result from faulty serotonin metabolism, then pharmacological interventions that elevate serotonin concentrations should be expected to reduce the severity of some SAD symptoms. Administration of the serotonin agonist δ-fenfluramine to patients with SAD reduces carbohydrate intake and the associated body mass gain. Delta-fenfluramine is also effective in reducing the depression associated with SAD (Wurtman et al., 1985).

Recall that serotonin is converted to melatonin in the pineal gland (see Chapter 2). Melatonin concentrations are higher during the night than during the day in both nocturnal and diurnal animals (see Chapter 10; Goldman, 1983). In humans, as in other mammals, phase-shifting of the light–dark cycle results in a comparable shift in the timing of the daily nighttime peak of melatonin secretion (Lewy et al., 1988). In a variety of mammals, including humans, the nocturnal synthesis and secretion of pineal melatonin can be rapidly inhibited by exposure to brief periods of light at night (Hoffmann et al., 1981; Illnerova and Vanecek, 1984; Lewy et al.,

1988). Thus light has two actions in humans, as it does in other mammals: (1) light can entrain, or synchronize, the daily melatonin rhythms, and (2) light can suppress daily melatonin secretion. Presumably, either or both effects of light might be involved in the therapeutic effects of bright light exposure in the treatment of SAD (Figure 13.7; Lewy et al., 1988, 1996; Wurtman and Wurtman, 1989).

Humans require high-intensity illumination to suppress nighttime melatonin secretion, in contrast to several other mammalian species, in which very low light intensities are capable of preventing pineal biosynthetic and secretory activity (see Chapter 10; Brainard et al., 1983). Illumination levels outdoors at temperate latitudes range between 12,000 and 100,000 lux (Benoit, 1964; Wurtman, 1975), while levels of artificial illumination indoors typically vary from 200 to 500 lux (Figure 13.8). The human visual system adapts rapidly to changing intensities of illumination; consequently, we may not perceive the light we encounter outdoors as being orders of magnitude brighter than indoor illumination. Physiologically, however, humans respond quite differently to the higher levels of illumination provided by exposure to sunlight. Exposure to 1500 lux or greater is necessary for the inhibition of human melatonin secretion (Lewy et al., 1980). This requirement may explain why normal indoor levels of artificial illumination are insufficient to relieve the symptoms of SAD; much brighter light must be used for effective treatment (Figure 13.9).

The depressive symptoms of SAD cause much human suffering. However, it must be emphasized that depression, however salient to the patient, physician, and family members, is only one of several foci of this seasonal disorder. Other

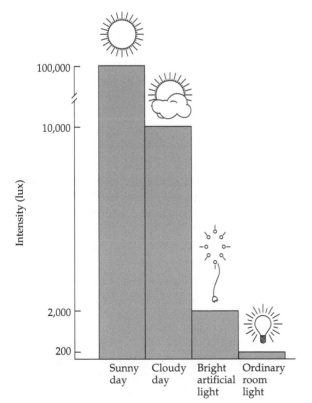

**13.8  Outdoor light is far brighter than artificial light.** Because our eyes adapt so quickly to different brightness levels, it is not apparent to us that outdoor light is generally several orders of magnitude brighter than that typically found indoors. Artificial indoor light is usually 200–500 lux, far below what is necessary to have a physiological effect on biological rhythms and mood. Bright sunlight in the mid-latitudes may be 100,000 lux in intensity. Even on a cloudy day, illumination levels outdoors usually exceed 10,000 lux. Source: OTA, 1991.

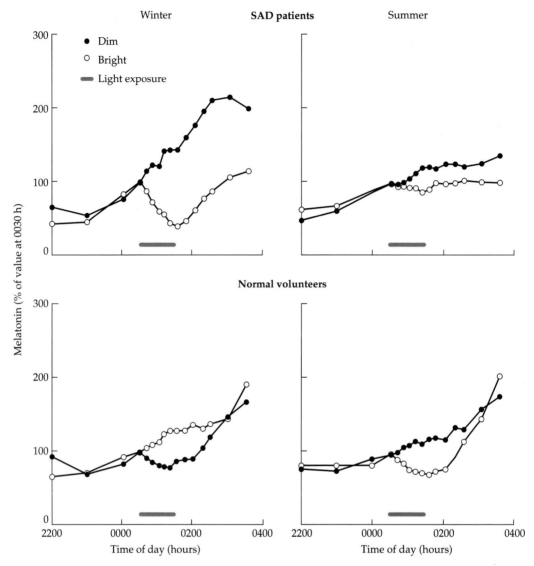

**13.9    Patterns of melatonin secretion in seasonal depression.** Melatonin secretion in winter and summer among SAD patients and normal volunteers in response to dim (500 lux; solid circles) and bright (2500 lux; open circles) illumination (shaded bars). Note that the elevated plasma levels of melatonin in SAD patients in winter are significantly reduced by bright illumination. Source: Thompson et al., 1990.

phenomena associated with the syndrome are increases in food intake, body mass, lethargy, and sleep bout length. A random sample of New York City residents indicated seasonal changes in all of these parameters, although these changes were less pronounced in the general population than in SAD patients (Terman, 1988). These seasonal changes may have evolved in order to provide for winter energy savings (e.g., Wirz-Justice et al., 1986). Thus, mild forms of depression may be part of an adaptive constellation of traits. In conjunction with this hypothesis, one might view SAD as an exaggerated form of this strategy.

It may be difficult to develop animal models for SAD. Because clinicians focus on the affective aspects of SAD, seasonally breeding animals may be an inappropriate model for SAD in humans (Zucker, 1988b). There have also been attempts to use other seasonal phenomena—hibernation, for example—as model systems to study the mechanisms of SAD (Mrosovsky, 1988). However, even among rodents, there are many different adaptive strategies for coping with seasonal environmental changes: some animals lose body mass in the autumn to reduce food requirements, while others increase autumnal body mass in order to create endogenous energy stores (see Chapter 9; Nelson, 1987). The nature and number of human seasonal cycles is still unknown; it may be prudent to reach a better understanding of human biological rhythms before animal models are developed.

As related above, it has been suggested that bright light therapy may relieve the symptoms of SAD via a mechanism that involves phase-shifting of circadian rhythms (Lewy et al., 1988, 1996). An alternative hypothesis is that supplementary light may act through a photoperiodic mechanism to alter a seasonal response (see Chapter 10; Kripke, 1981). This idea fits with the seasonal nature of SAD, particularly with the occurrence of the depression phase in the winter, when days are shortest. It is interesting to consider this hypothesis in conjunction with what is known about photoperiodic responses and seasonality in other mammals. First, in mammals, most overt responses to an abrupt change in day length require a period of several weeks (Goldman, 1983). This contrasts with the rapid ameliorative effect of bright light exposure in SAD patients. However, there are a few exceptions to this long time requirement in mammals; for example, immature Siberian hamsters exhibit changes in the rate of testis growth within 5 days after being shifted from long to short days (Carter and Goldman, 1983a). Second, several long-lived mammalian species exhibit the capacity for endogenous circannual rhythmicity, and in some of these animals photoperiod is an important synchronizer of circannual rhythms. Artificial manipulation of photoperiod can entrain circannual rhythms in these animals or induce them to display more than one complete cycle in a year (Gwinner, 1986). However, it is not possible to keep animals in one phase of the cycle indefinitely by manipulation of the photoperiod. Thus, if SAD is related to human circannual rhythmicity, it might be expected that light therapy would not eliminate or effectively reduce the total amount of depression experienced over the course of each annual cycle, but would rather rephase the onset of the depression.

Clearly, there are major gaps in our knowledge about SAD because there are virtually no data that bear directly on the question of whether humans are either photoperiodic or circannual. Nevertheless, the growing body of data from mammals with seasonal cycles may be useful in pointing the way to obtaining such information for humans and may eventually lead to effective pharmacological or behavioral treatments for SAD.

## Androgens and Affective Disorders

With the recent increase in anabolic steroid abuse, increasing reports of bizarre, hostile, and erratic behavior have been reported among men. Anabolic steroids enhance body tissue building processes and simultaneously retard or reverse tissue catabolism (see Chapter 9). The use of anabolic steroids by world-class athletes to improve their strength and performance has been widespread during the past two decades (Box 13.2) (Haupt and Rovere, 1984). This abuse has occurred despite the listing of anabolic steroids as "banned substances" by the United States Olympic Committee, the International Olympic Committee, the National Collegiate Athletic Association, and all North American professional sports organizations (Kibble and Ross, 1987). More recently, the abuse of anabolic steroids has become prevalent among recreational bodybuilders and competitive athletes in the 16–21-year-old cohort (Taylor and Black, 1987). More than a quarter of a million high school seniors in the United States are currently estimated to use anabolic steroids to enhance their athletic performance. Anabolic steroid abuse has also been reported among junior high school students (Moore, 1988). There is little evidence that anabolic steroids improve athletic performance or provide any sort of "competitive edge." Most individuals who use steroids begin to use them because they believe that their competitors are using them. People continue to use steroids because these substances cause psychological dependence and delusional thinking processes.

The health risks of chronic anabolic steroid use in adult men are well known. The adverse physiological effects of these steroids include liver, kidney, immune system, and endocrine dysfunction, as well as cardiovascular problems (Kibble and Ross, 1987; Wu, 1997). Many of the adverse effects of anabolic steroid use are irreversible. Notably, these adverse effects have been discovered primarily in patients using these substances for approved medical indications (such as anemia, congenital angioedema, senile or postmenopausal osteoporosis, corticosteroid-induced catabolism, or promotion of weight gain) at therapeutic doses (Limbird, 1985)—doses typically much lower than those taken by abusers of steroids.

Extrapolating the adverse consequences of therapeutic steroid use to predict the outcome of anabolic steroid abuse is difficult. Steroid abusers typically use several different agents simultaneously at doses many times higher than the maximum therapeutic doses. Also, the "stacking" and "cycling" treatment regimens used by many steroid abusers are quite different from the typical recommended therapeutic administration regimens (Perry et al., 1990). "Stacking" is bodybuilder's jargon for using two or more anabolic steroids at high dosages; usually a combination of oral and injectable forms is used (Kibble and Ross, 1987). Administration of the drugs is typically titrated upward, then downward over a 4–20 week period prior to a competitive event. Drug use is then suspended for several months; the drug-free and drug-use periods are called cycles (Strauss et al., 1985).

The adverse effects of steroid use are assumed to be worse among anabolic steroid abusers than among patients taking steroids at recommended therapeutic doses, but few data exist. Many ill effects of anabolic steroid abuse are probably never reported. Most steroids are obtained illegally, and users may fear legal penalties and competitive sanctions if their steroid use is discovered (Kibble and Ross, 1987). Some researchers have estimated that hundreds of millions of dollars are spent annually in the United States by over a million steroid abusers to obtain illegal anabolic steroids (Moore, 1988; Taylor and Black, 1987; Yesalis et al., 1997). The adverse medical effects of steroid abuse seem to increase as the age of abuse decreases (Moore, 1988; Middleman and DuRant, 1996; Yesalis et al., 1997). The most serious adverse medical consequence is cardiac hypertrophy. There have been several reports of young men with no previous medical complaints or histories of cardiac disease suffering fatal consequences; one report documents a 20-year-old

Box 13.2

# Anabolic Steroids: An Edge that Cuts Two Ways

According to a recent report issued by the National Institute on Drug Abuse, anabolic steroid abuse has reached epidemic proportions at all levels of athletic competition in North America. The problem came to public notice when Canadian sprinter Ben Johnson was stripped of his Olympic gold medal in 1988 after testing positive for anabolic steroids. His record-setting times for the 100-meter dash at the Seoul Olympics (9.79 seconds) and the 1987 World Track and Field Championship (9.83 seconds) were annulled. The current world record for the 100-meter is 9.84 seconds, set in 1996 by fellow Canadian sprinter Donovan Bailey. Johnson said that he did not believe he could run under 10 seconds without androgens. "If you've never used anything, just come to it natural, that's about my limit," said Johnson in a CNN interview shortly after American shot-putter Randy Barnes and sprinter Dennis Mitchell, as well as several Tour de France cyclists, tested positive for steroids.

More recently, it was disclosed that Mark McGwire, who hit a record 70 home runs during the 1998 professional baseball season, used androstenedione. Androstenedione, which can be converted to testosterone in the liver, is a legal over-the-counter strength enhancer. Although androstenedione is legal in professional baseball, it has been banned by the National Football League, the International Olympics Committee, and the National Collegiate Athletic Association. It is used in professional baseball to enhance performance and to speed healing after injury. McGwire defended his androgen use with the same arguments used by Ben Johnson: "Everybody that I know in the game of baseball uses the same stuff I use." The long-term effects of androstenedione on health are not known.

Lyle Alzado, one of the NFL's premier defensive players from the mid-1970s through the mid-1980s, was an imposing 150+ kg mass of muscle and mania. When he retired in 1986, he was recognized as one of the best ever at his position. Five years later, however, Alzado reappeared in the public eye with a startling admission—he had used anabolic steroids throughout his career, and had continued to use them after he retired from professional football, despite warnings from his physician. He also admitted that he had assaulted his wife while in a steroid-induced rage. Sadly, he announced that he was suffering from an incurable brain tumor that was probably caused by immunosuppression that resulted from anabolic steroid use. He crusaded against the use of anabolic steroids in amateur and professional sports during the remainder of his life. Alzado died on May 14, 1992, at the age of 43.

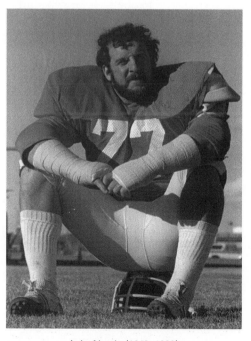

Lyle Alzado (1949–1992)

AP/Wide World Photos

bodybuilder who suffered sudden cardiac death after 1–2 years of anabolic steroid abuse (e.g., Dickerman et al., 1995; Huie, 1994; Mewis et al., 1996; Palfi et al., 1997). In young men abusing anabolic steroid hormones, sexual function is impaired (Moss et al., 1993), gynecomastia (breast development) occurs (Reyes et al., 1995), muscles can literally rupture (David et al., 1995), and immune function may become severely compromised, leading to cancer (e.g., Hughes et al., 1995, 1998).

Adverse behavioral effects of anabolic steroid abuse have also been reported (Malone et al., 1995). The best-known of these effects is the occurrence of extremely aggressive behavior, also known as "roids rage." Although some of the adverse physiological effects of steroid abuse may not be observed until many years after the cessation of steroid use, the onset of adverse behavioral effects may be relatively rapid, even at therapeutic doses. Oxymetholone is a 17-α-methyl testosterone derivative that is a common, orally administered treatment for anemia. One 18-year-old male treated with oxymetholone (150 mg/d) for idiopathic aplastic anemia developed a temporary elevation in aggression (Barker, 1987). Prior to treatment, the patient had not displayed any notable aggressive behavior. During the steroid treatment, however, he broke a friend's nose and also destroyed some personal property. As noted above, anabolic steroid abusers are exposed to much higher doses than those prescribed therapeutically. These high doses have been associated with violent aggression, often accompanied by affective and psychotic symptoms. The behavioral pathology of androgens can, for the most part, be avoided by avoiding pharmacological self-administration of anabolic steroids. However, the extent to which high endogenous androgen concentrations during adolescence evoke hyper-aggressiveness in human males remains unknown.

In one well-known study, researchers contacted gymnasiums and offered members using steroids a cash payment to engage in a confidential interview about their steroid use. The respondents reported routinely using doses 10–100 times higher than recommended therapeutic doses. Fifteen of the 41 individuals regularly using anabolic steroids reported experiencing major psychiatric symptoms; 13 other individuals became manic or near manic. One user, convinced of his immortality, drove a car into a tree at 65 kilometers per hour while a friend videotaped him (Pope and Katz, 1988). Most psychiatric symptoms subside when anabolic steroid use is discontinued. Unfortunately, no information is available on the long-term behavioral consequences of anabolic steroid abuse if the steroids were administered during puberty.

Anabolic steroid abuse has been associated with the perpetration of violent crimes (Canacher and Workman, 1989; Borowsky et al., 1997). Several individuals have impulsively committed homicides while taking anabolic steroids. Carefully structured interviews with the perpetrators suggest strongly that steroid abuse was an important, if not primary, factor in the manifestation of the extreme aggressive act in many such cases. Although the interviewed individuals may have emphasized the role of steroids in their violence to aid their legal positions, a consistent pattern of steroid-associated violence among previously nonaggressive individuals supports the possibility that these agents are involved in the mediation of violent behavior (Canacher and Workman, 1989; Orchard and Best, 1994).

Very few controlled studies of the effects of anabolic steroids on mood have been reported. In one study, healthy male volunteers consecutively received a placebo, a low dose (40 mg) of methyltestosterone, a high dose (240 mg) of methyltestosterone, and another placebo over the course of 3 days (Su et al., 1993). A number of neuropsychiatric measures were obtained, which showed that the high testosterone treatment caused positive changes in mood (e.g., euphoria, increased energy, and increased sexual arousal), as well as negative mood changes (e.g., irritability, mood swings, feelings of violence, and hostility) and cognitive impairments (e.g., distractability, confusion, and impaired memory) (Su et al., 1993). One of the 20 (i.e., 5% incidence) study participants became acutely manic, and another individual became hypomanic (i.e., 5% incidence). The results of this study indicate that even brief anabolic steroid use can affect mood in an adverse manner (Su et al., 1993). Elevated mood was not observed in another study using lower doses of anabolic steroids (50, 100, and 200 mg) (Fingerhood et al., 1997).

Recently, it has been suggested that a proportion of anabolic steroid abusers develop an addiction to steroids. This hypothesis is supported by the remarkable consistency with which anabolic steroid abusers fulfill the following commonly accepted criteria for psychoactive substance use disorder (Pope and Katz, 1990): (1) the steroids are used over longer periods than desired; (2) unsuccessful attempts to stop the steroid use occur; (3) substantial time is spent in procuring, using, or recovering from the effects of anabolic steroids; (4) use continues despite knowledge of the significant physical and behavioral problems it is causing; (5) characteristic withdrawal symptoms occur; and (6) more anabolic steroids are often taken to relieve the withdrawal symptoms (Kashkin and Kleber, 1989). These last two criteria in particular suggest that anabolic steroids might have direct reward properties similar to the reinforcing effects of drugs such as cocaine, amphetamines, morphine, and heroin (Shippenberg and Herz, 1987). Increasing reports of suicides in previously nondepressed young men who abruptly stop using anabolic steroids have been noted. These tragic events appear to be linked with the constellation of symptoms that resemble withdrawal symptoms. Thus, the withdrawal symptoms manifested by anabolic steroid abusers and the symptoms of PMS or postpartum depression may result from a common underlying cause; namely, dependence upon elevated steroid hormone concentrations. Additional research is required to ascertain the veracity of this hypothesis.

Recent studies have attempted to quantify the effects of prolonged androgen treatment in animals. In mice, male aggression was not affected by long-term pharmacological treatment with four different androgenic steroids; however, female aggression was significantly elevated by androgen treatment (Bronson, 1996). In an experiment that was designed to model the use of androgens by human teenagers, male hamsters were exposed to prolonged androgen treatment during adolescence. When these animals were tested in an intruder-resident aggression paradigm, they displayed elevated aggressiveness in the absence of elevated body mass (Melloni et al., 1997).

Importantly, exposure to anabolic steroids shortens the life span of male mice (Bronson and Matherne, 1997). Animals that received one of four anabolic steroids for 6 months were maintained in the laboratory for at least a year after the end of androgen treatment. Approximately 90% of control mice, which received no exogenous steroid treatment, survived to 20 months of age. About 50% and 65% of the mice receiving anabolic steroid treatment at 5 or 20 times normal androgen blood concentrations, respectively, survived to 20 months of age (Bronson and Matherne, 1997).

## Summary

- In addition to overt behavior, hormones also affect mood. Animal models are usually not useful for studying the effects of hormones on mood. Studies of humans that correlate mood changes with endocrine events are more useful for this purpose; the effects of endocrine manipulations on mood can then be assessed.

- Perimenstrual syndrome (PMS) is a cluster of physiological, behavioral, and mood symptoms that appear to be linked; these symptoms are associated with the normal changes in steroid hormone concentrations accompanying the menstrual cycle.

- PMS is a controversial research topic. Its prevalence, defining symptoms, and timing of symptoms, as well as its psychological and endocrinological correlates, remain unresolved. Feminist social scientists have noted that the medicalization of menstruation places women in a "sick" role and questions their competence. The vast majority of research has not detected any significant impairments in women's functioning due to PMS.

- The symptoms of PMS appear to cluster into four subtypes, and it is likely that different endocrine correlates underlie the different subtypes.

- Because most mood changes of PMS occur during the late luteal phase, when blood concentrations of progesterone are increasing, many studies have examined the role of progesterone in mediating PMS symptoms. Progesterone treatment does not consistently affect the prevalence of PMS symptoms. Estrogen treatment also does not consistently ameliorate PMS symptoms. Curiously, most medical treatments for PMS are aimed at correcting some putative endocrine "abnormality" associated with the late luteal phase of the menstrual cycle. However, even pharmacological elimination of the entire luteal phase does not affect PMS symptoms.

- Dietary factors, including carbohydrate and calcium intake, can interact with hormones to influence PMS symptoms.

- A significant minority of women report positive changes in mood associated with the perimenstrual phase. The endocrine correlates of these positive mood changes are poorly understood.

- Depression is often evoked by endocrine changes. The symptoms of depression include reduced mood, low self-esteem, general fatigue, feelings of guilt, sleep disturbances, anger, irritability, and reductions in sexual motivation and food consumption.

- TRH or TSH administration can ameliorate depressive symptoms. GH and prolactin are also linked to depression. Cortisol has also been implicated in depression; nearly half of depressed patients exhibit elevated cortisol production. These endocrine data suggest that depressed patients may have experienced an alteration in the neuroendocrine mechanisms underlying the hormone feedback control systems of the HPA axis. It remains unclear whether the changes in hormone concentrations are the cause or the result of the depressed mood.

• Estrogen deficits are also associated with depression. Estrogen replacement therapy can elevate mood in depressed women.

• Postpartum depression is a well-known subtype of depression that probably reflects adjustments to parenting rather than endocrine changes.

• Seasonal affective disorder (SAD) is characterized by depressed mood, lethargy, loss of libido, excess sleep, body mass increase, carbohydrate cravings, anxiety, and lack of concentration during autumn and winter. Bright lights have been used to alleviate depression; it is thought that they produce this effect by resetting biological clocks as well as providing a nonspecific "energizing" influence. Bright lights appear to work by affecting melatonin release patterns.

• Androgens are increasingly abused by men and boys to enhance body muscle mass and athletic performance. There is little evidence that anabolic steroids improve athletic performance or provide any sort of "competitive edge." Most individuals begin to use steroids because they believe that their competitors are probably using them. The health risks are very high; adverse medical effects of anabolic steroid abuse include liver, kidney, cardiovascular, and endocrine dysfunction.

• Adverse behavioral effects of anabolic steroid abuse include hyperaggressiveness (including murder) as well as a number of major psychiatric symptoms. Mania or hypomania is common among abusers of androgens.

• Anabolic steroid abusers may develop an addiction to these steroids. Characteristic withdrawal symptoms occur, and severe depression and suicide have been reported in individuals with no previous mental health problems who suddenly stopped using steroids. Exposure to high steroid concentrations may also account for some of the psychological symptoms associated with PMS and postpartum depression.

## Questions for Discussion

1. Given what you know about the effects of hormones on behavior, should people be able to use "hormonal state" (for example, anabolic steroid abuse, postpartum depression, PMS) as a defense against criminal behavior? Why or why not?

2. What are some minimum criteria that need to be established in order to describe and ultimately treat PMS?

3. Are the mood effects associated with menstruation any more dramatic than the mood swings that men experience? How would you address this question experimentally?

4. How is SAD like hibernation in nonhuman animals? How is it different? Are hibernation studies useful in understanding the mood changes associated with SAD?

## Suggested Readings

Brown-Parlee, M., 1982. Changes in moods and activation levels during the menstrual cycle. *Psychology of Women Quarterly*, 7: 119–131.

Demers, L. M., McGuire, J. L., Phillips, A., and Rubinow, D. R. 1989. *Premenstrual, Postpartum, and Menopausal Mood Disorders*. Urban and Schwarzenberg, Baltimore, MD.

Pearlstein, T. and Stone, A. B. 1998. Premenstrual syndrome. *Psychiatric Clinics of North America*, 21: 577–590.

Porcerelli, J. H. and Sandler, B. A. 1998. Anabolic–androgenic steroid abuse and psychopathology. *Psychiatric Clinics of North America*, 21: 829–833.

Rosenthal, N. E., Sack, D. A., Skwerer, R. G., Jacobsen, F. M., and Wehr, T. A. 1988. Phototherapy for seasonal affective disorder. *Journal of Biological Rhythms*, 3: 101–120.

Ruble, D. N. 1977. Premenstrual symptoms: A reinterpretation. *Science*, 187: 291–292.

Wurtman, R. J. and Wurtman, J. J. 1989. Carbohydrates and depression. *Scientific American*, 262: 68–75.

# Glossary

**Ablation**   Removal, especially by cutting.

**Active avoidance**   A type of learning in which an individual must perform an action to avoid a noxious situation.

**Adaptive function**   The role of any structural, physiological, or behavioral process that increases an individual's fitness to survive and reproduce as compared with other conspecifics.

**Adipose tissue**   Connective tissue in which fat is stored.

**Adrenal cortex**   The outer layer(s) of the endocrine organ that sits above the kidneys in vertebrates and secretes steroid hormones.

**Adrenal glands**   Paired, dual-compartment endocrine glands in vertebrates consisting of a medulla and a cortex. Epinephrine and norepinephrine are secreted from the medulla, and steroid hormones are released from the cortex.

**Adrenal medulla**   The inner portion of the endocrine organ that sits above the kidneys in vertebrates and secretes epinephrine and norepinephrine.

**Affiliation**   A form of social behavior that involves an individual's motivation to approach and remain in close proximity with a conspecific.

**Aggression**   A form of social interaction that includes threat, attack, and fighting.

**Agonist**   A chemical substance that binds to receptors for a hormone or neurotransmitter and causes a biological response that is indistinguishable from the response elicited by the natural hormone or neurotransmitter. Also called a mimic.

**Agonistic**   Any behavior associated with fighting including aggression, submission, or retreat.

**Aldosterone**   A mineralocorticoid that causes the kidneys to retain sodium.

**Allelle**   A specific version of a gene.

**Alloparents**   Parental assistants; in birds, older male siblings that do not disperse, but remain at the nest site to assist the parents with the rearing of the current young.

**Altricial**   Born or hatched at an early stage of development. Altricial offspring are generally quite helpless, and require substantial parental care to survive.

**Amnestic**   A substance or event that causes forgetting.

**Amplitude**   In biological rhythms, the amount of change in the rhythm above (to the peak) or below (to the nadir) the average value.

**Amygdala**   An almond-shaped structure located near the base of each temporal lobe of the brain. The amygdala is critical for the integration of sensory information that is important in sexual behavior.

**Anastomosis**   The joining together of two circulatory systems.

**Androgen insensitivity**   *See* Testicular feminization mutation.

**Androgens**   Any of the $C_{19}$ class of steroid hormones, so named because of their andros- (male) generating effects. Androgens are the primary steroidal product secreted from the testes. Testosterone and dihydrotestosterone are biologically important androgens.

**Androstenedione**   The primary sex hormone secreted by the human adrenal cortex.

**Anestrus (n); anestrous (adj)**   The reproductive condition of a female mammal that is not in estrus, or mating condition.

**Angiotensin II**   A parahormone that is produced in the blood by the actions of renin and angiotensinogen; it may be involved in the regulation of water balance and thirst.

**Anlage**   The primordial substrate in a developing individual.

**Antagonist**   A chemical substance that binds to receptors for a hormone or neurotransmitter, but does not cause a biological response. Also called a blocker.

**Anterior pituitary**   Front part of the endocrine gland that extends from the base of the brain and secretes a number of tropic hormones in response to hormonal signals from the hypothalamus.

**Antiamnestic**   A substance that protects against forgetting.

**Antidiuretic hormone (ADH)**   A hormone secreted from the anterior pituitary that regulates removal of water from the blood via the kidneys. Also called vasopressin.

**Apoptosis**   Programmed, orderly cell death that avoids immune system activation.

**Appetitive learning**   Reinforcement of a behavior by a positive outcome.

**Appetitive phase**   An ethological term, roughly equivalent to "courtship." All the behaviors an individual displays when attempting to gain access to an individual of the opposite sex for the purpose of mating.

**Arcuate nucleus**   A hypothalamic nucleus located near the base of the hypothalamus that contains the cell bodies of many neurons that secrete hypothalamic releasing hormones.

**Aromatase**   An enzyme that converts androgens into estrogens.

**Aromatization**   The process of converting an androgen molecule to an estrogen molecule via the enzyme aromatase. The removal of the carbon at position 19 from the androgen precursors results in an estrogen with a phenolic A-ring, which is known as an aromatic compound.

**Associated reproductive pattern**   The breeding pattern observed in most vertebrate species, in which reproductive behavior, maximal gonadal size and activity, high steroid concentrations, and gamete production coincide.

**Attractivity**   The stimulus value of a female for a particular male. Attractivity is a hypothetical construct that must be inferred by observation of a conspecific's behavior.

**Autocrine**   Pertaining to a signal secreted by a cell into the environment that affects the transmitting cell.

**Autoradiography**   A technique used to detect a radiolabeled substance, such as a hormone, in a cell or organism, by placing a thin slice of the material in contact with a photographic emulsion, which displays darkened silver grains in response to the radioactive emissions.

**Aversive learning**   A change in behavior to avoid some noxious outcome.

**Basal metabolic rate (BMR)**   Rate of metabolism at rest.
**Base**   A building block of DNA or RNA molecules. DNA contains four different bases (adenine, thymine, guanine, and cytosine), which form pairs that link the two strands of DNA together. The order of the bases provides the genetic information of the DNA molecule.
**Behavioral sex**   The sex of an individual as discriminated on the basis of male-typical and female-typical behaviors.
**Bioassay**   The use of a biological response to determine the presence or amount of a particular substance in a sample.
**Biochronometry**   *See* Chronobiology.
**Biological half-life**   The amount of time required to remove half of a hormone or other substance from the blood.
**Blastocyst**   A fluid-filled sphere of cells that develops from a zygote. The embryo usually develops from the cluster of cells in the center of the blastocyst, whereas the external wall of the blastocyst develops into the placenta.
**Blocker**   *See* Antagonist.
**Blood–brain barrier (BBB)**   The mechanism of blood vessels in the brain that prevents toxic substances from diffusing into the brain.
**Blot tests**   Techniques used to fractionate mixtures of proteins (Western), DNAs (Southern), or RNAs (Northern) so they can hybridize with markers that travel different distances in an electrophoretic gel based on their size.
**Bruce effect**   The interruption of pregnancy caused by the odors of a strange male.

**Cannulation**   A technique in which hollow electrodes or fine tubes (cannulas) are inserted into specific brain regions or into specific blood vessels, so that substances can be introduced precisely into a particular place or a blood sample obtained from a specific location.
**Castration**   The surgical removal of the gonads. Synonymous with gonadectomy in both sexes, and with orchidectomy in males and ovariectomy or oophorectomy in females.
**Catecholamines**   Hormones (e.g., epinephrine, norepinephrine) that are derived from tyrosine and secreted primarily from the adrenal medulla.
**Chimera**   An animal whose tissues are composed of two or more genetically distinct cell types; also called a mosaic.
**Cholecystokinin (CCK)**   A hormone released by the lining of the small intestine that may be involved in satiation of food intake.
**Chromosomal sex**   The sex of an individual as determined by the sex chromosomes that individual receives at fertilization.
**Chronobiology**   The study of biological clocks and their associated rhythms. Also called biochronometry.
**Circadian rhythm**   A biological rhythm with a period of about 24 hours.
**Circalunar rhythm**   A biological rhythm with a period of about 29.5 days that is closely tied to phases of the moon.
**Circannual rhythm**   A biological rhythm with a period of about 12 months.
**Circatidal rhythm**   A biological rhythm with a period of about 12.4 hours that is closely tied to changes in tides.
**Cloaca**   The external sexual organ in birds. Males discharge sperm through the cloaca; female lay eggs through it.
**Colloid**   A relatively large molecule that cannot pass through cell membranes. When injected under the skin or into the perineum, it draws in fluids by osmotic pressure.

**Concaveation**   The process of becoming sensitized to newborn animals so that full maternal behavior is expressed. Also called pup induction or sensitization.
**Congenital adrenal hyperplasia (CAH)**   A genetic deficiency that results in the overproduction of androgens by the adrenal glands. This syndrome has no reported ill effects in males, but causes various degrees of masculinization of the external genitalia in females, which may lead to erroneous assignment of sex at birth.
**Consummatory phase**   An ethological term that encompasses the completion of a motivated behavior. In terms of sexual behavior, copulation represents the consummatory phase.
**Corpus luteum**   An endocrine structure that forms from the remnants of the ovarian follicle after the egg is released. The corpus luteum secretes progestins, which support the uterine lining in preparation for blastocyst implantation.
**Corticoids**   A class of $C_{21}$ steroid hormones secreted primarily from the adrenal cortices. There are two main types of corticoids: glucocorticoids and mineralocorticoids.
**Corticosterone**   Glucocorticoid produced in the adrenal cortices of most rodents and birds.
**Courtship**   A system of communication that is used by one sex to induce mating in a receiving conspecific. Information about species, sex, physiological condition, and readiness to mate is exchanged during courtship.
**Crepuscular**   Active at dawn and dusk.
**Crop milk**   A prolactin-dependent substance discharged from the epithelial cells lining the crop in pigeons and doves, which is regurgitated to feed the young.
**Cytokine**   A protein chemical messenger that evokes the proliferation of other cells, especially in the immune system. Examples of cytokines are interleukins and interferons.

**Decidual reaction**   The formation of a deciduomata in the uterine wall. This process indicates that the corpora lutea are producing sufficient progestins to support implantation of blastocysts and it provides good evidence of pseudopregnancy.
**Deciduomata**   A small vascular structure that forms in the uterine wall to support an implanting blastocyst.
**Defeminization**   The removal of the potential for female traits.
**Demasculinization**   The removal of the potential for male traits.
**2-deoxyglucose (2-DG)**   A molecular mimic of glucose that provides no nutritional value. Cells that are actively working accumulate more 2-DG than inactive cells. If 2-DG is marked with a radioactive or immunoreactive tag, active neurons can be visualized.
**Deoxyribonucleic acid (DNA)**   A nucleic acid that codes hereditary information.
**Detection threshold**   The concentration at which an individual can tell the difference between two substances or stimuli.
**Diabetes insipidus**   A condition characterized by the failure of the kidneys to retain water because of a lack of antidiuretic hormone. Symptoms include excessive urination, thirst, and water intake.
**Diabetes mellitus**   A condition characterized by impaired glucose regulation because of reduced insulin secretion. Symptoms include high blood sugar levels and excessive urination, thirst, and water intake.
**Dimorphic**   Having two different forms; usually used regarding differences between the two sexes.

**Dissociated reproductive pattern**    A breeding pattern observed in some vertebrate species in which reproductive behavior does not coincide with maximal gonadal size and activity. Instead, copulation occurs when steroid levels and gamete production are low.

**Diurnal**    Active during the day.

**Dopamine**    A neurotransmitter produced primarily in the forebrain and diencephalon that acts in the basal ganglia, olfactory system, and some parts of the cerebral cortex.

**Down-regulation**    A process that is similar to negative feedback in which the overproduction of a hormone causes occupation of virtually all available receptors so that subsequent high levels of hormones cannot have a biological effect.

**Ejaculation**    The forceful expulsion of semen from a male's body via the urethra.

**Electrical stimulation**    Activation of nerve cells by electrical current.

**Embryo**    A term used to describe the stage of development in mammals from implantation of the blastocyst until organ function begins to specialize. Embryonic development begins 1 week after conception in humans and continues until 9 weeks after conception.

**Endocrine gland**    A ductless gland from which hormones are released into the blood system in response to specific physiological signals.

**Endocrinology**    The scientific study of the endocrine glands and their hormones.

**Endogenous**    Relating to a substance or process within the organism.

**Endometrium**    The tissue lining the uterus into which a blastocyst implants.

**Endorphin**    A hormone that acts as an endogenous opioid and binds the same receptors as morphine.

**Entrainment**    The synchronization of biological rhythms to a periodic environmental cue.

**Enzymoimmunoassay (EIA)**    An assay that uses the principle of competitive binding of an antibody to its antigen to determine the presence or quantity of a biological substance such as a hormone.

**Epinephrine**    A catecholamine produced in the adrenal medulla that increases cardiac tone and glucose levels.

**Estradiol**    The primary estrogenic steroid hormone produced by mammalian ovaries.

**Estrogen**    Any of the $C_{18}$ class of steroid hormones, so named because of their estrus-generating properties in female mammals. Biologically important estrogens include estradiol, estrone, and estriol.

**Estrous cycle**    A recurrent cycle between mating and non-mating conditions.

**Estrus**    The period during which female mammals will permit copulation.

**Eutherian mammal**    The subclass of mammals that possess a placenta during pregnancy.

**Evolutionary approach**    The perspective(s) adopted by biologists who assume that evolutionary processes are central to issues in ecology, systematics, and behavior.

**Exocrine gland**    A gland that has a duct through which its product is secreted into adjacent organs or the environment. Examples of exocrine glands include the salivary, sweat, and mammary glands.

**Exocytosis**    The extrusion or secretion of substances from a cell by the fusion of a vesicle membrane with the cell membrane. The vesicle contains the material to be extruded from the cell. This process occurs during hormone secretion and neurotransmitter release.

**Exogenous**    Relating to a subject or process outside the organism.

**Extirpation**    The complete surgical removal of a gland or other organ.

**Fallopian tubes**    Tubes that connect the ovary to the uterus. Ova travel down the fallopian tubes after ovulation, and fertilization normally occurs in these tubes.

**False negative**    A testing error in which an affected individual is reported to be unaffected.

**False positive**    A testing error in which an unaffected individual is reported to be affected.

**Feminization**    The induction of female traits.

**Fertilization**    The penetration of an egg by a sperm with the subsequent combination of paternal and maternal DNA.

**Fetus**    In humans, the stage of development that begins about 9 weeks after conception and continues until birth. The process of sexual differentiation begins in humans as embryos become fetuses.

**Flehmen response**    A stereotyped behavior exhibited by males of many ungulate (hoofed) species when sexually excited. This response is observed after the male investigates a female's anogenital region and consists of extending the neck and curling the upper lip to reveal the upper gums, which allows the female chemosignal to be delivered to the vomeronasal organ.

**Follicle**    An epithelial cell-lined sac or compartment of the thyroid gland, ovary, or other structure. Thyroid follicles are filled with colloidal material that contains thyroid hormones. In the ovary, each follicle contains an ovum. As the follicle and ovum mature, cells lining the follicle produce estrogens that regulate ovulation; after ovulation, the follicle develops into another endocrine structure called the corpus luteum.

**Follicle-stimulating hormone (FSH)**    A gonadotropic hormone from the anterior pituitary that stimulates follicle development in females and sperm production in males.

**Follicular phase**    The portion of the primate menstrual cycle that begins at the end of menstruation and ends at ovulation, characterized by high blood levels of estrogens and the development of follicles.

**Freemartin**    A (usually) sterile female calf that is born as a twin to a male.

**Free-running rhythm**    A biological rhythm that is not synchronized to its natural zeitgeber and expresses its own endogenous rhythm.

**Frequency**    The number of completed cycles per unit of time; for example, two cycles per month.

**G proteins**    A class of proteins located adjacent to the intracellular part of a hormone or neurotransmitter receptor that are activated when an appropriate ligand binds to the receptor.

**Gametic sex**    The sex of an individual as determined by the production of ova by females and sperm by males.

**Gender identity**    The psychological self-perception of being either male or female.

**Gender role**    The collection of behaviors and attitudes that are considered appropriate or normal within a specific culture for each sex.

**Genital tubercle**    The region of the embryo that develops into male or female genitalia. Because there is a single anlage for the genitalia, development of one type of genitalia is at the expense of the other. In humans, this developmental process begins about 6 weeks after conception.

**Genotype**   The sum of all the genetic information that an individual has inherited.

**Germinal ridge**   A thickened ridge of tissue on the ventro-medial surface of each mesonephros of an embryo that has the potential to develop into either a testis or an ovary. If the cortex of the ridge develops, an ovary forms; if the medulla develops, a testis is produced.

**Glucocorticoids**   One of the two types of corticoids secreted from the adrenal cortices. Glucocorticoids are involved in carbohydrate metabolism and are often released in response to stressful stimuli.

**Gluconeogenesis**   The production of glucose from amino acids, a process that occurs in the liver in response to mild fasting.

**Glycogenolysis**   The breakdown of stored glycogen in the liver or muscles to provide a steady supply of glucose for energy.

**Gonad**   An endocrine organ that produces sex steroids and gametes; the ovaries and testes are gonads.

**Gonadal sex**   The sex of an individual as determined by the possession of either ovaries or testes. Females have ovaries, whereas males have testes.

**Gonadectomy**   The surgical removal of the gonads; also known as castration.

**Gonadotropin**   A hormone from the anterior pituitary (luteinizing hormone and follicle-stimulating hormone) or placenta (human chorionic hormone) that stimulates steroid production and gamete maturation in the gonads.

**Gonadotropin-releasing hormone (GnRH)**   A decapeptide hormone from the hypothalamus that regulates FSH and LH release from the anterior pituitary.

**Granulosa cells**   The monolayer of flattened epithelial cells that surrounds the immature ova.

**Growth hormone (GH)**   A protein hormone that stimulates somatic (body) growth. GH, however, does not directly induce growth of the skeleton; it stimulates the production of growth-regulating substances called somatomedins by the liver, kidneys, and other tissues. Somatomedins cause bone to take up sulfates, leading to growth. GH and somatomedins also stimulate protein synthesis.

**Habituation**   A simple type of learning that involves a loss of response after repeated exposures to a stimulus.

**Hermaphrodite**   An individual who possesses both ovaries and testes. In some species, the possession of both types of gonads occurs simultaneously, whereas in other species it occurs sequentially.

**Hippocampus**   A paired structure of the cerebral hemispheres, found curled in the basal medial area of the temporal lobes, which is thought to be involved in learning and memory.

**Homeostasis**   The maintenance of a steady state within an organism by means of physiological or behavioral feedback control mechanisms.

**Hormone**   An organic chemical messenger released from endocrine cells that travels through the blood system to interact with cells at some distance away and causes a biological response.

**Hypophysectomy**   Surgical removal of the hypophysis, or pituitary gland.

**Hypothalamus**   A part of the diencephalon located just below the thalamus that is important in the regulation of autonomic and endocrine functions. The hypothalamus consists of several collections of nerve cell bodies, called nuclei, and regulates endocrine function by releasing neu-rohormones into the hypothalamic–pituitary portal system and by releasing hormones into the circulation of the posterior pituitary gland.

**Hypovolemia**   The state of low blood volume.

**Immediate causation**   The physiological mechanism(s) underlying behavior.

**Immunocytochemistry**   A technique that uses antibodies to determine the location of a hormone or hormone receptor in the body. Antibodies linked to marker molecules, such as fluorescent dyes, are introduced into tissues dissected from animal, where they bind to the hormone or neurotransmitter of interest.

**Impotence**   A sexual dysfunction characterized by the inability to achieve or maintain a penile erection sufficient for intercourse. Also called erectile dysfunction.

**In situ hybridization**   A technique in which nucleic acid probes are used to locate specific nucleic acids (DNA in chromosomes and RNA in cells). The probes form a hybrid with the nucleic acid of interest and can be visualized by autoradiography or by chemical means.

**Infradian rhythm**   A biological rhythm that has a period greater than a day, but shorter than a month (or a frequency greater than once per day).

**Insulin**   A protein hormone that regulates glucose uptake by all cells in the body (except the brain).

**Internal desynchronization**   The loss of synchronization among biological rhythms within an organism.

**Interstitial nuclei of the anterior hypothalamus (INAH)**   Four regions of neuronal cell bodies in the anterior hypothalamus and preoptic area of humans. Sex differences have been reported in INAH-2 and INAH-3. INAH-1 has been considered to be equivalent to the SDN-POA in rats.

**Intromission**   The entrance of the penis into the vagina.

**Islets of Langerhans**   Islands of endocrine tissue nested throughout the exocrine tissue of the pancreas. There are four different cell types among the islets of Langerhans, each of which secretes a different type of protein hormone.

**Kallmann syndrome**   A congenital condition in humans characterized by the inability to smell and lack of gonadal development, caused by a lack of olfactory bulb development and GnRH cell migration from the bulbs to their normal location in the hypothalamus during early development.

**Klinefelter syndrome**   A congenital condition in humans in which individuals possess an extra X chromosome (XXY) and are externally and internally masculinized. Klinefelter syndrome occurs approximately once in every 600 live births in North America.

**Knockout**   An individual, usually a mouse, in which a specific gene has been inactivated.

**Lactation**   The process of making milk in female mammals.

**Latency**   The time delay before the onset of the behavior of interest.

**Lateralization**   The tendency for the neural substrate for cognitive skills to be confined to one cerebral hemisphere; also called cerebral specialization.

**Learning**   An adaptive change in behavior that results from experience.

**Lee–Boot effect**   A suppression of estrous cycles in mice due to overcrowding that is mediated by olfactory information.

**Legal sex** The official designation of sex, which is heavily influenced by morphological sex at birth, but is also influenced by chromosomal and gonadal sex.

**Leptin** A protein hormone secreted by fat cells that may communicate information to the brain about body fat content.

**Lesion** Damage to an area, such as a brain region, that is caused by accident, disease, or experimental procedure.

**Levels of analysis** The set of overlapping and interacting questions about behavior that span different types of approaches, including immediate causation, development, evolution, and adaptive function.

**Leydig cells** The interstitial cells between the seminiferous tubules in the testes that produce androgens in response to luteinizing hormone from the anterior pituitary.

**Ligand** A substance that binds to a receptor molecule.

**Lipolysis** The breakdown of adipose tissue into free fatty acids.

**Lordosis** A female sexually receptive posture in which the hindquarters are raised and the tail is deflected to facilitate copulation.

**Luteal phase** The portion of the primate menstrual cycle that begins at ovulation and continues until the onset of menstruation, and is characterized by corpora luteal function and high blood levels of progesterone.

**Luteinizing hormone (LH)** A gonadotropin from the anterior pituitary that promotes formation of the corpora lutea in females and testosterone production in males.

**Lux** A unit of illumination equal to the direct illumination of a 1-meter surface by a uniform point source of 1 candle intensity.

**Marsupial** A mammal belonging to the subclass Metatheria that lacks a placenta, such as opossums and most Australian mammals. Most marsupials have a pouch (marsupium) in which the mammary glands are located and the young are transported.

**Masculinization** The induction of male traits.

**Maternal aggression** A type of aggressive behavior observed among new mothers when they fiercely defend their young from intruders.

**Maternal behavior** Parental behavior performed by the mother or another female.

**Mating** The behavioral process of bringing the two sex gamete types together for fertilization; i.e., copulation.

**Medial preoptic area** *See* Preoptic area.

**Meiosis** The process of gamete formation, in which each new haploid cell receives half of the chromosomes in the somatic cells.

**Melatonin** An indole amine hormone released by the pineal gland.

**Memory** The encoding, storage, and retrieval of information about past experience.

**Menopause** The cessation of menstrual cycles in women following the depletion of eggs from the ovary.

**Menstrual cycle** The cyclic changes in hormone levels observed in women and other female primates that are associated with changes in ovarian follicular and luteal activity.

**Menstruation** The sloughing off of the endometrial lining of the uterus in women during a nonpregnant menstrual cycle. The corkscrew-shaped blood vessels that remain after the endometrial lining is shed leak blood into the uterine lumen.

**Metabolic fuels** The normal sources of energy for individuals, usually consisting of simple sugars (e.g., glucose), fatty acids, ketone bodies, and amino acids.

**Mineralocorticoids** One of the two types of corticoids secreted from the adrenal cortices. Aldosterone is the most important mineralocorticoid secreted by terrestrial vertebrates, and is important in ion exchange and water metabolism.

**Mitosis** The process of division of somatic cells that involves the duplication of DNA.

**Monotreme** A primitive egg-laying mammal, such as the duck-billed platypus and spiny anteater.

**Morphological sex** The sex of an individual as determined by body form.

**Mounting** A behavior observed among males of many species with internal fertilization in which the male assumes a copulatory position, but does not insert his penis (or other intromittive organ) into the female's vagina (or urogenital opening). This behavior is androgen-dependent.

**Müllerian ducts** A duct system present in both sexes during embryonic development that connects the gonads to the exterior. During normal development, the Müllerian duct system develops into the accessory sex organs in females and regresses in males.

**Negative feedback** A regulatory system that tends to stabilize a process when its effects are pronounced by reducing its rate or output. A thermostat works on the principle of negative feedback to keep temperature within a certain range.

**Neuroendocrinology** The scientific study of the interaction between the nervous system and the endocrine system.

**Neurohormone** A hormone that is released into the blood from a neuron rather than from an endocrine gland.

**Nocturnal** Active at night.

**Nucleus (pl. nuclei)** A collection of nerve cell bodies in the brain.

**Ontogeny** The development or course of development of an individual.

**Opiates** A class of compounds that exert opium-like effects, including pain insensitivity.

**Opioids** Peptide hormones located throughout the brain that bind to opiate receptors.

**Orexinics** Protein hormones found in the lateral hypothalamus that may trigger feeding.

**Organizational/activational hypothesis** The proposal that early androgen exposure permanently organizes the nervous system of mammals in a male-like manner. After pre- or perinatal organization by androgens, these hormones more readily activate male-typical postpubertal behaviors by acting upon the organized structures.

**Oscillator** A self-sustained biological timekeeper that functions in constant conditions.

**Osmolality** The concentration of solutes in a solution.

**Osmoregulation** The physiological and behavioral control of osmolality.

**Osmosis** Process of movement of a solvent through a semipermeable membrane (e.g., a living cell) into a solution of higher solute concentration that tends to equalize the concentrations of solute on the two sides of the membrane.

**Osmotic thirst** Motivation to consume water caused by increased osmolality in the brain.

**Ovariectomy** The surgical removal of the ovaries.

**Ovary** The female gonad, which produces estrogens, progestins, and ova.

**Ovulation**   The release of a mature egg (ovum) from the ovary. Ovulation may occur spontaneously in response to a specific hormonal milieu or as a direct result of stimuli associated with copulation.

**Ovum**   A haploid female gamete.

**Oxytocin**   A peptide hormone secreted by the posterior pituitary that triggers milk letdown in lactating females and may be involved in other reproductive behaviors.

**Pacemaker**   An oscillator that regulates some physiological or behavioral function.

**Pancreas**   A composite vertebrate gland with both endocrine and exocrine functions. In humans, the pancreas is located within the curve of the duodenum behind the stomach and liver, and secretes digestive enzymes (exocrine function), insulin, glucagon, and somatostatin (endocrine function), as well as bicarbonate.

**Parathyroid gland**   In humans and most other eutherian mammals, four to eight islands of separate endocrine tissue associated with the thyroid gland. The parathyroid gland secretes parathyroid hormone, which increases blood calcium levels and decreases blood phosphate levels.

**Paraventricular nucleus**   A collection of cell bodies in the hypothalamus that produce vasopressin and oxytocin. These hormones are transported down the cells' axons for release from the posterior pituitary.

**Parental behavior**   Behaviors performed in relation to one's offspring that contribute directly to the survival of fertilized eggs or offspring that have left the body of the female.

**Parthenogenesis**   A type of asexual reproduction in which eggs can develop into offspring without fertilization.

**Parturition**   The process of giving birth in mammals.

**Passive avoidance**   A type of learning in which an individual must suppress some behavior that would otherwise be exhibited.

**Paternal behavior**   Parental behavior performed by the father or another male.

**Perception**   The transduction of sensory information entering the nervous system into biologically useful information.

**Perimenstrual syndrome (PMS)**   A constellation of symptoms, including anxiety, depression, moodiness, and fatigue, that recurs on a cyclical basis and is associated with menstruation.

**Period**   The length of time required to complete one cycle of a rhythm, such as the amount of time between peaks in a cycle.

**Permissive effect**   The process by which one hormone induces the production of receptors for a second hormone, or otherwise brings about the conditions necessary for the second hormone to be effective.

**Phase**   A point in a rhythm relative to some objective time point during the cycle, or during the cycle of another rhythm.

**Phase-response curve**   A graphic representation of the differential effects that a periodic environmental cue (usually light) has on the timing of biological rhythms

**Pheromone**   A chemical signal produced in one individual (the sender) that can alter the physiology and/or the behavior of another individual (the receiver).

**Photoperiod**   Day length, or the amount of light per day.

**Photoperiodism**   The use of photoperiod to time annual cycles.

**Photorefractoriness**   The loss of responsiveness to changes in photoperiod.

**Pineal gland**   An endocrine gland (also called the epiphysis), located in mammals between the telencephalon and diencephalon, that secretes melatonin, a hormone important in the regulation of daily and seasonal cycles.

**Pituitary gland**   An endocrine gland that has two distinct anatomical components in humans, the anterior pituitary and the posterior pituitary, which have different embryological origins and different functional roles in the endocrine system. The pituitary gland (also called the hypophysis) is connected to the median eminence of the hypothalamus by the pituitary stalk, or infundibulum.

**Placenta**   A specialized organ produced by the mammalian embryo that is attached to the uterine wall and serves to provide nutrients, hormones, and energy to the fetus.

**Plasma**   The clear, straw-colored fluid in which the blood cells are suspended.

**Polypeptide**   An unbranched string of amino acids linked together by peptide bonds.

**Portal system**   A special closed blood circuit in which two beds of capillaries are connected by a vein; thus, the flow of blood is in one direction only. The hypothalamus–pituitary portal system comprises the hypothalamic capillary bed and the anterior pituitary capillary bed, connected by a vein. The majority of blood flow, and hence endocrine information, is from the hypothalamus to the anterior pituitary.

**Positive feedback**   A regulatory process that tends to accelerate an ongoing process by increasing production in response to the end product.

**Posterior pituitary**   The rear part of the endocrine gland that extends from the base of the brain and stores and releases oxytocin and vasopressin (or some variant of these two nanopeptide hormones) which are produced in the hypothalamus.

**Postpartum depression**   A decrease in mood that occurs within a few days of giving birth. Symptoms can range from mild (maternity blues) and brief (24–48 hours) to severe. Hormones associated with parturition may be involved in postpartum depression, but social and psychological factors may be as important as biological factors in the mediation of this syndrome.

**Precocial**   Born or hatched at an advanced stage of development so that little or no parental intervention is required for survival.

**Preference threshold**   The first detectable preference displayed by an individual for any substance or solution.

**Pregnancy**   The state of a female mammal when she is carrying a developing fetus in her uterus.

**Pregnenolone**   A $C_{21}$ steroid prohormone that is the obligatory precursor for all other steroid hormones in vertebrates.

**Preoptic area**   A region of the brain anterior to the hypothalamus. This region is usually divided into the lateral and medial preoptic areas.

**Preoptic medial nucleus (POM)**   A collection of cell bodies in the songbird preoptic area that stains positively for estrogen receptors as well as for aromatase, and is thought to be critical in male avian copulatory behavior.

**Proceptivity**   The extent to which females initiate copulation.

**Proestrus**   The vaginal cellular condition coincident with mating behavior (estrus) in female rodents.

**Progestins**   A class of $C_{21}$ steroid hormones, so named for their "progestational," or pregnancy-maintaining, effects in mammals. Progesterone is a common progestin.

**Prohormone**   A molecule that can act as a hormone itself or can be converted into another hormone with different properties.

**Prolactin**   A protein hormone that is highly conserved throughout vertebrate evolution and has many physiological functions, which can be broken down into five basic classes: (1) reproduction, (2) growth and development, (3) water and electrolyte balance, (4) maintenance of integumentary structures, and (5) actions on steroid-dependent target tissues or synergisms with steroid hormones to affect target tissues.

**Prostaglandins**   A family of lipid-based hormones that possess a basic 20-carbon fatty acid skeleton called prostanoic acid; prostaglandins are involved in several aspects of reproductive function.

**Protandry**   A form of sequential hermaphroditism in which individuals begin life as males, then change into females.

**Protein hormone**   A hormone that consists of one or more polypeptide chains of amino acids, the sequence of which is specified by DNA.

**Protein kinase**   An enzyme that transfers a phosphate group from adenine triphosphate (ATP) to the protein substrate of the enzyme. The activation of specific protein kinases represents the mechanism by which most protein hormones initially exert their effects on cellular function.

**Protogyny**   A form of sequential hermaphroditism in which individuals begin life as females, then change into males.

**Pseudohermaphrodite**   An individual, especially a human, born with ambiguous external genitalia.

**Pseudopregnancy**   The luteal phase of the estrous cycle, or any period when there is a functional corpus luteum and buildup of the endometrial uterine layer in the absence of pregnancy.

**Puberty**   The process of sexual maturation during which an individual becomes fertile.

**Pulsatile secretion**   The episodic secretion of hormones in periodic bursts or spurts.

**Radioimmunoassay (RIA)**   A technique used to measure hormones or other biological substances by using antibodies and purified radiolabeled ligands.

**Receptivity**   The stimulus value of a female for eventually eliciting an intravaginal ejaculation from a male conspecific.

**Receptor**   A chemical structure on the cell surface or inside the cell that has an affinity for a specific chemical configuration of a hormone, neurotransmitter, or other chemical compound.

**5α-reductase**   An enzyme necessary to convert testosterone to 5α-dihydrotestosterone.

**Releasing hormone**   One of several polypeptides released from the hypothalamus that increase or decrease the release of hormones from the anterior pituitary gland.

**Rhythm**   A recurrent event that is characterized by its period, frequency, amplitude, and phase.

**Ribonucleic acid (RNA)**   A nucleic acid that implements the information stored in DNA. Two forms of RNA are transfer RNA and messenger RNA.

**Seasonal affective disorder (SAD)**   A psychological and physical syndrome, characterized by reduced mood, lethargy, loss of libido, hypersomnia, excessive weight gain, carbohydrate cravings, anxiety, and inability to concentrate or focus attention, that recurs during the late autumn and winter and subsides in the spring.

**Second messenger**   A biological molecule released when a hormone binds to its receptor; the second messenger activates the cellular machinery of the target cell (the hormone is the first messenger).

**Seminiferous tubules**   The long, convoluted tubes in which spermatogenesis occurs.

**Sensation**   The initial processing of sensory information as it enters the nervous system through sensory receptors.

**Sensitization**   *See* concaveation.

**Sequential hermaphrodite**   An animal that begins life as one sex, then changes to the other sex as an adult in response to environmental or genotypic factors.

**Sertoli cells**   Cells located along the basement membrane of the seminiferous tubules in which sperm cells are embedded while they mature.

**Set point**   A reference value for a regulated physiological variable.

**Sex determination**   The point at which an individual begins to develop as either a male or a female. In animals with sex chromosomes, sex determination occurs at fertilization; in animals that lack sex chromosomes, sex determination coincides with the presence of a specific environmental or social condition.

**Sex drive**   The powerful motivational forces propelling individuals to seek copulation; in humans, often referred to as libido.

**Sexual differentiation**   The process by which individuals develop the characteristics associated with being male or female. Among vertebrates, differential exposure to gonadal steroid hormones after sex determination causes sexual dimorphism in several structures, including the brain.

**Sexual orientation**   The process of developing an erotic sexual attraction for other people. This term suggests that the process is mediated primarily by biological factors.

**Sexual preference**   The process of developing an erotic sexual attraction for other people. This term suggests that the process is mediated primarily by learning and conscious choices.

**Sexual selection**   A subset of natural selection that occurs when individuals within a population differ in their abilities to compete with members of the same sex for mates (intrasexual selection) or to attract mates of the opposite sex (intersexual selection).

**Sexually dimorphic nucleus of the preoptic area (SDN-POA)**   A set of cell bodies anterior to the hypothalamus that is larger in male than in female humans and rodents. The functional significance of this brain dimorphism is unknown.

**Simultaneous hermaphrodite**   An animal that possesses ovotestes that produce both eggs and sperm, and alternates between two behavioral roles in providing eggs or sperm during spawning.

**Single-unit recording**   A technique that involves the placement of very small electrodes in or near one nerve cell to record changes in its neural activity before, during, and after some experimental treatment.

**Sperm**   A haploid male gamete.

**SRY gene**   Sex-determining region of the Y chromosome; the gene that is responsible for the transformation of the undifferentiated gonad into a testis.

**Steroid hormones**   A class of structurally related fat-soluble chemicals that are derived from cholesterol and are characterized by three six-carbon rings plus one conjugated five-carbon ring.

**Stress**   Any significant disturbance of homeostasis, as by extreme temperatures or psychological factors.

**Stroma**   The nonendocrine connective tissue of endocrine glands.

**Subfornical organ**   A small brain region located in the confluence of the lateral ventricles beneath the fornix. Neurons located in the subfornical organ detect the presence of angiotensin in the blood and activate neural circuits involved in water intake.

**Suprachiasmatic nuclei (SCN)**    A collection of cell bodies in the hypothalamus, located above the optic chiasm, that contains one or more biological clocks responsible for the temporal organization of many physiological and behavioral parameters.

**Supraoptic nuclei (SON)**    A collection of cell bodies in the hypothalamus, located above the optic nerve, that produces vasopressin, which is transported to the axon terminals in the posterior pituitary gland for release into the general circulation.

**Target cell**    A cell that has specific receptors for, and is affected by, a particular chemical messenger.

**Temperature-dependent sex determination**    A process that occurs in animals without sex chromosomes in which sex is determined solely on the basis of the temperature at which the egg incubates.

**Testicular feminization mutation (TFM)**    A condition in males, also called androgen insensitivity syndrome, in which functional androgen receptors are absent. TFM is caused by a genetic mutation on the X chromosome; genetic females have an additional X chromosome to code for androgen receptors and are not affected, but males develop male internal sex organs and a female external morphology.

**Testis determination factor (TDF)**    A protein product arising from a gene on the Y chromosome that instructs the medulla of the germinal ridge to develop into a testis.

**Testis**    The male gonad, which produces steroid hormones and sperm.

**Testosterone**    The primary androgen secreted by most vertebrate animals.

**Theca externa**    A concentric ring of cells that forms around the theca interna cells during follicular maturation. These cells also secrete estrogens, but transform along with other cell types into the corpus luteum after ovulation.

**Theca interna**    A concentric ring of cells that forms around the granulosa cells during follicular maturation. These cells secrete estrogens, but transform along with other cellular types into the corpus luteum after ovulation.

**Thyroid gland**    A double-lobed endocrine gland located on or near the trachea or esophagus in vertebrates that secretes several hormones important in metabolism, including triiodothyronine and thyroxine.

**Thyroxine (T4)**    The primary hormone secreted from the thyroid gland; it acts to increase oxidation rates in tissue. Also known as tetraiodothyronine.

**Transcription factor**    Substance that starts or blocks the process whereby a single strand of complementary RNA nucleotides is produced from a single strand of DNA.

**Transgenic**    Relating to an animal in which a gene has been inserted, altered, or deleted. Knockout mice are one type of transgenic mice.

**Translation**    The synthesis of a linear sequence of amino acids from an RNA sequence; occurs on ribosomes.

**Tropic hormones**    Hormones from the anterior pituitary that stimulate various physiological processes, either by acting directly on target tissues or by causing other endocrine glands to release hormones.

**Turner syndrome**    A congenital condition in which individuals lack an X chromosome (X0). These individuals have a female external appearance, but ovarian development is usually limited, and they do not attain puberty without medical attention.

**Ultradian rhythm**    A biological rhythm that has a period less than 24 hours (or a frequency greater than once per day).

**Up-regulation**    A process similar to positive feedback in which a hormone causes an increase in the production of receptors for that hormone.

**Vagus nerve**    The largest of the cranial nerves, the vagus nerve is made up of efferent fibers of the parasympathetic division of the autonomic nervous system that travel to the organs in the thorax and abdomen via specific branches. The vagus nerve also carries sensory fibers from these organs back to the brain.

**Vandenbergh effect**    The delay or acceleration of puberty in young females by exposure to chemosignals of adult females or males, respectively.

**Vasopressin**    A nanopeptide released from the posterior pituitary gland that reduces blood pressure during serious blood loss. Also called antidiuretic hormone (ADH) because it also stimulates reabsorption of water in the kidney.

**Ventromedial nucleus (VMH)**    A collection of cell bodies in the hypothalamus, located near the walls of the third ventricle, that is important in the regulation of sexual behavior in female rodents.

**Vesicle**    A secretory granule or sac within a cell in which hormone or neurotransmitter molecules are stored.

**Volemic thirst**    Motivation to consume water caused by a reduction in blood plasma volume.

**Vomeronasal organ**    An encapsulated sensory receptive organ located near the floor of the nasal cavity in mammals that receives chemosensory information, which then travels to the accessory olfactory bulbs.

**Whitten effect**    The suspension of estrous cycles in group-housed females and the subsequent induction of estrus when exposed to a male or his odors.

**Wolffian ducts**    A duct system present in both sexes during embryonic development that connects the gonads to the exterior. During normal development, the Wolffian duct system develops into the accessory sex organs in males and regresses in females.

**Zeitgeber**    A potent environmental time cue, or temporal synchronizer.

**Zona fasciculata**    The middle (and largest) zone of the adrenal cortex, consisting of orderly bands of epithelial cells. Glucocorticoid hormones are released from these cells in response to ACTH stimulation from the anterior pituitary.

**Zona glomerulosa**    The outermost zone of the adrenal cortex, consisting of whorls of epithelial cells. Aldosterone is released from these cells as an indirect response to low blood sodium levels.

**Zona pellucida**    The outer layer of cells surrounding the cell membranes of the maturing ovum.

**Zona reticularis**    The innermost zone of the adrenal cortex, consisting of a disorganized arrangement of epithelial cells. Sex steroid hormones are often released from this zone.

**Zygote**    A fertilized egg that contains both maternal and paternal DNA. A zygote develops into a blastocyst within days of conception.

# References

Abbott, D. H. 1984. Differentiation of sexual behaviour in female marmoset monkeys. Effects of neonatal testosterone or a male co-twin. In G. J. DeVries (ed.), *Prog. Brain Res.,* Vol. 61, pp. 349–358. Elsevier, Amsterdam.

Abbott, D. H., Saltzman, W., Schultz-Darken, N. J., Smith, T. E. 1997. Specific neuroendocrine mechanisms not involving generalized stress mediate social regulation of female reproduction in cooperatively breeding marmoset monkeys. *Ann. N. Y. Acad. Sci.,* 807:219–38

Abel, G. G., Barlow, D. H., Blanchard, E. B., and Arnold, D. 1977. The components of rapists' sexual arousal. *Arch. Gen. Psychiatry,* 34:895–903.

Abitbol, M. L. and Inglis, S. R. 1997. Role of amniotic fluid in newborn acceptance and bonding in canines. *J. Matern. Fetal Med.,* 6:49–52.

Abraham, G. E. 1980. The premenstrual tension syndromes. In L. K. McNall (ed.), *Contemp. Obstet. Gynecol. Nurs.,* Vol. 3, pp. 170–184. Mosby, St. Louis.

Adams, D. B., Gold, A. R., and Burt, A. D. 1978. Rise in female-initiated sexual activity at ovulation and its suppression by oral contraceptives. *N. Engl. J. Med.,* 229:1145–1150.

Adels, L. E., and Leon, M. 1986. Thermal control of mother–young contact in Norway rats: Factors mediating the chronic elevation of maternal temperature. *Physiol. Behav.,* 36:183–196.

Adkins, E. K. 1975. Hormonal basis of sexual differentiation in the Japanese quail. *J. Comp. Physiol. Psychol.,* 89:61–71.

Adkins, E. K. 1976. Embryonic exposure to an anti-estrogen masculinizes behavior of female quail. *Physiol. Behav.,* 17:357–359.

Adkins, E. K. 1978. Sex steroids and the differentiation of avian reproductive behavior. *Am. Zool.,* 18:501–509.

Adkins, E. K., and Adler, N. T. 1972. Hormonal control of behavior in the Japanese quail. *J. Comp. Physiol. Psychol.,* 81:27–36.

Adkins, E. K., and Nock, B. L. 1976. The effects of the antiestrogens C1-628 on sexual behavior activated by androgen or estrogen in quail. *Horm. Behav.,* 7:417–429.

Adkins, E. K., and Pniewski, E. E. 1978. Control of reproductive behavior by sex steroids in male quail. *J. Comp. Physiol. Psychol.,* 92:1169–1178.

Adkins-Regan, E. 1987. Sexual differentiation in birds. *Trends Neurosci.,* 10:517–522.

Adkins-Regan, E. 1988. Sex hormones and sexual orientation in animals. *Psychobiology,* 16:335–347.

Adkins-Regan, E. 1996. Neuroanatomy of sexual behavior in the male Japanese quail from top to bottom. *Poultry Avian Biol. Rev.,* 7:193–204.

Adkins-Regan, E. 1998. Hormonal mechanisms of mate choice. *Am. Zoologist,* 38:166–178.

Adkins-Regan, E., and Ascenzi, M. 1987. Social and sexual behavior of male and female zebra finches treated with estradiol during the nestling period. *Anim. Behav.,* 35:1100–1112.

Adkins-Regan, E., and Ascenzi, M. 1990. Sexual differentiation of behavior in the zebra finch: Effect of early gonadectomy or androgen treatment. *Horm. Behav.,* 24:114–127.

Adkins-Regan, E., Mansukhani, V., Thompson, A., and Yang, S. 1997. Organizational actions of sex hormones on sexual partner preference. *Brain Res. Bull.,* 44:497–502.

Adkins-Regan, E., Orgeur, P., and Signoret, J. P. 1989. Sexual differentiation of reproductive behavior in pigs: Defeminizing effects of prepubertal estradiol. *Horm. Behav.,* 23:290–303.

Agarwal, S. K., and Haney, A. F. 1994. Does recommending timed intercourse really help the infertile couple? *Obstet. Gynecol.,* 84:307–310.

Ågmo, A. 1997. Male rat sexual behavior. *Brain Res. Brain Res. Protoc.,* 1:203–209.

Agranoff, B. W., and Davis, R. E. 1968. The use of fishes in studies of memory formation. In D. Ingle (ed.), *The Central Nervous System and Fish Behavior,* pp. 193–202. University of Chicago Press, Chicago.

Aguzzi, A., Brandner, S., Sure, U., Ruedi, D., and Isenmann, S. 1994. Transgenic and knock-out mice: Models of neurological disease. *Brain Pathol.,* 4, 3–20.

Ahlenius, S., and Larsson, K. 1984. Apomorphine and haloperidol-induced effects on male sexual behavior: No evidence for actions due to stimulation of central dopamine autoreceptors. *Pharmacol. Biochem. Behav.,* 21:463–466.

Ahren, B., Mansson, S., Gingerich, R. L., and Havel, P. J. 1997. Regulation of plasma leptin in mice: influence of age, high-fat diet, and fasting. *Am. J. Physiol.,* 273: R113–R120.

Ainsworth, M. D. S. 1972. Attachment and dependency: A comparison. In J. L. Gerwirtz, *Attachment Dependency,* pp. 97–137. V. H. Winston, Washington, D.C.

Albers, H. E. 1981. Gonadal hormones organize and modulate the circadian system of the rat. *Am. J. Physiol.,* 241:R62–R66.

Albers, H. E., Hennessey, A. C., and Whitman, D. C. 1992. Vasopressin and the regulation of hamster social behavior. *Ann. N. Y. Acad. Sci.,* 652:227–242.

Albers, H. E., Pollock, J., Simmons, W. H., and Ferris, C. F. 1986. A V1-like receptor mediates vasopressin-induced flank marking behavior in hamster hypothalamus. *J. Neurosci.,* 6:2085–2089.

Albert, D. J., and Walsh, M. L. 1984. Neural systems and the inhibitory modulation of agonistic behavior: A comparison of mammalian species. *Neurosci. Biobehav. Rev.,* 8:5–24.

Albert, D. J., Petrovic, D. M., Walsh, M. L., and Jonik, R. H. 1990. Medial accumbens lesions attenuate testosterone-dependent aggression in male rats. *Physiol. Behav.,* 46:625–631.

Alberts, J. R. 1974. Producing and interpreting experimental olfactory deficits. *Comp. Biochem. Physiol.,* 40A:971–974.

Alberts, J. R., and Brunjes, P. C. 1978. Ontogeny of thermal and olfactory determinants of huddling in the rat. *J. Comp. Physiol. Psychol.,* 92:897–906.

Alberts, J. R., and Galef, B. G. 1971. Acute anosmia in the rat: A behavioral test of a peripherally induced olfactory deficit. *Physiol. Behav.,* 12:657–670.

Alberts, J. R., and Gubernick, D. J. 1990. Functional organization of dyadic and triadic parent–offspring systems. In N. A. Krasnegor and R. S. Bridges (eds.), *Mammalian Parenting,* pp. 416–440. Oxford University Press, Oxford.

Alcock, J. 1997. *Animal Behavior: An Evolutionary Approach* (5th ed.). Sinauer Associates, Sunderland, MA.

Alexander, G. M., and Sherwin, B. B. 1993. Sex steroids, sexual behavior, and selection attention for erotic stimuli in women using oral contraceptives. *Psychoneuroendocrinology,*18:91–102.

Alexander, G. M., Sherwin, B. B., Bancroft, J., and Davidson, D. W. 1990. Testosterone and sexual behavior in oral contraceptive users and nonusers: A prospective study. *Horm. Behav.,* 24:388–402.

Alexander, G. M., Swerdloff, R. S., Wang, C., Davidson, T., McDonald, V., Steiner, B., and Hines, M. 1998. Androgen-behavior correlations in hypogonadal men and eugonadal men. II. Cognitive abilities. *Horm. Behav.,* 33:85–94.

Alexander, R. D., Hoogland, J. L., Howard, R. D., Noonan, K. M., and Sherman, P. W. 1979. Sexual dimorphisms and breeding systems in pinnipeds, ungulates, primates and humans. In N. A. Chagnon and W. Irons (eds.), *Evolutionary Biology and Human Social Behavior,* pp. 402–435. Duxbury Press, North Scituate, MA.

Allada, R., White, N. E., So, W. W., Hall, J. C., and Rosbash, M. 1998. A mutant *Drosophila* homolog of mammalian Clock disrupts circadian rhythms and transcription of period and timeless. *Cell,* 93:791–804.

Allen, E. 1922. The oestrus cycle in the mouse. *Am. J. Anat.,* 30:297–325.

Allen, E., and Doisy, E. A. 1923. An ovarian hormone: Preliminary report of its localization, extraction and partial purification, and action in test animals. *J.A.M.A.,* 81:819–821.

Allen, E., Francis, B. F., Robertson, L. L., Colgate, C. E., Johnston, C. G., Doisy, E. A., Kountz, W. B., and Gibson, H. V. 1924. The hor-

mone of the ovarian follicle: Its localization and action in test animals, and additional points bearing upon the internal secretion of
the ovary. *Am. J. Anat.,* 34:133–182.

Allen, L. S., Hines, M., Shryne, J. E., and Gorski, R. A. 1989. Two sexually dimorphic cell groups in the human brain. *J. Neurosci.,*
9:497–506.

Allen, L. S., Richey, M. F., Chai, Y. M., and Gorski, R. A. 1991. Sex differences in the corpus callosum of the living human being. *J.
Neurosci.,* 11:933–942.

Altmann, J. 1980. *Baboon Mothers and Infants.* Harvard University
Press, Cambridge, MA.

Altshuler, L. L., Hendrick, V., and Parry, B. 1995. Pharmacological
management of premenstrual disorder. *Harv. Rev. Psychiatry,*
2:233–245.

Amalric, M., Cline, E. J., Martinez, J. L., Bloom, F. E., and Koob, G. F.
1987. Rewarding properties of b-endorphin as measured by conditioned place preference. *Psychopharmacology,* 91:14–19.

American Psychiatric Association. 1994. *Diagnostic and Statistical
Manual of Mental Disorders: DSM-IV.* (4th ed.) American
Psychiatric Association, Washington, D.C.

Anagnostaras, S. G., Maren, S., DeCola, J. P., Lane, N. I., Gale, G. D.,
Schlinger, B. A., and Fanselow, M. S. 1998. Testicular hormones
do not regulate sexually dimorphic Pavlovian fear conditioning or
perforant-path long-term potentiation in adult male rats. *Behav.
Brain Res.,* 92:1–9.

Anand, B. K., and Brobeck, J. R. 1951. Localization of a feeding center in the hypothalamus of the rat. *Proc. Soc. Exp. Biol. Med.,*
77:323–324.

Anastasi, A., Erspamer, V., and Bucci, M. 1971. Isolation and structure of bombesin and alytesin, 2 analogous active peptides from
the skin of the European amphibians Bombina and Alytes.
*Experientia,* 27:123–140.

Andersson, B., Eriksson, S., and Rundgren, M. 1995. Angiotensin and
the brain. *Acta Physiol. Scand.* 155:117–125.

Andersson, M. 1994. *Sexual Selection.* Princeton University Press,
Princeton.

Anonymous. 1970. Effects of sexual activity on beard growth in man.
*Nature,* 226:869–870.

Applezweig, M. H., and Baudry, F. D. 1955. The pituitary–adrenocortical system in avoidance learning. *Psychol. Rep.,* 1:417–420.

Applezweig, M. H., and Moeller, G. 1959. The pituitary–adrenocortical system and anxiety in avoidance learning. *Acta Psychol.,*
15:602–603.

Arai, A., Taniguchi, I., and Saito, N. 1989. Correlation between the
size of song control nuclei and plumage color change in orange
bishop birds. *Neurosci. Lett.,* 98:144–148.

Arase, K., York, D. A., Shimizu, H., Shargill, N., and Bray, G. A. 1988.
Effects of corticotropin-releasing factor on food intake and
brown adipose tissue thermogenesis in rats. *Am. J. Physiol.,* 255:
E255–E259.

Arena, B., Maffulli, N., Maffulli, F., and Morleo, M. A. 1995.
Reproductive hormones and menstrual changes with exercise in
female athletes. *Sports Med.,* 19:278–287.

Arendash, G. W., and Gorski, R. A. 1983. Effects of discrete lesions of
the sexually dimorphic nucleus of the preoptic area or other
medial preoptic regions on the sexual behavior of male rats.
*Brain Res. Bull.,* 10:147–150.

Arendt, J. 1997. Safety of melatonin long-term use. *J. Biol. Rhythms,*
12:673–681.

Arendt, J. 1998. Melatonin and the pineal gland: Influence on mammalian seasonal and circadian physiology. *Rev. Reprod.,* 3:13–22.

Argyriou, A., Prast, H., and Philippu, A. 1998. Melatonin facilitates
short-term memory. *Eur. J. Pharmacol.,* 349:159–162.

Aristotle. 1910. *Historia Animalium.* Translated by D. W. Thompson.
Clarendon Press, Oxford.

Arnold, A. P. 1996. Genetically triggered sexual differentiation of
brain and behavior. *Horm. Behav.,* 30:495–505.

Arnold, A. P. 1997. Experimental analysis of sexual differentiation of
the zebra finch brain. *Brain Res. Bull.,* 44:503–508.

Arnold, A. P., and Breedlove, S. M. 1985. Organizational and activational effects of sex steroid hormones on vertebrate brain and
behavior: A re-analysis. *Horm. Behav.,* 19:469–498.

Arnold, A. P., and Gorski, R. A. 1984. Gonadal steroid induction of
structural sex differences in the CNS. *Annu. Rev. Neurosci.,*
7:413–442.

Arnold, A. P., and Jordan, C. L. 1988. Hormonal organization of neural
circuits. *Frontiers in Neuroendocrinology,* 10:185–214.

Arnold, A. P., and Matthews, G. 1988. Sexual differentiation of brain
and behavior in birds. In J. M. A. Sitsen (ed.), *Handbook of*

*Sexology, Vol. 6: The Pharmacology and Endocrinology of Sexual
Function,* pp. 122–144. Elsevier, New York.

Arnold, A. P., and Schlinger, B. A. 1993. Sexual differentiation of
brain and behavior: The zebra finch is not just a flying rat. *Brain
Behav. Evol.,* 42: 231–241.

Arnold, A. P., Bottjer, S. W., Brenowitz, E. A., Nordeen, E. J., and
Nordeen, K. W. 1987. Sexual dimorphisms in the neural vocal
control system in song birds: Ontogeny and phylogeny. *Brain
Behav. Evol.,* 28:22–31.

Aschoff, J. 1965. Circadian rhythms in man: A self-sustained oscillator with an inherent frequency underlies human 24-hour periodicity. *Science,* 148: 1427–1432.

Aschoff, J. 1981. Annual rhythms in man. In J. Aschoff (ed.),
*Handbook of Behavioral Neurobiology,* Vol. 4, pp. 475–490.
Plenum Press, New York.

Asdell, S. A. 1964. *Patterns of Mammalian Reproduction.* Cornell
University Press, Ithaca, NY.

Auger, A. P., Moffatt, C. A., and Blaustein, J. D. 1996.
Reproductively-relevant stimuli induce Fos-immunoreactivity
within progestin receptor-containing neurons in localized regions
of female rat forebrain. *J. Neuroendocrinol.,* 8:831–838.

Avitsur, R., Pollak, Y., and Yirmiya, R. 1997b. Administration of inter-
leukin-1 into the hypothalamic paraventricular nucleus induces
febrile and behavioral effects. *Neuroimmunomodulation,*
4:258–265.

Avitsur, R., Pollak, Y., and Yirmiya, R. 1998. Administration of inter-
leukin-1 into the hypothalamic paraventricular nucleus induces
febrile and behavioral effects. *Neuroimmunomodulation,*
4:258–265.

Bachman, G. A., and Kemmann, E. 1982. Prevalence of oligomenor-
rhea and amenorrhea in a college population. *Am. J. Obstet.
Gynecol.,* 117:80–86.

Backstrom, T., Sanders, D., Leask, R., Davidson, D., Warner, P., and
Bancroft, J. 1983. Mood, sexuality, hormones, and the menstrual
cycle. II. Hormone levels and their relationship to the premenstrual syndrome. *Psychosomat. Med.,* 45:503–507.

Badura, L. L., and Nunez, A. A. 1989. Photoperiodic modulation of
sexual and aggressive behavior in female golden hamsters
(*Mesocricetus auratus*): Role of the pineal gland. *Horm. Behav.,*
23:27–42.

Badura, L. L., Yant, W. R., and Nunez, A. A. 1987. Photoperiodic modulation of steroid-induced lordosis in golden hamsters. *Physiol.
Behav.,* 40:551–554.

Bailey, J. M., and Pillard, R. C. 1991. A genetic study of male sexual
orientation. *Arch. Gen. Psychiatry,* 48:1089–1096.

Baker, J. R. 1938. The evolution of breeding seasons. In J. DeBeer
(ed.), *Evolution,* pp. 161–177. Clarendon Press, Oxford.

Baker, M. C., Bottjer, S. W., and Arnold, A. P. 1984. Sexual dimorphism and lack of seasonal changes in vocal control regions of
the white-crowned sparrow brain. *Brain Res.,* 295:85–89.

Baldwin, J. D. 1968. The social behavior of adult male squirrel monkeys (*Saimiri sciureus*) in a semi-natural environment. *Folia
Primatol.,* 9:281–314.

Ball, G. F. 1991. Endocrine mechanisms and the evolution of avian
parental care. *Acta XX Congressus Internationalis Ornithologici,*
984–991.

Ball, J. 1934a. Normal sex behavior in the rat after total extirpation of
the vasa deferentia. *Anat. Rec.,* 58:49.

Ball, J. 1934b. Sex behavior in the rat after removal of the uterus and
vagina. *J. Comp. Psychol.,* 18:419–422.

Ball, J. 1937. Sex activity of castrated male rats increased by estrin
administration. *J. Comp. Psychol.,* 24:135–144.

Ball, J. 1941. Effect of progesterone upon sexual excitability in the
female monkey. *Psychol. Bull.,* 38:533–534.

Ball, J., and Hartman, C. G. 1935. Sexual excitability as related to the
menstrual cycle in the monkey. *Am. J. Obstet. Gynecol.,*
29:117–119.

Balthazart, J. 1989. Steroid metabolism and the activation of social
behavior. In J. Balthazart (ed.), *Advances in Comparative and
Environmental Physiology,* Vol. 3, pp. 105–159. Springer, Berlin.

Balthazart, J., and Ball, G. F. 1992. Is dopamine interacting with aromatase to control sexual behavior in male quail? *Poultry Sci.
Rev.,* 4:217–233.

Balthazart, J., and Ball, G. F. 1993. Neurochemical differences in two
steroid sensitive areas mediating reproductive behaviors. In R.
Gilles (ed.), *Advances in Comparative and Environmental
Physiology,* pp. 133–161. Springer-Verlag, New York.

Balthazart, J., and Ball, G. F. 1995. Sexual differentiation of brain and
behavior in birds. *Trends Endocrinol. Metab.* 6:21–29.

Balthazart, J., and Ball, G. F. 1998. New insights into the regulation and function of brain estrogen synthase (aromatase). *Trends Neurosci.*, 21:243–249.

Balthazart, J., and Foidart, A. 1993. Neural bases of behavioral sex differences in the quail. In M. Haug (ed.), *The Development of Sex Differences and Similarities in Behavior*, pp. 51–75. Kluwer Academic Publishers, Amsterdam.

Balthazart, J., Foidart, A., Surlemont, C., and Harada, N. 1991. Neuroanatomical specificity in the co-localization of aromatase and estrogen receptors. *J. Neurobiol.*, 22:143–157.

Balthazart, J., Foidart, A., Wilson, E. M., and Ball, G. F. 1992. Immunocytochemical localization of androgen receptors in the male songbird and quail brain. *J. Comp. Neurol.*, 317:407–420.

Balthazart, J., Schumacher, M., and Malacarne, G. 1985. Interaction of androgens and estrogens in the control of sexual behavior in male Japanese quail. *Physiol. Behav.*, 35:157–166.

Balthazart, J., Schumacher, M., and Ottinger, M. A. 1983. Sexual differences in the Japanese quail: Behavior, morphology, and nonneural intracellular metabolism of testosterone. *Gen. Comp. Endocrinol.*, 51:191–207.

Balthazart, J., Tlemcani, O., and Ball, G. F. 1996. Do sex differences in the brain explain sex differences in the hormonal induction of reproductive behavior? What 25 years of research on Japanese quail tells us. *Horm. Behav.*, 30:627–661.

Bambino, T. H., and Hseuh, A. J. 1981. Direct inhibitory effect of glucocorticoids upon testicular luteinizing hormone receptors and steroidogenesis in vivo and in vitro. *Endocrinology*, 108:2142–2148.

Bamshad, M., and Albers, H. E. 1996. Neural circuitry controlling vasopressin-stimulated scent marking in Syrian hamsters (*Mesocricetus auratus*). *J. Comp. Neurol.*, 369:252–263.

Bancroft, J. 1978. The relationship between hormones and sexual behaviour in humans. In J. B. Hutchison (ed.), *Biological Determinants of Sexual Behaviour*, pp. 493–519. New York, Wiley.

Bancroft, J. 1984. Hormones and human sexual behavior. *J. Sex Marital Ther.*, 10:3–21.

Bancroft, J., Sherwin, B. B., Alexander, G. M., Davidson, D. W., and Walker, A. 1991. Oral contraceptives, androgens, and the sexuality of young women: I. A comparison of sexual experience, sexual attitudes, and gender role in oral contraceptive users and nonusers. *Arch. Sex. Behav.*, 20:105–120.

Bancroft, J., Sherwin, B. B., Alexander, G. M., Davidson, D. W., and Walker, A. 1991. Oral contraceptives, androgens, and the sexuality of young women: II. The role of androgens. *Arch. Sex. Behav.*, 20:121–135.

Barbarino, A., DeMarinis, L., and Mancini, A. 1983. Estradiol modulation of basal and gonadotropin-releasing hormone–induced gonadotropin release in intact and castrated men. *Neuroendocrinology*, 36: 105–111.

Barbazanges, A., Piazza, P. V., Le Moal, M., and Maccari, S. 1996. Maternal glucocorticoid secretion mediates long-term effects of prenatal stress. *J. Neurosci.*, 16: 3943–3949.

Bard, P. 1936. Oestrual behavior in surviving decorticate cats. *Am. J. Physiol.*, 116:4–5.

Barfield, R. J. 1971. Activation of sexual and aggressive behavior by androgen implanted into the male ring dove brain. *Endocrinology*, 89:1470–1476.

Barfield, R. J., and Chen, J. J. 1977. Activation of estrous behavior in ovariectomized rats by intracerebral implants of estradiol benzoate. *Endocrinology*, 101: 1716–1725.

Barker, S. 1987. Oxymethalone and aggression. *Br. J. Psychiatry*, 151:564–565.

Barkley, M. S., and Goldman, B. D. 1977. A quantitative study of serum testosterone, sex accessory organ weight growth and the development of intermale aggression in the mouse. *Horm. Behav.*, 9:21–48.

Barkley, M. S., Geschwind, I. I., and Bradford, G. E. 1979. The gestational pattern of estradiol, testosterone, and progesterone secretion in selected strains of mice. *Biol. Reprod.*, 20:733–738.

Barnes, B. M., and York, A. D. 1990. Effect of winter high temperatures on reproduction and circannual rhythms in hibernating ground squirrels. *J. Biol. Rhythms*, 5:119–130.

Barr GA, Gibbons JL, Moyer KE. 1975. The relationship between mouse killing and intraspecific fighting in the albino rat. *Behav. Biology*, 14: 201–208.

Bartke, A., Goldman, B. D., Bex, F., and Dalterio, S. 1977b. Effects of prolactin on pituitary and testicular function in mice with hereditary prolactin deficiency. *Endocrinology*, 101:1760–1766.

Bartke, A., Smith, M. S., Michael, S. D., Peron, F. G., and Dalterio, S. 1977a. Effects of experimentally-induced chronic hyperpro-

lactinemia on testosterone and gonadotropin levels in male rats and mice. *Endocrinology*, 100:182–186.

Bartness, T. J., and Goldman, B. D. 1988a. Peak duration of serum melatonin and short-day responses in adult Siberian hamsters. *Am. J. Physiol.*, 255:R812–R822.

Bartness, T. J., and Goldman, B. D. 1988b. Effects of melatonin on long-day responses in short-day housed adult Siberian hamsters. *Am. J. Physiol.*, 255:R823–R830.

Bartness, T. J., and Goldman, B. D. 1989. Mammalian pineal melatonin: A clock for all seasons. *Experientia*, 45:939–945.

Bartness, T. J., and Wade, G. N. 1984. Photoperiodic control of body weight and energy metabolism in Syrian hamsters (Mesocricetus auratus): Role of pineal gland, melatonin, gonads and diet. *Endocrinology*, 114:492–498.

Bartness, T. J., and Wade, G. N. 1985. Photoperiodic control of seasonal body weight cycles in hamsters. *Neurosci. Biobehav. Rev.*, 9:599–612.

Bartness, T. J., Powers, J. B., Hastings, M. H., Bittman, E. L., and Goldman, B. D. 1993. The timed infusion paradigm for melatonin delivery: what has it taught us about the melatonin signal, its reception, and the photoperiodic control of seasonal responses? *J. Pineal Res.*, 15:161–190.

Bass, A. H. 1986. A hormone-sensitive communication system in an electric fish. *J. Neurobiol.*, 17:131–156.

Bass, A. H. 1993. From brains to behaviour: Hormonal cascades and alternative mating tactics in teleost fishes. *Rev. Fish Biol. Fish.*, 3:181–186.

Bass, A. H. 1995. Alternative life history strategies and dimorphic males in an acoustic communication system. Fifth International Symposium on Reproductive Physiology in Fish, pp. 258–260. Austin, TX.

Bass, A. H. 1996. Shaping brain sexuality. *Am. Sci.*, 84: 352–364.

Bass, A. H. 1998. Behavioral and evolutionary neurobiology: A pluralistic approach. *Am. Zool.*, 38:97–107.

Bass, A. H., and Hopkins, C. 1984. Shifts in frequency tuning in electroreceptors in androgen-treated mormyrid fish. *J. Comp. Physiol. [A]*, 155:713–724.

Bass, A. H., Horvath, B. J., and Brothers, E. B. 1996. Nonsequential developmental trajectories lead to dimorphic vocal circuitry for males with alternative reproductive tactics. *J. Neurobiol.*, 30:493–504.

Bass, F. 1947. L'amenorrhee au camp de concentration de Terezin. *Gynaecologia*, 123:211–218.

Bast, J. D., and Greenwald, G. S. 1977. Acute and chronic elevation in serum levels of FSH after unilateral ovariectomy in the cyclic hamster. *Endocrinology*, 100:955–966.

Bateman, A. J. 1948. Intra-sexual selection in *Drosophila*. *Heredity*, 2:349–368.

Batty, J. 1978. Acute changes in plasma testosterone levels and their relation to measures of sexual behaviour in the male house mouse (*Mus musculus*). *Anim. Behav.*, 26:349–357.

Baum, M. J., Brand, T., Ooms, M., Vreeburg, J. T. M., and Slob, A. K. 1988. Immediate postnatal rise in whole body androgen content in male rats: Correlation with increased testicular content and reduced body clearance of testosterone. *Biol. Reprod.*, 38:980–986.

Baum, M. J., Carroll, R. S., Cherry, J. A., and Tobet, S. A. 1990. Steroidal control of behavioural, neuroendocrine and brain sexual differentiation: Studies in a carnivore, the ferret. *J. Neuroendocrinol.*, 2:401–418.

Beach, F. A. 1937. The neural basis of innate behavior: I. Effects of cortical lesions upon the maternal behavior pattern in the rat. *J. Comp. Psychol.*, 24:393–436.

Beach, F. A. 1942a. Analysis of factors involved in the arousal, maintenance and manifestation of sexual excitement in male animals. *Psychosom. Med.*, 4: 173–198.

Beach, F. A. 1942b. Analysis of the stimuli adequate to elicit mating behavior in the sexually inexperienced male rat. *J. Comp. Psychol.*, 33:163–207.

Beach, F. A. 1942c. Copulatory behavior in prepuberally castrated male rats and its modification by estrogen administration. *Endocrinology*, 31:679–683.

Beach, F. A. 1942d. Importance of progesterone to induction of sexual receptivity in spayed female rats. *Proc. Soc. Exp. Biol. Med.*, 51:369–371.

Beach, F. A. 1944. Relative effects of androgen upon mating behavior in male rats subjected to castration or forebrain injury. *J. Exp. Zool.*, 97:249–285.

Beach, F. A. 1947. Evolutionary changes in the physiological control of mating behavior in mammals. *Psychol. Rev.*, 54:297–315.

Beach, F. A. 1948. *Hormones and Behavior.* Paul B. Hoeber, New York.

Beach, F. A. 1967. Cerebral and hormonal control of reflexive mechanisms involved in copulatory behavior. *Physiol. Rev.,* 47:289–316.

Beach, F. A. 1968. Factors involved in the control of mounting behavior by female mammals. In M. Diamond (ed.), *Perspectives in Reproduction and Sexual Behavior: A Memorial to William C. Young,* pp. 83–131, Indiana University Press, Bloomington.

Beach, F. A. 1970. Hormonal effects on socio-sexual behavior in dogs. In M. Gibian and E. J. Plotz (eds.), *Mammalian Reproduction,* pp. 437–466. Springer-Verlag, Berlin.

Beach, F. A. 1971. Hormonal factors controlling the differentiation, development, and display of copulatory behavior in the ramstergig and related species. In E. Tobach, L. R. Aronson, and E. Shaw (eds.), *The Biopsychology of Development,* pp. 249–296. Academic Press, New York.

Beach, F. A. 1974a. Behavioral endocrinology and the study of reproduction. *Biol. Reprod.,* 10:2–18.

Beach, F. A. 1974b. Effects of gonadal hormones on urinary behavior in dogs. *Physiol. Behav.,* 12:1005–1013.

Beach, F. A. 1975. Hormonal modification of sexually dimorphic behavior. *Psychoneuroendocrinology,* 1:3–23.

Beach, F. A. 1976. Sexual attractivity, proceptivity, and receptivity in female mammals. *Horm. Behav.,* 7: 105–138.

Beach, F. A. 1981. Histological origins of modern research on hormones and behavior. *Horm. Behav.,* 15:325–376.

Beach, F. A. 1984. Hormone modulation of genital reflexes in male and masculinized female dogs. *Behav. Neurosci.,* 98, 325–332.

Beach, F. A., and Buehler, M. G. 1977. Male rats with inherited insensitivity to androgen show reduced sexual behavior. *Endocrinology,* 100:197–200.

Beach, F. A., and Gilmore, R. W. 1949. Response of male dogs to urine from females in heat. *J. Mammalogy,* 30:391–392.

Beach, F. A., and Holz-Tucker, M. 1949. Effects of different concentrations of androgen upon sexual behavior in castrated male rats. *J. Comp. Physiol. Psychol.,* 42:433–453.

Beach, F. A., and Inman, B. G. 1965. Effects of castration and androgen replacement on mating in male quail. *Proc. Natl. Acad. Sci. U.S.A.,* 54:1426–1431.

Beach, F. A., and Jordan, L. 1956. Sexual exhaustion and recovery in the male rat. *Q. J. Exp. Psychol.,* 8:121–133.

Beach, F. A., and LeBoeuf, B. J. 1967. Coital behaviour in dogs. I. Preferential mating in the bitch. *Anim. Behav.,* 15:546–558.

Beach, F. A., and Merari, A. 1968. Coital behavior in dogs. IV. Effects of progesterone in the bitch. *Proc. Natl. Acad. Sci. U.S.A.,* 61:442–444.

Beach, F. A., and Merari, A. 1970. Coital behavior in dogs. V. Effects of estrogen and progesterone on mating and other forms of social behavior in the bitch. *J. Comp. Physiol. Psychol. Monogr.,* 70:1–49.

Beach, F. A., Buehler, M. G., and Dunbar, I. F. 1983. Sexual cycles in female dogs treated with androgen during development. *Behav. Neural Biol.,* 38:1–31.

Beach, F. A., Kuehn, R. E., Sprague, R. H., and Anisko, J. J. 1972. Coital behavior in dogs. XI. Effects of androgen stimulation during development on masculine mating response in females. *Horm. Behav.,* 3:143–168.

Beasley, L. J., and Nelson, R. J. 1982. Thyroid gland influences the period of hamster circadian oscillations. *Experientia,* 38:870–871.

Beatty, W. W. 1979. Gonadal hormones and sex differences in nonreproductive behaviors in rodents: Organizational and activational influences. *Horm. Behav.,* 12:112–163.

Beauchamp, G. K., Magnus, J. G., Shmunes, N. T., and Durham, T. 1977. Effects of olfactory bulbectomy on social behavior of male guinea pigs (*Cavia porcellus*). *J. Comp. Physiol. Psychol.,* 91:336–346.

Becker, J. B. 1990. Estrogen rapidly potentiates amphetamine-induced striatal dopamine release and rotational behavior during microdialysis. *Neurosci. Lett.,* 118:169–171.

Becker, J. B., Breedlove, S. M., and Crews, D. (eds.). 1992. *Behavioral Endocrinology.* MIT Press, Cambridge, MA.

Becker, S. 1981. Seasonality of fertility in Matlab, Bangladesh. *J. Biosocial Sci.,* 13:97–105.

Beckhardt, S., and Ward, I. L. 1983. Reproductive functioning in the prenatally stressed female rat. *Dev. Psychobiol.,* 16:111–118.

Bell, R. and Hobson, H. 1994. 5-HT$_{1A}$ receptor influences on rodent social and agonistic behavior: A review and empirical study. *Neurosci. Biobehav. Rev.,* 18:325–338.

Bellastella, A., Pisano, G., Iorio, S., Pasquali, D., Orio, F., Venditto, T., and Sinisi, A. A. 1998. Endocrine secretions under abnormal light-dark cycles and in the blind. *Horm. Res.,* 49:153–157.

Benbow, C. P., and Stanley, J. C. 1983. Sex differences in mathematical reasoning ability: More facts. *Science,* 222:1029–1031.

Benloucif, S., and Dubocovich, M. L. 1996. Melatonin and light induce phase shifts of circadian activity rhythms in the C3H/HeN mouse. *J. Biol. Rhythms,* 11:113–125.

Benoit, J. 1964. The role of the eyes and of the hypothalamus in the photostimulation of gonads in the duck. *Ann. N. Y. Acad. Sci.,* 117:204–217.

Bentley, G. E., Demas, G. E., Nelson, R. J., and Ball, G. F. 1998. Melatonin, immunity and cost of reproductive state in male European starlings. *Proc. R. Soc. Lond. B,* 265:1191–1195.

Bentley, G. E., Van't Hof, T. J., and Ball, G. F. 1999. Seasonal neuroplasticity in the songbird telencephalon: A role for melatonin. *Proc. Natl. Acad. Sci. U.S.A.,* 96:4674–4679.

Benton, D., and Brain, P. F. 1988. The role of opioid mechanisms in social interaction and attachment. In R. J. Rodgers and S. J. Cooper (eds.), *Endorphins, Opiates, and Behavioural Processes,* pp. 217–235. Wiley, New York.

Berenbaum, S. A., and Hines, M. 1992. Early androgens are related to childhood sex-typed toy preferences. *Psychol. Sci.,* 3:203–206.

Berenbaum, S. A., and Resnick, S. M. 1997. Early androgen effects on aggression in children and adults with congenital adrenal hyperplasia. *Psychoneuroendocrinology,* 22:505–515.

Berga, S. L., Daniels, T. L., and Giles, D. E. 1997. Women with functional hypothalamic amenorrhea but not other forms of anovulation display amplified cortisol concentrations. *Fertil. Steril.,* 67:1024–1030.

Berger, N. C., Negus, N. C., and Rowsemitt, C. N. 1987. Effect of 6-methoxybenzoazolinone on sex ratio and breeding performance in Microtus montanus. *Biol. Reprod.,* 36:255–260.

Bermant, G. 1961. Response latencies of female rats during sexual intercourse. *Science,* 133:1771–1773.

Bermant, G., and Taylor, L. 1969. Interactive effects of experience and olfactory bulb lesions in male rat copulation. *Physiol. Behav.,* 4:13–17.

Bermant, G., and Westbrook, W. H. 1966. Peripheral factors in the regulation of sexual contact by female rats. *J. Comp. Physiol. Psychol.,* 61:244–250.

Bermant, G., Lott, D. F., and Anderson, L. 1968. Temporal characteristics of the Coolidge effect in male rat copulatory behavior. *J. Comp. Physiol. Psychol.,* 65: 447–452.

Bern, H. A. 1990. The "new" endocrinology: Its scope and its impact. *Am. Zool.,* 30:877–885.

Bernard, C. 1856. *Leçons de physiologie expérimentale appliquée à la médicine faites au Collège de France.* Vol. 2, Baillière, Paris.

Bernard, D. J., and Ball, G. F. 1993. Two independent markers demonstrate an increased volume of HVC in short-day photosensitive relative to long-day photorefractory European starlings. *Soc. Neurosci. Abstr.,* 19:1017.

Bernard, D., Wilson, F., and Ball, G. 1997. Testis-dependent and -independent effects of photoperiod on volumes of song control nuclei in American tree sparrows (*Spizella arborea*). *Brain Res.,* 760:163–9.

Berndtson, W. E., and Desjardins, C. 1974. Circulating LH and FSH levels and testicular function in hamsters during light deprivation and subsequent photoperiodic stimulation. *Endocrinology,* 95:195–205.

Bernhardt, P. C., Dabbs, J. M., Fielden, J. A., and Lutter, C. D. 1998. Testosterone changes during vicarious experiences of winning and losing among fans at sporting events. *Physiol. Behav.,* 65:59–62.

Bernstein, A., and Breitman, M. 1989. Genetic ablation in transgenic mice. *Mol. Biol. Med.,* 6, 523–530.

Bernstein, I. S. 1981. Dominance: The baby and the bathwater. *Behav. Brain Sci.,* 4:419–457.

Bernstein, I. S., Rose, R. M., and Gordon, T. P. 1974. Behavioral and environmental events influencing primate testosterone levels. *J. Hum. Evol.,* 3:517–525.

Bernstein, P. L., Zuo, M., and Cheng, M.-F. 1993. Social condition affects the courtship behavior of male ring doves with posterior medial hypothalamic lesions. *Behav. Neural Biol.,* 59:120–125.

Berta, P., Hawkins, J. R., Sinclair, A. H., Taylor, A., Griffiths, B. L., Goodfellow, P. N. 1990. Genetic evidence equating SRY and the testis-determining factor. *Nature,* 348:448–450.

Berthold, A. A. 1837. Einige Beobachtungen über den Winterschlaf der Thiere. *Arch. Anat. Physiol. Wissensch. Med.,* 11:63–68.

Berthold, A. A. 1849. Transplantation der hoden. *Arch. Anat. Physiol. Wissenschr. Med.,* 16:42–49.

Berthold, A. A. 1849. Transplantation of testes. Trans. by D. P. Quiring. *Bull. History Med.,* 16:42–46, 1944.

Bertolucci, C., and Foa, A. 1998. Seasonality and role of SCN in entrainment of lizard circadian rhythms to daily melatonin injections. *Am. J. Physiol.,* 274:R1004–1014.

Bex, F. J., and Goldman, B. D. 1975. Serum gonadotropins and follicular development in the Syrian hamster. *Endocrinology,* 96:928–933.

Beyer, C., and Feder, H. 1987. Sex steroids and afferent input: Their roles in brain differentiation. *Annu. Rev. Psychol.,* 49:349–364.

Beyer, C., Morali, G., Naftolin, F., Larsson, K., and Perez-Palacios, G. 1976. Effect of some antiestrogens and aromatase inhibitors on androgen induced sexual behavior in castrated male rats. *Horm. Behav.,* 7:353–363.

Bielak, T., and Pucek, Z. 1960. Season changes in the brain weight of the common shrew (*Sorez araneus araneus Linnaeus,* 1758). *Acta Theriol.,* 3:297–300.

Biessels, G. J., Kamal, A., Ramakers, G. M., Urban, I. J., Spruijt, B. M., Erkelens, D. W., and Gispen, W. H. 1996. Place learning and hippocampal synaptic plasticity in streptozotocin-induced diabetic rats. *Diabetes,* 45:1259–1266.

Biessels, G. J., Kamal, A., Urban, I. J., Spruijt, B. M., Erkelens, D. W., and Gispen, W. H. 1998. Water maze learning and hippocampal synaptic plasticity in streptozotocin-diabetic rats: Effects of insulin treatment. *Brain Res.,* 800:125–135.

Bird, E., Cardone, C. C., and Contreras, R. J. 1983. Area postrema lesions disrupt food intake induced by cerebroventricular infusions of 5-thioglucose in the rat. *Brain Res.,* 270:193–196.

Biron, D., Dauphin, C., and Di Paolo, T. 1992. Effects of adrenalectomy and glucocorticoids on rat brain dopamine receptors. *Neuroendocrinology,* 55:468–476.

Bishop, M. W. 1970. Aging and reproduction in the male. *J. Reprod. Fertil. (Suppl.),* 12:65–87.

Bitran, D. and Dowd, J. A. 1996. Ovarian steroids modify the behavioral and neurochemical responses of the central benzodiazepine receptor. *Psychopharmacology,* 125:65–73.

Bitran, D., Hull, E. M., Holmes, G. M., and Lookingland, K. J. 1988. Regulation of male rat copulatory behavior by preoptic incertohypothalamic dopamine neurons. *Brain Res. Bull.,* 20:323–331.

Bitran, D., Shiekh, M., and McLeod, M. 1995. Anxiolytic effect of progesterone is mediated by the neurosteroid allopregnanolone at brain GABA$_A$ receptors. *J. Neuroendocrinol.,* 7:171–177.

Bittman, E. L. 1993. Melatonin: A durational signal regulating steroid-dependent and -independent aspects of limbic and hypophyseal function. In Y. Touitou, J. Arendt, and P. Pevet (eds.), *Melatonin and the Pineal Gland: From Basic Science to Clinical Application,* pp. 151–158. Elsevier, Amsterdam.

Bittman, E. L., and Goldman, B. D. 1979. Serum levels of gonadotrophins in hamsters exposed to short photoperiods: Effects of adrenalectomy and ovariectomy. *J. Endocrinol.,* 83:113–118.

Bittman, E. L., and Karsch, F. J. 1984. Nightly duration of pineal melatonin secretion determines the reproductive response to inhibitory day length in the ewe. *Biol. Reprod.,* 30:585–593.

Bittman, E. L., and Weaver, D. R. 1990. The distribution of melatonin binding sites in neuroendocrine tissues of the ewe. *Biol. Reprod.,* 43:986–993.

Bittman, E. L., Jonassen, J. A., and Hegarty, C. M. 1992. Photoperiodic regulation of pulsatile luteinizing hormone secretion and adrenohypophyseal gene expression in female golden hamsters. *Biol. Reprod.,* 47:66–71.

Biver, F., Lotstra, F., Monclus, M., Wikler, D., Damhaut, P., Mendlewicz, J., and Goldman, S. 1996. Sex difference in 5HT2 receptor in the living human brain. *Neurosci. Letters,* 204:25–28.

Blair-West, J. R., Coghlan, J. P., Denton, D. A., Nelson, J. F., Ochard, E., Scoggins, B. A., Wright, R. D, Myers, K., and Junqueira, C. L. 1968. Physiological, morphological and behavioural adaptation to a sodium deficient environment by wild native Australian and introduced species of animals. *Nature,* 217:922–928.

Blanchard, D. C., Spencer, R. L., Weiss, S. M., Blanchard, R. J., McEwen, B., and Sakai, R. R. 1995. Visible burrow system as a model of chronic social stress: behavioral and neuroendocrine correlates. *Psychoneuroendocrinology,* 20:117–34.

Blandau, R. J., and Soderwall, A. L. 1941. Post-parturitional heat and the time of ovulation in the albino rat. *Anat. Rec.,* 81:419–429.

Blank, J. L., and Desjardins, C. 1985. Photic cues induce multiple neuroendocrine adjustments in testicular function. *Am. J. Physiol.,* 238:R181–R189.

Blask, D. E., Leadem, C. A., Orstead, M., and Larsen, B. R. 1986. Prolactin cell activity in female and male Syrian hamsters: An apparent sexually dimorphic response to light deprivation and pinealectomy. *Neuroendocrinology,* 42:15–20.

Blass, E. M., and Epstein, A. N. 1971. A lateral preoptic osmosensitive zone for thirst in the rat. *J. Comp. Physiol. Psychol.,* 76:378–394.

Blaustein, J. D. 1996. Ovarian steroid hormone receptors in the brain: Localization, action and behavioral function. In K. A. Ginsburg (ed.), *Infertility and Reproductive Medicine Clinics of North America, Premenstrual Syndrome and Related Disorders,* vol. 7: 243–265. W. B. Saunders, Ridley Park, PA.

Blaustein, J. D., and Olster, D. H. 1989. Gonadal steroid hormone receptors and social behaviors. *Adv. Comp. Env. Physiol.,* 3:31–104.

Blaustein, J. D., and Wade, G. N. 1976. Ovarian influences on the meal pattern of female rats. *Physiol. Behav.,* 17:201–208.

Bloch, G. J., and Gorski, R. A. 1988. Cytoarchitectonic analysis of the SDN-POA of the intact and gonadectomized rat. *J. Comp. Neurol.,* 275:604–612.

Bloom, S. R., and Polak, J. M. (eds.). 1981. *Gut Hormones.* (2nd ed.). Churchill-Livingstone, Edinburgh.

Blurton Jones, N. G. 1986. Bushman birth spacing: A test for optimal interbirth intervals. *Ethol. Sociobiol.,* 7:91–105.

Bluthe, R. M., Gheusi, G., and Dantzer, R. 1993. Gonadal steroids influence the involvement of arginine vasopressin in social recognition in mice. *Psychoneuroendocrinology,* 18:323–335.

Boccia, M. M., Kopf, S. R., and Baratti, C. M. 1998. Effects of a single administrationof oxytocin or vasopressin and their interactions with two selective receptor antagonists on memory storage in mice. *Neurobiol. Learn. Mem.,* 69:136–146.

Boden, G., Chen, X., Mozzoli, M., and Ryan, I. J. 1996. Effect of fasting on serum leptin in normal human subjects. *Clin. Endocrinol. Metab.,* 81:3419–3423.

Boggs, S. S. 1990. Targeted gene modification for gene therapy of stem cells. *Int. J. Cell Clon.,* 8, 80–96.

Bohus, B., Conti, L., Kovacs, G. L., and Versteeg, D. H. G. 1982. Modulation of memory processes by neuropeptides: Interaction with neurotransmitter systems. In C. A. Marsan and H. Matthies (eds.), *Neuronal Plasticity and Memory Formation,* pp. 75–87. Raven Press, New York.

Bolig, R., Price, C. S., O'Neill, P. L., and Suomi, S. J. 1992. Subjective assessment of reactivity level and personality traits of rhesus monkeys. *Int. J. Primatol.,* 13:287–306.

Boling, J. L., and Blandau, R. J. 1939. The estrogen–progesterone induction of mating responses in the spayed female rat. *Endocrinology,* 25:359–364.

Boling, J. L., Blandau, R. J., Soderwall, A. L., and Young, W. C. 1941. Growth of the Graafian follicle and the time of ovulation in the albino rat. *Anat. Rec.,* 79:313–325.

Bonsall, R. W., and Michael, R. P. 1992. Developmental changes in the uptake of testosterone by the primate brain. *Neuroendocrinology,* 55:84–91.

Bonsall, R. W., Rees, H. D., and Michael, R. P. 1985. The distribution, nuclear uptake and metabolism of [$^3$H]Dihydrotestosterone in the brain, pituitary gland and genital tract of the male rhesus monkey. *J. Steroid Biochem.,* 23:389–398.

Bonsall, R. W., Zumpe, D., and Michael, R. P. 1978. Menstrual cycle influences on operant behavior of female rhesus monkeys. *J. Comp. Physiol. Psychol.,* 92:846–855.

Bonsall, R. W., Zumpe, D., and Michael, R. P. 1990. Comparisons of the nuclear uptake of [3H]-testosterone and its metabolites by the brains of male and female macaque fetuses at 122 days of gestation. *Neuroendocrinology,* 51:474–480.

Booth, A., Shelley, G., Mazur, A., Tharp, G., and Kittok, R. 1989. Testosterone and wining and losing in human competition. *Horm. Behav.,* 23:556–571.

Booth, J. E. 1977. Sexual behavior of neonatally castrated rats injected during infancy with oestrogen and dihydrotestosterone. *J. Endocrinol.,* 72:135–142.

Borowsky, I. W., Hogan, M., and Ireland, M. 1997. Adolescent sexual aggression: Risk and protective factors. *Pediatrics,* 100:E7.

Bottjer, S. W., Glaessner, S. L., and Arnold, A. P. 1985. Ontogeny of brain nuclei controlling song learning and behavior in zebra finches. *J. Neurosci.,* 5:1556–1562.

Bottjer, S. W., Halsema, K. A., Brown, S. A., and Miesner, E. A. 1989. Axonal connections of a forebrain nucleus involved with vocal learning in zebra finches. *J. Comp. Neurol.,* 279:312–326.

Bottjer, S. W., Miesner, E. A., and Arnold, A. P. 1984. Forebrain lesions disrupt development but not maintenance of song in passerine birds. *Science*, 224:901–903.

Bottjer, S. W., Schoonmaker, J. N., and Arnold, A. P. 1986. Auditory and hormonal stimulation interact to produce neural growth in adult canaries. *J. Neurobiol.*, 17:605–612.

Bouissou, M. F. 1983. Androgens, aggressive behaviour and social relationships in higher mammals. *Horm. Res.*, 18:43–61.

Bowen, D. J., and Grunberg, N. E. 1990. Variations in food preference and consumption across the menstrual cycle. *Physiol. Behav.*, 47:287–291.

Bowlby, J. 1969. *Attachment and Loss. Vol. 1. Attachment.* Basic Books, New York.

Boyd, S. 1997. Brain, vasotocin pathways and the control of sexual behavior in the bullfrog. *Brain Res. Bull.*, 44:345–350.

Bozarth, M. A. and Wise, R. A. 1985. Toxicity associated with long-term intravenous heroin and cocaine self-administration in the rat. *J. A. M. A.*, 254:81–83.

Bozart, M. A., Murray, A., and Wise, R. A. 1989. Influence of housing conditions on the acquisition of intravenous heroin and cocaine self-administration in rats. *Pharmacol. Biochem. Behav.* 33:903–907.

Brain, P. F., and Nowell, N. W. 1969. Some endocrine and behavioral changes in the development of the albino laboratory mouse. *Commun. Behav. Biol.*, 4:203–220.

Brain, P. F., Haug, M., and Kamis, A. B. 1983. Hormones and different tests for aggression with particular reference to the effects of testosterone metabolites. In J. Balthazart, E. Prove, and R. Gilles (eds.), *Hormones and Behaviour in Higher Vertebrates*, pp. 3–25. Springer-Verlag, Berlin.

Brainard, G. C., Richardson, B. A., King, T. S., Matthews, S. A., and Reiter, R. J. 1983. The suppression of pineal melatonin content and N-acetyltransferase activity by different light irradiances in the Syrian hamster: A dose–response relationship. *Endocrinology*, 113:293–296.

Brantley, R. K., Wingfield, J., and Bass, A. H. 1993. Hormonal bases for male teleost dimorphisms: Sex steroid levels in *Porichthys notatus*, a fish with alternative reproductive tactics. *Horm. Behav.*, 27:332–347.

Breedlove, S. M. 1992. Sexual dimorphism in the vertebrate nervous system. *J. Neurosci.*, 12:4133–4142.

Breedlove, S. M. 1994. Sexual differentiation of the human nervous system. *Annu. Rev. Neurosci.* 45:389–418.

Breedlove, S. M. 1997. Sex on the brain. *Nature*, 389:801.

Breedlove, S. M., and Arnold, A. P. 1981. Sexually dimorphic motor nucleus in the rat lumbar spinal cord: Response to adult hormone manipulation, absence in androgen-insensitive rats. *Brain Res.*, 225:297–307.

Breedlove, S. M., and Arnold, A. P. 1983a. Hormonal control of a developing neuromuscular system: I. Complete demasculinization of the spinal nucleus of the bulbocavernosus in male rats using the anti-androgen flutamide. *J. Neurosci.*, 3:417–423.

Breedlove, S. M., and Arnold, A. P. 1983b. Hormonal control of a developing neuromuscular system: II. Sensitive periods for the androgen-induced masculinization of the rat spinal nucleus of the bulbocavernosus. *J. Neurosci.*, 3:424–432.

Bremner, J. D., Scott, T. M., Delaney, R. C., Southwick, S. M., Mason, J. W., Johnson, D. R., Innis, R. B., McCarthy, G., and Charney, D. S. 1993. Deficits in short-term memory in posttraumatic stress disorder. *Am. J. Psychiatry*, 150:1015–1019.

Brenowitz, E. A. 1991. Altered perception of species-specific song by female birds after lesions of a forebrain nucleus. *Science*, 251:303–305.

Brenowitz, E. A. 1997. Comparative approaches to the avian song system. *J. Neurobiol.*, 33:517–531.

Brenowitz, E. A., and Arnold, A. P. 1985. Lack of sexual dimorphism in the steroid accumulation in vocal control brain regions of duet-ting song birds. *Brain Res.*, 344:172–180.

Brenowitz, E. A., and Arnold, A. P. 1986. Interspecific comparison of the size in neural song control regions and song complexity in duetting birds: Evolutionary implications. *J. Neurosci.*, 6:2875–2879.

Brenowitz, E. A., and Arnold, A. P. 1989. Accumulation of estrogen in a vocal control brain region of a duetting song bird. *Brain Res.*, 359:364–367.

Brenowitz, E. A., and Arnold, A. P. 1992. Hormone accumulation in song regions of the canary brain. *J. Neurobiol.*, 23:871–880.

Brenowitz, E. A., Arnold, A. P., and Levin, R. N. 1985. Neural corre-lates of female song in tropical duetting birds. *Brain Res.*, 480: 119–125.

Brenowitz, E. A., Baptista, L., Lent, K., and Wingfield, J. 1998. Seasonal plasticity of the song control system in wild Nuttall's white-crowned sparrows. *J. Neurobiol.*, 34: 69–82.

Brenowitz, E. A., Nalls, B., Wingfield, J. C., and Kroodsma, D. E. 1991. Seasonal changes in avian song control nuclei without seasonal changes in song repertoire. *J. Neurosci.*, 11:1367–1374.

Bridges, R. S. 1975. Long-term effects of pregnancy and parturition upon maternal responsiveness in the rat. *Physiol. Behav.*, 14:245–249.

Bridges, R. S. 1977. Parturition: Its role in the long-term retention of maternal behavior in the rat. *Physiol. Behav.*,18:487–490.

Bridges, R. S. 1978. Retention of rapid onset of maternal behavior during pregnancy in primiparous rats. *Behav. Biology*, 24:113–117.

Bridges, R. S. 1990. Endocrine regulation of parental behavior in rodents. In N. A. Krasnegor and R. S. Bridges (eds.), *Mammalian Parenting*, pp. 93–117. Oxford University Press, Oxford.

Bridges, R. S. 1996. Biochemical basis of parental behavior in the rat. *Adv. Study Behav.*, 25:215–242.

Bridges, R. S., and Freemark, M. S. 1995. Human placental lactogen infusions into the medial preoptic area stimulate maternal behav-ior in steroid-primed, nulliparous female rats. *Horm. Behav.*, 29:216–226.

Bridges, R. S., and Goldman, B. D. 1975. Diurnal rhythms in gonado-tropins and progesterone in lactating and photoperiod induced acyclic hamsters. *Biol. Reprod.*, 13:617–622.

Bridges, R. S., Robertson, M. C., Shiu, R. P., Friesen, H. G., Stuer, A. M., and Mann, P. E. 1996. Endocrine communication between conceptus and mother: Placental lactogen stimulation of mater-nal behavior. *Neuroendocrinology*, 64:57–64.

Bridges, R. S., Rosenblatt, J. S., and Feder, H. 1978a. Serum proges-terone concentrations and maternal behavior in rats after preg-nancy termination: Behavioral stimulation following progesterone withdrawal and inhibition by progesterone maintenance. *Endo-crinology*, 102:258–267.

Bridges, R. S., Rosenblatt, J. S., and Feder, H. 1978b. Stimulation of maternal responsiveness after pregnancy termination in rats: Effect of time of onset of behavioral testing. *Horm. Behav.*, 10:235–245.

Brinkmann, A., Jenster, G., Ris-Stalpers, C., van der Korput, H., Bruggenwirth, H., Boehmer, A., and Trapman, J. 1996. Molecular basis of androgen insensitivity. *Steroids*, 61:172–5175.

Brinsmead, M., Smith, R., Singh, B., Lewin, T., and Owens, P. 1985. Peripartum concentrations of beta-endorphin and cortisol and maternal mood states. *Aust. N. Z. J. Obstet. Gynaecol.*, 12:194–197.

Brobeck, J. R., Wheatland, M., and Strominger, J. L. 1947. Variations in regulation of energy exchange associated with estrus, diestrus and pseudopregnancy in rats. *Endocrinology*, 40:65–72.

Broida, J., Michael, S., and Svare, B. 1981. Plasma prolactin is not related to the initiation, maintenance, and decline of maternal aggression in mice. *Behav. Neural Biol.*, 35:121–125.

Bronson, F. H. 1967. Effects of social stimulation on adrenal and reproductive physiology of rodents. In M. L. Conalty (ed.), *Husbandry of Laboratory Animals.* Academic Press, New York.

Bronson, F. H. 1979. The reproductive ecology of the house mouse. *Q. Rev. Biol.*, 54:265–299.

Bronson, F. H. 1988. Seasonal regulation of reproduction in mam-mals. In E. Knobil and J. D. Neill (eds.), *The Physiology of Reproduction*, Vol. 2, pp. 1831–1872. Raven Press, New York.

Bronson, F. H. 1989. *Mammalian Reproductive Biology.* University of Chicago Press, Chicago.

Bronson, F. H. 1996. Effects of prolonged exposure to anabolic steroids on the behavior of male and female mice. *Pharmacol. Biochem. Behav.* 53:329–334.

Bronson, F. H. 1999. Puberty and energy reserves: a walk on the wild side. In K. Wallen and J. E. Schneider (eds.), *Reproduction in Context.* MIT Press, Cambridge, MA.

Bronson, F. H. and Matherne, C. M. 1997. Exposure to anabolic-androgenic steroids shortens life span of male mice. *Med. Sci. Sports Exerc.*, 29:615–619.

Bronson, F. H., and Desjardins, C. 1982a. Endocrine responses to sexual arousal in male mice. *Endocrinology*, 111:1286–1291.

Bronson, F. H., and Desjardins, C. 1982b. Reproductive aging in male mice. In M. E. Reff (ed.), *Biological Markers of Aging*, pp. 87–93. NIH, Bethesda, MD. Publication no. 82-2221.

Bronson, F. H., and Heideman, P. D. 1994. Seasonal regulation of reproduction in mammals. In E. Knobil and J. D. Neill (eds.), *The Physiology of Reproduction*, Vol. 2, pp. 541–584. Raven Press, New York.

Brookhart, J. M., Dey, F. L., and Ranson, S. W. 1941. The abolition of mating behavior by hypothalamic lesions in guinea pigs. *Endocrinology,* 28:561–565.

Brooks-Gunn, J. 1986. Differentiating premenstrual syndromes. *Psychosomat. Med.,* 48:385–387.

Brown, C. S., Ling, F. W., Andersen, R. N., Farmer, R. G., and Arheart, K. L. 1994. Efficacy of depot leuprolide in premenstrual syndrome: Effect of symptom severity and type in a controlled trial. *Obstet. Gynecol.,* 84:77–786.

Brown, F. A. 1972. The clocks timing biological rhythms. *Am. Sci.,* 60:756–766.

Brown, J. R., Ye, H., Bronson, R. T., Dikkes, P., and Greenberg, M. E. 1996. A defect in nurturing in mice lacking the immediate early gene fosB. *Cell,* 86:297–309.

Brown, L. L., Siegel, H., and Etgen, A. M. 1996. Global sex differences in stress-induced activation of cerebral metabolism revealed by 2-deoxyglucose autoradiography. *Horm. Behav.,* 30:611–617.

Brown, M., Rivier, J., Kobayashi, R., and Vale, W. 1978. Cholecystokinin in feeding behavior. In S. R. Bloom (ed.), *Gut Hormones,* pp. 550–558. Raven Press, New York.

Brown, R. E. 1994. *An Introduction to Neuroendocrinology.* Cambridge University Press, Cambridge.

Brown, R. E., Murdoch, T., Murphy, P. R., and Moger, W. H. 1995. Hormonal responses of male gerbils to stimuli from their mate and pups. *Horm. Behav.,* 29:474–491.

Brown, R., and Kulik, J. 1977. Flashbulb memories. *Cognition,* 5:73–99.

Brown, T. J., Naftolin, F., and Maclusky, N. J. 1992. Sex differences in estrogen receptor binding in the rat hypothalamus: Effects of subsaturating pulses of estradiol. *Brain Res.,* 578: 129–134.

Brown, W. A., Monti, P. M., and Corriveau, D. P. 1978. Serum testosterone and sexual activity and interest in men. *Arch. Sex. Behav.,* 7:97–103.

Brown-Parlee, M. 1990. Integrating biological and social scientific research on menopause. *Ann. N. Y. Acad. Sci.,* 592:379–389.

Brown-Parlee, M. 1991. The social construction of premenstrual syndrome: A case study of scientific discourse as cultural contestation. Working paper presented at: *The Good Body: Asceticism in Contemporary Culture.* Institute for the Medical Humanities, University of Texas, Galveston, TX.

Brown-Séquard, C. E. 1899. The effects produced on man by subcutaneous injections of a liquid obtained from the testicles of animals. *Lancet,* 105–106, reprinted in Carter, C. S. (ed.), *Hormones and Sexual Behavior.* Stroudsburg, Dowden, Hutchinson and Ross, Inc.

Bruce, H. M. 1959. An exteroceptive block to pregnancy in the mouse. *Nature,* 184:105.

Bruce, H. M. 1960. A block to pregnancy in the mouse caused by the proximity of strange males. *J. Reprod. Fertil.,* 1:96–103.

Brunelli, S. A., and Hofer, M. A. 1990. Parental behavior in juvenile rats: Environmental and biological determinants. In N. A. Krasnegor and R. S. Bridges (eds.), *Mammalian Parenting,* pp. 372–399. Oxford University Press, Oxford.

Bryant, K. J. 1982. Personality correlates of sense of direction and geographic orientation. *J. Pers. Soc. Psychol.,* 43:1318–1324.

Bryant, K. J. 1991. Geographical/spatial orientation ability within real-world and simulated large-scale environments. *Multivar. Behav. Res.,* 26:109–136.

Buckman, M. T., and Kellner, R. 1985. Reduction of distress in hyperprolactinemia with bromocriptine. *Am. J. Psychiatry,* 142:242–244.

Buhrich, N., Bailey, J. M., and Martin, N. G. 1991. Sexual orientation, sexual identity, and sex-dimorphic behaviors in male twins. *Behav. Genet.,* 21:75–96.

Bull, J. J. 1980. Sex determination in reptiles. *Q. Rev. Biol.,* 55:3–21.

Bull, J. J. 1983. *Evolution of Sex Determining Mechanisms.* Benjamin/Cummings, Menlo Park, CA.

Bullock, D. W. 1970. Induction of heat in ovariectomized guinea pigs by brief exposure to estrogen and progesterone. *Horm. Behav.,* 1:137–143.

Bunnell, B. N., Boland, B. D., and Dewsbury, D. A. 1976. Copulatory behavior of the golden hamster (*Mescricetus auratus*). *Behaviour,* 61:180–206.

Buntin, J. D. 1996. Neural and hormonal control of parental behavior in birds. *Adv. Study Behav.,* 25:161–213.

Buntin, J. D., Ruzycki, E., and Witebsky, J. 1993. Prolactin receptors in dove brain: Autoradiographic analysis of binding characteristics in discrete brain regions and accessibility to blood-borne prolactin. *Neuroendocrinology,* 57:738–750.

Burgers, J. K., Nelson, R. J., Quinlan, D. M., and Walsh, P. C. 1991. Nerve growth factor, nerve grafts and amniotic membrane grafts restore erectile function in rats. *J. Urol.,* 146:463–468.

Burghardt, G. M. 1988. Precocity, play, and the ectotherm–endotherm transition: Profound reorganization or superficial adaptation? In E. M. Blass (ed.), *Handbook of Behavioral Neurobiology,* Vol. 9, pp. 107–148. Plenum, New York.

Burkhardt, R. W. 1987. The Journal of Animal Behavior and the early history of animal behavior in America. *J. Comp. Psychol.,* 101:223–230.

Burnett, A. L. 1995. Role of nitric oxide in the physiology of erection. *Biol. Reprod.,* 52:485–489.

Burnett, A. L., Johns, D. G., Kriegsfeld, L. J., Klein, S. L., Calvin, D. C., Demas, G. E., Schramm, L. P., Tonegawa, S., Nelson, R. J., Snyder, S. H., and Poss, K. D. 1998. Ejaculatory abnormalities in mice with targeted disruption of the gene for heme oxygenase-2. *Nat. Med.,* 4:84–87.

Burrows, W. 1945. Periodic spawning of the Palolo worms in Pacific waters. *Nature,* 155:47–48.

Butenandt, A. 1929. Uber "progynon," ein kristall-isiertes weibliches Sexualhormone. *Naturwiessenschaften,* 17:879. Abstract translated by E. W. Henry in *Biol. Abstr.,* 5:85 (881).

Butera, P. C., and Beikirch, R. J. 1989. Central implants of diluted estradiol: Independent effects on ingestive and reproductive behaviors of ovariectomized rats. *Brain Res.,* 491:266–273.

Buvat, J., Lemaire, A., Buvat-Herbaut, M., Fourlinnie, J. C., Racadot, A., and Fossati, P. 1985. Hyperprolactinemia and sexual function in men. *Horm. Res.,* 22:196–203.

Byne, W., and Parsons, B. 1993. Human sexual orientation: The biologic theories reappraised. *Arch. Gen. Psychiatry,* 50:228–239.

Cahill, G. M., Grace, M. S., and Besharse, J. C. 1991. Rhythmic regulation of retinal melatonin: Metabolic pathways, neurochemical regulation and the ocular circadian clock. *Cell. Mol. Neurobiol.,* 11: 529–560.

Cahill, L., Prins, B., Weber, M., and McGaugh, J. L. 1994. Beta-adrenergic activation and memory for emotional events. *Nature,* 271:702–704.

Cain, D. P. 1974. The role of the olfactory bulbs in limbic mechanisms. *Psychol. Bull.,* 81:654–671.

Caldji, C., Tannenbaum, B., Sharma, S., Francis, D., Plotsky, P. M., and Meaney, M. J. 1998. Maternal care during infancy regulates the development of neural systems mediating the expression of fearfulness in the rat. *Proc. Natl. Acad. Sci. U.S.A.,* 95:5335–5340.

Caldwell, G. S., Glickman, S. E., and Smith, E. R. 1984. Seasonal aggression is independent of seasonal testosterone in wood rats. *Proc. Natl. Acad. Sci. U.S.A.,* 81:5255–5257.

Calhoun, J. B. 1961. Phenomena associated with population density. *Proc. Natl. Acad. Sci. U.S.A.,* 47:428–49.

Calhoun, J. B. 1962a. *The Ecology and Sociology of the Norway Rat.* U. S. Government Printing Office, Washington, D.C.

Calhoun, J. B. 1962b. Population density and social pathology. *Sci. Am.,* 206:139–148.

Camazine, B., Gartska, W., Tokarz, R., and Crews, D. 1980. Effects of castration and androgen replacement on male courtship behaviour in the red-sided garter snake (*Thamnophis sirtalis parietalis*). *Horm. Behav.,* 14:358–372.

Cameron, J. L. 1997. Stress and behaviorally-induced reproductive dysfunction in primates. *Sem. Reprod. Endocrinol.,* 15:37–45.

Cameron, J. L., Helmreich, D. L., and Schreihofer, D. A. 1993. Modulation of reproductive hormone secretion by nutritional intake: Stress signals versus metabolic signals. *Hum. Reprod.,* 8:162–167.

Campbell, C. S., Finkelstein, J. S., and Turek, F. W. 1978. The interaction of photoperiod and testosterone on the development of copulatory behavior in male hamsters. *Physiol. Behav.,* 21:409–415.

Campbell, S. S., and Murphy, P. J. 1998. Extraocular circadian phototransduction in humans. *Science,* 279:396–399.

Campfield, L. A., Smith, F. J., and Burn, P. 1995. The OB protein (leptin) pathway—a link between adipose tissue mass and central neural networks. *Horm. Metab. Res.,* 28:619–632.

Campfield, L. A., Smith, F. J., Guisez, Y., Devos, R., and Burn, P. 1995. Recombinant mouse OB protein: Evidence for a peripheral signal linking adiposity and central neural networks. *Science,* 269:546–549.

Canacher, G. N., and Workman, D. G. 1989. Violent crime possibly associated with anabolic steroid use. *Am. J. Psychiatry,* 146:679.

Candolle, A. P. de 1832. *Physiologie Vegetale,* vol. 2. Bechet Jeune: Paris.

Cannon, W. B. 1929. *Bodily Changes in Pain, Hunger, Fear and Rage.* Appleton, New York.

Capitanio, J. P., Mendoza, S. P., Lerche, N. W., and Mason, W. A. 1998. Social stress results in altered glucocorticoid regulation and shorter survival in simian acquired immune deficiency syndrome. *Proc. Natl. Acad. Sci. U.S.A.,* 95:471–4719.

Carani, C., Bancroft, J., DelRio, G., Granata, A. R. M., Faccinetti, F., and Marrama, P. 1990. The endocrine effects of visual erotic stimuli in normal men. *Psychoneuroendocrinology,* 15:207–216.

Carboni, E., Imperato, A., Perezzani, L., and Di Chiara, G. 1989. Differential inhibitory effects of a 5-HT3 antagonist on drug-induced stimulation of dopamine release. *Eur. J. Pharmacol.,* 164:515–519.

Cardwell, J. R., and Liley, N. R. 1991a. Androgen control of social status in males of a wild population of stoplight parrot fish, *Sparisoma viride. Horm. Behav.,* 25:1–18.

Cardwell, J. R., and Liley, N. R. 1991b. Hormonal control of sex and color change in the stoplight parrot fish, *Sparisoma viride* (Scaridae). *J. Comp. Physiol.,* 115:299–317.

Cardwell, J. R., Sorensen, P. W., Van der Kraak, G. J., and Liley, N. R. 1996. Effect of dominance status on sex hormone levels in laboratory and wild-spawning male trout. *Gen. Comp. Endocrinol.,* 101:333–341.

Carlsen, E., Giwercman, A., Keiding, N., and Skakkebaek, N. E. 1992. Evidence for decreasing quality of semen during the past 50 years. *Br. Med. J.,* 305:609–613.

Carmichael, M. S., Nelson, R. J., and Zucker, I. 1981. Hamster activity and estrous cycles: Control by a single versus multiple circadian oscillator(s). *Proc. Natl. Acad. Sci. U.S.A.,* 78:7830–7834.

Carpenter, C. R. 1940. A field study of the behavior and social relations of howling monkeys. *Comp. Psychol. Monogr.,* 16:1–21.

Carpenter, C. R. 1942a. Sexual behavior of free ranging rhesus monkeys (*Macaca mulatta*). I. Specimens, procedures, and behavioral characteristics of estrus. *J. Comp. Psychol.,* 33:113–142.

Carpenter, C. R. 1942b. Sexual behavior of free ranging rhesus monkeys (*Macaca mulatta*). II. Periodicity of estrus, homosexual, autoerotic and non-conformist behavior. *J. Comp. Psychol.,* 33:143–162.

Carr, C. E. 1993. Processing of temporal information in the brain. *Annu. Rev. Neurosci.,* 16:223–243.

Carroll, B. J. 1980. Dexamethasone suppression test in depression. *Lancet,* 8206:1249.

Carroll, B. J., Curtis, G. C., and Mendels, J. 1976. Neuroendocrine regulation in depression. I. Limbic system-adrenocortical dysfunction. *Arch. Gen. Psychiatry,* 33:1039.

Carroll, B. J., Martin, F. I. R., and Davies, B. 1968. Resistance to suppression by dexamethasone of plasma 11-OHCS levels in severe depressive illness. *Br. Med. J.,* 3:285–290.

Carter, C. S. (ed.). 1974. *Hormones and Sexual Behavior.* Stroudsburg, Dowden, Hutchinson and Ross, Inc.

Carter, C. S., DeVries, A. C., and Getz, L. L. 1995. Physiological substrates of mammalian monogamy. *Neurosci. Biobehav. Rev.,* 19:303–314.

Carter, C. S., DeVries, A. C., Taymans, S. E., Roberts, R. L., Williams, J. R., and Getz, L. L. 1997a. Peptides, steroids, and pair bonding. *Ann. N. Y. Acad. Sci.,* 807:260–272.

Carter, C. S., Getz, L. L., and Cohen-Parsons, M. 1986. Relationship between social organization and behavioral endocrinology in a monogamous mammal. *Adv. Study Behav.,* 16:109–145.

Carter, C. S., Getz, L. L., Gavish, L., McDermott, J. L., and Arnold, P. 1980. Male-related pheromones and the activation of female reproduction in the prairie vole (*Microtus ochrogaster*). *Biol. Reprod.,* 23:1038–1045.

Carter, C. S., Lederhendler, I. I., and Kirkpatrick, B. 1997b. *Integrative Neurobiology of Affiliation.* Vol. 807. New York Academy of Sciences: New York.

Carter, C. S., Williams, J. R., Witt, D. M., and Insel, T. R. 1992. Oxytocin and social bonding. *Ann. N. Y. Acad. Sci.,* 652:204–211.

Carter, C. S., Witt, D. M., Auksi, T., and Casten, L. 1987. Estrogen and the induction of lordosis in female and male prairie voles (*Microtus ochrogaster*). *Horm. Behav.,* 21:65–73.

Carter, D. S., and Goldman, B. D. 1983a. Antigonadal effects of timed melatonin infusion in pinealectomized male Djungarian hamsters (*Phodopus sungorus sungorus*): Duration is the critical parameter. *Endocrinology,* 113:1261–1267.

Carter, D. S., and Goldman, B. D. 1983b. Progonadal role of the pineal in the Djungarian hamster (*Phodopus sungorus sungorus*): Mediation by melatonin. *Endocrinology,* 113:1268–1273.

Cascio, C., Yu, G. Z., Insel, T. R., and Wang, Z. X. 1998. Dopamine D$_2$ receptor-mediated regulation of partner preferences in female prairie voles. *Soc. Neurosci. Abstr.,* 24:372.13.

Cassone, V. M. 1998. Melatonin's role in vertebrate circadian rhythms. *Chronobiol. Int.,* 15:457–473.

Cawthorn, J. M., Morris, D. L., Ketterson, E. D., and Nolan, V. 1998. Influence of experimentally elevated testosterone on nest defense in dark-eyed juncos. *Anim. Behav.,* 56:617–621.

Cedrini, L., and Fasolo, A. 1970. Olfactory attractants in sex recognition of the crested newt: An electrophysiological research. *Monitore Zoology* (Italy), 5:223–229.

Celotti, F., Negri-Cesi, P., and Poletti, A. 1997. Steroid metabolism in the mammalian brain: 5 alpha-reduction and aromatization. *Brain Res. Bull.,* 44:365–375.

Chakraborty, S. 1995. Plasma prolactin and luteinizing hormone during termination and onset of photorefractoriness in intact and pinealectomized European starlings (*Sturnus vulgaris*). *Gen. Comp. Endocrinol.,* 99:185–91.

Challis, J. R. G., Davies, I. J., and Ryan, K. J. 1973. The concentrations of progesterone, estrone and estradiol-17β in the plasma of pregnant rabbits. *Endocrinology,* 93:971–976.

Chamley, W. A., Buckmaster, J. M., Cerini, M. R., Cumming, I. A., Goding, J. R., Obst, J. M., Williams, A., and Wingfield, C. 1973. Changes in the levels of progesterone, corticosteroids, estrone, estradiol-17β, luteinizing hormone, and prolactin in the peripheral plasma of the ewe during late pregnancy and at parturition. *Biol. Reprod.,* 9:30–35.

Chappel, S. C. 1985. Neuroendocrine regulation of luteinizing hormone and follicle stimulating hormone: A review. *Life Sci.,* 36:97–103.

Charles-Dominique, P. 1977. *Ecology and Behaviour of Nocturnal Primates.* Duckworth, London.

Chavez, M., Riedy, C. A., Van Dijk, G., and Woods, S. C. 1996. Central insulin and macronutrient intake in the rat. *Am. J. Physiol.,* 271:R727–R731.

Chehab, F. F., Lim, M. E., and Lu, R. 1996. Correction of the sterility defect in homozygous obese female mice by treatment with the human recombinant leptin. *Nat. Gen.,* 12:318–20.

Chen, G., Koyama, K., Yuan, X., Lee, Y., Zhou, Y.-T., O'Doherty, R., Newgard, C. B., and Unger, R. H. 1996. Disappearance of body fat in normal rats induced by adenovirus-mediated leptin gene therapy. *Proc. Natl. Acad. Sci. U.S.A.,* 93:14795–15799.

Cheng, M.-F. 1986. Individual behavioral response mediates endocrine changes induced by social interaction. In B. Komisaruk, H. Siegel, H. Feder, and M. F. Cheng (eds.), *Reproduction: A Behavioral and Neuroendocrine Perspective,* pp. 4–12. New York Academy of Sciences, New York.

Cheng, M.-F. 1992. For whom does the female dove coo? A case for the role of vocal self-stimulation. *Anim. Behav.,* 43:1035–1044.

Cheng, M.-F., and Lehrman, D. S. 1973. Relative effectiveness of diethylstilbestrol and estradiol benzoate in inducing female behavior patterns of ovariectomized ring doves (*Streptopelia risoria*). *Horm. Behav.,* 4:123–127.

Cheng, M.-F., and Silver, R. 1975. Estrogen–progesterone regulation of nest building behavior in ovariectomized ring doves (*Streptopelia risoria*). *J. Comp. Physiol. Psychol.,* 88:256–263.

Cheng, M.-F., and Zuo, M. 1994. Proposed pathways for vocal self-stimulation: met-enkephalinergic projections linking the midbrain vocal nucleus, auditory-responsive thalamic regions and neurosecretory hypothalamus. *J. Neurobiol.,* 25:361–379.

Cheng, M.-F., Peng, J. P., and Johnson, P. 1998. Hypothalamic neurons preferentially respond to female nest coo stimulation: demonstration of direct acoustic stimulation of luteinizing hormone release. *J. Neurosci.,* 18:5477–5489.

Cherry, J. A., and Baum, M. J. 1990. Effects of lesions of a sexually dimorphic nucleus in the preoptic/anterior hypothalamic area on the expression of androgen- and estrogen-dependent sexual behaviors in male ferrets. *Brain Res.,* 522:191–203.

Cherry, J. A., Basham, M. E., Weaver, C. E., Krohmer, R. W., and Baum, M. J. 1990. Ontogeny of the sexually dimorphic male nucleus in the preoptic/anterior hypothalamus of ferrets and its manipulation by gonadal steroids. *J. Neurobiol.,* 21:844–857.

Chester-Jones, I. 1955. Role of the adrenal cortex in reproduction. *Br. Med. J.,* 11:156–160.

Cheung, C. C., Thornton, J. E., Kuijper, J. L., Weigle, D. S., Clifton, D. K., and Steiner, R. A. 1997. Leptin is a metabolic gate for the onset of puberty in the female rat. *Endocrinology,* 138:855–858.

Chevalier, G., and Deniau, J. M. 1990. Disinhibition as a basic process in the expression of striatal functions. *Trends Neurosci.,* 13:277–290.

Childress, A. R., Ehrman, R., McLellan, A. T., MacRae, J., Natale, M., and O'Brien, C. P. 1994. Can induced moods trigger drug-related responses in opiate abuse patients? *J. Subst. Abuse Treat.,* 11:17–23.

Chitty, D. 1961. Variations in the weight of the adrenal glands of the field vole (*Microtus agrestis*). *J. Endocrinol.,* 22:287–293.

Christensen, L. W., and Clemens, L. G. 1975. Blockade of testosterone-induced mounting behavior in the male rat with intracranial application of the aromatization inhibitor, androst-1,4,6-triene-3,17-dione. *Endocrinology,* 97:1545–1551.

Christian, J. J. 1950. The adreno-pituitary system and population cycles in mammals. *J. Mammalogy,* 31:247–259.

Christian, J. J. 1959. The role of endocrine and behavioral factors in the growth of mammalian populations. In A. Gorbman (ed.), *Comparative Endocrinology,* pp. 71–97. Wiley, New York,

Christian, J. J., Lloyd, J. A., and Davis, D. E. 1965. The role of endocrines in the self-regulation of mammalian populations. *Rec. Prog. Horm. Res.,* 21:501–578.

Chrousos, G. P. 1998. Stressors, stress, and neuroendocrine integration of the adaptive response. The 1997 Hans Selye Memorial Lecture. *Ann. N.Y. Acad. Sci.,* 85:311–335

Chrousos, G. P., McCarty, R., Pacak, K., Cizza, G., Sternberg, E., Gold, P. W., and Kvetnansky, R. (eds.). 1995. *Stress: Basic Mechanisms Clinical Implications.* Vol. 771. New York Academy of Science, New York.

Chrousos, G. P., Torpy, D. J., and Gold, P. W. 1998. Interactions between the hypothalamic-pituitary-adrenal axis and the female reproductive system: Clinical implications. *Ann. Intern. Med.,* 129:229–240.

Cinti, S., Frederich, R. C., Zingaretti, M. C., De Matteis, R., Flier, J. S., and Lowell, B. B. 1997. Immunohistichemical localization of leptin and uncoupling protein in white and brown adipose tissue. *Endocrinology,* 138:797–804.

Clancy, A. N., Zumpe, D., and Michael, R. P. 1995. Intracerebral infusion of an aromatase inhibitor, sexual behavior and brain estrogen receptor-like immunoreactivity in intact male rats. *Neuroendocrinology,* 61:98–111.

Clare, A. W. 1985. Hormones, behavior, and the menstrual cycle. *J. Psychosom. Res.,* 29:225–233.

Clark, A. S., and Roy, E. J. 1983. Behavioral and cellular responses to pulses of low doses of estradiol-17 beta. *Physiol. Behav.,* 30:561–565.

Clark, A. S., Davis, L. A., and Roy, E. J. 1985. A possible physiological basis for the dud-stud phenomenon. *Horm. Behav.,* 19:227–230.

Clark, A. S., Pfeifle, J. K., and Edwards, D. A. 1981. Ventromedial hypothalamic damage and sexual proceptivity in female rats. *Physiol. Behav.,* 27:597–602.

Clark, M. M., Desousa, D., Vonk, J., Galef, B. G. 1997. Parenting and potency: Alternative routes to reproductive success in male Mongolian gerbils. *Anim. Behav.,* 54:635–62.

Clark, M. M., vom Saal, F. S., and Galef, B. G. 1992. Intrauterine positions and testosterone levels of adult male gerbils are correlated. *Physiol. Behav.,* 51:957–960.

Clarke, A. S. and Schneider, M. L. 1993. Prenatal stress has long-term effects on behavioral responses to stress in juvenile rhesus monkeys. *Dev. Psychobiol.,* 26:293–304.

Clarke, A. S., Wittwer, D. J., Abbott, D. H., and Schneider, M. L. 1994. Long-term effects of prenatal stress on HPA axis activity in juvenile rhesus monkeys. *Dev. Psychobiol.,* 27:257–269.

Clemens, L. G., and Weaver, D. R. 1985. The role of gonadal hormones in the activation of feminine sexual behavior. In N. T. Adler, D. W. Pfaff, and R. W. Goy (eds.), *Handbook of Behavioral Neurobiology,* Vol. 7, pp. 183–227. Plenum Press, New York.

Clemens, L. G., Gladue, B. A., and Coniglio, L. P. 1978. Prenatal endogenous androgenic influences on masculine sexual behavior and genital morphology in male and female rats. *Horm. Behav.,* 10:40–53.

Clough, G. C. 1965. Lemmings and population problems. *Am. Sci.,* 53:99–112.

Clutton-Brock, T. H. 1991. *The Evolution of Parental Care.* Princeton University Press, Princeton.

Clutton-Brock, T. H., Albon, S. D., Gibson, R. J., and Guinness, F. E. 1979. The logical stag: Adaptive aspects of fighting in red deer (*Cervus elaphus* L.). *Anim. Behav.,* 27:211–225.

Coccaro, E. F., Kavoussi, R. J., Hauger, R. L., Cooper, T. B., and Ferris, C. F. 1998. Cerebrospinal fluid vasopressin levels: Correlates with aggression and serotonin function in personality-disordered subjects. *Arch. Gen. Psychiatry,* 55:708–714.

Cochran, C. G. 1979. Proceptive patterns of behavior throughout the menstrual cycle in female rhesus monkeys. *Behav. Neural Biol.,* 27:342–253.

Coe, C. L. 1990. Psychobiology of maternal behavior in nonhuman primates. In N. A. Krasnegor and R. S. Bridges (eds.), *Mammalian Parenting,* pp. 157–183. Oxford University Press, Oxford.

Coe, C. L., Mendoza, S. P., Somtherman, W. P., and Levine, S. 1978. Mother-infant attachment in the squirrel monkey: Adrenal response to separation. *Behav. Biology,* 22:256–263.

Cohen, I. T., Sherwin, B. B., and Fleming, A. S. 1987. Food cravings, mood, and the menstrual cycle. *Horm. Behav.,* 21:457–470.

Cohen, J. 1977. *Statistical Power Analysis for the Behavioral Sciences.* Academic Press, New York.

Cohen, R. A., and Albers, H. E. 1991. Disruption of human circadian and cognitive regulation following a discrete hypothalamic lesion: A case study. *Neurology,* 41:726–729.

Cohen, S. L., Halaas, J. L., Friedman, J. M., Chait, B. T., Bennet, L., Chang, D., Hecht, R., and Collins, F. 1996. Human leptin characterization. *Nature,* 382:589.

Colborn, T., Myers, J. P., and Dumanoski, D. 1997. *Our Stolen Future: Are We Threatening Our Own Fertility, Intelligence, and Survival? A Scientific Detective Story.* E. F. Dutton, New York.

Coleman, R. M. 1986. *Awake at 3:00 A.M. By Choice or by Chance?* W. H. Freeman, New York.

Collaer, M. L., and Hines, M. 1995. Human behavioral sex differences: A role for gonadal hormones during early development? *Psychol. Bull.,* 118:55–107.

Collier, T. J., Quirk, G. J., and Routtenberg, A. 1987. Separable roles of hippocampal granule cells in forgetting and pyramidal cells in remembering spatial information. *Brain Res.,* 409:316–328.

Cologer-Clifford, A., Smoluk, S. A., and Simon, N. G. 1996. Effects of serotonergic 1A and 1B agonists and androgenic versus estrogenic systems for aggression. *Ann. N. Y. Acad. Sci.,* 794:339–342.

Coltheart, M., Hull, E., and Slater, D. 1975. Sex differences in imagery and reading. *Nature,* 253:438–440.

Commins, D., and Yahr, P. 1984. Adult testosterone levels influence the morphology of a sexually dimorphic area in the Mongolian gerbil brain. *J. Comp. Neurol.,* 224:132–140.

Commins, D., and Yahr, P. 1985. Autoradiographic localization of estrogen and androgen receptors in the sexually dimorphic area and other regions of the gerbil brain. *J. Comp. Neurol.,* 231:473–489.

Commins, W. D. 1932. The effect of castration at various ages upon learning ability of male albino rats. *J. Comp. Psychol.,* 14:29–53.

Compaan, J. C., Buijs, R. M., Pool, C. W., DeRuiter, A. J., and Koolhaus, J. M. 1993. Differential lateral septal vasopressin innervation in aggressive and nonaggressive male mice. *Brain Res. Bull.,* 30:1–6.

Conaway, C. H. 1971. Ecological adaptation and mammalian reproduction. *Biol. Reprod.,* 1:239–247.

Conaway, C. H., and Wight, H. M. 1962. Onset of reproductive season and first pregnancy of the season in cottontails. *J. Wildlife Mgmt.,* 26:278–290.

Connor, J. R., and Davis, H. N. 1980a. Postpartum estrus in Norway rats. I. Behavior. *Biol. Reprod.,* 23:994–999.

Connor, J. R., and Davis, H. N. 1980b. Postpartum estrus in Norway rats. II. Physiology. *Biol. Reprod.,* 23:1000–1006.

Conrad, C., and Roy, E. 1992. Selective loss of hippocampal granule cells following adrenalectomy: Implications for spatial memory. *J. Neurosci.,* 13:2582–2590.

Constantini, N. W., and Warren, M. P. 1994. Special problems of the female athlete. *Baillieres Clin. Rheumatol.,* 8:199–219.

Conte, C. O., Rosito, G. B. A., Palmini, A. L. F., Lucion, A. B., and de Almeida, A. M. R. 1986. Pre-training adrenaline recovers the amnestic effect of Met-enkephalin in demedullated rats. *Behav. Brain Res.,* 21:163–166.

Contreras, R. J., Fox, E., and Drugovich, M. L. 1982. Area postrema lesions produce feeding deficits in the rat: Effects of preoperative dieting and 2-deoxy-D-glucose. *Physiol. Behav.,* 29:875–884.

Cooper, A. J. 1986. Progestins in the treatment of male sex offenders: A review. *Can. J. Psychiatry,* 31:73–79.

Cooper, J. R., Bloom, F. E, and Roth, R. H. 1986. *The Biochemical Basis of Neuropharmacology.* Oxford University Press, New York.

Coopersmith, C., Candurra, C., and Erskine, M. S. 1996. Effects of paced mating and intromissive stimulation on feminine sexual behavior and estrus termination in the cycling rat. *J. Comp. Psych.,* 110:176–186.

Cordoba-Montoya, D. A., and Carrer, H. F. 1997. Estrogen facilitates induction of long term potentiation in the hippocampus of awake rats. *Brain Res.,* 778:430–438.

Cormack, M., and Sheldrake, P. 1974. Menstrual cycle variations in cognitive ability: A preliminary report. *Int. J. Chronobiol.,* 2:53–55.

Corner, G. W., and Allen, W. M. 1929. Physiology of the corpus luteum. II. Production of a special uterine reaction (progestational proliferation) by extracts of the corpus luteum. *Am. J. Physiol.,* 88:326–339.

Corsini, R. J. 1984. *Encyclopaedia of Psychology.* Vol. 1. Wiley, New York.

Corso, J. F. 1959. Age and sex differences in thresholds. *J. A. S. A.,* 31:489–507.

Cortin, C. M., and Fleming, A. S. 1995. Psychobiology of maternal behavior in human beings. In M. H. Bornstein (ed.), *Handbook of Parenting*, Vol. 2, pp. 87–132. Erlbaum Associates.

Couse, J. F., Lindzey, J., Grandien, K., Gustafsson, J. A., and Korach, K. S. 1997. Tissue distribution and quantitative analysis of estrogen receptor-alpha (ERalpha) and estrogen receptor-beta (ERbeta) messenger ribonucleic acid in the wild-type and Eralpha-knockout mouse. *Endocrinology*, 138:4613–4621.

Crawford, S. G., Kaplan, B. J., and Field, L. L. 1995. Absence of an association between insulin-dependent diabetes mellitus and developmental learning difficulties. *Hereditas*, 122:73–78.

Creel, S., Creel, N. M., and Monfort, S. L. 1996. Social stress and dominance. *Nature*, 379:212.

Creel, S., Creel, N. M., Mills, M. G. L., and Monfort, S. L. 1997. Rank and reproduction in cooperatively breeding African wild dogs: Behavioral and endocrine correlates. *Behav. Ecol.*, 8:298–306.

Crews, D. 1984. Gamete production, sex hormone secretion, and mating behavior uncoupled. *Horm. Behav.*, 18:22–28.

Crews, D. 1987. Diversity and evolution of behavioral controlling mechanisms. In D. Crews (ed.), *Psychobiology of Reproductive Behavior*, pp. 88–119. Prentice Hall, Englewood Cliffs, NJ.

Crews, D. 1991. Trans-seasonal action of androgen in the control of spring courtship behavior in male red-sided garter snakes. *Proc. Natl. Acad. Sci. U.S.A.*, 88:3545–3548.

Crews, D. 1997. Species diversity and the evolution of behavioral controlling mechanisms. *Ann. N. Y. Acad. Sci.*, 807:1–21.

Crews, D., and Bergeron, J. M. 1994. Role of reductase and aromatase in sex determination in the red-eared slider (*Trachemys scripta*), a turtle with temperature-dependent sex determination. *J. Endocrinol.*, 143:279–289.

Crews, D., and Bull, J. J. 1987. Evolutionary insights from reptilian sexual differentiation. In F. P. Haseltine, M. E. McClure, and E. H. Goldberg (eds.), *Genetic Markers of Sex Differentiation*, pp. 11–26. Plenum, New York.

Crews, D., and Fitzgerald, K. 1980. "Sexual" behavior in parthenogenetic lizards (*Cnemidophorus*). *Proc. Natl. Acad. Sci. U.S.A.*, 77:499–502.

Crews, D., and Gartska, W. R. 1982. The ecological physiology of a garter snake. *Sci. Am.*, Nov., 158–168.

Crews, D., and Silver, R. 1985. Reproductive physiology and behavior interactions in nonmammalian vertebrates. In N. T. Adler, D. Pfaff, and R. W. Goy (eds.), *Handbook of Behavioral Neurobiology*, Vol. 7, Reproduction, pp. 101–182. Plenum Press, New York.

Crews, D., Bull, J. J., and Billy, A. J. 1988a. Sex determination and sexual differentiation in reptiles. In J. M. A. Sitsen (ed.), *Handbook of Sexology, Vol. 6: The Pharmacology and Endocrinology of Sexual Function*, pp. 98–121. Elsevier, New York.

Crews, D., Camazine, M., Diamond, R., Mason, R. T., Tokarz, R. R., and Garstka, W. R. 1984. Hormonal independence of courtship behavior in the male garter snake. *Horm. Behav.*, 18:29–41.

Crews, D., Diamond, M. A., Whittier, J., and Mason, R. 1985. Small male body size in garter snake depends on testes. *Am. J. Physiol.*, 249:R62–R66.

Crews, D., Hingorani, V., and Nelson, R. J. 1988b. Role of the pineal gland in the control of annual reproductive behavioral and physiological cycles in the red-sided garter snake (*Thamnophis sirtalis parietalis*). *J. Biol. Rhythms*, 3:293–302.

Crichton-Browne, J. 1880. On the weight of the brain and its component parts in the insane. *Brain*, 2:42–67.

Critchlow, V., Liebelt, A., Bar-Sela, M., Mountcastle, W., and Lipscomb, H. S. 1963. Sex differences in resting pituitary-adrenal function in the rat. *Am. J. Physiol.*, 205:807–815.

Cummings, D. C., Quigley, M. E., and Yen, S. S. 1983. Acute suppression of circulating testosterone levels by cortisol in men. *J. Clin. Endocrinol. Metab.*, 57:671–673.

Cunningham, J. T. 1900. *Sexual Dimorphisms in the Animal Kingdom*. Black, London.

Czaja, J. A. 1978. Ovarian influences on primate food intake: Assessment of progesterone actions. *Physiol. Behav.*, 21:923–928.

Czaja, J. A., and Goy, R. W. 1975. Ovarian hormones and food intake in female guinea pigs and rhesus monkeys. *Horm. Behav.*, 6:923–928.

Czeisler, C. A., Kronauer, R. E., Allan, J. S., et al. 1989. Bright light induction of strong (Type 0) resetting of the human circadian pacemaker. *Science*, 244:1328–1332.

Czeisler, C. A., Zimmerman, J. C., Ronda, J. M., et al. 1980. Timing of REM sleep is coupled to the circadian rhythm of body temperature in man. *Sleep*, 2:329–346.

Daan, S. 1981. Adaptive daily strategies in behavior. *Handbook of Behavioral Neurobiology*, Vol. 4, pp. 275–298.

Daan, S., Damassa, D., Pittendrigh, C. S., and Smith, E. R. 1975. An effect of castration and testosterone replacement on a circadian pacemaker in mice (*Mus musculus*). *Proc. Natl. Acad. Sci. U.S.A.*, 72:3744–3747.

Dabbs, J. M. 1990. Age and seasonal variation in serum testosterone concentrations among men. *Chronobiol. Int.*, 7:245–249.

Dabbs, J. M., and Hargrove, M. F. 1997. Age, testosterone, and behavior among female prison inmates. *Psychosom. Med.*, 59:477–480.

Dabbs, J. M., and Mohammed, S. 1992. Male and female salivary testosterone concentrations before and after sexual activity. *Physiol. Behav.*, 52:195–197.

Dabbs, J. M., and Morris, R. 1990. Testosterone, social class, and antisocial behavior in a sample of 4,462 men. *Psychol. Sci.*, 1:209–211.

Dabbs, J. M., Frady, R. L., Carr, T. S., and Besch, N. F. 1987. Saliva testosterone and criminal violence in young adult prison inmates. *Psychosom. Med.*, 49:174–182.

Dabbs, J. M., LaRue, D., and Williams, P. M. 1990. Testosterone and occupational choice: Actors, ministers, and other men. *J. Pers. Soc. Psychol.*, 59:1261–1265.

Dabbs, J. M., Ruback, R. B., Frady, R. L., Hopper, C. H., and Sgoutas, D. S. 1989. Saliva testosterone and criminal violence among women. *Pers. Indiv. Diff.*, 9:269–275.

DaCosta, A. P., Guevara-Guzman, R. G., Ohkura, S., Goode, J. A., and Kendrick, K. M. 1996. The role of oxytocin release in the paraventricular nucleus in the control of maternal behaviour in the sheep. *J. Neuroendocrinol.*, 8:163–177.

Dalvit, S. P. 1981. The effect of the menstrual cycle on patterns of food intake. *Am. J. Clin. Nutr.*, 34:1811–1815.

Dalvit-McPhillips, S. P. 1983. The effect of the human menstrual cycle on nutrient intake. *Physiol. Behav.*, 31:209–212.

Daly, M., and Wilson, M. 1983. *Sex, Evolution, and Behavior*. Weber and Schmidt, Boston.

Damassa, D. A., Davidson, J. M., and Smith, E. R. 1977. The relationship between circulating testosterone levels and male sexual behavior in rats. *Horm. Behav.*, 8:275–286.

Daniel, J. M., Fader, A. J., Spencer, A. L., and Dohanich, G. P. 1997. Estrogen enhances performance of female rats during acquisition of a radial arm maze. *Horm. Behav.*, 32:217–225.

Dark, J., and Zucker, I. 1984. Gonadal and photoperiodic control of seasonal body weight changes in male voles. *Am. J. Physiol.*, 247:R84–R88.

Dark, J., and Zucker, I. 1985. Circannual rhythms of ground squirrels: Role of the hypothalamic paraventricular nucleus. *J. Biol. Rhythms*, 1:17–23.

Dark, J., and Zucker, I. 1986. Photoperiodic regulation of body mass and fat reserves in the meadow vole. *Physiol. Behav.*, 38:851–854.

Dark, J., Dark, K. A., and Zucker, I. 1987a. Long day lengths increase brain weight and DNA content in the meadow vole, *Microtus pennsylvanicus*. *Brain Res.*, 409:302–307.

Dark, J., Pickard, G. E., and Zucker, I. 1985. Persistence of circannual rhythms in ground squirrels with lesions of the suprachiasmatic nuclei. *Brain Res.*, 332:201–07.

Dark, J., Spears, N., Whaling, C. S., Meyer, J. S., Wade, G. N., and Zucker, I. 1990. Long day lengths promote brain growth in meadow voles. *Dev. Brain Res.*, 53:264–269.

Dark, J., Stern, J., and Zucker, I. 1989. Adipose tissue dynamics during cyclic weight loss and weight gain of ground squirrels. *Am. J. Physiol.*, 256:R1286–1292.

Dark, J., Whaling, C. S., and Zucker, I. 1987b. Androgens exert opposite effects on body mass of heavy and light meadow voles. *Horm. Behav.*, 21:471–477.

Dark, J., Zucker, I., and Wade, G. N. 1983. Photoperiodic regulation of body mass, food intake, and reproduction in meadow voles. *Am. J. Physiol.*, 245:R334–R338.

Darlington, T. K., Wagner-Smith, K., Ceriani, M. F., Staknis, D., Gekakis, N., Steeves, T. D. L., Weitz, C. J., Takahashi, J. S., and Kay, S. A. 1998. Closing the circadian loop: CLOCK-induced transcription of its own inhibitors *per* and *tim*. *Science*, 280:1599–1603.

Darrow, J. M., and Goldman, B. D. 1986. Circadian regulation of pineal melatonin and reproduction in the Djungarian hamster. *J. Biol. Rhythms*, 1:39–53.

Darrow, J. M., Duncan, M. J., Bartke, A., Bona-Gallo, A., and Goldman, B. D. 1988. Influence of photoperiod and gonadal steroids on hibernation in the European hamster. *J. Comp. Physiol.,* 163:339–48.

Darrow, J. M., Yogev, L., and Goldman, B. D. 1987. Patterns of reproductive hormone secretion in hibernating Turkish hamsters. *Am. J. Physiol.,* 253:R329–R336.

Daugherty, J. E. 1998. Treatment strategies for premenstrual syndrome. *Am. Fam. Physician,* 58:197–198.

David, H. G., Green, J. T., Grant, A. J., and Wilson, C. A. 1995. Simultaneous bilateral quadriceps rupture: A complication of anabolic steroid abuse. *J. Bone Joint Surg. Br.,* 77:159–160.

David, K., Dingemanse, E., Freud, J., and Lanquer, E. 1935. Crystalline male hormone from testes (testosterone) are more active than androsterone prepared from urine or cholesterol. *J. Physiol. Chem.,* 233:281–282.

Davidson, J. M. 1966a. Activation of the male rat's sexual behavior by intracerebral implantation of androgen. *Endocrinology,* 84:1365–1372.

Davidson, J. M. 1966b. Characteristics of sex behaviour in male rats following castration. *Anim. Behav.,* 14:266–272.

Davidson, J. M. 1969. Effects of estrogen on the sexual behavior of male rats. *Endocrinology,* 84:1365–1372.

Davidson, J. M., Camargo, C. A., and Smith, E. R. 1979. Effects of androgen on sexual behavior in hypogonadal men. *J. Clin. Endocrinol. Metab.,* 48:955–958.

Davidson, J. M., Kwan, M., and Greenleaf, W. J. 1982. Hormonal replacement and sexuality in men. *J. Clin. Endocrinol. Metab.,* 11:599–623.

Davidson, J. M., Stefanick, M. L., Sachs, B. D., and Smith, E. R. 1978. Role of androgen in sexual reflexes of the male rat. *Physiol. Behav.,* 21:141–146.

Davis, G. J., and Meyer, R. K. 1973. Seasonal variation in LH and FSH of bilaterally castrated snowshoe hares. *Gen. Comp. Endocrinol.,* 20:61–68.

Davis, H. P., and Squire, L. R. 1984. Protein synthesis and memory: A review. *Psychol. Bull.,* 96:518–559.

Davis, J. D., and Campbell, C. S. 1973. Peripheral control of meal size in the rat: Effect of sham feeding on meal size and drinking rate. *J. Comp. Physiol. Psychol.,* 83:379–387.

Davis, J. D., Gallagher, R. J., Ladove, R. F., and Turavasky, A. J. 1969. Inhibition of food intake by a humoral factor. *J. Comp. Physiol. Psychol.,* 67:407–417.

Davis, P. G., and Barfield, R. J. 1979. Activation of masculine sexual behavior by intracranial estradiol benzoate implants in male rats. *Neuroendocrinology,* 28:217–227.

Dawson, A. 1983. Plasma gonadal steroid levels in wild starlings (*Sturnus vulgaris*) during the annual cycle and in relation to the stages of breeding. *Gen. Comp. Endocrinol.,* 49:286–94.

Dawson, T. M., and Snyder, S. H. 1994. Gases as biological messengers: nitric oxide and carbon monoxide in the brain. *J. Neurosci.,* 14:5147–5159.

De Kloet, E. R., Joels, M., Oitzl, M., and Sutanto, W. 1991. Implication of brain corticosteroid receptor diversity for the adaptation syndrome concept. In G. Jasmin and M. Cantin (eds.), *Stress Revisited: Neuroendocrinology of Stress. Methods and Achievements in Experimental Pathology,* Vol 14:104–132. Karger, Basel.

De Mairan, J. J. 1729. *Observation Botanique.* L'Academie Royale des Sciences Paris, 35–36.

De Quervain, D. J., Roozendaal, B., and McGaugh, J. L. 1998. Stress and glucocorticoids impair retrieval of long-term spatial memory. *Nature,* 394:787–790.

de Waal, F. B. M. 1987. Tension regulation and nonreproductive functions of sex among captive bonobos (*Pan paniscus*). *Natl. Geogr. Res.,* 3:318–335.

de Waal, F. B. M. 1995. Bonobo sex and society. *Sci. Am.,* 272:82–88.

de Waal, F. B. M., and Lanting, F. 1997. *Bonobo: The Forgotten Ape,* University of California Press, Berkeley.

Deakin, J. F. W. 1988. Relevance of hormone–CNS interactions to psychological changes in the puerperium. In R. Kumar and I. F. Brockington (eds.), *Motherhood and Mental Illness 2: Causes and Consequences,* pp. 113–132. Wright, Boston.

DeBold, J. F., and Frye, C. A. 1994. Progesterone and the neural mechanisms of hamster sexual behavior. *Psychoneuroendocrinology,* 19:563–579.

DeJonge, F. H., Louwerse, A. L., Ooms, M. P., Evers, P., Endert, E., and Van de Poll, N. E. 1989. Lesions of the SDN–POA inhibit sexual behavior of male Wistar rats. *Brain Res. Bull.,* 23:483–492.

del Abril, A., Segovia, S., and Guillamon, A. 1987. The bed nucleus of the stria terminalis in the rat: regional sex differences controlled by gonadal steroids early after birth. *Brain Res.,* 429:295–300.

deLacoste, M.-C., Holloway, R. L., and Woodward, D. J. 1986. Sex differences in the fetal human corpus callosum. *Hum. Neurobiol.,* 5:1–5.

deLacoste-Utamsing, C., and Holloway, R. L. 1982. Sexual dimorphism in the human corpus callosum. *Science,* 216:1431–1432.

Delfs, J. M., Schreiber, L., and Kelley, A. E. 1990. Microinjection of cocaine into the nucleus accumbens elicits locomotor activation in the rat. *J. Neurosci.,* 10:303–310.

Delville, Y., and Blaustein, J. D. 1991. A site for estradiol priming of progesterone-facilitated sexual receptivity in the ventrolateral hypothalamus of female guinea pigs. *Brain Res.,* 559(2):191–199.

Delville, Y., Mansour, K. M., and Ferris, C. F. 1996. Testosterone facilitates aggression by modulating vasopressin receptors in the hypothalamus. *Physiol. Behav.,* 60:25–29.

Delville, Y., Melloni, R. H., and Ferris, C. F. 1998. Behavioral and neurobiological consequences of social subjugation during puberty in golden hamsters. *J. Neurosci.,* 18:2667–2672.

Demas, G. E., Eliasson, M. J. L., Dawson, T. M., Dawson, V. L., Kriegsfeld, L. J., Nelson, R. J. and Snyder, S. H. 1997. Inhibition of neuronal nitric oxide synthase increases aggressive behavior in mice. *Mol. Med.,* 3: 611–617.

Deminiere, J. M., Piazza, P. V., Guegan, G., Abrous, N., Maccari, S., Le Moal, M., and Simon, H. 1992. Increased locomotor response to novelty and propensity to intravenous amphetamine self-administration in adult offspring of stressed mothers. *Brain Res.,* 586:135–139.

Dempsey, E. W. 1968. William Caldwell Young. An appreciation. In M. Diamond (ed.), *Perspectives in Reproduction and Sexual Behavior,* pp. 453–458. University of Indiana Press, Bloomington.

Dempsey, E. W., Hertz, R., and Young, W. C. 1936. The experimental induction of oestrus (sexual receptivity) in the normal and ovariectomized guinea pig. *Am. J. Physiol.,* 116:201–209.

Demski, L. S. 1987. Diversity in reproductive patterns and behavior in teleost fishes. In D. Crews (ed.), *Psychobiology of Reproductive Behavior,* pp. 2–27. Prentice Hall, Englewood Cliffs, NJ.

Dennis, R. 1992. Cultural change and the reproductive cycle. *Social Sci. Med.,* 34:485–489.

Denton, D. 1982. *The Hunger for Salt.* Springer-Verlag, Berlin.

Desmond, N. L., and Levy, W. B. 1997. Ovarian steroid control of connectivity in the female hipppocampus: An overview of recent experimental findings and speculations on its functional consequences. *Hippocampus,* 7:239–245.

Dessypris, A., Kuoppasalmi, K., and Adlercreutz, H. 1976. Plasma cortisol, testosterone, androstenedione and luteinizing hormone (LH) in a non-competitive marathon run. *J. Steroid Biochem.,* 7:33–37.

Dethier, V. G. 1976. *The Hungry Fly: A Physiological Study of the Behavior Associated with Feeding.* Harvard University Press, Cambridge, MA.

Deutch, A. Y., and Roth, R. H. 1990. The determinants of stress-induced activation of the prefrontal cortical dopamine system. *Progr. Brain Res.,* 85:367–402.

Deutsch, J. A. 1982. Controversies in food intake regulation. In B. G. Hoebel and D. Novin (eds.), *The Neural Basis of Feeding and Reward,* pp. 137–148. Haer Institute, Brunswick, ME.

DeVries, A. C., DeVries, M. B., Taymans, S. E., and Carter, C. S. 1995a. The effects of social stress on social preferences are sexually dimorphic in prairie voles. *Proc. Natl. Acad. Sci. U.S.A.,* 93:11980–11984.

DeVries, A. C., DeVries, M. B., Taymans, S. E., and Carter, C. S. 1995b. Modulation of pair bonding by corticosterone in female prairie voles (*Microtus ochrogaster*). *Proc. Natl. Acad. Sci. U.S.A.,* 92:7744–7748.

DeVries, A. C., Johnson, C.L., and Carter, C. S. 1996. Characterization of partner preference in male and female prairie voles (*Microtus ochrogaster*). *Can. J. Zool.,* 75:295–301.

DeVries, A. C., Taymans, S. E., Sundstrom, J. M., and Pert, A. 1998. Conditioned release of corticosterone by contextual stimuli associated with cocaine is mediated by corticotropin-releasing factor. *Brain Res.,* 786:39–46.

DeVries, A. C., Young, W. S., Nelson, R. J. 1997. Reduced aggressiveness in mice with targeted disruption of the gene for oxytocin. *J. Neuroendocrinol.,* 9:363–368.

DeVries, G. J., Best, W., and Sluiter, A. A. 1983. The influence of androgens on the development of a sex difference in the vasopressinergic innervation of the rat lateral septum. *Brain Res.,* 284:377–380.

DeVries, G. J., Buijs, R. M., Van Leeuwen, F. W., Caffe, A. R., and Swaab, D. F. 1985. The vasopressinergic innervation of the brain in normal and castrated rats. *J. Comp. Neurol.,* 233:236–254.

DeVries, G. J., Crenshaw, B. J., and Al-Shamma, H. A. 1995. Gonadal steroid modulation of vasopressin pathways. *Ann. N. Y. Acad. Sci.*, 652:387–396.

DeWied, D. 1964. Influence of anterior pituitary on avoidance learning and escape behavior. *Am. J. Physiol.*, 207:255–259.

DeWied, D. 1969. Effects of peptide hormones on behavior. In W. F. Ganong and L. Martini (eds.), *Front. Neuroendocrinol.*, pp. 97–140. Oxford Press, New York.

DeWied, D. 1974. Pituitary–adrenal system hormones and behavior. In F. O. Schmidt and F. G. Worden (eds.), *The Neurosciences: Third Study Program*, pp. 653–666. MIT Press, Cambridge, MA.

DeWied, D. 1977. Peptides and behavior. *Life Sci.*, 20:195–204.

DeWied, D. 1980. Hormonal influences on motivation, learning, memory, and psychosis. In D. T. Krieger and J. C. Hughes (eds.), *Neuroendocrinology*, pp. 194–204. Sinauer Associates, Sunderland, MA.

DeWied, D. 1984. Neurohypophyseal hormone influences on learning and memory processes. In G. Lynch, J. L. McGaugh, and N. M. Weinberger (eds.), *Neurobiology of Learning and Memory*, pp. 289–312. Guilford, New York.

DeWied, D. 1997. The neuropeptide story. *Front. Neuroendocrinol.*, 18:101–118.

DeWied, D., Diamant, M., and Fodor, M. 1993. Central nervous system effects of the neurohypophyseal hormones and related peptides. *Front. Neuroendocrinol.*, 14:251–302.

Dewsbury, D. A. 1972. Patterns of copulatory behavior in male mammals. *Q. Rev. Biol.*, 47:1–33.

Dewsbury, D. A. 1979. *Comparative Animal Behavior*. McGraw-Hill, New York.

Dewsbury, D. A. 1984. *Comparative Psychology in the Twentieth Century*. Hutchinson Ross, Stroudsburg, PA.

Di Chiara, G. 1995. The role of dopamine in drug abuse viewed from the perspective of its role in motivation. *Drug Alcohol Dependency*, 38:95–137.

Diakow, C. 1974. Motion picture analysis of rat mating behavior. *J. Comp. Physiol. Psychol.*, 88:704–712.

Diamond, A. W. 1976. Subannual breeding and moult cycles in the bridled tern *Sterna anaethetus* in the Seychelles. *Ibis*, 114:395–398.

Diamond, M. 1970. Intromission pattern and species vaginal code in relation to induction of pseudopregnancy. *Science*, 169:995–997.

Diamond, M. 1984. *Sex Watching*. Macdonald and Company, London.

Diamond, M. 1996. Prenatal predisposition and the clinical management of some pediatric conditions. *J. Sex Marital Ther.*, 22:139–147.

Diamond, M., and Sigmundson, H. K. 1997. Sex reassignment at birth. *Arch. Pediatr. Adolesc. Med.*, 151:298–304.

Diaz, R., Ogren, S. O., Blum, M., and Fuxe, K. 1995. Prenatal corticosterone increases spontaneous and d-amphetamine induced locomotor activity and brain dopamine metabolism in prepubertal male and female rats. *Neuroscience*, 66:467–473.

Dickerman, R. D., Schaller, F., Prather, I., and McConathy, W. J. 1995. Sudden cardiac death in a 20-year-old bodybuilder using anabolic steroids. *Cardiology*, 86:172–173.

Dickinson, R. L. 1949. *Atlas of Human Sex Anatomy*. Williams & Wilkins, Baltimore.

Dietrich, A., and Allen, J. D. 1997a. Vasopressin and memory. I. The vasopressin analogue AVP4–9 enhances working memory as well as reference memory in the radial arm maze. *Behav. Brain Res.*, 87:197–200.

Dietrich, A., and Allen, J. D. 1997b. Vasopressin and memory. II. Lesions to the hippocampus block the memory enhancing effects of a AVP4–9 in the radial maze. *Behav. Brain Res.*, 87:201–208.

Dinan, T. G. 1998. Psychoneuroendocrinology of depression. Growth hormone. *Psychiatr. Clin. North Am.*, 21:325–339.

Dinges, D. F. 1984. The nature and timing of sleep. *Trans. Stud. Coll. Physicians Phila.* 6:177–206.

Disney, H. J., Lofts, B., and Murton, A. J. 1959. Duration of the regeneration period of the internal reproductive rhythm in a xerophilous equatorial bird, *Quelea quelea*. *Nature*, 184:1659–1660.

Dixson, A. F. 1980. Androgens and aggressive behavior in primates: A review. *Aggressive Behav.*, 6:37–67.

Dixson, A. F. 1997. Evolutionary perspectives on primae mating systems and behavior. *Ann. N. Y. Acad. Sci.*, 807:42–61.

Dixson, A. F., and George, L. 1982. Prolactin and parental behaviour in a male New World primate. *Nature*, 299:551–553.

Dixson, A. F., Everitt, G. J., Herbert, J., Rugman, S. J., and Scruton, D. M. 1973. Hormonal and other determinants of sexual attractiveness and receptivity in rhesus and talapoin monkeys. IVth

International Congress of Primatology. Vol. 2. *Primate Reproductive Behavior*, pp. 36–63. Karger, Basel.

Dluzen, D. E., and Ramirez, V. D. 1983. Localized and discrete changes in neuropeptide (LHRH and TRH) and neurotransmitter (NE and DA) concentrations within the olfactory bulbs of male mice as a function of social interaction. *Horm. Behav.*, 17:139–145.

Dluzen, D. E., Ramirez, V. D., Carter, C. S., and Getz, L. L. 1981. Male vole urine changes luteinizing hormone-releasing hormone and norepinephrine in female olfactory bulb. *Science*, 212:573–575.

Doering, C. H., Brodie, H. K. H., Kraemer, H. C., Moos, R. H., Becker, H. B., and Hamburg, D. A. 1975. Negative affect and plasma testosterone: A longitudinal human study. *Psychosom. Med.*, 37:484–491.

Döhler, K. D., and Hancke, J. L. 1978. Thoughts on the mechanism of sexual brain differentiation. In K. D. Döhler and M. Kawakami (eds.), *Hormones and Brain Development*, pp. 153–157. Elsevier, Amsterdam.

Döhler, K. D., Hines, M., Coquelin, A., Davis, F., Shryne, J. E., and Gorski, R. A. 1982. Pre- and postnatal influence of diethylstilbestrol on differentiation of the sexually dimorphic nucleus in the preoptic area of the female rat brain. *Neuroendocrinol. Lett.*, 4:361–365.

Doisy, E. A., and MacCorquodale, D. W. 1936. The hormones. *Annu. Rev. Biochem.*, 5:315–354.

Doisy, E. A., Veler, C. D., and Thayer, S. 1929. Folliculin from urine of pregnant women. *Am. J. Physiol.*, 90:329–330.

Doty, R. L. 1978. Gender and reproductive state correlates of taste perception in humans. In T. McGill, D. A. Dewsbury, and B. Sachs (eds.), *Sex and Behavior: Status and Prospects*, pp. 337–362. Plenum, New York.

Doty, R. L. 1986. Odor-guided behaviour in mammals. *Experientia*, 42:257–271.

Doty, R. L., and Anisko, J. J. 1973. Procaine hydrochloride olfactory block eliminated mounting in the golden hamster. *Physiol. Behav.*, 10:395–397.

Doty, R. L., Applebaum, S., Zusho, H., and Settle, R. G. 1985. Sex differences in odor identification ability: A crosscultural analysis. *Neurophysiologia*, 23:667–672.

Doty, R. L., Shaman, P., Applebaum, S. L., et al. 1984. Smell identification ability: Changes with age. *Science*, 226:1441–1443.

Dowell, S. F., and Lynch, G. R. 1987. Duration of the melatonin pulse in the hypothalamus controls testicular function in pinealectomized mice (*Peromyscus leucopus*). *Biol. Reprod.*, 36:1095–1101.

Dreger, A. D. 1998. *Hermaphrodites and the Medical Invention of Sex*. Harvard University Press, Cambridge, MA.

Drickamer, L. C. and Vessey S. H. 1982. *Animal Behavior: Concepts, Processes, Methods*. PWS, Boston.

Du, J., Lorrain, D. S., and Hull, E. M. 1998. Castration decreases extracellular, but increases intracellular, dopamine in medial preoptic area of male rats. *Brain Res.*, 782:11–17.

Dunbar, I. 1975. Behaviour of castrated animals. *Vet. Rec.*, 96:92–93.

Duncan, M. J. 1998. Photoperiodic regulation of hypothalamic neuropeptide messenger RNA expression: Effect of pinealectomy and neuroanatomical location. *Mol. Brain Res.*, 57:142–148.

Dunlap, J. 1998. Circadian rhythms: An end in the beginning. *Science*, 280:1548–1549.

Dunn, A. J., Steelman, S., and Delanoy, R. 1980. Intraventricular ACTH and vasopressin cause regionally specific changes in cerebral deoxyglucose uptake. *J. Neurosci. Res.*, 5:485–495.

Dworkin, S. I., Goeders, N. E., Grabowski, J., and Smith, J. E. 1987. The effects of 12-hour limited access to cocaine: reduction in drug intake and mortality. *NIDA Res. Monogr.*, 76:221–225.

Eakin, R. M. 1973. *The Third Eye*. University of California Press, Berkeley.

Ebbinghaus, H. 1908. *Psychology: An Elementary Textbook*. D. C. Heath, Boston.

Eberhart, J. A. 1988. Neural and hormonal correlates of primate sexual behavior. *Comp. Primate Biol. Neurosci.*, 4:675–705.

Eckhardt, C. 1863. Untersuchungen uber die erektion des penis beim hund. *Beitr. Anat. Phisiol.*, 3:123–147.

Eddy, E. M., Washburn, T. F., Bunch, D. O., Goulding, E. H., Gladen, B. C., Lubahn, D. B., and Korach, K. S. 1996. Targeted disruption of the estrogen receptor gene in male mice causes alternation of spermatogenesis and infertility. *Endocrinology*, 137:4796–4805.

Edwards, D. A. 1969. Early androgen stimulation and aggressive behavior in male and female mice. *Physiol. Behav.*, 4:333–338.

Edwards, D. A. 1970. Post-neonatal androgenization and adult aggressive behavior in female mice. *Physiol. Behav.,* 5:465–467.

Egawa, M., Yoshimatsu, H., and Bray, G. A. 1990. Effect of corticotropin releasing hormone and neuropeptide Y on electrophysiological activity of sympathetic nerves to interscapular brown brown adipose tissue. *Neuroscience,* 34:771–775.

Ehrenkranz, J., Bliss, E., and Sheard, M. H. 1974. Plasma testosterone: Correlation with aggressive behavior and social dominance in man. *Psychosom. Med.,* 36:469–475.

Ehrensing, R. H., Kastin, A. J., Schalch, D. S., Friesen, H. G., Vargas, J. R., and Schally, A. V. 1974. Affective state and thyrotropin and prolactin responses after repeated injections of thyrotropin-releasing hormone in depressed patients. *Am. J. Psychiatry,* 131:714–718.

Ehrhardt, A. A., and Baker, S. W. 1974. Fetal androgens, human central nervous system differentiation and behavioral sex differences. In R. C. Friedman, R. M. Richart, and R. L. VandeWiele (eds.), *Sex Differences in Behavior,* pp. 33–51. Wiley and Sons, New York.

Ehrhardt, A. A., and Meyer-Bahlburg, H. F. L. 1981. Effects of prenatal sex hormones on gender-related behavior. *Science,* 1312–1318.

Ehrhardt, A. A., and Money, J. 1967. Progestin-induced hermaphroditism: IQ and psychosexual identity in a study of ten girls. *J. Sex Res.,* 3:83–100.

Ehrhardt, A. A., Epstein, R., and Money, J. 1968a. Fetal androgens and female gender identity in the early-treated adrenogenital syndrome. *Johns Hopkins Med. J.,* 122:160–167.

Ehrhardt, A. A., Evers, K., and Money, J. 1968b. Influence of androgen on some aspects of sexually dimorphic behavior in women with the late-treated adrenogenital syndrome. *Johns Hopkins Med. J.,* 123:115–122.

Ehrhardt, A. A., Grisanti, G. C., and Meyer-Bahlburg, H. F. L. 1977. Prenatal exposure to medroxyprogesterone acetate (MPA) in girls. *Psychoneuroendocrinology,* 2:391–398.

Ehrhardt, A. A., Meyer-Bahlburg, H. F. L., Rosen, L. R., Feldman, J. F., Veridiano, N. P., Zimmerman, I., and McEwen, B. S. 1985. Sexual orientation after prenatal exposure to exogenous estrogen. *Arch. Sex Behav.,* 14:57–78.

Elias, M. 1981. Cortisol, testosterone and testosterone-binding globulin responses to competitive fighting in human males. *Aggressive Behav.,* 7:215–219.

Elliot, C. D. 1971. Noise tolerance and extraversion in children. *Br. J. Psychol.,* 62:375–380.

Elliott, A. S., and Nunez, A. A. 1992. Photoperiod modulates the effects of steroids on sociosexual behaviors of hamsters. *Physiol. Behav.,* 51:1189–1193.

Elliott, J. A., and Goldman, B. D. 1981. Seasonal reproduction: Photoperiodism and biological clocks. In N. T. Adler (ed.), *Neuroendocrinology of Reproduction,* pp. 377–423. Plenum Press, New York.

Ellis, A. 1945. The sexual psychology of human hermaphrodites. *Psychosom. Med.,* 7:108–125.

Ellis, G. B., and Turek, F. W. 1979. Changes in locomotor activity associated with the photoperiodic response of testes in male golden hamsters. *J. Comp. Physiol.,* 132:277–284.

Ellis, G. B., and Turek, F. W. 1980a. Photoperiod-induced change in responsiveness of the hypothalamic-pituitary axis to exogenous 5-alpha-dihydrotestosterone and 17β-estradiol in castrated male hamsters. *Neuroendocrinology,* 31:205–209.

Ellis, G. B., and Turek, F. W. 1980b. Photoperiodic regulation of serum luteinizing hormone and follicle-stimulating hormone in castrated and castrated-adrenalectomized male hamsters. *Endocrinology,* 106:1338–1344.

Ellis, G. B., and Turek, F. W. 1983. Testosterone and photoperiod interact to regulate locomotor activity in male hamsters. *Horm. Behav.,* 17:66–75.

Elwood, R. W. 1983. Paternal care in rodents. In R. W. Elwood (ed.), *Parental Behaviour in Rodents,* pp. 235–257. Wiley, New York.

Elwood, R. W., and Mason, C. 1994. The couvade and the onset of paternal care: A biological perspective. *Ethol. Sociobiol.,* 15:145–156.

Emery, D. E., and Moss, R. L. 1984. Lesions confined to the ventromedial hypothalamus decrease the frequency of coital contacts in female rats. *Horm. Behav.,* 18:313–329.

Emlen, S. T. 1978. The evolution of cooperative breeding in birds. In J. R. Krebs and N. B. Davies (eds.), *Behavioural Ecology: An Evolutionary Approach,* pp. 245–281. Blackwell Scientific Publications, Oxford.

Endicott, J., and Halbreich, U. 1982. Retrospective report of premenstrual depressive changes: Factors affecting confirmation by daily ratings. *Psychopharm. Bull.,* 18:109–112.

Endicott, J., Halbreich, U., Schacht, S., and Nee, J. 1981. Premenstrual changes and affective disorders. *Psychosom. Med.,* 43:519–529.

Engelmann, M., Ebner, K., Wotjak, C. T., and Landgraf, R. 1998. Endogenous oxytocin is involved in short-term olfactory memory in female rats. *Behav. Brain Res.,* 90:89–94.

Engelmann, M., Wotjak, C. T., Neumann, I., Ludwig, M., and Landgraf, R. 1996. Behavioral consequences of intracerebral vasopressin and oxytocin: Focus on learning and memory. *Neurosci. Biobehav. Rev.,* 20:341–358.

Englander-Golden, P., Change, H., Whitmore, M. R., and Dienstbier, R. A. 1980. Female sexual arousal and the menstrual cycle. *J. Hum. Stress,* 6:42–48.

Erickson, J. C., Ahima, R. S., Hollopeter, G., Flier, J. S., and Palmiter, R. D. 1997. Endocrine function of neuropeptide Y knockout mice. *Regul. Pept.,* 70:199–202.

Erikson, C. J., and Hutchison, J. B. 1977. Induction of nest-material collecting in male Barbary Doves by intracerebral androgen. *J. Reprod. Fertil.,* 50:9–16.

Erkinaro, E. 1961. The seasonal change of the activity of Microtus agrestis. *Oikos,* 12:157–63.

Erskine, M. S. 1985. Effects of paced coital stimulation on estrus duration in intact cycling rats and ovariectomized and ovariectomized-adrenalectomized hormone-primed rats. *Behav. Neurosci.,* 99:151–161.

Erskine, M. S. 1989. Solicitation behavior in the estrous female rat: A review. *Horm. Behav.,* 23:473–502.

Erskine, M. S., and Hanrahan, S. B. 1997. Effects of paced mating on c-fos gene expression in the female rat brain. *J. Neuroendocrinol.,* 9:903–912.

Erskine, M. S., Barfield, R. J., and Goldman, B. D. 1980a. Postpartum aggression in rats: Effects of hypophysectomy. *J. Comp. Physiol. Psychol.,* 94:484–494.

Erskine, M. S., Barfield, R. J., and Goldman, B. D. 1980b. Postpartum aggression in rats: II. Dependence on maternal sensitivity to young and effects of experience with pregnancy and parturition. *J. Comp. Physiol. Psychol.,* 94:495–505.

Espmark, Y. 1964. Rutting behaviour in reindeer (*Rangifer tarandus* L.). *Anim. Behav.,* 12:159–163.

Evans, D. L., Leserman, J., Perkins, D. O., Stern, R. A., Murphy, C., Zheng, B., Gettes, D., Longmate, J. A., Silva, S. G., van der Horst, C. M., Hall, C. D., Folds, J. D., Golden, R. N., and Petitto, J. M. 1997. Severe life stress as a predictor of early disease progression in HIV infection. *Am. J. Psychiatry,* 154:630–634.

Evans-Pritchard, E. E. 1963. *The Nuer.* Clarendon Press, Oxford.

Everett, J. W. 1961. The mammalian female reproductive cycle and its controlling mechanisms. In W. C. Young (ed.), *Sex and Internal Secretions,* Vol. 1, pp. 497–555. Williams & Wilkins, Baltimore.

Everitt, B. J. 1990. Sexual motivation: A neural and behavioral analysis of male rats. *Neurosci. Biobehav. Rev.*14:217–232.

Everitt, B. J., and Herbert, J. 1971. The effects of dexa-methasone and androgens on sexual receptivity of female rhesus monkeys. *J. Endocrinol.,* 51:575–588.

Ewald, P. W. 1994. *Evolution of Infectious Diseases.* Oxford University Press, Oxford.

Ewer, J., Gammie, S. C., and Truman, J. W. 1997. Control of insect ecdysis by a positive-feedback endocrine system: Roles of eclosion hormone and ecdysis triggering hormone. *J. Exp. Biol.,* 200:869–881.

Fader, A. J., Hendricson, A. W., and Dohanich, G. P. 1998. Estrogen improves performance of reinforced T-maze alteration and prevents the amnestic effects of scopolamine administered systemically or intrahippocampally. *Neurobiol. Learn. Mem.,* 69:225–240.

Fahrbach, S. E., and Pfaff, D. W. 1986. Effects of preoptic region implants of dilute estradiol on the maternal behavior of ovariectomized, nulliparous rats. *Horm. Behav.,* 20:957–959.

Fahrbach, S. E., Morrell, J. I., and Pfaff, D. W. 1986. Effect of varying the duration of pre-test cage habituation on oxytocin induction of short-latency maternal behavior. *Physiol. Behav.,* 37:135–139.

Fava, G. A., Fava, M., Kellner, R., Serafini, E., and Mastrogiacomo, I. 1981. Depression, hostility and anxiety in hyperprolactinemic amenorrhea. *Psychother. Psychosom.,* 36:122–128.

Favreau, O. E. 1993. Do the Ns justify the means? Null hypothesis testing applied to sex and other differences. *Can. Psych.,* 34: 64–78.

Feare, C. 1984. *The Starling.* Oxford University Press, New York.

Feder, H. H. 1971. The comparative action of testosterone propionate and 5α-androstan-17β-ol-3-one propionate on the reproductive behaviour, physiology and morphology of male rats. *J. Endocrinol.,* 51:242–252.

Feder, H. H. 1981. Estrous cyclicity in mammals. In N. T. Adler (ed.), *Neuroendocrinology of Reproduction,* pp. 279–348. Plenum Press, New York.

Feder, H. H., and Whalen, R. E. 1965. Feminine behavior in neonatally castrated and estrogen-treated male rats. *Science,* 147:306–307.

Feder, H. H., Naftolin, F., and Ryan, K. J. 1974. Male and female sexual responses in male rats given estradiol benzoate and 5α-androstan-17β-ol-3-one propionate. *Endocrinology,* 94:136–141.

Fee, A. R., and Parkes, A. S. 1930. Studies on ovulation. III. Effect of vaginal anaesthesia on ovulation in the rabbit. *J. Physiol. (Lond.),* 70:385–397.

Ferin, M. 1984. Endogenous opioid peptides and the menstrual cycle. *Trends Neurosci.,* 7:194–196.

Ferkin, M. H. 1988. Seasonal differences in social behavior among adult and juvenile meadow voles, *Microtus pennsylvanicus.* *Ethology,* 79:116–125.

Ferkin, M. H., and Seamon, J. O. 1987. Odor preference and social behavior in meadow voles, *Microtus pennsylvanicus:* Seasonal differences. *Can. J. Zool.,* 65:2931–2937.

Ferris, C. F. 1992. Role of vasopressin in aggressive and dominant/subordinate behaviors. *Ann. N. Y. Acad. Sci.,* 652:212–226.

Ferris, C. F., Axelson, J. F., Shinto, L. H., and Albers, H. E. 1987. Scent marking and the maintenance of dominant/subordinate status in male golden hamsters. *Physiol. Behav.,* 40:661–664.

Ferris, C. F., Delville, Y., Grzonka, Z., Luber-Narod, J., and Insel, T. R. 1993. An iodinated vasopressin (V1) antagonist blocks flank marking and selectively labels neural binding sites in golden hamsters. *Physiol. Behav.,* 54:737–747.

Ferris, C. F., Melloni, R. H., Koppel, G., Perry, K. W., Fuller, R. W., and Delville, Y. 1997. Vasopressin/serotonin interactions in the anterior hypothalamus control aggressive behavior in golden hamsters. *J. Neurosci.,* 17:4331–4340.

Fikentscher, R., Rosenberg, B., Spinar, H., and Bruckmuller, W. 1977. Loss of taste in the elderly: Sex differences. *Clin. Otolaryngol.,* 2:183–189.

Fingerhood, M. I., Sullivan, J. T., Testa, M., and Jasinski, D. R. 1997. Abuse liability of testosterone. *J. Psychopharmacol.,* 11:59–63.

Fink, G. 1988. Gonadotropin secretion and its control. In E. Knobil and J. Neill (eds.), *Physiology of Reproduction,* pp. 1349–1378. Raven Press, New York.

Fink, G., Sumner, B. E., Rosie, R., Grace, O., and Quinn, J. P. 1996. Estrogen control of central neurotransmission: Effect of mood, mental state, and memory. *Cellular Molecular Neurobiology,* 16:325–344.

Fiorino, D. F., Coury, A., and Phillips, A. G. 1997. Dynamic changes in nucleus accumbens dopamine efflux during the Coolidge effect in male rats. *J. Neurosci.,* 17: 4849–4855

Fishman, R. B., and Breedlove, S. M. 1987. Androgen blockade of bulbocavernosus muscle inhibits testosterone-dependent masculinization of spinal motoneurons in newborn female rats. *Soc. Neurosci. Abstr.,* 13:1520.

Fishman, R. B., Chism, L., Firestone, G. L., and Breedlove, S. M. 1990. Evidence for androgen receptors in sexually dimorphic perineal muscles of neonatal male rats: Absence of androgen accumulation by the perineal motoneurons. *J. Neurobiol.,* 21:694–705.

Fitzgerald, K. M., and Zucker, I. 1976. Circadian organization of the estrous cycle of the golden hamster. *Proc. Natl. Acad. Sci. U.S.A.,* 73:2923–2927.

Fitzsimons, J. T. 1961. Drinking by rats depleted of body fluid without increase in osmotic pressure. *J. Physiol. (Lond.),* 159:297–309.

Fitzsimons, J. T. 1998. Angiotensin, thirst, and sodium appetite. *Physiol. Rev.,* 78:583–686.

Fitzsimons, J. T., and Simons, B. J. 1969. The effect on drinking in the rat of intravenous infusion of angiotensin, given alone or in combination with other stimuli of thirst. *J. Physiol.,* 203:45–57.

Fivizzani, A. J., and Oring, L. W. 1986. Plasma steroid hormones in relation to behavioral sex role reversal in the spotted sandpiper, *Actitis macularia. Biol. Reprod.,* 35:1195–1201.

Fivizzani, A. J., Colwell, M. A., and Oring, L. W. 1986. Plasma steroid hormone levels in free-living Wilson's Phalaropes (*Phalaropus tricolor*). *Gen. Comp. Endocrinol.,* 62:137–144.

Flanagan-Cato, L. M., and Fluharty, S. J. 1997. Emerging mechanisms of the behavioral effects of steroids. *Curr. Opin. Neurobiol.,* 7:844–848.

Fleming, A. S. 1986. Psychobiology of rat maternal behavior. How and where hormones act to promote maternal behavior at parturition. *Ann. N. Y. Acad. Sci.,* 474:234–251.

Fleming, A. S. 1988. Factors influencing maternal responsiveness in humans: Usefulness of an animal model. *Psychoneuroendocrinology,* 13:189–212.

Fleming, A. S. 1990. Hormonal and experimental correlates of maternal responsiveness in human mothers. In N. A. Krasnegor and R. S. Bridges (eds.), *Mammalian Parenting,* pp. 184–208. Oxford University Press, Oxford.

Fleming, A. S., and Corter, C. M. 1995. Psychobiology of maternal behavior in nonhuman mammals. In M. H. Bornstein (ed.), *Handbook of Parenting,* Vol. 2, pp. 59–85. Erlbaum Associates.

Fleming, A. S., and Korsmit, M. 1996. Plasticity in the maternal circuit: Effects of maternal experience on Fos-Lir in hypothalamic, limbic, and cortical structures in the postpartum rat. *Behav. Neurosci.,* 110:567–582.

Fleming, A. S., and Luebke, C. 1981. Timidity prevents the nulliparous female from being a good mother. *Physiol. Behav.,* 27:863–868.

Fleming, A. S., and Pliner, P. 1983. Food intake, body weight, and sweetness preferences over the menstrual cycle in humans. *Physiol. Behav.,* 30:663–666.

Fleming, A. S., and Rosenblatt, J. S. 1974. Olfactory regulation of maternal behavior in rats: II. Effects of peripherally induced anosmia and lesions of the lateral olfactory tract in pup-induced virgins. *J. Comp. Physiol. Psychol.,* 86:233–246.

Fleming, A. S., Cheung, U. S., and Barry, M. 1990a. Cyclohexamide blocks the retention of maternal experience in postpartum rats. *Behav. Neural Biol.,* 53:64–73.

Fleming, A. S., Corter, C., Franks, P., Surbey, M., Schneider, B., and Steiner, M. 1993. Postpartum factors related to mother's attraction to newborn infant odors. *Dev. Psychobiol.,* 26:115–132.

Fleming, A. S., Corter, C., Surbey, M., Franks, P., and Steiner, M. 1995. Postpartum factors related to mother's recognition of newborn infant odours. *J. Reprod. Infant Psychol.,* 13:197–210.

Fleming, A. S., Krieger, H., and Wong, P. Y. 1990b. Affect and nurturance in first-time mothers: Role of psychobiological influences. In B. Lerer and S. Gershon (eds.), *New Directions in Affective Disorders,* pp. 388–392, Springer-Verlag, New York.

Fleming, A. S., Miceli, M., and Morretto, D. 1983. Lesions of the medial preoptic area prevent the facilitation of maternal behavior produced by amygdaloid lesions. *Physiol. Behav.,* 31:502–510.

Fleming, A. S., Morgan, H. D., and Walsh, C. 1996. Experiential factors in postpartum regulation of maternal care. In J. S. Rosenblatt and C. T. Snowdon (eds.), *Parental Care: Evolution, Mechanisms, Adaptive Significance,* pp. 295–332. Academic Press, San Diego.

Fleming, A. S., Ruble, D. N., Krieger, H., and Wong, P. Y. 1997a. Hormonal and experiential correlates of maternal responsiveness during pregnancy and the puerperium in human mothers. *Horm. Behav.,* 31:145–158.

Fleming, A. S., Steiner, M., and Anderson, V. 1987. Hormonal and attitudinal correlates of maternal behavior during the early postpartum period in first-time mothers. *J. Reprod. Infant Psychol.,* 5:193–205.

Fleming, A. S., Steiner, M., and Corter, C. 1997b. Cortisol, hedonics, and maternal responsiveness in human mothers. *Horm. Behav.,* 32:85–98.

Fleming, A. S., Suh, E. J., Korsmit, M., and Rusak, B. 1994. Activation of Fos-like immunoreactivity in the medial preoptic area and limbic structures by maternal and social interactions in rats. *Behav. Neurosci.,* 108:724–734.

Fleming, A. S., Vaccarino, F., and Luebke, C. 1980. Amygdaloid inhibition of maternal behavior in the nulliparous rat. *Physiol. Behav.,* 25:731–743.

Fleming, A. S., Vaccarino, F., Tambosso, L., and Chee, P. 1979. Vomeronasal and olfactory system modulation of maternal behavior in the rat. *Science,* 203:372–374.

Flood, J. F., and Morley, J. E. 1991. Increased food intake by neuropeptide Y is due to an increased motivation to eat. *Peptides,* 12:1329–1332.

Flood, J. F., Smith, G. E., and Morley, J. E. 1987. Modulation of memory processing by cholecystokinin: Dependence on the vagus nerve. *Science,* 236:832–834.

Florant, G. L., Tokuyama, K., and Rintoul, D. A. 1989. Carbohydrate and lipid utilization in hibernators. In A. Malan and B. Canguilhem (eds.), *Living in the Cold,* pp. 137–145. John Libbey, London.

Fluharty, S. J., and Sakai, R. R. 1995. Behavioral and cellular analysis of adrenal steroid and angiotensin interactions mediating salt appetite. *Progr. Psychobiol. Physiol. Psychol.,* 16:177–212.

Follett, B. K. 1991. The physiology of puberty in seasonally breeding birds. In M. Hunzicker-Dunn and N. B. Schwartz (eds.), *Follicle*

*Stimulating Hormone: Regulation of Secretion and Molecular Mechanisms of Action,* pp. 54–65. Springer-Verlag, New York.

Folman, Y., and Drori, D. 1966. Effects of social isolation and of female odours on the reproductive system, kidneys and adrenals of unmated male rats. *J. Reprod. Fertil.,* 11:43–50.

Forbes, T. R. 1949. A. A. Berthold and the first endocrine experiment: Some speculations as to its origin. *Bull. Hist. Med.,* 23:263–267.

Ford, C. S., and Beach, F. A. 1951. *Patterns of Sexual Behavior.* Harper and Row, New York.

Forest, M. G., and Cathiard, A. M. 1975. Pattern of plasma testosterone and androstenedione in normal newborns: Evidence for testicular activity at birth. *J. Clin. Endocrinol. Metab.,* 41:977–980.

Forger, N. G. 1998. Sex differentiation, psychological. In E. Knobil and J. D. Neill (eds.), *Encyclopedia of Reproduction,* vol. 4., pp. 421–430. Academic Press, San Diego.

Forger, N. G. 1999. Sexual differentiation, psychological. In E. Knobil and J. D. Neill (eds.), *Encyclopedia of Reproduction.* Vol. 4, pp. 421–430. Academic Press, New York.

Forger, N. G., and Breedlove, S. M. 1986. Sexual dimorphism in human and canine spinal cord: Role of early androgen. *Proc. Natl. Acad. Sci. U.S.A.,* 83:7527–7531.

Formby, D. 1967. Maternal recognition of infant's cry. *Dev. Med. Child Neurol.,* 9:293–298.

Fossey, D. 1974. Observations on the home range of one group of mountain gorillas (*Gorilla gorilla beringei*). *Anim. Behav.,* 22:568–581.

Fox, C. A., Ismail, A. A., Love, D. N., Kirkham, K. E., and Loraine, J. A. 1972. Studies on the relationship between plasma testosterone levels and human sexual activity. *J. Endocrinol.,* 52:51–58.

Fraile, I. G., Pfaff, D. W., and McEwen, B. S. 1987. Progestin receptors with and without estrogen induction in male and female hamster brain. *Neuroendocrinology,* 45:487–491.

Frank, L. G. 1983. Reproduction and intra-sexual dominance in the spotted hyena (*Crocuta crocuta*). Ph.D. Dissertation, University of California, Berkeley, CA.

Frank, L. G. 1986. Social organisation of the spotted hyaena: II. Dominance and reproduction. *Anim. Behav.,* 35:1510–1527.

Frank, L. G., Davidson, J. M., and Smith, E. R. 1985. Androgen levels in the spotted hyena *Crocuta crocuta*: The influence of social factors. *J. Zool. (Lond.),* 206:525–531.

Frank, R. T. 1931. The hormonal causes of premenstrual tension. *Arch. Neurol. Psychiatry,* 26:1053–1057.

Frankenhaeuser, M. 1978. Psychoneuroendocrine approaches to the study of emotion as related to stress and coping. *Neb. Symp. Motiv.,* 26:123–162.

Friedman, M. I. 1978. Hyperphagia in rats with experimental diabetes mellitus: A response to a decreased supply of utilizable fuels. *J. Comp. Physiol. Psychol.,* 92:109–117.

Friedman, M. I. 1990. Body fat and the metabolic control of food intake. *Int. J. Obesity,* 14:53–66.

Friedman, M. I., and Granneman, J. 1983. Food intake and peripheral factors after recovery from insulin-induced hypoglycemia *Am. J. Physiol.,* 244:R374–R382.

Friedman, M. I., and Stricker, E. M. 1976. The physiological psychology of hunger: A physiological perspective. *Psychol. Rev.,* 83:409–431.

Friedman, M. I., and Tordoff, MG. 1986. Fatty acid oxidation and glucose utilization interact to control food intake in rats. *Am. J. Physiol.,* 251:R840–845.

Friedman, M. I., Ramirez, I., Edens, N. K., and Granneman, J. 1985. Food intake in diabetic rats: Isolation of primary metabolic effects of rat feeding. *Am. J. Physiol.,* 249:R44–R51.

Fry, D. M., and Toone, C. K. 1981. DDT-induced feminization of gull embryos. *Science,* 213:922–924.

Frye, C. A. 1995. Estrus-associated decrements in a water maze task are limited to acquisition. *Physiol. Behav.,* 57:5–14.

Frye, C. A., and DeBold, J. F. 1993. 3 alpha-OH-DHP and 5 alpha-THDOC implants to the ventral tegmental area facilitate sexual receptivity in hamsters after progesterone priming to the ventral medial hypothalamus. *Brain Res.,* 612:130–137.

Frye, C. A., Mermelstein, P. G., and DeBold, J. F. 1992. Evidence for a non-genomic action of progestins on sexual receptivity in hamster ventral tegmental area but not hypothalamus. *Brain Res.,* 578:87–93.

Fuchs, A.-R., and Dawood, M. Y. 1980. Oxytocin release and uterine activation during parturition in rabbits. *Endocrinology,* 107:1117–1126.

Fuchs, A.-R., and Fuchs, F. 1984. Endocrinology of human parturition: A review. *Br. J. Obstet. Gynaecol.,* 91:948–967.

Gahr, M. 1990. Delineations of a brain nucleus: Comparisons of cytochemical, hodological, and cytoarchitectural views of the song control nucleus HVc of the adult canary. *J. Comp. Neurol.,* 294:30–36.

Gahr, M., and Kosar, E. 1996. Identification, distribution, and developmental changes of a melatonin binding site in the song control system of the zebra finch. *J. Comp. Neurol.,* 367:308–18.

Gahr, M., Flügge, G., and Güttinger, H.-R. 1987. Immunocytochemical localization of estrogen-binding neurons in the songbird brain. *Brain Res.,* 402:173–177.

Gahr, M., Güttinger, H.-R., and Kroodsma, D. A. 1993. Estrogen receptors in the avian brain: Survey reveals general distribution and forebrain areas unique to songbirds. *J. Comp. Neurol.,* 327:112–122.

Gaines, M. S., Fugate, C. L., Johnson, M. L., Johnson, D. C., Hisey, J. R., and Quadagno, D. M. 1985. Manipulation of aggressive behavior in male prairie voles (*Microtus ochrogaster*) implanted with testosterone in Silastic tubing. *Can. J. Zool.,* 63:2525–2528.

Galea, L. A., Kavaliers, M., and Ossenkopp, K. P. 1996. Sexually dimorphic spatial learning in meadow voles (*Microtus pennsylvanicus*) and deer mice (*Peromyscus maniculatus*). *J. Exp. Biol.,* 199:195–200.

Galea, L. A., Kavaliers, M., Ossenkopp, K. P., and Hampson, E. 1995. Gonadal hormone levels and spatial learning performance in the Morris water maze in male and female meadow voles, *Microtus pennsylvanicus. Horm. Behav.,* 29:106–125.

Gallagher, M., Kapp, B. S., Pascoe, J. P., and Rapp, P. R. 1981. A neuropharmacology of amygdaloid systems which contribute to learning and memory. In I. Ben Ari (ed.), *The Amygdaloid Complex,* pp. 343–354. Elsevier, Amsterdam.

Galli-Taliadoros, L. S., Sedgwick, J. D., Wood, S. A., and Korner, H. 1995. Gene knock-out technology: A methodological overview for the interested novice. *J. Immunol. Meth,* 181, 1–15.

Gammie, S. C., and Truman, J. W. 1997. An endogenous elevation of cGMP increases the excitability of identified insect neurosecretory cells. *J. Comp. Physiol. A:* 180:329–338.

Ganong, W. F. 1993. *Review of Medical Physiology.* (16th ed.). Appleton & Lange, Norwalk, CT.

Ganong, W. F. 1995. Review of Medical Physiology. (17th ed.). Appleton & Lange, Norwalk, CT.

Ganong, W. F. 1997. *Review of Medical Physiology.* (18th ed.). Lange, Los Altos, CA.

Garcia, M. C., and Ginther, O. J. 1976. Effects of ovariectomy and season on plasma luteinizing hormone in mares. *Endocrinology,* 98:958–962.

Gary, K. A., Sollars, P. J., Lexow, N., Winokur, A., and Pickard, G. E. 1996. Thyrotropin-releasing hormone phase shifts circadian rhythms in hamsters. *Neuroreport,* 7:1631–1634.

Garza-Trevino, E. S. 1994. Neurobiological factors in aggressive behavior. *Hosp. Comm. Psychiatry,* 45:690–699.

Gass, G. H., and Kaplan, H. M. 1996. *Handbook of Endocrinology.* CRC Press, Boca Raton, FL.

Gatchel, R. J., Baum, A., and Krantz, D. S. 1989. *An Introduction to Health Psychology.* (2nd ed.). Newberry, New York.

Gauer, O. H., and Henry, J. P. 1963. Circulatory basis of fluid volume control. *Physiol. Rev.,* 43:423–481.

Gaulin, S. J. C., and FitzGerald, R. W. 1986. Sex differences in spatial ability: An evolutionary hypothesis and test. *Am. Nat.,* 127:74–88.

Gaulin, S. J. C., and FitzGerald, R. W. 1989. Sexual selection for spatial-learning ability. *Anim. Behav.,* 37:322–331.

Gavish, L., Carter, C. S., and Getz, L. L. 1983. Male-female interactions in prairie voles. *Anim. Behav.,* 31:511–517.

Ge, R. S., Hardy, D. O., Catterall, J. F., and Hardy, M. P. 1997. Developmental changes in glucocorticoid receptor and 11-hydroxysteroid dehydrogenase oxidative and reductive activities in rat Leydig cells. *Endocrinology,* 138:5089–5095.

Geist, V. 1971. *Mountain Sheep.* University of Chicago Press, Chicago.

Gekakis, N., Staknis, D., Nguyen, H. B., Davis, F. C., Wilsbacher, L. D., King, D. P., Takahashi, J. S., and Weitz, C. J. 1998. Role of the CLOCK protein in the mammalian circadian mechanism. *Science,* 280:1564–1569.

Genazzani, A. R., and Petraglia, F. 1989. Opioid control of luteinizing hormone secretion in humans. *J. Steroid Biochem.,* 33:751–755.

Gentry, R. T., and Wade, G. N. 1976. Androgenic control of food intake and body weight in male rats. *J. Comp. Physiol. Psychol.,* 90:18–25.

George, A. J., and Sandler, M. 1988. Endocrine and biochemical studies in puerperal mental disorders. In R. Kumar and I. F.

Brockington (eds.), *Motherhood and Mental Illness 2: Causes and Consequences,* pp. 78–112. Wright, Boston.

Gerall, A. A., and Givon, L. 1992. Early androgen and age-related modifications in female rat reproduction. In A. A. Gerall, H. Moltz, and I. L. Ward (eds.), *Sexual Differentiation.* Vol. 11. *Handbook of Behavioral Neurobiology,* pp. 313–354. Plenum Press, New York.

Gerall, A. A., Moltz, H., and Ward, I. L. 1992. *Sexual Differentiation: Handbook of Behavioral Neurobiology,* Vol. 11. Plenum, New York.

Gessa, G. L., Paglietti, E., and Quarantotti, B. P. 1979. Induction of copulatory behavior in sexually inactive rats by naloxone. *Science,* 204:203–205.

Getz, L. L., and Carter, C. S. 1996. Prairie vole partnerships. *Am. Sci.,* 84:56–62.

Getz, L. L., Hofmann, J. E., and Carter, C. S. 1987. Mating system and population fluctuation of the prairie vole (*Microtus ochrogaster*). *Am. Zool.,* 27:909–920.

Giantonio, G. W., Lund, N. L., and Gerall, A. A. 1970. Effect of dien-cephalic and rhinencephalic lesions on the male rat's sexual behavior. *J. Comp. Physiol. Psychol.,* 73:38–46.

Gibbs, J., Fauser, D. J., Rowe, E. A., Rolls, B. J., Rolls, E. T., and Maddison, S. P. 1979. Bombesin suppresses feeding in rats. *Nature,* 282:208–210.

Gibbs, J., Young, R. C., and Smith, G. P. 1973. Cholecystokinin elicits satiety in rats with open gastric fistulas. *Nature,* 245:323–325.

Gibbs, R. B. 1997. Effects of estrogen on basal forebrain cholinergic neurons vary as a function of dose and duration of treatment. *Brain Res.,* 757:10–16.

Gilbeau, P. M., and Smith, C. G. 1985. Naloxone reversal of stress-induced reproductive effects in the male rhesus monkey. *Neuropeptides,* 5:335–338.

Gillespie, C. F., Huhman, K. L., Babagbemi, T. O., and Albers, H. E. 1996. Bicuculline increases and muscimol reduces the phase-delaying effects of light and VIP/PHI/GRP in the suprachiasmatic region. *J. Biol. Rhythms,* 11:137–144.

Gingrich, B. S., Cascio, C., Young, L. J., Liu, Y.,Wang, Z. X., and Insel, T. R. 1998. Oxytocin, dopamine, and enkephalin in the nucleus accumbens: A neurochemical cascade for pair bonding. *Soc. Neurosci. Abstr.,* 24:372.14.

Ginsberg, B., and Allee, W. C. 1942. Some effects of conditioning of social dominance and subordination in inbred strains of mice. *Physiol. Zool.,* 15:485–506.

Ginton, A., and Merari, A. 1977. Long range effects of MPOA lesions on mating behavior in the male rat. *Brain Res.,* 120:158–163.

Giordano, A. L., Ahdieh, H. B., Mayer, A. D., Siegel, H. I., and Rosenblatt, J. S. 1990. Cytosol and nuclear estrogen receptor binding in the preoptic area and hypothalamus of female rats during pregnancy and ovariectomized, nulliparous rats after steroid priming: correlation with maternal behavior. *Horm. Behav.,* 24:232–255.

Giordano, A. L., and Rosenblatt, J. S. 1986. Relationship between maternal behavior and nuclear estrogen receptor binding in pre-optic area and hypothalamus during pregnancy in rats. *Soc. Neurosci. Abstr.,* p. 17.

Giovenardi, M., Padoin, M. J.,Cadore, L. P., and Lucion, A. B. 1998. Hypothalamic paraventricular nucleus modulates maternal aggression in rats: Effects of ibotenic acid lesion and oxytocin antisense. *Physiol. Behav.,* 63:351–359.

Giros, B., Jaber, M., Jones, S. R., Wightman, R. M., and Caron, M. G. 1996. Hyperlocomotion and indifference to cocaine and ampheta-mine in mice lacking the dopamine transporter. *Nature.* 379:606–612.

Gitlin, M. J., and Pasnau, R. O. 1989. Psychiatric syndromes linked to reproductive function in women: A review of current knowledge. *Am. J. Psychiatry,* 146:1414–1422.

Giwercman, A., and Skakkebaek, N. E. 1992. The human testis—an organ at risk? *Int. J. Androl.* 15:373–375.

Gladue, B. A., Beatty, W. W., Larson, J., and Staton, R. D. 1990. Sexual orientation and spatial ability in men and women. *Psychobiology,* 18:101–108.

Gladue, B. A., Green, R., and Hellman, R. E. 1984. Neuroendocrine response to estrogen and sexual orientation. *Science,* 225:1496–1499.

Glaser, J. H., Rubin, B. S., and Barfield, R. J. 1983. Onset of the receptive and proceptive components of feminine sexual behav-ior in rats following the intravenous administration of progester-one. *Horm. Behav.,* 17:18–27.

Gleason, P. E., Michael, S. D., and Christian, J. J. 1981. Prolactin-induced aggression in female Peromyscus leucopus. *Behav. Neural Biol.,* 33:243–248.

Glickman, S. E., Frank, L. G., Davidson, J. M., Smith, E. R., and Siiteri, P. K. 1987. Androstenedione may organize or activate sex-reversed traits in female spotted hyenas. *Proc. Natl. Acad. Sci. U.S.A.,* 84:3444–3447.

Glickman, S. E., Frank, L. G., Licht, P., Yalcinkaya, T., Siiteri, P. K., and Davidson, J. 1992. Sexual differentiation of the female spotted hyena. One of nature's experiments. *Ann. N. Y. Acad. Sci.,* 662:135–159.

Go, V. L. E., DiMagno, E. P., Gardner, J. D., Lebenthal, E., Reber, H. A., and Scheely, G. A. 1993. *The Pancreas: Biology, Pathobiology and Disease.* Raven Press, New York.

Godwin, J., Hartman, V., Grammer, M., and Crews, D. 1996. Progesterone inhibits female-typical receptive behavior and decreases hypothalamic estrogen and progesterone receptor messenger ribonucleic acid levels in whiptail lizards (genus Cnemidophorus). *Horm. Behav.,* 30:138–144.

Goeders, N. E. 1997. A neuroendocrine role in cocaine reinforce-ment. *Psychoneuroendocrinology,* 22:237–259.

Goeders, N. E. and Guerin, G. F. 1996a. Role of corticosterone in intravenous cocaine self-administration in rats. *Neuroendo-crinology,* 64:337–348.

Goeders, N. E., and Guerin, G. F. 1994. Non-contingent electric foot-shock facilities the acquisition of intravenous cocaine self-administration in rats. *Psychopharmacology,* 114:63–70.

Goeders, N. E., and Guerin, G. F. 1996. Effects of surgical and phar-macological adrenalectomy on the initiation and maintenance of intravenous cocaine self-administration in rats. *Brain Res.,* 722:145–152.

Goeders, N. E., and Guerin, G. F. 1996. Role of corticosterone in intra-venous cocaine self-administration in rats. *Neuroendocrinology,* 64:337–348.

Goeders, N. E., and Guerin, G. F. 1997.Tolerance and sensitization to the behavioral effects of cocaine in rats: relationship to benzodi-azepine receptors. *Pharmacol. Biochem. Behav.,* 57:43–56.

Gold, P. E. 1986. Glucose modulation of memory storage processing. *Behav. Neural Biol.,* 45:342–349.

Gold, P. E. 1987. Sweet memories. *Am. Sci.,* 75:151–155.

Gold, P. E., and Van Buskirk, R. B. 1975. Facilitation of time-depen-dent memory processes with post-trial epinephrine injections. *Behav. Biol.,* 13:145–153.

Goldfoot, D. A., Wiegand, S. J., and Scheffler, G. 1978. Continued copulation in ovariectomized adrenal-suppressed stumptail macaques (Macaca artoides). *Horm. Behav.,* 11:89–99.

Goldman, B. D. 1983. The physiology of melatonin in mammals. In R. J. Reiter (ed.), *Pineal Research Reviews,* pp. 145–182. Alan R. Liss, New York.

Goldman, B. D., and Darrow, J. M. 1983. The pineal gland and mam-malian photoperiodism. *Neuroendocrinology,* 37:386–396.

Goldman, B. D., and Elliott, J. A. 1988. Photoperiodism and seasonali-ty in hamsters: Role of the pineal gland. In M. H. Stetson (ed.), *Processing of Environmental Information in Vertebrates,* pp. 203–218. Springer-Verlag, New York.

Goldman, B. D., and Nelson, R. J. 1993. Melatonin and seasonality in mammals. In H. S. Yu and R. J. Reiter (eds.), *Melatonin: Biosyn-thesis, Physiological Effects, and Clinical Applications,* pp. 225–252. CRC Press, Boca Raton, FL.

Goldman, B. D., Matt, K. S., Roychoudhury, P., and Stetson, M. H. 1981. Prolactin release in golden hamsters: Photoperiod and gonadal influences. *Biol. Reprod.,* 24:287–292.

Goldsmith, A. R. 1983. Prolactin in avian reproductive cycles. In J. Balthazart, J. E. Prove, and R. Gilles (eds.), *Hormones and Behaviour in Higher Vertebrates,* pp. 375–387. Springer-Verlag, Berlin.

Gonzàlez-Mariscal, G., and Rosenblatt, J. S. 1996. Maternal behavior in rabbits: A historical and multidisciplinary perspective. *Adv. Study Behav.,* 25:333–360.

Gonzàlez-Mariscal, G., Cuamatzi, E., and Rosenblatt, J. S. 1998. Hormones and external factors: Are they "on/off" signals for maternal nest-building in rabbits? *Horm. Behav.,* 33:1–8.

Good, D. J., Porter, F. D., Mahon, K. A., Parlow, A. F., Westphal, H., and Kirsch, I. R. 1997. Hypogonadism and obesity in mice with a targeted deletion of the Nh1h2 gene. *Nat. Gen.,* 15:397–401.

Goodale, H. D. 1918. Feminized male birds. *Genetics,* 3:276–299.

Goodfellow, P. N., and Lovell-Badge, R. 1993. SRY and sex determi-nation in mammals. *Annu. Rev. Genet.,* 27:71–92.

Goodson, J. L. 1998. Territorial aggression and dawn song are modu-lad by septal vasotocin and vasoactive intestinal polypeptide in male field sparrows (Spizella pusilla). *Horm. Behav.,* 34:67–77.

Gooren, L. 1990. Biomedical theories of sexual orientation: A critical examination. In D. P. McWhirter, S. A. Sanders, and J. M.

Reinisch (eds.), *Homosexuality/Heterosexuality: Concepts of Sexual Orientation*, pp. 71–87. Oxford University Press, New York.

Gooren, L. J. 1985. Human male sexual functions do not require aromatization of testosterone: A study using tamoxifern, testolactone, and dihydrotestosterone. *Arch. Sex Behav.,* 14:539–548.

Gooren, L. J. G. 1986. The neuroendocrine response of luteinizing hormone to estrogen administration in heterosexual, homosexual, and transsexual subjects. *J. Clin. Endocrinol. Metab.,* 63:583–588.

Gooren, L. J. G., Rao, B. R., Van Kessel, H., and Harmsen-Louman, W. 1984. Estrogen positive feedback on LH secretion in transsexuality. *Psychoneuroendocrinology,* 9:249–260.

Gordon, G. G., Southren, A. L., Tochimoto, S., Olivo, J., Altman, K., Rand, J., and Lemberger, L. 1970. Effect of medroxyprogesterone acetate (Provera) on the metabolism and biological activity of testosterone. *J. Clin. Endocrinol. Metab.,* 30:449–456.

Gordon, H. W., and Galatzer, A. 1980. Cerebral organization in patients with gonadal dysgenesis. *Psychoneuroendocrinology,* 5:235–244.

Gorman, M. R. 1994. Male homosexual desire: Neurological investigations and scientific bias. *Perspect. Biol. Med.,* 38:61–81.

Gorman, M. R., Ferkin, M. H., Nelson, R. J., and Zucker, I. 1993. Reproductive status influences odor preferences of the meadow vole, Microtus pennsylvanicus, in winter day lengths. *Can. J. Zool.,* 71:1748–1754.

Gorski, R. A. 1984. Critical role for the medial preoptic area in the sexual differentiation of the brain. *Prog. Brain Res.,* 61:129–146.

Gorski, R. A. 1993. Editorial: Estradiol acts via the estrogen receptor in the sexual differentiation of the rat brain, but what does this complex do? *Endocrinology,* 133:431–432.

Gorski, R. A., Gordon, J. H., Shryne, J. E., and Southam, A. M. 1978. Evidence for a morphological sex difference within the medial preoptic area of the rat brain. *Brain Res.,* 143:333–346.

Goss, R. J. 1980. Photoperiodic control of antler cycles in deer. *J. Exp. Zool.,* 211:101–105.

Goss, R. J. 1984. Photoperiodic control of antler cycles in deer. VI. Circannual rhythms on altered day lengths. *J. Exp. Zool.,* 230:265–271.

Goss, R. J., and Rosen, J. K. 1973. The effects of latitude and photoperiod on the growth of antlers. *J. Reprod. Fertil. (Suppl.),* 19:111–118.

Gotlib, I. H., Whiffen, V. E., Mount, J. H., Milne, K., and Cordy, N. I. 1989. Prevalence rates and demographic characteristics associated with depression in pregnancy and the postpartum. *J. Consult. Clin. Psychol.,* 57:269–274.

Gouchie, C., and Kimura, D. 1991. The relationship between testosterone levels and cognitive ability patterns. *Psychoneuroendocrinology* 16:323–334.

Gould, E., Tanapat, P., McEwen, B. S., Flugge, G., and Fuchs, E. 1998. Proliferation of granule cell precursors in the dentate gyrus of adult monkeys is diminished by stress. *Proc. Natl. Acad. Sci. U.S.A.,* 95:3168–3171.

Gould, E., Woolley, C. S., and McEwen, B. S. 1991. The hippocampal formation: Morphological changes induced by thyroid, gonadal, and adrenal hormones. *Psychoneuroendocrinology,* 16:67–84.

Gould, E., Woolley, C. S., Frankfurt, M., and McEwen, B. S. 1990. Gonadal steroids regulate dendritic spine density in hippocampal pyramidal cells in adulthood. *J. Neurosci.,* 10:1286–1291.

Gowaty, P. A. 1996. Field studies of parental care in birds: New data focus questions on variation among females. *Adv. Study Behav.,* 25:477–532.

Goy, R. W. 1966. Role of androgens in the establishment and regulation of behavioral sex differences in mammals. *J. Anim. Sci.,* 25:21–31.

Goy, R. W. 1967. William Caldwell Young. *Anat. Rec.,* 157:4–11.

Goy, R. W. 1978. Development of play and mounting behaviour in female rhesus virilized prenatally with esters of testosterone or dihydrotestosterone. In D. J. Chivers and J. Herbert (eds.), *Recent Advances in Primatology,* Vol. 1, pp. 449–462. Academic Press, London.

Goy, R. W. 1979. Sexual compatibility in rhesus monkeys: Predicting sexual behavior of oppositely sexed pairs of adult. In *Sex, Hormones, and Behavior,* pp. 227–255. CIBA Foundation Symposium. Elsevier, Amsterdam.

Goy, R. W., and Phoenix, C. H. 1971. Gonadal hormones and behavior of normal and pseudohermaphroditic female primates. In C. H. Sawyer and R. S. Gorski (eds.), *Steroids, Hormones and Brain Function,* pp. 193–202. University of California Press, Berkeley.

Goy, R. W., and Phoenix, C. H. 1972. The effects of testosterone propionate administered before birth on the development of behav-

ior in genetic female rhesus monkeys. In C. Sawyer and R. Gorski (eds.), *Steroid Hormones and Brain Function,* pp. 193–201. University of California Press, Berkeley.

Goy, R. W., and Resko, J. A. 1972. Gonadal hormones and behavior of normal and pseudohermaphroditic nonhuman female primates. *Rec. Prog. Horm. Res.,* 28:707–733.

Goy, R. W., and Young, W. C. 1956/1957. Strain differences in the behavioral responses of female guinea pigs to alpha-estradial benzoate and progesterone. *Behaviour,* 10:340–355.

Goy, R. W., Bercovitch, F. B., and McBrair, M. C. 1988. Behavioral masculinization is independent of genital masculinization in prenatally androgenized female rhesus macaques. *Horm. Behav.,* 22:552–571.

Goy, R. W., Bridson, W. E., and Young, W. C. 1964. The period of maximal susceptibility of the prenatal female guinea pig to masculinizing actions of testosterone propionate. *J. Comp. Physiol. Psychol.,* 57:166–174.

Grady, K. L., Phoenix, C. H., and Young, W. C. 1965. Role of the developing rat testis in differentiation of the neural tissues mediating mating behavior. *J. Comp. Physiol. Psychol.,* 59:176–182.

Graham, J. M., and Desjardins, C. 1980. Classical conditioning: Induction of luteinizing hormone and testosterone secretion in anticipation of sexual activity. *Science,* 210:1039–1041.

Grandi, M., and Celani, M. F. 1990. Effects of football on the pituitary-testicular axis (PTA): Differences between professional and non-professional soccer players. *Exp. Clin. Endocrinol.,* 96:253–259.

Granneman, J., and Friedman, M. I. 1980. Hepatic modulation of insulin-induced gastric acid secretion and EMB activity in rats. *Am. J. Physiol.,* 238:R346–R352.

Gray, G. D., and Dewsbury, D. A. 1973. A quantitative description of copulatory behavior in prairie voles (*Microtus ochrogaster*). *Brain Behav. Ecol.,* 8:837–852.

Gray, G. D., Smith, E. R., and Davidson, J. M. 1980. Hormonal regulation of penile erection in castrated male rats. *Physiol. Behav.,* 24:463–468.

Gray, J. A., and Lalljee, B. 1974. Sex differences in emotional behavior in the rat: Correlation between open field, defecation, and active avoidance. *Anim. Behav.,* 22:856–861.

Gray, J. M., and Wade, G. N. 1979. Cytoplasmic progestin binding in rat adipose tissues. *Endocrinology,* 104:1377–1382.

Gray, T. S., and Morley, J. E. 1986. Neuropeptide Y: Anatomical distribution and possible function in mammalian nervous system. *Life Sci.,* 38:389–401.

Greef, W. J. de, and Merkx, J. A. M. 1982. Receptivity, proceptivity and attractivity of pregnant and pseudopregnant rats. *Behav. Brain Res.,* 4:203–208.

Green, R. 1987. *The "Sissy-Boy Syndrome" and the Development of Homosexuality.* Yale University Press, New Haven, CT.

Greenberg, R. 1986. Competition in migrant birds in the nonbreeding season. In R. J. Johnson (ed.), *Curr. Ornithol.,* pp. 281–307. Plenum, New York.

Greenfield, D. A. 1997. Does psychological support and counseling reduce the stress experienced by couples involved in assisted reproductive technology? *J. Assist. Reprod. Gen.,* 14:186–188.

Griffin, J. E., and Ojeda, S. R. 1988. *Textbook of Endocrine Physiology.* Oxford University Press, New York.

Grill, H. J., and Kaplan, J. M. 1990. Caudal brainstem participates in the distributed neuronal control of feeding. In E. M. Stricker (ed.), *Handbook of Behav. Neurobiology: Neurobiology of Food Fluid Intake,* pp. 125–150. Plenum Press, New York.

Grill, H. J., Donahey, J. C. K., King, L, and Kaplan, J. M. 1997. Contribution of caudal brainstem to δ-fenfluramine anorexia. *Psychopharmacology,* 130:375–381.

Grill, H. J., Ginsberg, A. B., Seeley, R. J., and Kaplan, J. M. 1998. Brainstem application of melanocortin receptor ligands produces long-lasting effects on feeding and body weight. *J. Neurosci.,* 18:10128–10135.

Grimes, L. J., Melnyk, R. B., Martin, J. M., and Mrosovsky, N. 1981. Infradian cycles in glucose utilization and lipogenic enzyme activity in dormouse (*Glis glis*) adipocytes. *Gen. Comp. Endocrinol.,* 45:21–25.

Grisham, W., Kerchner, M., and Ward, I. L. 1991. Prenatal stress alters sexually dimorphic nuclei in the spinal cord of male rats. *Brain Res.,* 551:126–131.

Groos, G. 1982. The comparative physiology of extraocular photoreception. *Experientia,* 38:989–1128.

Grosse, J., Maywood, E. S., Ebling, F. J., and Hastings, M. H. 1993. Testicular regression in pinealectomized Syrian hamsters following infusions of melatonin delivered on non-circadian schedules. *Biol. Reprod.,* 49:666–674.

Gruder-Adams, S., and Getz, L. L. 1985. Comparison of the mating system and paternal behavior in *Microtus ochrogaster* and *M. pennsylvanicus. J. Mammalogy*, 66:165–167.

Grunt, J. A., and Young, W. C. 1952. Differential reactivity of individuals and the response of the male guinea pig to testosterone propionate. *Endocrinology*, 51:237–248.

Grunt, J. A., and Young, W. C. 1953. Consistency of sexual behavior patterns in individual male guinea pigs following castration and androgen therapy. *J. Comp. Physiol. Psychol.*, 46:138–144.

Gu, Q., and Moss, R. L. 1996. 17 beta-Estradiol potentiates kainate-induced currents via activation of the cAMP cascade. *J. Neurosci.*, 16:3620–3629.

Guardiola-Lemaitre, B. 1997. Toxicology of melatonin. *J. Biol. Rhythms*, 12:697–706.

Gubernick, D. J., and Alberts, J. R. 1987. The biparental care system of the California mouse, *Peromyscus californicus. J. Comp. Psychol.*, 101:169–177.

Gubernick, D. J., and Klopfer, P. H. (eds.). 1981. *Parental Care in Mammals*. Plenum Press, New York.

Gubernick, D. J., and Nelson, R. J. 1989. Prolactin and paternal behavior in the biparental California mouse, *Peromyscus californicus. Horm. Behav.*, 23:203–210.

Gubernick, D. J., Winslow, J. T., Jensen, P., Jeanotte, L., and Bowen, J. 1995. Oxytocin changes in males over the reproductive cycle in the monogamous, biparental California mouse, *Peromyscus californicus. Horm. Behav.*, 29:5/1–/23.

Guillamón, A., and Segovia, S. 1997. Sex differences in the vomeronasal system. *Brain Res. Bull.*, 44:377–382.

Guinness, F. E., Albon, S. D., and Clutton-Brock, T. H. 1978. Factors affecting reproduction in red deer *(Cervus elaphus L.). J. Reprod. Fertil.*, 54:325–334.

Gulledge, C., and Deviche, P. 1997. Androgen control of vocal control region volumes in a wild migratory songbird (*Junco hyemalis*) is region and possibly age dependent. *J. Neurobiol.*, 32:391–402.

Gunnet, J. W., and Freeman, M. E. 1983. The mating-induced release of prolactin: A unique neuroendocrine response. *Endocrinol. Rev.*, 4:44–61.

Gurney, M. E., and Konishi, M. 1980. Hormone induced sexual differentiation of brain and behavior in zebra finches. *Science*, 208:1380–1383.

Gustafson, M. L., and Donahoe, P. K. 1994. Male sex determination: Current concepts of male sexual differentiation. *Annu. Rev. Med.*, 45:505–524.

Gutzke, W. H. N., and Crews, D. 1988. Embryonic temperature determines adult sexuality in a reptile. *Nature*, 332:832–834.

Gutzke, W. H. N., and Paukstis, G. L. 1983. Influence of the hydric environment on sexual differentiation of turtles. *J. Exp. Zool.*, 226:467–469.

Gwinner, E. 1986. *Circannual Rhythms*. Springer-Verlag, Berlin.

Gwinner, E., Hau, M., and Heigl, S. 1997. Melatonin: Generation and modulation of avian circadian rhythms. *Brain Res. Bull.*, 44:439–444.

Haaren, F. van, Hest, A., and Heinsbroek, R. P. W. 1990. Behavioral differences between male and female rats: Effects of gonadal hormones on learning and memory. *Neurosci. Biobehav. Rev.*, 14: 23–33.

Hadley, M. E. 1996. *Endocrinology.* (4th ed.). Prentice Hall, Englewood Cliffs, NJ.

Haffen, K., and Wolff, E. 1977. Natural and experimental modification of ovarian development. In L. Z. Zuckerman and B. J. Wier (eds.), *The Ovary*, pp. 393–423. Academic Press, New York.

Hagedorn, M. 1986. The ecology, courtship and mating of gymnotiform electric fish. In T. Bullock and W. Heiligenberg (eds.), *Electroreception*, pp. 497–527. Wiley, New York.

Halaas, J. L., Gajiwala, K. S., Maffei, M., Cohen, S. L., Chait, B. T., Rabinowitz, D., Lallone, R. L., Burley, S. K., and Friedman, J. M. 1995. Weight-reducing effects of the plasma protein encoded by the obese gene. *Science*, 269:543–546.

Halberg, F. 1959. Physiologic 24-hour periodicity in human beings and mice, the lighting regimen and daily routine. In R. B. Withrow (ed.), *Photoperiodism and Related Phenomena in Plants and Animals*, pp. 803–878. American Association for the Advancement of Science, Washington, D.C.

Halberg, F. 1977. Implications of biological rhythms for clinical practice. *Hosp. Prac.*, 12:139–149.

Halbreich, U. 1997. Role of estrogen in postmenopausal depression. *Neurology*, 48:S16-S19.

Halbreich, U., Endicott, J., Schacts, D., and Nee, J. 1982. The diversity of premenstrual changes as reflected in the premenstrual assessment form. *Acta Psychiatrica Scand.*, 65:46–65.

Hall, J. C., and Rosbash, M. 1987. Genetic and molecular analysis of biological rhythms. *J. Biol. Rhythms*, 2:153–178.

Hall, J. L, Gonder-Frederick, L. A., Chewning, W. W., Silveira, J., and Gold, P. E. 1989. Glucose enhancement of performance on memory tests in young and aged humans. *Neuropsychologia*, 27:1129–1138.

Hall, J. L, Reilly, R. T., Cottrill, K. L, Stone, W. S., and Gold, P. E. 1992. Phlorizin enhancement of memory in rats and mice. *Pharmacol. Biochem. Behav.*, 41:295–299.

Hall, R. C., Popkin, M. K., Stickney, S. K., and Gardner, E. R. 1979. Presentation of steroid the psychoses. *J. Nerv. Ment. Dis.*, 167:229–236.

Hall, V. D., and Goldman, B. D. 1980. Effects of gonadal steroid hormones on hibernation in the Turkish hamster (*Mesocricetus brandti). J. Comp. Physiol.*, 135:107–114.

Hall, V. D., Bartke, A., and Goldman, B. D. 1982. Role of the testes in regulating the duration of hibernation in the Turkish hamster (*Mesocricetus brandti). Biol. Reprod.*, 27:802–810.

Hamilton, J. A., Parry, B. L., and Blumenthal, S. J. 1988. The menstrual cycle in context. I. Affective syndromes associated with reproductive hormonal changes. *J. Clin. Psychiatry*, 49:474–480.

Hamilton, J. B., and Gardner, W. U. 1937. Effects in female young born of pregnant rats injected with androgens. *Proc. Soc. Exp. Biol. Med.*, 37:570–572.

Hamilton, M. 1960. A rating scale for depression. *J. Neurol. Neurosurg. Psychiatry*, 23: 56–61.

Hampton, J. K., Hampton, S. H., and Landwehr, B. T. 1966. Observations on a successful breeding colony of the marmoset, *Oedipomidas oedipus. Folia Primatol.*, 4:265–287.

Handa, R. J., Burgess, L. H., Kerr, J. E., and O'Keefe, J. A. 1994. Gonadal steroid hormone receptors and sex differences in the hypothalamo-pituitary-adrenal axis. *Horm. Behav.*, 28:464–476.

Hansen, J. T., and Karasek, M. 1982. Neuron or endocrine cell? The pinealocyte as a paraneuron. In R. J. Reiter (ed.), *The Pineal and Its Hormones*, pp. 1–9. Alan R. Liss, New York.

Hansen, S., Ferreira, A., and Selart, M. E. 1985. Behavioural similarities between mother rats and benzodiazepine-treated non-maternal animals. *Psychopharmacology*, 86:344–347.

Hansen, S., Köhler, C., and Ross, S. B. 1982. On the role of the dorsal mesencephalic tegmentum in the control of masculine sexual behavior in the rat: Effects of electrolytic lesions, ibotenic acid and DSP4. *Brain Res.*, 240:311–320.

Hansen, S., Stanfield, E. J., and Everitt, B. J. 1980. The role of the ventral bundle noradrenergic neurones in sensory components of sexual behaviour and coitus-induced pseudopregnancy. *Nature*, 286:152–154.

Hansen, S., Stanfield, E. J., and Everitt, B. J. 1981. The effects of lesions of lateral tegmental noradrenergic neurons on components of sexual behavior and pseudopregnancy in female rats. *Neuroscience*, 6:1105–1117.

Harasty, J, Double, K. L., Halliday, G. M., Kril, J. J., and McRitchie, D. A. 1997. Language-associated cortical regions are proportionally larger in the female brain. *Arch. Neurol.*, 54:171–176.

Hardie, L. J., Rayner, D. V., Holmes, S., and Trayhurn, P. 1996. Circulating leptin levels are modulated by fasting, cold exposure and insulin administration in lean, but not Zucker (*fa/fa*) rats as measured by ELISA. *Biochem. Biophys. Res. Commun.*, 223:660–665.

Hardin, P. E., Hall, J. C., and Rosbash, M. 1990. Feedback of the Drosophila period gene product on circadian cycling of its messenger RNA levels. *Nature*, 343:536–540.

Harding, C. F., and Follett, B. K. 1979. Hormone changes triggered by aggression in a natural population of blackbirds. *Science*, 203:918–920.

Harding, C. F., Sheridan, K., and Walters, M. J. 1983. Hormonal specificity and activation of sexual behavior in male zebra finches. *Horm. Behav.*, 17:111–113.

Harding, C. F., Walters, M. J., Collado, M., and Sheridan, K. 1988. Hormonal specificity and activation of social behavior in male red-winged blackbirds. *Horm. Behav.*, 22:402–418.

Hardy, D. F., and DeBold, J. F. 1971. Effects of mounts without intromission upon the behavior of female rats during the onset of estrogen-induced heat. *Physiol. Behav.*, 7:643–645.

Harley, V. R., and Goodfellow, P. N. 1995. The biochemical role of SRY in sex determination. *Mol. Reprod. Dev.*, 39:184–193.

Harlow, H. F. 1959. Love in infant monkeys. *Sci. Am.*, (June), 100–106

Harlow, H. F., and Harlow, M. K. 1965. The affectional systems. In A. N. Schrier, H. F. Harlow, and F. Stollnitz (eds.), *Behavior of Nonhuman Primates.* Vol. 2, pp. 287–334. Academic Press, New York.

Harlow, H. F., Harlow, M. K., and Suomi, S. 1971. From thought to therapy: Lessons from a primate laboratory. *Am. Sci.,* 59:538–549.

Harris, G. W. 1937. The induction of ovulation in the rabbit by electrical stimulation of the hypothalamo-hypophysial mechanism. *Proc. R. Soc. Lond.,* B122:374–394.

Harris, G. W. 1948. Electrical stimulation of the hypothalamus and the mechanism of neural control of the adenohypophysis. *J. Physiol.,* 107:418–429.

Harris, G. W. 1955. *Neural Control of the Pituitary Gland.* E. Arnold, London.

Harris, G. W., and Jacobsohn, D. 1952. Functional grafts of the anterior pituitary gland. *Proc. R. Soc. Lond. B,* 139:263–276.

Harris, L. J. 1980. Lateralized sex differences: Substrates and significance. *Behav. Brain Sci.,* 3:236–237.

Harris, M. P. 1969. Breeding seasons of sea-birds in the Galapagos Islands. *J. Zool. (Lond.),* 159:145–165.

Hart, B. L. 1974. Gonadal androgen and sociosexual behavior of male mammals: A comparative analysis. *Psychol. Bull.,* 7:383–400.

Hart, B. L. 1979. Activation of sexual reflexes of male rats by dihydrotestosterone but not estrogen. *Physiol. Behav.,* 23:107–109.

Hart, B. L. 1988. Biological basis of the behavior of sick animals. *Neurosci. Biobehav. Rev.,* 12:123–137.

Hart, B. L., and Leedy, M. G. 1985. Neurological bases of sexual behavior. A comparative analysis. In N. Adler, D. Pfaff, and R. W. Goy (eds.), *Handbook of Behavioral Neurobiology,* Vol. 7, pp. 372–422. Plenum, New York.

Hart, B. L., Wallach, S. J. R., and Melese-d'Hospital, P. Y. 1983. Differences in responsiveness to testosterone of penile reflexes and copulatory behavior of male rats. *Horm. Behav.,* 17:274–283.

Hartung, T. G., and Dewsbury, D. A. 1979. Paternal behaviour in six species of muroid rodents. *Behav. Neural Biol.,* 26:466–478.

Harvey, S. M. 1987. Female sexual behavior: fluctuations during the menstrual cycle. *J. Psychosom. Res.,*31:101–110.

Hastings, J. W., Rusak, B., and Boulos, Z. 1991. The physiology of biological timing. In C. L. Prosser (ed.), *Neural and Integrative Animal Physiology,* pp. 435–546. Wiley-Liss, New York.

Hastings, M. H., Duffield, G. E., Ebling, F. J., Kidd, A., Maywood, E. S., Schurov, I. 1998. Non-photic signalling in the suprachiasmatic nucleus. *Biol. Cell,* 89:495–503.

Hatton, D.C., and Meyer, M. E. 1973. Paternal behavior in cactus mice (*Peromyscus eremicus). Bull. Psychonom. Soc.,* 2:330.

Hatton, J. D., and Ellisman, M. H. 1982. A restructuring of hypothalamic synapses is associated with motherhood. *J. Neurosci.,* 2:704–707.

Haug, M., Brain, P. F., and Kamis, A. B. 1986. A brief review comparing the effects of sex steroids on two forms of aggression in laboratory mice. *Neurosci. Biobehav. Rev.,* 10:463–468.

Haupt, H. A., and Rovere, G. D. 1984. Anabolic steroids: A review of the literature. *Am. J. Sports Med.,* 12:469–484.

Heeb, M. M., and Yahr, P. 1996. C-fos immunoreactivity in the sexually dimorphic area of the hypothalamus and related brain regions of male gerbils after exposure to sex-related stimuli or performance of specific sexual behaviors. *Neurosci.,* 72:1049–1071.

Hegner, R. E., and Wingfield, J. C. 1987. Social status and circulating levels of hormones in flocks of house sparrows, *Passer domesticus. Ethology,* 76:1–14.

Heid, P., Güttinger, H.-R., and Prove, E. 1985. The influence of castration and testosterone replacement on the song architecture of canaries (*Serinus canarius). Z. Tierpsychol.,* 69:224–236.

Heigl, S., and Gwinner, E. 1995. Synchronization of circadian rhythms of house sparrows by oral melatonin: effects of changing period. *J. Biol. Rhythms,* 10:225–33.

Heim, N., and Hursch, C. J. 1979. Castration for sex offenders: Treatment or punishment? A review and critique of recent European literature. *Arch. Sex Behav.,* 8:281–304.

Heimer, L., and Larsson, K. 1964. Drastic changes in the mating behaviour of male rats following lesions in the junction of diencephalon and mesencephalon. *Experientia,* 20:460–461.

Heimer, L., and Larsson, K. 1966. Impairment of mating behavior in male rats following lesions in the preoptic-anterior hypothalamic continuum. *Brain Res.,* 3:248–263.

Heinrichs, S. C., Cole, B. J., Pich, E. M., Menzaghi, F., Koob, G. F., and Hauger, R. L. 1992. Endogenous corticotropin-releasing factor modulates feeding induced by neuropeptide Y or a tail-pinch stressor. *Peptides,* 13:879–884.

Heinsbroek, R. P., van Haaren, F, and van de Poll, N. E. 1988. Sex differences in passive avoidance behavior in rats: Sex-dependent susceptibility to shock-induced behavioral depression. *Physiol. Behav.,* 43:201–206.

Helkala, E. L.,Niskanen, L., Viinamaki, H., Partanen, J., and Uusitupa, M. 1995. Short-term and long-term memory in elderly patients with NIDDM. *Diabetes Care,* 18:681–685.

Heller, H. C., and Poulson, T. L. 1970. Circannian rhythms: II. Endogenous and exogenous factor controlling reproduction and hibernation in chipmunks (*Eutamias*) and ground squirrels (*Spermophilus*). *Comp. Biochem. Physiol.,* 33:357–383.

Helvacioglu, A., Yeoman, R. R., Hazelton, J. M., and Aksel, S. 1993. Premenstrual syndrome and related hormonal changes. Longlasting gonadotropin releasing hormone agonist treatment. *J. Reprod. Med.,* 38:864–870.

Henderson, B. A., and Berenbaum, S. A. 1997. Sex-typed play in opposite-sex twins. *Dev. Psychobiol.,* 31:115–123.

Hendrick, V., Altshuler, L. L., and Suri, R. 1998. Hormonal changes in the postpartum and implications for postpartum depression. *Psychosomatics,* 39:93–101.

Hendricks, S. E., Graber, B., and Rodriguez-Sierra, J. F. 1989. Neuroendocrine response to estrogen: No differences between heterosexual and homosexual men. *Psychoneuroendocrinology,* 14:177–185.

Henn, W., and Zang, K. D. 1997. Mosaicism in Turner's syndrome. *Nature,* 390:569.

Hennessey, A. C., Huhman, K. L., and Albers, H. E. 1994. Vasopressin and sex differences in hamster flank marking. *Physiol. Behav.,* 55:905–911.

Hennessy, M. B. 1997. Hypothalamic-pituitary-adrenal responses to brief social separation. *Neurosci. Biobehav. Rev.* 21:11–29.

Hennessy, M. B., Mendoza, S. P., Kaplan, J. N. 1982. Behavior and plasma cortisol following brief peer separation in juvenile squirrel monkeys. *Am. J. Primatol.,* 3:143–151.

Henry, C., Kabbaj, M., Simon, H., Le Moal, M., and Maccari, S. 1994. Prenatal stress increases the hypothalamo-pituitary-adrenal axis response in young and adult rats. *J. Neuroendocrinol.,* 6:341–345.

Herbert, J. 1970. Hormones and reproductive behavior in rhesus and talapoin monkeys. *J. Reprod. Fertil., (Suppl.)* 11:119–140.

Herbert, J., and Trimble, M. R. 1967. Effect of oestradiol and testosterone on the sexual receptivity and attractiveness of the female rhesus monkey. *Nature,* 216:165–166.

Herdt, G. H., and Davidson, J. 1988. The Sambia "turnim-man": Sociocultural and clinical aspects of gender formation in male pseudohermaphrodites with 5α-reductase deficiency in Papua New Guinea. *Arch. Sex. Behav.,* 17:33–56.

Heriot, A. 1974. *The Castrati in Opera.* DaCapo, New York.

Herman, T. B. 1977. Activity patterns and movements of subarctic voles. *Oikos,* 29:434–444.

Herrenkohl, L. R. 1986. Prenatal stress disrupts reproductive behavior and physiology in offspring. *Ann. N. Y. Acad. Sci.,*474:120–128.

Hervey, E., and Hervey, G. R. 1967. The effects of progesterone on body weight and composition in the rat. *J. Endocrinol.,* 37:361–384.

Heske, E. J., and Nelson, R. J. 1984. Pregnancy interruption in Microtus ochrogaster: Laboratory artifact or field phenomenon? *Biol. Reprod.,* 31:97–103.

Hetherington, A. W., and Ranson, S. W. 1940. Hypothalamic lesions and adiposity in the rat. *Anat. Rec.,* 78:149–172.

Heuser, I. 1998. Anna-Monika-Prize paper. The hypothalamus-pituitary-adrenal system in depression. *Pharmacopsychiatry,* 31:10–13.

Hews, D. K., Thompson, C. W., Moore, I. T., and Moore, M. C. 1997. Population frequencies of alternative male phenotypes in tree lizards: Microgeographic variation and common-garden rearing studies. *Behav. Ecol.Sociobiol.,* 41:371–380.

Higley, J. D., Hasert, M. F., Suomi, S. J., and Linnoila, M. 1991. Nonhuman primate model of alcohol abuse: Effects of early experience, personality, and stress on alcohol consumption. *Proc. Natl. Acad. Sci. U.S.A.,* 88:7261–7265.

Hinde, R. A. 1966. *Animal Behaviour.* McGraw-Hill, New York.

Hinde, R. A. 1970. *Animal Behaviour: A Synthesis of Ethology and Comparative Psychology.* McGraw-Hill, New York.

Hines, M. 1982. Prenatal gonadal hormones and sex differences in human behavior. *Psychol. Bull.,* 92:56–80.

Hines, M. 1991. Gonadal hormones and human cognitive development. In J. Balthazart (ed.), *Hormones, Brain and Behavior in Vertebrates,* pp. 51–63. Karger, Basel.

Hirschberg, A. L. 1998. Hormonal regulation of appetite and food intake. *Ann. of Med.,* 30:7–20.

Hodges, J. K., and Hearne, J. P. 1978. A positive feedback effect of oestradiol on LH release in the male marmoset monkey. *J. Reprod. Fertil.,* 52:83–86.

Hoffman, K. A., Mendoza, S. P., Hennessy, M. B., and Mason, W. A. 1996. Responses of infant titi monkeys, *Callicebus moloch*, to removal of one or both parents: Evidence for paternal attachment. *Dev. Psychobiol.*, 28:399–407.

Hoffman, R. A., and Reiter, R. J. 1965. Pineal gland: Influence on gonads of male hamsters. *Science*, 148:1609–1615.

Hoffmann, K., Illnerova, H., and Vanecek, J. 1981. Effect of photoperiod and of one minute light at night-time on the pineal rhythm on N-acetyltransferase activity in the Djungarian hamster, *Phodopus sungorus*. *Biol. Reprod.*, 24:551–556.

Hofman, M. A., Zhou, J. N., and Swaab, D. F. 1996. Suprachiasmatic nucleus of the human brain: An immunocytochemical and morphometric analysis. *Anatomical Record*, 244:552–562.

Holekamp, K. E. 1986. Proximal causes of natal dispersal in Belding's ground squirrels (*Spermophilus beldingii*). *Ecol. Monogr.*, 56:365–391.

Holekamp, K. E., and Sherman, P. W. 1989. Why male ground squirrels disperse. *Am. Sci.*, 77:232–239.

Holman, S. D., and Goy, R. W. 1980. Behavioral and mammary responses of adult female rhesus to strange infants. *Horm. Behav.*, 14:348–357.

Holtzman, S. G. 1975. Effects of narcotic antagonists on fluid intake in the rat. *Life Sci.*, 16:1465–1470.

Hook, E. B. 1973. Behavioral implications of the human XYY genotype. *Science*, 179:139–149.

Hopkins, C. 1972. Sex differences in signalling in an electric fish. *Science*, 176:1035–1037.

Hopkins, C. 1984. Behavior of mormyridae. In T. Bullock and W. Heiligenberg (eds.), pp. 527–576. *Electroreception*, Wiley, New York.

Hopkins, C. 1988. Neuroethology of electric communication. *Annu. Rev. Neurosci.*, 11:497–536.

Hopkins, J., Marcues, M., and Campbell, S. B. 1984. Postpartum depression: A critical review. *Psychol. Bull.*, 95:498–515.

Horn, C. C., and Friedman, M. I. 1998. Metabolic inhibition increases feeding and brain Fos-like immunoreactivity as a function of diet. *Am. J. Physiol.*, 275: R448–R459.

Horseman, N. D., and Buntin, J. D. 1995. Regulation of pigeon crop-milk secretion and parental behaviors by prolactin. *Annu. Rev. Nutr.*, 15:213–238.

Hostetler, A. M., McHugh, P. R., and Moran, T. H. 1989. Bombesin affects feeding independent of a gastric mechanism or site of action. *Am. J. Physiol.*, 257:R1219–R1224.

Hotta, M., Shibasaki, T., Yamauchi, N., Ohno, H., Benoit, R., Ling, N., and Demura, H. 1991. The effects of chronic central administration of corticotropin-releasing factor on food intake, body weight, and hypothalamic-pituitary-adrenocortical hormones. *Life Sci.*, 48:1483–1491.

Howard, R. A., and Lively, C. M. 1994. Parasitism, mutation accumulation, and the maintenance of sex. *Nature*, 367:554–557.

Huck, U. M., Lisk, R. D., and Gore, A. C. 1985. Scent marking and mate choice in the golden hamster. *Physiol. Behav.*, 35:389–393.

Huck, U. W., Labov, J. B., and Lisk, R. D. 1986. Food restricting young hamsters (*Mesocricetus auratus*) alters sex ratio and growth of subsequent offspring. *Biol. Reprod.*, 36:592–598.

Hudson, R., and Distel, H. 1982. The pattern of behaviour of rabbit pups in the nest. *Behaviour*, 79:255–271.

Hudson, R., and Distel, H. 1989. Temporal pattern of suckling in rabbit pups: A model of circadian synchrony between mother and young. In S. M. Reppert (ed.), *Research in Perinatal Medicine*, Vol. 9, *Development of Circadian Rhythmicity and Photoperiodism in Mammals*, pp. 83–102. Perinatology Press, Ithaca.

Hufeland, C. W. 1797. The Art of Prolonging Life. J. Bell, London.

Hughes, T. K., Fulep, E., Juelich, T., Smith, E. M., and Stanton, G. J. 1995. Modulation of immune responses by anabolic androgenic steroids. *Int. J. Immunopharmacol.*, 17:857–863.

Hughes, T. K., Rady, P. L., and Smith, E. M. 1998. Potential for the effects of anabolic steroid abuse in the immune and neuroendocrine axis. *J. Neuroimmunol.*, 83:162- 167.

Huhman, K. L., and Albers, H. E. 1993. Estradiol increases the behavioral response to arginine vasopressin (AVP) in the medial preoptic-anterior hypothalamus. *Peptides*, 14:1049–1054.

Huhman, K. L., Gillespie, C. F., Marvel, C. L., and Albers, H. E. 1996. Neuropeptide Y phase shifts circadian rhythms in vivo via a $Y_2$ receptor. *NeuroReport*, 7:1249–1252.

Huhman, K. L., Gillespie, C. F., Marvel, C. L., and Albers, H. E. 1997. Peptidergic mechanisms of action in the suprachiasmatic nucleus. *Ann. N. Y. Acad. Sci.*, 814:300–304.

Huie, M. J. 1994. An acute myocardial infarction occurring in an anabolic steroid user. *Med. Sci. Sports Exer.*, 26:408–413.

Hull, E. M., Du, J., Lorrain, D. S., and Matuszewich, L. 1995. Extracellular dopamine in the medial preoptic area: Implications for sexual motivation and hormonal control of copulation. *J. Neurosci.*, 15:7465–7471.

Hull, E. M., Du, J., Lorrain, D. S., and Matuszewich, L. 1997. Testosterone, preoptic dopamine, and copulation in male rats. *Brain Res. Bull.*, 44:327–334.

Hulse, G. K., and Coleman, G. J. 1983. The role of endogenous opioids in the blockade of reproductive function in the rat following exposure to acute stress. *Pharmacol. Biochem. Behav.*, 19:795–799.

Hurn, P. D., Littleton-Kearny, M. T., Kirsch, J. R., Dharmarajan, A. M., and Traystman, R. J. 1995. Post-ischemic cerebral blood flow recovery in the female: Effect of 17β-estradiol. *J. Cereb. Blood Flow Metab.*,15:666–672.

Hutchison, J. B. 1970. Differential effects of testosterone and oestradiol on male courtship in Barbary doves (*Streptopelia risoria*). *Anim. Behav.*, 18:41–51.

Hutchison, J. B., and Steimer, T. 1983. Hormone-mediated behavioural transitions: A role for brain aromatase. In J. Balthazart, E. Prove, and R. Gilles (eds.), *Hormones and Behaviour in Higher Vertebrates*, pp. 261–274. Springer Verlag, Berlin.

Hyde, T. M., and Miselis, R. R. 1983. Effects of area postrema/caudal medial nucleus of solitary tract lesions on food intake and body weight. *Am. J. Physiol.*, 244:R577–R587.

Ieni, J. R., and Thurmond, J. B. 1985. Maternal aggression in mice: Effects of treatments with PCPA, 5-HTP and 5-HT receptor antagonists. *Eur. J. Pharmacol.*, 111:211–220.

Illnerova, H., and Vanecek, J. 1984. Circadian rhythm in inducibility of rat pineal N-acetyltransferase after brief light pulses at night: Control by a morning oscillator. *J. Comp. Physiol. A*, 154:739–744.

Illnerova, H., Hoffmann, K., and Vanecek, J. 1986. Adjustments of the rat pineal N-acetyltransferase rhythm to change from long to short photoperiod depends on the direction of the extension of the dark period. *Brain Res.*, 362:403–408.

Illnerova, H., Zvolsky, P., and Vanecek, J. 1985. The circadian rhythm in plasma melatonin concentration of the urbanized man: The effect of summer and winter time. *Brain Res.*, 328:186–192.

Imperato-McGinley, J., Guerrero, L., Gautier, T., and Peterson, R. E. 1974. Steroid 5-alpha-reductase deficiency in man: An inherited form of male pseudohermaphroditism. *Science*, 1:1213–1215.

Imperato-McGinley, J., Peterson, R. E., Gautier, T., and Sturla, E. 1979a. Androgens and the evolution of male-gender identity among male pseudohermaphrodites with 5-alpha-reductase deficiency. *N. Engl. J. Med.*, 300:1233–1237.

Imperato-McGinley, J., Peterson, R. E., Stoller, R., and Goodwin, W. E. 1979b. Male pseudohermaphroditism secondary to 17 beta-hydroxysteroid dehydrogenase deficiency: gender role change with puberty. *J. Clin. Endocrinol. Metab.*, 49:391–395.

Inouye, S. T., and Kawamura, H. 1979. Persistence of circadian rhythmicity in a mammalian hypothalamic "island" containing the suprachiasmatic nucleus. *Proc. Natl. Acad. Sci. U.S.A.*, 76:5962–5966.

Insel, T. R. 1990a. Oxytocin and maternal behavior. In N. A. Krasnegor and R. S. Bridges (eds.), *Mammalian Parenting*, pp. 260–280. Oxford University Press, Oxford.

Insel, T. R. 1990a. Regional changes in brain oxytocin receptors postpartum: Time-course and relationship to maternal behaviour. *J. Neuroendocrinol.*, 2:539–545.

Insel, T. R. 1990b. Regional changes in brain oxytocin receptors postpartum: Time-course and relationship to maternal behaviour. *J. Neuroendocrinol.*, 2:539–545.

Insel, T. R. 1997. A neurobiological basis of social attachment. *Am. J. Psychiatry*, 154:726–735.

Insel, T. R., and Hulihan, T. J. 1995. A gender-specific mechanism for pair bonding: oxytocin and partner preference formation in monogamous voles. *Behav. Neurosci.*, 109: 782–789.

Insel, T. R., and Shapiro, L. E. 1992. Oxytocin receptor distribution reflects social organization in monogamous and polygamous voles. *Proc. Natl. Acad. Sci. U.S.A.*, 89:5981–5985.

Insel, T. R., and Winslow, J. T. 1998. Serotonin and neuropeptides in affiliative behaviors. *Biol. Psychiatry*, 44:207–219.

Insel, T. R., Gilhard, R., and Shapiro, L. E. 1991. The comparative distribution of forebrain receptors for neurohypophyseal peptides in monogamous and polygamous mice. *Neuroscience*, 43:623–630.

Insel, T. R., Wang, Z. X., and Ferris, C. F. 1994. Patterns of brain vasopressin receptor distribution associated with social organization in microtine rodents. *J. Neurosci.*, 14:5381–5392.

Introini-Collison, I. B., and Baratti, C. M. 1986. Opioid peptidergic systems modulate the activity of beta-adrenergic mechanisms during memory consolidation processes. *Behav. Neural Biol.*, 46:227–241.

Isgor, C., and Sengelaub, D. R. 1998. Prenatal gonadal steroids affect adult spatial behavior, CA1 and CA3 pyramidal cell morphology in rats. *Horm. Behav.,* 34:183–198.

Jacobs, L. F., Gaulin, S. J. C., Sherry, D. F., and Hoffman, G. E. 1990. Evolution of spatial cognition: Sex-specific patterns of spatial behavior predict hippocampal size. *Proc. Natl. Acad. Sci. U.S.A.,* 87:6349–6352.

Jacobs, M., and Lightman, S. L. 1980. Studies in the opioid control of anterior pituitary hormones. *J. Physiol. (Lond.),* 300:53–60.

Jacobs, P. A., Brunton, M., Melville, M. M., Brittain, R. P., and McClemont, W. F. 1965. Aggressive behavior, mental subnormality and the XYY male. *Nature,* 208:1351–1352.

Jacobson, C. D. 1980. The characterization, ontogeny and influence of androgen on the sexually dimorphic nucleus of the preoptic area. Ph.D. dissertation, University of California, Los Angeles.

Jacobson, C. D., and Gorski, R. A. 1981. Neurogenesis of the sexually dimorphic nucleus of the preoptic area in the rat. *J. Comp. Neurol.,* 196:519–529.

James, V. H. T. 1992. *The Adrenal Gland.* Raven Press, New York.

Janowitz, H. D., and Grossman, M. I. 1949. Some factors affecting the food intake of normal dogs and dogs with esophagostomy and gastric fistula. *Am. J. Physiol.,* 159:143–148.

Janowsky, D. S., Berens, S. C., and Davis, J. M. 1973. Correlations between mood, weight, and electrolytes during the menstrual cycle: A renin-angiotensin-aldosterone hypothesis of premenstrual tension. *Psychosom. Med.,* 35:143–154.

Jensen, B. K. 1982. Menstrual cycle effects on task performance examined in the context of stress research. *Acta Psychol.,* 50:159–178.

Jensen, T. S., Genefke, I. K., Hyldebrandt, N., Pedersen, H., Petersen, H. D., Weile, B.1982. Cerebral atrophy in young torture victims. *N. Engl. J. Med.,* 307:1341.

Jilge, B. 1993. The ontogeny of circadian rhythms in the rabbit. *J. Biol. Rhythms,* 8:247–260.

Johanson, C. E., Balster, R. L., and Bonese, K. 1976. Self-administration of psychomotor stimulant drugs: the effects of unlimited access. *Pharmacol. Biochem. Behav.,* 4:45–51.

Johnson, F., and Bottjer, S. W. 1993. Hormone-induced changes in identified cell populations of the higher vocal center in male canaries. *J. Neurobiol.,* 24:400–418.

Johnson, F., and Whalen, R. E. 1988. Testicular hormones reduce individual differences in the aggressive behavior of male mice: A theory of hormone action. *Neurosci. Biobehav. Rev.,* 12:93–99.

Johnston, A. L., and File, S. E. 1991. Sex differences in animal tests of anxiety. *Physiol. Behav.,* 49:245–250.

Johnston, P. G., and Davidson, J. M. 1979. Priming action of estrogen: Minimum duration of exposure for feedback and behavioral effects. *Neuroendocrinology,* 28:155–159.

Johnston, R. E. 1985. Communication. In H. I. Siegel (ed.), *The Hamster: Reproduction Behavior,* pp. 121–154. Plenum Press, New York.

Jolly, A. 1966. *Lemur Behavior.* University of Chicago Press, Chicago.

Jones, H. E., Ruscio, M. A., Keyser, L. A., Gonzalez, C., Billack, B., Rowe, R., Hancock, C., Lambert, K. G., and Kinsley, C. H. 1997. Prenatal stress alters the size the rostral anterior commissure in rats. *Brain Res. Bull.,* 42:341–346.

Jost, A. 1979. Basic sexual trends in the development of vertebrates. In *Sex, Hormones and Behavior.* CIBA Foundation Symposium, No. 62. Elsevier, Amsterdam.

Judson, O. P. 1997. A model of asexuality and clonal diversity: Cloning the red queen. *J. Theoret. Biol.,* 186:33–40.

Julian, T., and McKenry, P. C. 1989. Relationship of testosterone to men's family functioning at mid-life: A research note. *Aggressive Behav.,* 15:281–289.

Kaitz, M. 1992. Recognition of familiar individuals by touch. *Physiol. Behav.,* 52:565–567.

Kalin, N. H., Shelton, S. E., and Barksdale, C. M. 1988. Opiate modulation of separation-induced distress in non-human primates. *Brain Res.,* 440:285–292.

Kalra, P. S., Fuentes, M., Sahu, A., and Kalra, S. P. 1990. Endogenous opioid peptides mediate the interleukin-1-induced inhibition of the release of luteinizing hormone (LH)-releasing hormone and LH. *Endocrinology,* 127:2381–2386.

Kalra, S. P., Dube, M. G., Sahu, A., Phelps, C. P., and Kalra, P. S. 1991. Neuropeptide Y secretion increases in the paraventricular nucleus in association with increased appetite for food. *Proc. Natl. Acad. Sci. U.S.A.,* 88:10931–10935.

Kannan, C. R. 1987. *The Pituitary Gland.* Plenum Medical Book, New York.

Kano, T. 1992. *The Last Ape: Pygmy Chimpanzee Behav. Ecology.* Stanford University Press. Stanford, CA.

Kaplan, J. M., Seeley, R. J., and Grill, H. J. 1993. Daily caloric intake in intact and chronic decerebrate rats. *Behav. Neurosci.,* 107:876–881.

Kaplan, J. M., Song, S., and Grill, H. J. 1998. Serotonin receptors in the caudal brainstem are necessary and sufficient for the anorectic effect of peripherally administered mCPP. *Psychopharmacology,* 137:43–49.

Karp, J. D., and Powers, J. B. 1993. Photoperiodic and pineal influences on estrogen-stimulated behaviors in female Syrian hamsters. *Physiol. Behav.,* 54:19–28.

Karsch, F. J. 1987. Central actions of ovarian steroids in the feedback regulation of pulsatile secretion of luteinizing hormone. *Annu. Rev. Physiol.,* 49:365–382.

Karsch, F. J., Bittman, E. L., Foster, D. L., Goodman, R. L., Legan, S. J., and Robinson, J. E. 1984. Neuroendocrine basis of seasonal reproduction. *Rec. Prog. Horm. Res.,* 40:185–232.

Karsch, F. J., Dierschke, D. J., and Knobil, E. 1973. Sexual differentiation of pituitary function: Apparent difference between primates and rodents. *Science,* 179:484–486.

Kashkin, K. B., and Kleber, H. D. 1989. Hooked on hormones? An anabolic steroid addiction hypothesis. *J. A. M. A.,* 262:3166–3170.

Kask, A., Rago, L., Harro, J. 1998. Evidence for involvement of neuropeptide Y receptors in the regulation of food intake: Studies with Y1-selective antagonist BIBP3226. *Br. J. Pharmacol.,* 124:1507–1515.

Kasper, S., Wehr, T., Bartko, J., Gaist, P., and Rosenthal, N. 1989. Epidemiological findings of seasonal changes in mood and behavior. A telephone survey of Montgomery County, Maryland. *Arch. Gen. Psychiatry,* 46:823–833.

Kastin, A. J., Ehrensing, R. H., Schalch, D. S., and Anderson, M. S. 1972a. Improvement in mental depression with decreased thyrotropin response after administration of thyrotropin-releasing hormone. *Lancet,* 780:740–742.

Kastin, A. J., Sandman, C. A., Stratton, L. O., Schally, A. V., and Miller, L. H. 1975. Behavioral and electrographic changes in rat and man after MSH. *Prog. Brain Res.,* 42:143–150.

Kastin, A. J., Schally, A. V., Gaul, C., Midgley, A. R., Miller, M. C., and Flores, P. 1972b. Increased release of LH after administration of LHRH to men pretreated with clomiphene. *J. Clin. Endocrinol. Metab.,* 34:753–756.

Katona, C., Rose, S., and Smale, L. 1998. The expression of Fos with the suprachiasmatic nucleus of the diurnal rodent *Arvicanthis niloticus. Brain Res.,* 791:27–34.

Ke, F. C., and Ramirez, V. D. 1990. Binding of progesterone to nerve cell membranes of rat brain using progesterone conjugated to 125I-bovine serum albumin as a ligand. *J. Neurochem.,* 54:467–472.

Kendrick, K. M., Levy, F., and Keverne, E. B. 1992. Changes in the sensory processing of olfactory signals induced by birth in sleep. *Science,* 256:833–836.

Kendrick, K. M., Fabre-Nys, C., Blache, D., Goode, J. A., and Broad, K. D. 1993. The role of oxytocin release in the mediobasal hypothalamus of the sheep in relation to female sexual receptivity. *J. Neuroendocrinol.,* 5:13–21.

Kennedy, G. C. 1964. Hypothalamic control of the endocrine and behavioural changes associated with oestrus in the rat. *J. Physiol. (Lond),* 166:395–407.

Kent, S., Tom, C., and Levine, S. 1997. Effect of interleukin-1 on pituitary-adrenal responses and body weight in neonatal rats: Interaction with maternal deprivation. *Stress,* 1:213–230.

Kerchner, M., and Ward, I. L. 1992. SDN-MPOA volume in male rats is decreased by prenatal stress, but is not related to ejaculatory behavior. *Brain Res.,* 581:244–251.

Kerchner, M., Malsbury, C. W., Ward, O. B., and Ward, I. L. 1995. Sexually dimorphic areas in the rat medial amygdala: Resistance to the demasculinizing effect of prenatal stress. *Brain Res.,* 20:251–260.

Keverne, E. B. 1978. Olfactory cues in mammalian sexual behaviour. In J. B. Hutchison (ed.), *Biological Determinants of Sexual Behaviour,* pp. 727–764. Wiley and Sons, New York.

Keverne, E. B., and Kendrick, K. M. 1992. Oxytocin facilitation of maternal behavior in sheep. *Ann. N. Y. Acad. Sci.,* 652:83–101.

Keverne, E. B., and Kendrick, K. M. 1994. Maternal behaviour in sheep and its neuroendocrine regulation. *Acta Paediatr.* 397:47–56.

Keverne, E. B., Levy, F., Poindron, P., and Lindsay, D. R. 1983. Vaginal stimulation: An important determinant of maternal bonding in sheep. *Science,* 219:81–83.

Kibble, M. W., and Ross, M. B. 1987. Adversive effects of anabolic steroids in athletes. *Clin. Pharm.*, 6:686–692.

Kikuyama, S., Toyoda, F., Ohmiya, Y., Matsuda, K., Tanaka, S., Hayashi, H. 1995. Sodefrin: A female-attracting peptide pheromone in newt cloacal glands. *Science,* 267:1643–1645.

Kikuyama, S., Toyoda, F., Yamamoto, K., Tanaka, S., and Hayashi, H. 1997. Female-attracting pheromone in newt cloacal glands. *Brain Res. Bull.,* 44:415–422.

Kimura, D. 1992. Sex Differences in the Brain. *Sci. Am.,* September 1992, 119–125.

Kimura, D., and Harshman, R. A. 1984. Sex differences in brain organization for verbal and non-verbal functions. *Prog. Brain Res.,* 61:423–441.

King, J. M. 1979. Effects of lesions of the amygdala, preoptic area, and hypothalamus on estradiol-induced activity in the female rat. *J. Comp. Physiol. Psychol.,* 93:360–367.

Kinsey, A. C., Pomeroy, W. B., and Martin, C. E. 1948. *Sexual Behavior in the Human Male.* W. B. Saunders, Philadelphia.

Kinsey, A. C., Pomeroy, W. B., Martin, C. E., and Gebhard, P. 1953. *Sexual Behavior in the Human Female.* Saunders, Philadelphia.

Kinsley, C. H. 1990. Prenatal and postnatal influences on parental behavior in rodents. In N. A. Krasnegor and R. S. Bridges (eds.), *Mammalian Parenting,* pp. 347–371. Oxford University Press, Oxford.

Kinsley, C. H. 1994. Developmental psychobiological influences on rodent parental behavior. *Neurosci. Biobehav. Rev.*18:269–280.

Kinsley, C. H., Mann, P. E., and Bridges, R. S. 1989. Alterations in stress-induced prolactin release in adult female and male rats exposed to stress, *in utero. Physiol. Behav.,* 45:1073–1076.

Kirn, J. R., Clower, R. P., Kroodsma, D. E., and DeVoogd, T. J. 1989. Song-related brain regions in the red-winged blackbird are affected by sex and season but not repertoire size. *J. Neurobiol.,* 11:139–163.

Kitay, J. I. 1963. Pituitary-adrenal function in the rat after gonadectomy and gonadal hormone replacement. *Endocrinology,* 73:253–260.

Klaiber, E. L., Broverman, D. M., Vogel, W., and Kobayski, V. 1979. Estrogen therapy for severe persistent depressions in women. *Arch. Gen. Psychiatry,* 36:550–554.

Klaus, M. H., and Kennell, J. H. 1976. *Maternal-Infant Bonding.* Mosby: St. Louis.

Kleiman, D. G., and Malcolm, J. R. 1981. The evolution of male parental investment. In D. J. Gubernick and P. H. Klopfer (eds.), *Parental Care in Mammals,* pp. 347–387. Plenum, New York.

Klein, D.C., Reppert, S. M., and Moore, R. Y. (eds.). 1991. *The Suprachiasmatic Nucleus: The Mind's Clock,* Elsevier, New York.

Klein, D.C., Smoot, R., Weller, J. L., Higa, S., Markey, S. P., Creed, G. H., and Jacobowitz, D. M. 1983. Lesions of the paraventricular nucleus area of the hypothalamus disrupt the suprachiasmatic–spinal cord circuit in the melatonin rhythm generating system. *Brain Res. Bull.,* 10:647–652.

Klein, K. E., and Wegmann, H. M. 1974. The resynchronization of human circadian rhythms after transmeridian flights as a result of flight direction and mode of activity. In L. E. Scheving, F. Halberg, and J. E. Pauley (eds.), *Chronobiology,* pp. 564–570. Igaku, Tokyo.

Klein, S. L., and Nelson, R. J. 1998. Adaptive immune responses are linked to the mating systems of arvicoline rodents. *Am. Nat.,* 151:59–67.

Klemfuss, H. 1992. Rhythms and the pharmacology of lithium. *Pharmacol. Ther.,* 56:53–78.

Klerman, E. B., Rimmer, D. W., Dijk, D. J., Kronauer, R. E., Rizzo, J. F., and Czeisler, C. A. 1998. Nonphotic entrainment of the human circadian pacemaker. *Am. J. Physiol.,* 274:R991–R996.

Kluger, M. J. 1978. The evolution and adaptive value of fever. *Am. Sci.,* 66:38–43.

Kluger, M. J. 1986. Is fever beneficial? *Yale J. Biol. Med.,* 59:89–95.

Kluger, M. J. 1989. Body temperature changes during inflammation: Their mediation and nutritional significance. *Proc. Nutr. Soc.,* 48:337–345.

Kluver, H. N., and Tinbergen, N. 1953. Territory and the regulation of density of titmice. *Arch. Neerlandaises de Zool.,* 10:265–289.

Klüver, H., and Bucy, P. C. 1939. Preliminary analysis of functions of the temporal lobes in monkeys. *Arch. Neurol. Psychiatry,* 42:979–1000.

Knobil, E., and Hotchkiss, J. 1988. The menstrual cycle and its neuroendocrine control. In E. Knobil and, J. D. Neill (eds.), *The Physiology of Reproduction,* Vol. 2, pp. 1971–1994. Raven, New York.

Knobil, E., and Neill, J. D. 1994. *The Physiology of Reproduction.* (2nd ed.). Raven Press, New York.

Koelega, H. S., and Koster, E. P. 1974. Some experiments on sex differences in odor perception. *Ann. N. Y. Acad. Sci.,* 27:234–246.

Koeske, R. K. D. 1980. Theoretical perspectives on menstrual cycle research: The relevance of attributional approaches for the perception and explanation of premenstrual emotionality. In A. J. Dan, E. A. Graham, and C. P. Beecher (eds.), *The Menstrual Cycle,* pp. 161–181. Springer Verlag, New York.

Kolaczynski, J. W., Considine, R. V., Ohannesian, J., Marco, C., Opentanova, I., Nyce, M. R., Myint, M., and Caro, J. F. 1996. Responses of leptin to short-term fasting and refeeding in humans: a link with ketogenesis but not ketones themselves. *Diabetes,* 45:1511–1515.

Komisaruk, B. R. 1967. Effects of local brain implants of progesterone on reproductive behavior in ring doves. *J. Comp. Physiol. Psychol.,* 64:219–224.

Komisaruk, B. R., Terasawa, E., and Rodriguez-Sierra, J. F. 1981. How the brain mediates ovarian responses to environmental stimuli. In N. T. Adler (ed.), *Neuroendocrinology of Reproduction,* pp. 349–376. Plenum Press, New York.

Konopka, R. J. 1987. Genetics of biological rhythms in *Drosophila. Annu. Rev. Genet.,* 21:227–236.

Konopka, R. J., and Benzer, S. 1971. Clock mutants of *Drosophila melanogaster. Proc. Natl. Acad. Sci. U.S.A.,* 68:2112–2116.

Koob, G. F. 1992 . Drugs of abuse:anatomy, pharmacology and function of reward pathways. *Trends Pharmacol. Sci.,* 13:177–184.

Koob, G. F., and Bloom, F. E. 1988. Cellular and molecular mechanisms of drug dependence. *Science,* 242:715–723.

Koopmans, H. S. 1983. A stomach hormone that inhibits food intake. *J. Autonomic Nerv. Syst.,* 9:157–171.

Kopin, I. J. 1995. Definitions of stress and sympathetic neuronal responses. *Ann. N. Y. Acad. Sci.,*771:19–30.

Korach, K. S. 1994. Insights from the study of animals lacking functional estrogen receptor. *Science,* 266:1524–1527.

Kornhauser, J. M., Nelson, D. E., Mayo, K. E., and Takahashi, J. S. 1990. Photic and circadian regulation of c-fos gene expression in the hamster suprachiasmatic nucleus. *Neuron,* 5:127–134.

Korol, D. L., and Gold, P. E. 1998. Glucose, memory, and aging. *Am. J. Clin. Nutr.,* 67:764S–771S.

Korol, D. L., Unick, K., Goosens, K., Crane, C., Gold, P. E., and Foster, T. C. 1994. Estrogen effects on spatial performance and hippocampal physiology in female rats. *Soc. Neurosci. Abstr.,* 20:1436.

Korpelainen, H. 1990. Sex ratios and conditions required for environmental sex determination in animals. *Biol. Rev.,* 65:147–184.

Kosman, M. E., and Gerard, R. W. 1955. The effect of adrenaline on a conditioned avoidance response. *J. Comp. Physiol. Psychol.,* 48:506–508.

Kotrschal, K., Hirschenhauser, K., and Möstl, E. 1998. The relationship between social stress and dominance is seasonal in greylag geese. *Anim. Behav.,* 55:171–176.

Kow, L.-M., and Pfaff, D. W. 1998. Mapping of neural and signal transduction pathways for lordosis in the search for estrogen actions on the central nervous system. *Behav. Brain Res.,* 92:169–180.

Kow, L.-M., Montgomery, M. O., and Pfaff, D. W. 1979. Triggering of lordosis reflex in female rats with somatosensory stimulation: Quantitative determination of stimulus parameters. *J. Neurophysiol.,* 42:195–202.

Krasnegor, N. A., and Bridges, R. S. (eds.). 1990. *Mammalian Parenting.* Oxford University Press, Oxford.

Krecek, J. 1973. Sex differences in salt taste: The effect of testosterone. *Physiol. Behav.,* 10:683–688.

Kreuz, L. E., and Rose, R. M. 1972. Assessment of aggressive behavior and plasma testosterone in a young criminal population. *Psychosom. Med.,* 34:321–332.

Kriegsfeld, L. J., Dawson, T. M., Dawson, V. L., Nelson, R. J. & Snyder, S. H. 1997. Aggressive behavior in male mice lacking the gene for nNOS is testosterone-dependent. *Brain Res.,* 769:66–70.

Kripke, D. F. 1981. Photoperiodic mechanisms for depression and its treatment. In C. Perris, G. Struwe, and B. Jansson (eds.), *Biological Psychiatry,* pp. 1249–1252. Elsevier, Amsterdam.

Kripke, D. F., Elliott, J. A., Youngstedt, S. D., and Smith, J. S. 1998. Melatonin: Marvel or marker? *Ann. Med.,* 30:81–87.

Krohmer, R. W., and Crews, D. 1987. Temperature activation of courtship behavior in the male red-sided garter snake (*Thamnophis sirtalis parietalis*): Role of the anterior hypothalamus-preoptic area. *Behav. Neurosci.,* 101:228–236.

Kruuk, H. 1972. *The Spotted Hyena: A Study of Predation and Social Behavior.* University of Chicago Press, Chicago.

Kuederling, I., Evans, C. S., Abbott, D. H., Pryce, C. R., and Epple, G. 1995. Differential excretion of urinary oestrogen by breeding females and daughters in the red-bellied tamarin (*Saguinus labiatus*). *Fol. Primatol.*, 64:140–145.

Kuevi, V., Causon, R., Dixson, A. F., Everard, D. M., Hall, J. M., Hole, D., Whitehead, S. A., Wilson, C. A., and Wise, J. C. M. 1983. Plasma amine and hormone changes in 'post-partum' blues. *Clin. Endocrinol.*, 19:39–46.

Kuiper, G. C., Enmark, E., Pelto-Huikko, M., Nilsson, S., and Gustafsson, J. A. 1996. Cloning of a novel estrogen receptor expressed in rat prostate and ovary. *Proc. Natl. Acad. Sci. U.S.A.*, 93:5925–5930.

Kuhn, H. F., and Reiter, E. O. 1976. Gonadotropin and testosterone measurements after estrogen administration to adult men, prepubertal and pubertal boys, and men with hypogonadotropism: Evidence for maturation of positive feed-back in the male. *Pediatr. Res.*, 10:46–51.

Kupfer, D. J., Monk, T. H., and Barchas, J. D. (eds.). 1988. *Biological Rhythms and Mental Disorders*. Guilford Press, New York.

Kurzer, M. S. 1997. Women, food, and mood. *Nutr. Rev.*, 55:268–276.

Labov, J. B. 1981. Pregnancy blocking in rodents: Adaptive advantages for females. *Am. Nat.*, 118:361–371.

Lack, D. 1954. *The Natural Regulation of Animal Numbers*. Clarendon Press, Oxford.

Lacroix, A., McKenna, T., and Rabinowitz, D. 1979. Sex steroid modulation of gonadotropins in normal men and in androgen insensitivity syndrome. *J. Clin. Endocrinol. Metab.*, 48:235–240.

Ladle, R. J., Johnstone, R. A., and Judson, O. P. 1993. Coevolutionary dynamics of sex in a metapopulation-Escaping the red queen. *Proc. R. Soc. Lond. B.*, 253:155–160.

LaFerla, J. J., Anderson, D. L., and Schalch, D. S. 1978. Psychoendocrine response to sexual arousal in human males. *Psychosom. Med.*, 40:166–172.

Lahr, G., Maxson, S., Mayer, A., Just, W., Pilgrim, C., and Reisert, I. 1995. Transcription of the Y chromosomal gene, Sry, in adult mouse brain. *Mol. Brain Res.*, 33:179–182.

Lal, S., Ackman, D., Thavundayil, J. X., Kiely, M. E., and Etienne, P. 1984. Effect of apomorphine, a dopamine receptor agonist, on penile tumescence in normal subjects. *Prog. Neuropsychopharmacol. Biol. Psychiatry*, 8:695–699.

Lal, S., Laryea, E., Thavundayil, J. X., Nair, N. P. V., Negrete, J., Ackman, D., Blundell, P., and Gardiner, R. J. 1987. Apomorphine-induced penile tumescence in impotent patients—preliminary findings. *Prog. Neuropsychopharmacol. Biol. Psychiatry*, 11:235–242.

Lance, S. L., and Wells, K. D. 1993. Are spring peeper satellite males physiologically inferior to calling males? *Copeia*, 1993:1162–1166.

Landsman, R. E. 1991. Captivity affects behavioral physiology: Plasticity in signaling sexual identity. *Experientia*, 47:31–38.

Landsman, R. E., and Moller, P. 1988. Testosterone changes the electric organ discharge and external morphology of the mormyrid fish *Gnathonemus petersii* (Mormyriformes). *Experientia*, 44:900–903.

Landsman, R. E., Harding, C. F., Moller, P., and Thomas, P. 1990. The effects of androgens and estrogen on the external morphology and electric organ discharge waveform of *Gnathonemus petersii* (Mormyridae, Teleostei). *Horm. Behav.*, 24:532–553.

Lane, A. J. P., and Wathes, D.C. 1998. An electronic nose to detect changes in perineal odors associated with estrus in the cow. *J. Dairy Sci.*, 81:2145–2150.

Langevin, R., Paitich, D., Hucker, S., Newman, S., Ramsay, G., Pope, S., Geller, G., and Anderson, C. 1979. The effect of assertiveness training, Provera and sex of therapist in the treatment of genital exhibitionism. *J. Behav. Ther. Exp. Psychiatry*, 10:275–282.

Langhans, W., and Scharrer, E. J. 1987. Evidence for a vagally mediated satiety signal derived from hepatic fatty acid oxidation. *Autonomic Nerv. Sys.*, 18:13–18.

Lank, D. B., Smith, C. M., Hanotte, O., Burke, T., and Cooke, F. 1995. Genetic polymorphism for alternative mating behaviour in lekking male ruff *Philomachus pugnax*. *Nature*, 378:59–62.

Larsson, K. 1962. Mating behavior in male rats after cerebral cortex ablation. I. Effects of lesions in the dorsolateral and the median cortex. *J. Exp. Zool.*, 151:167–176.

Larsson, K. 1966. Individual differences in reactivity to androgen in male rats. *Physiol. Behav.*, 1:255–258.

Larsson, K. 1969. Failure of gonadal and gonadotrophic hormones to compensate for an impaired sexual function in anosmic male rats. *Physiol. Behav.*, 4:733–737.

Larsson, K. 1979. Features of the neuroendocrine regulation of masculine sexual behavior. In C. Beyer (ed.), *Endocrine Control of Sexual Behavior*, pp. 77–163. Raven Press, New York.

Lashley, K. S. 1938. Experimental analysis of instinctive behavior. *Psychol. Rev.*, 45:445–471.

Lavie, P. 1985. Ultradian rhythms: Gates of sleep and wakefulness. In H. Schulz and P. Lavie (eds.), *Ultradian Rhythms in Physiology and Behavior*, pp. 148–164. Springer-Verlag, Berlin.

Le Mouellic, H., Lallemand, Y., and Brulet, P. 1990. Targeted replacement of the homeobox gene Hox-3.1 by the *Escherischia coli* lacZ in mouse chimeric embryos. *Proc. Natl. Acad. Sci. U.S.A.*, 87, 4712–4716.

Lea, R. W., Vowels, D. M., and Dick, H. R. 1986. Factors affecting prolactin secretion during the breeding cycle of the ring dove (*Streptopelia risoria*) and its possible role in incubation. *J. Endocrinol.*, 110: 447–458.

LeBlond, C. P. 1938. Extra-hormonal factors in maternal behavior. *Proc. Soc. Exp. Biol.*, 38:66–70.

LeBoeuf, B. J. 1967. Interindividual associations in dogs. *Behaviour*, 29:268–295.

LeBoeuf, B. J. 1970. Copulatory and aggressive behavior in the prepubertally castrated male dog. *Horm. Behav.*, 1:127–136.

LeBoeuf, B. J. 1974. Male-male competition and reproductive success in elephant seals. *Am. Zool.*, 14:163–176.

Leboucher, G., Richard-Yris, M.-A., Williams, J. A., and Chadwick, A. 1990. Incubation and maternal behaviour in domestic hens: Influence of the presence of chicks on circulating luteinising hormone, prolactin, and oestradiol and on behaviour. *Br. Poultry Sci.*, 31:851–862.

Lee, R., Jaffe, R., and Midgley, A. 1974. Lack of alteration of serum gonadotropins in men and women following sexual intercourse. *Am. J. Obstet. Gynecol.*, 120:985–987.

Lee, T. M., Carmichael, M. S., and Zucker, I. 1986. Circannual variations in circadian rhythms of ground squirrels. *Am. J. Physiol.*, 244:R607–R610.

Leedom, L. J., Meehan, W. P., and Zeidler, A. 1987. Avoidance responding in mice with diabetes mellitus. *Physiol. Behav.*, 40:447–451.

Lefebvre, L., Viville, S., Barton, S. C., Ishino, F., Keverne, E. B., and Surani, M. A. 1998. Abnormal maternal behaviour and growth retardation associated with loss of the imprinted gene Mest. *Nat. Genet.*, 20:163–169.

Lehman, M. N., and Winans, S. S. 1982. Vomeronasal and olfactory pathways to the amygdala controlling male hamster sexual behavior: Autoradiographic and behavioral analyses. *Brain Res.*, 240:27–41.

Lehman, M. N., Silver, R., Gladstone, W. R., Kahn, R. M., Gibson, M., and Bittman, E. L. 1987. Circadian rhythmicity restored by neural transplant. Immunocytochemical characterization of the graft and its integration with the host brain. *J. Neurosci.*, 7:1626–1638.

Lehne, G. K. 1988. Treatment of sex offenders with medroxyprogesterone acetate. In J. B. A. Sitsen (ed.), *Handbook of Sexology*, Vol. 6, *The Pharmacology and Endocrinology of Sexual Function*, pp. 516–525. Elsevier Science Publishers, Amsterdam.

Lehrman, D. S. 1953. A critique of Konrad Lorenz's theory of instinctive behavior. *Q. Rev. Biol.*, 28:337–363.

Lehrman, D. S. 1961. Hormonal regulation of parental behavior in birds and infrahuman mammals. In W. C. Young (ed.), *Sex and Internal Secretions*, Vol. 2, pp. 1268–1382. Williams & Wilkins, Baltimore.

Lehrman, D. S. 1965. Interaction between internal and external environments in the regulation of the reproductive cycle of the ring dove. In F. A. Beach (ed.), *Sex and Behavior*, pp. 335–380. Wiley, New York.

Lehrman, D. S., and Brody, P. 1961. Does prolactin induce incubation behavior in the ring dove? *J. Endocrinol.*, 22:369–375.

Leinhart, R. 1927. Contribution a l'étude de l'incubation. *C. R. Soc. Biol.* (*Paris*), 97:1296–1297.

Leipheimer, R. E., and Sachs, B. D. 1993. Relative androgen sensitivity of the vascular and striated-muscle systems regulating penile erection in rats. *Physiol. Behav.*, 54:1085–1090.

Leon, M. 1980. Development of olfactory attraction by young Norway rats. In D. Müller-Schwarze and R. M. Silverstein (eds.), *Chemical Signals*, pp. 193–209. Plenum, New York.

Leon, M. 1992. Neuroethology of olfactory preference development. *J. Neurobiol.*, 23:1557–1573.

Leon, M., and Moltz, H. 1972. The development of the pheromonal bond in the albino rat. *Physiol. Behav.*, 8:683–686.

Leon, M., Coopersmith, R., Beasley, L. J., and Sullivan, R. M. 1990. Thermal aspects of parenting. In N. A. Krasnegor and R. S. Bridges (eds.), *Mammalian Parenting*, pp. 400–415. Oxford University Press, Oxford.

Leon, M., Croskerry, P. G., and Smith, G. K. 1978. Thermal control of mother-young contact in rats. *Physiol. Behav.*, 21:793–811.

Lepri, J. J., and Wysocki, C. J. 1987. Removal of the vomeronasal organ disrupts the activation of reproduction in female voles. *Physiol. Behav.*, 40:349–355.

Lepri, J. J., Wysocki, C. J., and Vandenbergh, J. G. 1985. Mouse vomeronasal organ: Effects on chemosignal production and maternal behavior. *Physiol. Behav.*, 35:809–814.

LeSauter, J., Romero, P., Cascio, M., and Silver, R. 1997. Attachment site of grafted SCN influences precision of restored circadian rhythm. *J. Biol. Rhythms,* 12:327–338.

Leshner, A. 1978. *An Introduction to Behavioral Endocrinology.* Oxford University Press, New York.

Leshner, A. I., and Collier, G. 1973. The effects of gonadectomy on the sex differences in dietary self-selection patterns and carcass compositions of rats. *Physiol. Behav.*, 11:671–676.

Leshner, A. I., and Moyer, J. A. 1975. Androgens and agonistic behavior in mice: Relevance to aggression and irrelevance to avoidance-of-attack. *Physiol. Behav.*, 15:695–699.

LeVay, S. 1993. *The Sexual Brain.* MIT Press, Cambridge, MA.

LeVay, S. 1991. A difference in hypothalamic structure between heterosexual and homosexual men. *Science,* 253:1034–1037.

Levine, A. S., and Morley, J. E. 1984. Neuropeptide Y: A potent inducer of consummatory behavior in rats. *Peptides,* 5:1025–1029.

Levine, S. 1993. The psychoendocrinology of stress. *Ann. N. Y. Acad. Sci.,* 697:61–69.

Levine, S., Haltmeyer, G. C., and Karas, G. G. 1967. Physiological and behavioral effects of infantile stimulation. *Physiol. Behav.,* 2:55–59.

Levine, S., Huchton, D. M., Wiener, S. G., and Rosenfeld, P. 1991. Time course of the effect of maternal deprivation on the hypothalamic-pituitary-adrenal axis in the infant rat. *Dev. Psychobiol.,* 24:547–558.

Levy, A. D., Baumann, M. H., and Van De Kar, L. D. 1994. Monoaminergic regulation of neuroendocrine function and its modification by cocaine. *Front. Neuroendocrinol.,* 15:85–156.

Levy, A., and Lightman, S. L. 1997. *Endocrinology.* Oxford University Press, Oxford.

Lévy, F., Porter, R. H., Kendrick, K. M., Keverne, E. B., and Romeyer, A. 1996. Physiological, sensory, and experiential factors of parental care in sheep. *Adv. Study Behav.,* 25:385–422.

Levy, J. V., and King, J. A. 1953. The effects of testosterone propionate on fighting behaviour in young male C57BL/10 mice. *Anat. Rec.,* 117:562–563.

Lewy, A. J., Ahmed, S., and Sack, R. L. 1996. Phase shifting the human circadian clock using melatonin. *Behav. Brain Res.,* 73:131–134.

Lewy, A. J., Bauer, V. K., Cutler, N. L., Sack, R. L., Ahmed, S., Thomas, K. H., Blood, J. L., and Jackson, J. M. 1998. Morning vs evening light treatment of patients with winter depression. *Arch. Gen. Psychiatry,* 55:890–896.

Lewy, A. J., Sack, R. L., and Singer, C. M. 1985. Melatonin, light and chronobiological disorders. In D. Evered and S. Clark. (eds.), *Photoperiodism, Melatonin and the Pineal.* Ciba Foundation Symposium, 117, pp. 231–252. Pitman, London.

Lewy, A. J., Sack, R. L., Miller, S., et al. 1987. Antidepressant and circadian phase-shifting effects of light. *Science,* 235:352–354.

Lewy, A. J., Sack, R. L., Singer, C. M., White, D. M., and Hoban, T. M. 1988. Winter depression and the phase-shift hypothesis for bright light's therapeutic effects: History, theory, and experimental evidence. *J. Biol. Rhythms,* 3:121–134.

Lewy, A. J., Wehr, T. A., Goodwin, F. K., Newsome, D. A., and Markey, S. P. 1980. Light suppresses melatonin secretion in humans. *Science,* 210:1267–1269.

Liberzon, I., Trujillo, K. A., Akil, H., and Young, E. A. 1997. Motivational properties of oxytocin in the conditioned place preference paradigm. *Neuropsychopharmacology,* 17:353–359.

Licht, P., McCreery, B. R., Barnes, B. R., Pang, R. 1983. Seasonal and stress related changes in plasma gonadotropins, sex steroids, and corticosterone in the bullfrog, *Rana catesbeiana. Gen. Comp. Endocrinol.,* 50:124–145.

Lillie, F. R. 1917. The freemartin: A study of the action of sex hormones in the foetal life of cattle. *J. Exp. Zool.,* 23:371–385.

Limbird, T. J. 1985. Anabolic steroids in the training and treatment of athletes. *Compr. Ther.,* 11:25–30.

Lincoln, G. 1974. Lutinising hormone and testosterone in man. *Nature,* 252:232–233.

Lincoln, G. A., Guinness, F., and Short, R. V. 1972. The way in which testosterone controls the social and sexual behavior of the red deer stag (*Cervus elaphus*). *Horm. Behav.,* 3:375–396.

Ling, M. H. M., Perry, P. J., and Tsuang, M. T. 1981. Side effects of corticosteroid therapy. *Arch. Gen. Psychiatry,* 38:471–477.

Lisk, R. D. 1962. Diencephalic placement of estradiol and sexual receptivity in the female rat. *Am. J. Physiol.,* 203:493–502.

Lisk, R. D. 1971. Oestrogen and progesterone synergism and elicitation of maternal nest-building in the *mouse (Mus musculus*). *Anim. Behav.,* 19:606–616.

Liu, D., Diorio, J., Tannenbaum, B., Caldji, C., Francis, D., Freedman, A., Sharma, S., Pearson, D., Plotsky, P. M., and Meaney, M. J. 1997. Maternal care, hippocampal glucocorticoid receptors, and hypothalamic-pituitary-adrenal responses to stress. *Science,* 277:1659–1662.

Liu, Y-C., Salamonee, J. D., and Sachs, B. D. 1997a. Impaired sexual response after lesions of the paraventricular nucleus of the hypothalamus in male rats. *Behav. Neurosci.,* 111:1–7.

Liu, Y-C., Salamonee, J. D., and Sachs, B. D. 1997b. Lesions in medial preoptic area and bed nucleus of stria terminalis: Differential effects on copulatory behavior and noncontact erection in male rats. *J. Neurosci.,* 17:5245–5253.

Llewellyn, A. M., Stone, Z. N., and Nemeroff, C. B. 1997. Depression during pregnancy and the puerperium. *J. Clin. Psychiatry,* 58:S26–32.

Lloyd, J. A. 1971. Weights of testes, thymi and accessory reproductive glands in relation to rank in paired and grouped housed mice (*Mus musculus*). *Proc. Soc. Exp. Biol. Med.,* 137:19–22.

Lockley, S. W., Skene, D. J., Thapan, K., English, J., Ribeiro, D., Haimov, I., Hampton, S., Middleon, B., von Schantz, M., and Arendt, J. 1998. Extraocular light exposure does not suppress plasma melatonin in humans. *J. Clin. Endocrinol. Metab.,* 83:3369–3372.

Logue, C. M., and Moos, R. H. 1986. Perimenstrual symptoms: Prevalence and risk factors. *Psychosom. Med.,* 48:388–414.

Logue, C. M., and Moos, R. H. 1988. Positive perimenstrual changes: Toward a new perspective on the menstrual cycle. *J. Psychosom. Res.,* 32:31–40.

Long, J. A., and Evans, H. M. 1922. The oestrus cycle in the rat and its associated phenomena. *Memoirs of the University of California,* 6:1–148.

Lonstein, J. S., Simmons, D. A., Swann, J. M., and Stern, J. M. 1998. Forebrain expression of c-fos due to active maternal behaviour in lactating rats. *Neuroscience,* 82:267–281.

Lorens, S. 1978. Some behavioral effects of serotonin depletion depend on method: A comparison of 5,7-dihydroxytrptamine, p-chlorophenylalanine, p-chloroamphetamine, and electrolytic raphe lesions. *Ann. N. Y. Acad. Sci.,* 305:532–555.

Loundes, D. D., and Bridges, R. S. 1986. Length of prolactin priming differentially affects maternal behavior in female rats. *Biol. Reprod.,* 34:495–501.

Loy, R. J., Gerlach, J. L., and McEwen, B. S. 1988. Autoradiographic location of estradiol-binding neurons in the rat hippocampal formation and entorhinal cortex. *Dev. Brain Res.,* 39:245–251.

Lu, K. H., Chen, H. T., Huang, H. H., Grandison, L., Marshall, S., and Meites, J. 1976. Relation between prolactin and gonadotropin secretion in postpartum lactating rats. *J. Endocrinol.,* 68:241–250.

Lubahn, D. B., Moyer, J. S., Golding, T. S., Couse, J. F., Korach, K. S., and Smithies, O. 1993. Alteration of reproductive function but not prenatal sexual development after insertional disruption of the mouse estrogen receptor gene. *Proc. Natl. Acad. Sci. U.S.A.* 90:11162–11166.

Lubin, M., Leon, M., Moltz, H., and Numan, M. 1972. Hormones and maternal behavior in the male rat. *Horm. Behav.,* 3:369–374.

Lucas, B. K., Ormandy, C. J., Binart, N., Bridges, R. S., and Kelly, P. A. 1998. Null mutation of the prolactin receptor gene produces a defect in maternal behavior. *Endocrinology,* 139:4102–4107.

Luger, A., Deuster, P. A., Kyle, S. B., Gallucci, W. T., Montgomery, L. C., Gold, P. W., Loriaux, L. D., and Chrousos, G. P. 1987. Acute hypothalamic-pituitary-adrenal responses to the stress of treadmill exercise: Physiological adaptations to physical training. *N. Engl. J. Med.,* 316:1309–1315.

Lugg, J. A., Rajfer, J., and González-Cadavid, N. F. 1995. Dihydrotestosterone (DHT) is the active androgen in the maintenance of nitric oxide-mediated penile erection in the rat. *Endocrinology,* 136:1495–501.

Luine, V. 1994. Steroid hormone influences on spatial memory. *Ann. N. Y. Acad. Sci.,* 743: 201–211.

Luine, V. N., Spencer, R. L., and McEwen, B. S. 1993. Effects of chronic corticosterone ingestion on spatial memory performance and hippocampal serotonergic function. *Brain Res.,* 616:65–70.

Luine, V., and Rodriguez, M. 1994. Effects of estradiol on radial arm maze performance of young and aged rats. *Behav. Neural Biol.,* 62:230–236.

Luine, V., Richards, S. T., Wu, V. Y., and Beck, K. D. 1998. Estradiol enhances learning and memory in a spatial memory task and effects [sic] levels of monoaminergic neurotransmitters. *Horm. Behav.,* 34:149–162.

Luine, V., Villegas, M., Martinez, C., and McEwen, B. S. 1994. Repeated stress causes impairments of spatial memory performance. *Brain Res.,* 639:167–170.

Lydon, J. P., DeMayo, F. J., Conneely, O. M., and O'Malley, B. W. 1996. Reproductive phenotpes of the progesterone receptor null mutant mouse. *J. Steroid Biochem. Mol. Biol.* 56:67–77.

Lynn, R. B., Cao, G-Y., Considine, R. V., Hyde, T. M., and Caro, J. F. 1996. Autoradiographic localization of leptin binding in the choroid plexus of *ob/ob* and *db/db* mice. *Biochem. Biophys. Res. Commun.,* 219:884–889.

Ma, L-Y., Itharat, P., Fluharty, S. J., and Sakai, R. R. 1997. Intracerebroventricular administration of mineralocorticoid receptor antisense oligonucleotides attenuates salt appetite in the rat. *Stress,* 2:37–50.

Maccari, S., Piazza, P. V., Deminiere, J. M., Leminaire, V., Mormede, P., Simon, H., Angelucci, L., and Le Moal, M. 1991. Life events-induced decrease of corticosterone type I receptors is associated with reduced corticosterone feedback and enhanced vulnerability to amphetamine self-administration. *Brain Res.,* 547:7–12.

Maccoby, E. E., and Jacklin, C. N. 1974. *The Psychology of Sex Differences.* Stanford University Press, Stanford, CA.

MacConnie, S. E., Barkan, A., Lampman, R. M., Schorok, M. A., and Beitins, I. Z. 1986. Decreased hypothalamic gonadotropin-releasing hormone secretion in male marathon runners. *N. Engl. J. Med.,* 315:411–417.

MacLean, P. D., and Ploog, D. W. 1962. Cerebral representation of penile erection. *J. Neurophysiol.,* 25:29–55.

MacLusky, N. J., Yuan, H., Elliott, J., and Brown, T. J. 1996. Sex differences in corticosteroid binding in the rat brain: An in vitro autoradiographic study. *Brain Res.,* 708:71–81.

Maddocks, S., Hahn, P., Moller, F., and Reid, R. L. 1986. A double-blind placebo-controlled trial of progesterone vaginal suppositories in the treatment of premenstrual syndrome. *Am. J. Obstet. Gynecol.,* 154:573–581.

Madison, D. M. 1984. Group nesting and its ecological and evolutionary significance in overwintering microtine rodents. *Bull. Carnegie Museum Nat. Hist.,* 10:267–274.

Madlafousek, J., and Hlinak, Z. 1977. Sexual behaviour of the laboratory rat: Inventory, patterning, and measurement. *Behaviour,* 63:129–174.

Maeda, K., Kato, Y., Ohgo, S., Chihara, K., Yoshimoto, Y., Yamaguchi, N., Kuromaru, S., and Imura, H. 1975. Growth hormone and prolactin release after injection of thyrotropin-releasing hormone in patients with depression. *J. Clin. Endocrinol. Metab.,* 40:501–505.

Maehlen, J., and Torvik, A. 1990. Necrosis of granule cells of hippocampus in adrenocortical failure. *Acta Neuropathol.,* 80:85–87.

Maggi, A., Bettini, S. E., Mantero, G., and Zucchi, I. 1989. Hippocampus: A target for estrogen action in mammalian brain. *Mol. Endocrinol.,* 3:1165–1170.

Mahmoud, I. Y., and Licht, P. 1997. Seasonal changes in gonadal activity and the effects of stress on reproductive hormones in the common snapping turtle, *Chelydra serpentina. Gen. Comp. Endocrinol.,* 107:359–372.

Majewska, M. D. 1987. Actions of steroids on reward: Role of personality, mood, stress, and disease. *Integr. Psychiatry,* 5:258–273.

Majewska, M. D., Harrison, N. L., Schwartz, R. D., Barker, J. L., and Paul, S. M. 1986. Steroid hormone metabolites are barbiturate-like modulators of the GABA receptor. *Science,* 232:1004–1007.

Malacarne, G., Bottoni, L, Massa, R., and Vellano, C. 1984. The abdominal gland of the crested: A possible source of courtship pheromones. Preliminary ethological and biochemical data. *Monitore Zool.* (Italy), 18:33–39.

Malamuth, N. M., Heim, M., and Feshbach, S. 1980. Sexual responsiveness of college students to rape depictions: Inhibitory and disinhibitory effects. *J. Pers. Soc. Psychol.,* 38:399–408.

Malone, D. A., Dimef, R. J., Lombardo, J. A., and Sample, R. H. 1995. Psychiatric effects and psychoactive substance use in anabolic-androgenic steroid users. *Clin. J. Sports Med.,* 5:25–31.

Malsbury, C. W. 1971. Facilitation of male rat copulatory behavior by electrical stimulation of the medial preoptic area. *Physiol. Behav.,* 7:797–805.

Mangat, H. K., Chhina, G. S., Singh, B., and Anand, B. K. 1978a. Effect of testosterone proprionate on electrical activity of brain in intact and gonadectomized rhesus monkeys. *Indian J. Exp. Biol.,* 16:893–896.

Mangat, H. K., Chhina, G. S., Singh, B., and Anand, B. K. 1978b. Influence of gonadal hormones and genital afferents on EEG activity of the hypothalamus in adult male rhesus monkeys. *Physiol. Behav.,* 20:377–384.

Mani, S. K., Allen, J. M., Clark, J. H., Blaustein, J. D., and O'Malley, B. W. 1995. Convergent pathways for steroid hormone- and neurotransmitter-induced rat sexual behavior. *Science* 265:1246–1249.

Mani, S. K., Blaustein, J. D., and O'Malley, B. W. 1997. Progesterone receptor function from a behavioral perspective. *Horm. Behav.,* 31:244–255.

Mann, M. A., Konen, C., and Svare, B. 1984. The role of progesterone in pregnancy-induced aggression in mice. *Horm. Behav.,* 18:140–160.

Mann, M. A., Michael, S., and Svare, B. 1980. Ergot drugs suppress prolactin and lactation but not aggressive behavior in parturient mice. *Horm. Behav.,* 14:319–328.

Manning, C. A., Honn, V. J., Stone, W. S., Jane, J. S., and Gold, P. E. 1998b. Glucose effects on cognition in adults with Down's syndrome. *Neuropsychology,* 12:479–484.

Manning, C. A., Parsons, M. W., and Gold, P. E. 1992. Anterograde and retrograde enhancement of 24-h memory by glucose in elderly humans. *Behav. Neural Biol.,* 58:125–130.

Manning, C. A., Stone, W. S., Korol, D. L., and Gold, P. E. 1998a. Glucose enhancement of2-h memory retrieval in healthy elderly humans. *Behav. Brain Res.,* 93:71–76.

Mansukhani, V., Adkins-Regan, E., and Yang, S. 1996. Sexual partner preference in female zebra finches: the role of early hormones and social environment. *Horm. Behav.,* 30:506–13.

Marler, C. A., and Moore, M. C. 1988. Evolutionary costs of aggression revealed by testosterone manipulations in free-living male lizards. *Behav. Ecol. Sociobiol.,* 23:21–26.

Marler, C. A., and Moore, M. C. 1991. Supplementary feeding compensates for testosterone-induced costs of aggression in male mountain spiny lizards, *Sceloporus jarrovi. Anim. Behav.,* 42:209–219.

Marler, C. A., and Moore, M. C. 1995. Time and energy costs of aggression in testosterone-implanted free-living male mountain spiny lizards (*Sceloporus jarrovi*). *Physiol. Zool.,* 62:1334–1350.

Marler, C. A., Walsberg, G., White, M. L., and Moore, M. 1995. Increased energy expenditure due to increased territorial defense in male lizards after phenotypic manipulation. *Behav. Ecol. Sociobiol.,* 37:225–231.

Marques, D. M., and Valenstein, E. S. 1976. Another hamster paradox: More males carry pups and fewer kill and cannibalize young than do females. *J. Comp. Physiol. Psychol.,* 90:653–657.

Marra, P. A., Hobson, K. A., and Holmes, R. T. 1998. Linking winter and summer events in a migratory bird by using stable-carbon isotopes. *Science,* 282:1884–1886.

Marshall, J. F., Turner, B. H., and Teitelbaum, P. 1971. Sensory neglect produced by lateral hypothalamic damage. *Science,* 174:523–525.

Marshall, J. R., and Henkin, R. I. 1971. Olfactory acuity, menstrual abnormalities, and oocyte status. *Ann. Intern. Med.,* 75:207–211.

Marstellar, F. A., and Lynch, C. B. 1987. Reproductive responses to variation in temperature and food supply by house mice: II. Lactation. *Biol. Reprod.,* 37:844–850.

Martin, R. D., and May, R. M. 1981. Outward signs of breeding. *Nature,* 293:7–9.

Martinet, L., Allair, D., and Weine, C. 1982. Role of prolactin in the photoperiodic control of the molting in the mink (*Mustela vison*). *J. Endocrinol.* 103:9–15.

Martins, T., and Valle, J. R. 1948. Hormonal regulation of the micturition behavior of the dog. *J. Comp. Physiol. Psychol.,* 41:301–311.

Mas, M. 1995. Neurobiological correlates of masculine sexual behavior. *Neurosci. Biobehav. Rev.,* 19:261–277.

Mason, J. 1968. A review of psychoendocrine research on the pituitary adrenal cortical system. *Psychosom. Med.,* 30:576–583.

Mason, J. W. 1975. A historical view of the stress field. *J. Hum. Stress,* 1:6–12.

Mason, R. T. 1987. Sex pheromones and the mediation of reproduction in the red-sided garter snake *Thamnophis sirtalis parietalis.* Ph.D. Dissertation. University of Texas, Austin.

Mason, R. T., Fales, H. M., Jones, T. H., Pannell, L. K., Chinn, J. W., and Crews, D. 1989. Sex pheromones in snakes. *Science,* 245:290–293.

Mason, W. A., and Capitanio, J. P. 1988. Formation and expression of filial attachment oin rhesus monkeys raised with living and inanimate mother substitutes. *Dev. Psychobiol.,* 21:401–430.

Mason, W. A., and Kenney, W. D. 1974. Redirection of filial attachments in rhesus monkeys raised with living and inanimate mother substitutes. *Science,* 183:1209–1211.

Masters, W., and Johnson, V. 1966. *Human Sexual Response.* Little, Brown, Boston.

Mastrogiacomo, I., Fava, M., Fava, G. A., Kellner, R., Grismondi, G., and Cetera, C. 1982/1983. Postpartum hostility and prolactin. *Int. J. Psychiatry Med.,* 12:289–294.

Matsumoto, T. 1992. Familial association, nymphal development and population density of the Australian giant burrowing cockroach, *Macropanesthia rhinoceros* (Blattaria: Blaberidae). *Zool. Sci.,* 9:835–842.

Matteo, S., and Rissman, E. F. 1984. Increased sexual activity during the midcycle portion of the human menstrual cycle. *Horm. Behav.,* 18:249–255.

Matthews, R. 1979. Testosterone levels in aggressive offenders. In M. Sandler (ed.), *Psychopharmacology of Aggression,* pp. 123–130. Raven Press, New York.

Matthews, T. J., Grigore, M., Tang, L., Doat, M., Kow, L. M., and Pfaff, D. W. 1997. Sexual reinforcement in the female rat. *J. Exp. Anal. Behav.,* 68:399–410.

Mayer, A. D., Freeman, N. C., and Rosenblatt, J. S. 1979. Ontogeny of maternal behavior in the laboratory rat: factors underlying changes in responsiveness from 30 to 90 days. *Dev. Psychobiol.,* 12:425–439.

Mayer, A. D., Freeman, N. C., and Rosenblatt, J. S. 1979. Ontogeny of maternal behavior in the laboratory rat: factors underlying changes in responsiveness from 30 to 90 days. *Dev. Psychobiol.,* 12:425–439.

Mazur, A., and Lamb, T. A. 1980. Testosterone, status, and mood in human males. *Horm. Behav.,* 14:236–246.

Mazur, A., Booth, A., and Dabbs, J. M. 1992. Testosterone and chess competition. *Soc. Psychol. Q.,* 55:70–77.

McAllister-Williams, R. H., Ferrier, I. N., and Young, A. H. 1998. Mood and neuropsychological function in depression: The role of corticosteroids and serotonin. *Psychol. Med.,* 28:573–584.

McCann, S. M., and Ramirez, V. D. 1964. The neuroendocrine regulation of hypophyseal luteinizing hormone secretion. *Rec. Prog. Horm. Res.,* 20:131–170.

McCarthy, M. M., and Pfaus, J. G. 1996. Steroid modulation of neurotransmitter function to alter female reproductive behavior. *Trends Endocrinol. Metab.,* 7:327–333.

McCarthy, M. M., Brooks, P. J., Pfaus, J. G., Brown, H. E., Flanagan, L. M., Schwartz-Giblin, S., and Pfaff, D. W. 1993a. Antisense oligodexoxynucleotides in behavioral neuroscience. *Neuroprotocols,* 2:67–74.

McCarthy, M. M., Schlenker, E. H., and Pfaff, D. W. 1993b. Enduring consequences of neonatal treatment with antisense oligodeoxynucleotides to estrogen receptor messenger ribonucleic acid on sexual differentiation of rat brain. *Endocrinology,* 133:433–439.

McCarty, R., and Southwick, C. H. 1977. Paternal care and the development of behavior in the southern grasshopper mouse, *Onychomys torridus. Behav. Biol.,* 19:476–490.

McClintock, M. K. 1971. Menstrual synchrony and suppression. *Nature,* 229:244–245.

McClintock, M. K. 1978. Estrous synchrony and its mediation by airborne chemical communication (*Rattus norvegicus*). *Horm. Behav.,* 10:264–276.

McClintock, M. K. 1984. Group mating in the domestic rat as a context for sexual selection: Consequences for the analysis of sexual behavior and neuroendocrine responses. *Adv. Study Behav.,* 14:1–50.

McClintock, M. K. 1987. A functional approach to the behavioral endocrinology of rodents. In D. Crews (ed.), *Psychobiology of Reproductive Behavior: An Evolutionary Perspective,* pp. 176–203. Prentice Hall, Englewood Cliffs, NJ.

McClintock, M. K., and Adler, N. T. 1978. The role of the female during copulation in wild and domestic Norway rats (*Rattus norvegicus*). *Behaviour,* 67:67–96.

McClintock, M. K., and Herdt, G. 1996. Rethinking puberty: The development of sexual attraction. *Curr. Dir. Psychol. Sci.,* 5.

McCloskey, M., Wible, C. G., and Cohen, N. J. 1988. Is there a special flashbulb-memory mechanism? *J. Exp. Psychol. General,* 117:171–181.

McConnell, J., Benson, G. S., and Wood, J. G. 1982. Autonomic innervation of the urogenital system: Adrenergic and cholinergic elements. *Brain Res. Bull.,* 9:679–694.

McCormack, J. T., and Greenwald, G. S. 1974. Progesterone and oestradiol-17b concentrations in the peripheral plasma during pregnancy in the mouse. *J. Endocrinol.,* 62:101–107.

McCormick, C. M., Smythe, J. W., Sharma, S., and Meaney, M. J. 1995. Sex-specific effects of prenatal stress on hypothalmic-pitu-

itary-adrenal responses to stress and brain glucocorticoid receptor density in adult rats. *Brain Res. Dev. Brain Res.,* 84:55–61.

McElreavey, K., Barbaux, S., Ion, A., and Fellous, M. 1995. The genetic basis of murine and human sex determination: A review. *Heredity,* 75:599–611.

McEwen, B. S., Gould, E., Orchinik, M., Weiland, N. G., and Woolley, C. S. 1995. Oestrogens and the structural and functional plasticity of neurons: Implications for memory, ageing and neurodegenerative processes. *Ciba Found. Symp.,* 191:52–66.

McEwen, B. S., Pfaff, D. W., Chaptal, C., and Luine, V. N. 1975. Brain cell nuclear retention of [3H]estradiol doses able to promote lordosis: Temporal and regional aspects. *Brain Res.,* 86:155–161.

McFadden, D., and Loehlin, J. C. 1995. On the heritability of spontaneous otoacoustic emissions: A twins study. *Hearing Res.,* 85:181–198.

McFadden, D., and Pasanen, E. G. 1998. Comparison of the auditory systems of heterosexuals and homosexuals: Click-evoked otoacoustic emissions. *Proc. Natl. Acad. Sci. U.S.A.,* 95:2709–2713.

McGaugh, J. L. 1983. Hormonal influences on memory. *Annu. Rev. Psychol.,* 34:297–323.

McGaugh, J. L. 1989. Involvement of hormonal and neuromodulatory systems in the regulation of memory storage. *Annu. Rev. Neurosci.,* 12:255–287.

McGaugh, J. L., and Gold, P. E. 1976. Modulation of memory by electrical stimulation of the brain. In M. R. Rosenzweig and E. L. Bennett (eds.), *Neural Mechanisms of Learning and Memory,* pp. 549–560. MIT Press, Cambridge, MA.

McGaugh, J. L., Bennett, M. C., Liang, K. C., Juler, R. G., and Tam, D. 1987. Memory-enhancing effect of posttraining epinephrine is not blocked by dexa-methasone. *Psychobiology,* 15:343–344.

McGee, L. C., Juhn, M., and Domm, L. V. 1928. The development of secondary sex characters by injection of bull testes. *Am. J. Physiol.,* 87:406–435.

McGee, M. G. 1979. Human spatial abilities: Psychometric studies and environmental, genetic, hormonal and neurological influences. *Psychol. Bull.,* 80:889–918.

McGill, T. E. 1962. Sexual behavior in three inbred strains of mice. *Behaviour,* 19:341–350.

McGill, T. E. 1977. Reproductive isolation, behavioral genetics, and function of sexual behavior in rodents. In J. S. Rosenblatt and B. R. Komisaruk (eds.), *Reproductive Behavior and Evolution,* pp. 73–109. Plenum Press, New York.

McGinnis, M. Y., Parsons, B., Rainbow, T. C., Krey, L. C., and McEwen, B. S. 1981. Temporal relationship between cell nuclear progestin receptor levels and sexual receptivity following intravenous progesterone administration. *Brain Res.,* 218:365–371.

McGinnis, M. Y., Williams, G. W., and Lumia, A. R. 1996. Inhibition of male sex behavior by androgen receptor blockade in preoptic area or hypothalamus, but not amygdala or septum. *Physiol. Behav.,* 60:783–789.

McGlone, J. 1980. Sex differences in human brain asymmetry: A critical survey. *Behav. Brain Sci.,* 3:215–263.

McGowan, M. K., Andrews, K., Kelly, J., and Grossman, S. P. 1990. Effects of chronic intrahypothalamic infusion of insulin on food intake and diurnal meal patterning in the rat. *Behav. Neurosci.,* 104:373–385.

McGregor, G. P., Desaga, J. F., Ehlenz, K., Fischer, A., Heese, F., Hegele, A., Lammer, C., Peiser, C., and Lang, R. E. 1996. Radioimmunological measurement of leptin in plasma of obese and diabetic human subjects. *Endocrinology,* 137:1501–1504.

McGuinness, D. 1972. Hearing: Individual differences in perceiving. *Perception,* 1:465–473.

McGuinness, D. 1976. Away from a unisex psychology: Individual differences in visual sensory and perceptual processes. *Perception,* 5:279–294.

McKinney, T. D., and Desjardins, C. 1973. Intermale stimuli and testicular function in adult and immature house mice. *Biol. Reprod.,* 9:370–378.

McLay, R. N., Freeman, S. M., and Zadina, J. E. 1998. Chronic corticosterone impairs memory performance in the Barnes maze. *Physiol. Behav.,* 63:933–937.

McMinn, J. E., Seeley, R. J., Wilkinson, C. W., Havel, P. J., Woods, S. C., and Schwartz, M. W. 1998. NPY-induced overfeeding suppresses hypothalamic NPY mRNA expression: Potential roles of plasma insulin and leptin. *Regul. Pept.,* 25:75–76.

McNeilly, A. S., Sharpe, R. M., and Fraser, H. M. 1983. Increased sensitivity to the negative feedback effect of testosterone induced by hyperprolactinemia in the adult male rat. *Endocrinology,* 112:22–28.

McNemar, Q., and Stone, C. P. 1932. The sex difference in rats on three learning tasks. *J. Comp. Psychol.,* 14:171–180.

McShea, W. J. 1990. Social tolerance and proximate mechanisms of dispersal among winter groups of meadow voles (*Microtus pennsylvanicus*). *Anim. Behav.*, 39:346–351.

Meaney, M. J. 1988. The sexual differentiation of social play. *Trends Neurosci.*, 11:54–58.

Meaney, M. J., and McEwen, B. S. 1986. Testosterone implants into the amygdala during the. neonatal period masculinize the social play of juvenile female rats. *Brain Res.*, 398:324–328.

Meaney, M. J., Diorio, J., Francis, D., Widdowson, J., LaPlante, P., Caldji, C., Sharma, S., Seckl, J. R., and Plotsky, P. M. 1996. Early environmental regulation of forebrain glucocorticoid receptor gene expression: Implications for adrenocortical responses to stress. *Dev. Neurosci.*, 18:49–72.

Meijer, J. H., and Rietveld, W. J. 1989. Neurophysiology of the suprachiasmatic circadian pacemaker in rodents. *Physiol. Rev.*, 69:671–707.

Meisel, R. L., and Sachs, B. D. 1994. The physiology of male sexual behavior. In E. Knobil and J. D. Neill (eds.), *The Physiology of Reproduction*, Vol. 2, pp. 3–105. Raven Press, New York.

Meisel, R. L., Lumia, A. R., and Sachs, B. D. 1980. Effects of olfactory bulb removal and flank shock on copulation in male rats. *Physiol. Behav.*, 25:383–387.

Meisel, R. L., O'Hanlon, J. K., and Sachs, B. D. 1984. Differential maintenance of penile responses and copulatory behavior by gonadal hormones in castrated male rats. *Horm. Behav.*, 18:56–64.

Meisel, R., and Pfaff, D. W. 1984. RNA and protein synthesis inhibitors: Effects on sexual behavior in female rats. *Brain Res. Bull.*, 12:187–193.

Melis, M. R., and Argiolas, A. 1995. Dopamine and sexual behavior. *Neurosci. Biobehav. Rev.*19:19–38.

Meliska, C. J., Burke, P. A., Bartke, A., and Jensen, R. A. 1997. Inhibitory avoidance and appetitive learning in aged normal mice: Comparison with transgenic mice having elevated plasma growth hormone levels. *Neurobiol. Learn. Mem.*, 68:1–12.

Melloni, R. H., Connor, D. F., Hang, P. T., Harrison, R. J., and Ferris, C. F. 1997. Anabolic-androgenic steroid exposure during adolescence and aggressive behavior in golden hamsters. *Physiol. Behav.*, 61:359–364.

Melniczek, J. R., and Ward, I. L. 1994. Patterns of ano-genital licking mother rats exhibit toward prenatally-stressed neonates. *Physiol. Behav.*, 56:457–461.

Melnyk, R. B., Mrosovsky, N., and Martin, J. M. 1983. Spontaneous obesity and weight loss: insulin action in the dormouse. *Am. J. Physiol.*, 245:R396–402.

Menaker, M. 1968. Extraretinal light perception in the sparrow. I. Entrainment of the biological clock. *Proc. Natl. Acad. Sci. U.S.A.*, 59: 414–21.

Menaker, M., Moreira, L. F., and Tosini, G. 1997. Evolution of circadian organization in vertebrates. *Brazilian J. Med. Biol. Res.*, 30:305–313.

Mendelson, J. H., and Mello, N. K. 1982. Hormones and psycho-sexual development in young men following chronic heroin use. *Neurobehav. Toxicol. Teratol.*, 4:441–445.

Mendonca, M. T., and Licht, P. 1986. Seasonal cycles in gonadal activity and plasma gonadotropin in the musk turtle, *Sternotherus odoratus. Gen. Comp. Endocrinol.*, 62:459–469.

Mendoza, S. P., and Mason, W. A. 1986. Parental division of labour and differentiation of attachments in a monogamous primate (*Callicebus moloch*). *Anim. Behav.*, 34:1336–1347.

Mendoza, S. P., and Mason, W. A. 1997. Attachment relationships in New World primates. *Ann. N. Y. Acad. Sci.*,807:203–209.

Mendoza, S. P., Lowe, E. L., and Resko, J. A. 1978. Seasonal variations in gonadal hormones and social behavior in squirrel monkeys. *Physiol. Behav.*, 20:515–522.

Mendoza, S. P., Lyons, D. M., and Saltzman, W. 1991. Sociophysiology of squirrel monkeys. *Am. J. Primatol.*, 23:37–54.

Menzel, R. 1983. Neurobiology of learning and memory: The honeybee as a model system. *Naturwissenschaften*, 70:504–511.

Menzel, R., and Michelsen, B. 1986. Neuropharmacology of associative learning in bees. In H. Matthies (ed.), *Learning and Memory: Mechanisms of Information Storage in the Nervous System*, pp. 273–275. Pergamon, Oxford.

Mercer, J. G., Hoggard, N., Williams, L. M., Lawrence, C. B., Hannah, L. T., and Trayhurn, P. 1996. Localization of leptin receptor mRNA and the long form splice variant (Ob-Rb) in mouse hypothalamus and adjacent brain regions by in situ hybridization. *FEBS Lett.*, 387:113–116.

Messier, C., and White, N. M. 1987. Memory improvement by glucose, fructose, and two glucose analogs: A possible effect on peripheral glucose transport. *Behav. Neural Biol.*, 48:104–127.

Mewis, C., Spyridopoulos, I., Kuhlkamp, V., and Seipel, L. 1996. Manifestation of severe coronary heart disease after anabolic drug abuse. *Clin. Cardiol.*, 19:153–155.

Meyer, W. J., Walker, P. A., Emory, L. E., and Smith, E. R. 1985. Physical, metabolic, and hormonal effects on men of long-term therapy with medroxyprogesterone acetate. *Fertil. Steril.*, 43:102–106.

Meyer-Bahlburg, H. F. L. 1984. Psychoendocrine research on sexual orientation. Current status and future options. In G. J. DeVries, J. P. C. De Bruin, H. B. M. Uylings, and M. A. Corner (eds.), *Progress in Brain Research: Sex Differences in the Brain*, pp. 375–398. Elsevier Science Publishers, Amsterdam.

Meyer-Bahlburg, H. F. L., Grisanti, G. C., and Ehrhardt, A. A. 1977. Prenatal effects of sex hormones on human male behavior: Medroxyprogesterone acetate (MPA). *Psychoneuroendocrinology*, 2:383–390.

Miceli, M. O., and Malsbury, C. W. 1982a. Availability of a food hoard facilitates maternal behaviour in virgin female hamsters. *Physiol. Behav.*, 28:855–856.

Miceli, M. O., and Malsbury, C. W. 1982b. Sagittal knife cuts in the near and far lateral preoptic area–hypothalamus disrupt maternal behavior in female hamsters. *Physiol. Behav.*, 28:857–867.

Micevych, P. E., Eckersell, C. B., Brecha, N., and Holland, K. L. 1997. Estrogen modulation of opioid and cholecystokinin systems in the limbic-hypothalamic circuit. *Brain Res. Bull.*, 44:335–343.

Michael, R. P. 1972. Determinants of primate reproductive behaviour. In E. Diczfalusy and C. C. Standley (eds.), *The Use of Non-human Primates in Research on Human Reproduction*. WHO Symposium, Karolinska Institute, Stockholm.

Michael, R. P., and Zumpe, D. 1978. Annual cycles of aggression and plasma testosterone in captive male rhesus monkeys. *Psychoneuroendocrinology*, 3:217–220.

Michael, R. P., Zumpe, D., and Bonsall, R. W. 1992. The interaction of testosterone with the brain of the orchidectomized primate fetus. *Brain Res.*, 570:68–74.

Michael, R. P., and Zumpe, D. 1993. A review of hormonal factors influencing the sexual and aggressive behavior of macaques. *Am. J. Primatol.*, 30:213–241.

Michael, R. P., and Zumpe, D. 1996. Biological factors in the organization and expression of sexual behaviour. In I. Rosen (ed.), *Sexual Deviation*, pp. 452–287. Oxford University Press, Oxford.

Michael, R. P., Clancy, A. N., and Zumpe, D. 1995. Distribution of androgen receptor-like immunoreactivity in the brains of Cynomolgus monkeys. *J. Neuroendocrinol.*, 7:713–719.

Michael, R. P., Zumpe, D., Kerverne, E. B., and Bonsall, R. W. 1972. Neuroendocrine factors in the control of primate behavior. *Rec. Prog. Horm. Res.*, 28:665–706.

Michel, G. F., and Moore, C. L. 1995. *Developmental Psychobiology: An Interdisciplinary Science*. MIT Press: Cambridge, MA.

Michiels, N. K., and Newman, L. J. 1998. Sex and violence in hermaphrodites. *Nature*, 391:647.

Middleman, A. B., and DuRant, R. H. 1996. Anabolic steroid use and associated health risk behaviours. *Sports Med.*, 21:251–225.

Miernicki, M., Pospichal, M., Karg, J., and Powers, J. B. 1988. Photoperiodic effects on male sexual behavior. *Conference on Reproductive Behavior*, pp. 64, Omaha, NE.

Migeon, C. J., and Wisniewski, A. B. 1998. Sexual differentiation: from genes to gender. *Horm. Res.*, 50:245–251.

Miles, C., Green, R., Sanders, G., and Hines, M. 1998. Estrogen and memory in a transsexual population. *Horm. Behav.*, 34:199–208.

Milette, J. J., and Turek, F. W. 1986. Circadian and photoperiodic effects of brief light pulses in male Djungarian hamsters. *Biol. Reprod.*, 35:327–335.

Mills, M. J., and Stunkard, A. J. 1976. Behavioral changes following surgery for obesity. *Am. J. Psychiatry*, 133:527–531.

Milner, P., and Zucker, I. 1965. Specific hunger for potassium in the rat. *Psychonom. Sci.*, 2:17–18.

Mitani, J. C. 1985. Mating behavior of male orangutans in the Kutai Game Reserve, Indonesia. *Anim. Behav.*, 33:392–402.

Mitchell, A. J. 1998. The role of corticotropin releasing factor in depressive illness: A critical review. *Neurosci. Biobehav. Rev.*, 22:635–651.

Mitchell, J. S., and Keesey, R. E. 1974. The effects of lateral hypothalamic lesions and castration upon the body weight and composition of male rats. *Behav. Biol.*, 11:69–82.

Mizukami, S., Nishizuka, M., and Arai, Y. 1983. Sexual difference in nuclear volume and its ontogeny in the rat amygdala. *Exp. Neurol.*, 79:569–575.

Moberg, G. P. 1991. How behavioral stress disrupts the endocrine control of reproduction in domestic animals. *J. Dairy Sci.*, 74:304–311.

Modney, B. K., and Hatton, G. I. 1990. Motherhood modifies magnocellular neuronal interrelationships in functionally meaningful ways. In N. A. Krasnegor and R. S. Bridges (eds.), *Mammalian Parenting*, pp. 305–323. Oxford University Press, Oxford.

Moffatt, C. A. 1994. Seasonal and Social Regulation of Reproductive Behavior in Female Prairie Voles, *Microtus ochrogaster*. Dissertation, Johns Hopkins University, Baltimore, MD.

Moffatt, C. A., and Nelson, R. J. 1993. Day length influences proceptive behavior of female prairie voles (*Microtus ochrogaster*). *Physiol. Behav.*, 55:1163–1165.

Moffatt, C. A., DeVries, A. C., and Nelson, R. J. 1993. Winter adaptations of male deer mice (*Peromyscus maniculatus*) and prairie voles (*Microtus ochrogaster*) that vary in reproductive responsiveness to photoperiod. *J. Biol. Rhythms*, 8:221–232.

Mogenson, G. J., Jones, D. L., and Yim, C. Y. 1980. From motivation to action: Functional interface between the limbic system and the motor system. *Prog. Neurobiol.*, 14:69–97.

Moltz, H., and Kilpatrick, S. J. 1978. Response to the maternal pheromone in the rat as protection against necrotizing enterocolitis. *Neurosci. Biobehav. Rev.*, 2:277–280.

Moltz, H., Lubin, M., Leon, M., and Numan, M. 1970. Hormonal induction of maternal behavior in the ovariectomized nulliparous rat. *Physiol. Behav.*, 5:1373–1377.

Monder, C., Hardy, M. P., Blanchard, R. J., and Blanchard, D.C. 1994. Comparative aspects of 11-hydroxysteroid dehydrogenase. Testicular 11-hydroxysteroid dehydrogenase: Development of a model for the mediation of Leydig cell function by corticosteroids. *Steroids*, 59:69–73.

Money, J. 1961. Sex hormones and other variables in human eroticism. In W. C. Young (ed.), *Sex and Internal Secretions*, pp. 1383–1400. Williams & Wilkins, Baltimore.

Money, J. 1988. The ethics of pornography in the era of AIDS. *J. Sex Marital Ther.*, 14:177–183.

Money, J., and Bennett, R. G. 1981. Postadolescent paraphilic sex offenders: Antiandrogenic and counseling therapy follow-up. *Int. J. Ment. Health*, 10:122–133.

Money, J., and Dalery, J. 1976. Iatrogenic homosexuality: Gender identity in seven 46 XX chromosomal females with hyperadrenocortical hermaphroditism born with a penis, three reared as boys, four reared as girls. *J. Homosexuality*, 1:357–371.

Money, J., and Ehrhardt, A. A. 1972. *Man and Woman, Boy and Girl*. Johns Hopkins University Press, Baltimore.

Money, J., and Norman, B. F. 1987. Gender identity and gender transposition: Longitudinal outcome study of 24 male hermaphrodites assigned as boys. *J. Sex Marital Ther.*, 13:75–92.

Money, J., and Ogunro, C. 1974. Behavioral sexology: Ten cases of genetic male intersexuality with impaired prenatal and pubertal androgenization. *Arch. Sex. Behav.*, 3:181–205.

Money, J., Devore, H., and Norman, B. F. 1986. Gender identity and gender transposition: Longitudinal outcome study of 32 male hermaphrodites assigned as girls. *J. Sex Marital Ther.*, 12:165–180.

Money, J., Schwartz, M., and Lewis, V. G. 1984. Adult heterosexual status and fetal hormonal masculinization and demasculinization: 46XX congenital virilizing adrenal hyperplasia and 46XY androgen insensitivity syndrome compared. *Psychoneuroendocrinology*, 9:405–414.

Monfort, S. L., Mashburn, K. L., Brewer, B. A., and Creel, S. R. 1998. Evaluating adrenal activity in African wild dogs (*Lycaon pictus*) by fecal corticosteroid analysis. *J. Zoo Wildlife Med.*, 29:129–133.

Monk, T. H. 1980. Traffic accident increases as a possible indicant of desynchronosis. *Chronobiologia*, 7:527–529.

Monk, T. H., and Aplin, L. C. 1980. Spring and autumn Daylight Savings Time changes: Studies of adjustment in sleep timings, mood, and efficiency. *Ergonomics*, 23:167–178.

Montague, C. T., Farooqi, I. S., Whitehead, J. P., Soos, M. A., Rau, H., Wareham, N. J., Sewter, C. P., Digby, J. E., Mohammed, S. N., Hurst, J. A., Cheetham, C. H., Earley, A. R., Barnett, A. H., Prins, J. B., and O'Rahilly, S. 1997. Congenital leptin deficiency is associated with severe early-onset obesity in humans. *Nature*, 387:903–908.

Monti, P. M., Brown, W. A., and Corriveau, D. P. 1977. Testosterone and components of aggressive and sexual behavior in man. *Am. J. Psychiatry*, 134:692–694.

Mook, D. G., Kenney, N. J., Roberts, S., Nussbaum, A. I., and Rodier, W. I. 1972. Ovarian-adrenal interactions in regulation of body weight in female rats. *J. Comp. Physiol. Psychol.*, 81:198–211.

Moore, C. L. 1984. Maternal contributions to the development of masculine sexual behavior in laboratory rats. *Dev. Psychobiol.*, 17:347–356.

Moore, C. L. 1986. Interaction of species-typical environmental and hormonal factors in sexual differentiation of behavior. *Ann. N. Y. Acad. Sci.*, 474:108–119.

Moore, C. L., and Morelli, G. A. 1979. Mother rats interact differently with male and female offspring. *J. Comp. Physiol. Psychol.*, 93:677–684.

Moore, C. L., Dou, H., and Juraska, J. M. 1992. Maternal stimulation affects the number of motor neurons in a sexually dimorphic nucleus of the lumbar spinal cord. *Brain Res.*, 572:52–56.

Moore, C. R., and Price, D. 1932. Gonad hormone functions and the reciprocal influence between gonads and hypophysis with its bearing on the problem of sex-hormone antagonism. *Am. J. Anat.*, 50:13–71.

Moore, C. R., and Price, D. 1938. Some effects of testosterone and testosterone propionate in the rat. *Anat. Rec.*, 71:59–78.

Moore, F. L., and Orchinik, M. 1994. Membrane receptors for corticosterone: a mechanism for rapid behavioral responses in an amphibian. *Horm. Behav.*, 28:512–519.

Moore, F. L., Orchinik, M., and Lowry, C. 1995. Functional studies of corticosterone receptors in neuronal membranes. *Receptor*, 5:21–28.

Moore, M. C. 1984. Changes in territorial defense produced by changes in circulating levels of testosterone: A possible hormonal basis for mate-guarding in white-crowned sparrows. *Behaviour*, 88:215–226.

Moore, M. C. 1987. Castration affects territorial and sexual behavior of free-living male lizards, *Sceloporus jarrovi*. *Anim. Behav.*, 35:1193–1199.

Moore, M. C. 1991. Application of organization-activation theory to alternative male reproductive strategies: A review. *Horm. Behav.*, 25:154–179.

Moore, M. C., and Kranz, R. 1983. Evidence for androgen independence of male mounting behavior in white-crowned sparrows (*Zonotrichia leucophrys gambelli*). *Horm. Behav.*, 17:414–423.

Moore, M. C., and Marler, C. A. 1987. Effects of testosterone manipulations on nonbreeding season territorial aggression in free-living male lizards, *Sceloporus jarrovi*. *Gen. Comp. Endocrinol.*, 65:225–232.

Moore, M. C., Hews, D. K., and Knapp, R. 1998. Hormonal control and evolution of alternative male phenotypes: Generalizations of models for sexual differentiation. *Am. Zool.*, 38:133–151.

Moore, R. M., and Eichler, V. B. 1972. Loss of a circadian adrenal corticosterone rhythm following suprachiasmatic lesions in the rat. *Brain Res.*, 42:201–206.

Moore, R. Y. 1997. Circadian rhythms: Basic neurobiology and clinical applications. *Annu. Rev. Med.*, 48:253–266.

Moore, W. V. 1988. Anabolic steroid use in adolescence. *J.A.M.A.*, 260:3484–3486.

Moore-Ede, M. C., Sulzman, F. M., and Fuller, C. A. 1982. *The Clocks That Time Us*. Harvard University Press, Cambridge.

Moran, T. H., Ameglio, P. J., Schwartz, G. J., and McHugh, P. R. 1992. Blockade of type A, not type B, CCK receptors attenuates satiety actions of exogenous and endogenous CCK. *Am. J. Physiol.*, 262:R46–R50.

Moran, T. H., and McHugh, P. R. 1979. Cholecystokinin: Gastric emptying and feeding in *Macaca mulatta*. *Fed. Proc.*, 38:1131.

Moran, T. H., and McHugh, P. R. 1982. Cholecystokinin suppresses food intake by inhibiting gastric emptying. *Am. J. Physiol.*, 242:R491–R497.

Morin, L. P. 1988. Propylthiouracil, but not other antithyroid treatments, lengthens hamster circadian period. *Am. J. Physiol.*, 255:R1–R5.

Morin, L. P., and Cummings, L. A. 1981. Effect of surgical or photoperiodic castration, testosterone replacement or pinealectomy on male hamster running rhythmicity. *Physiol. Behav.*, 26:825–38.

Morin, L. P., and Zucker, I. 1978. Photoperiodic regulation of copulatory behavior in the male hamster. *J. Endocrinol.*, 77:249–258.

Morin, L. P., Fitzgerald, K. M., and Zucker, I. 1977. Estradiol shortens the period of hamster circadian rhythms. *Science*, 196:305–307.

Morin, L. P., Gavin, M. L., and Ottenweller, J. E. 1986. Propylthiouracil causes phase delays and circadian period lengthening in male and female hamsters. *Am. J. Physiol.*, 250:R151–R160.

Morin, M. P., DeMarchi, P., Champagnat, J., Vanderhaeghen, J. J., Rossier, J., and Denavit-Staubie, M. 1983. Inhibitory effect of cholecystokinin octapeptide on neurons in the nucleus tractus solitarius. *Brain Res.*, 265:333–338.

Morley, J. E., Bartness, T. J., Gosnell, B. A., and Levine, A. S. 1985a. Peptidergic regulation of feeding. *Int. Rev. Neurobiol.*, 27:207–298.

Morley, J. E., Levine, A. S., Bartness, T. J., Nizielski, S. E., Shaw, M. J., and Hughes, J. J. 1985b. Species differences in the response to cholecystokinin. *Ann. N. Y. Acad. Sci.*, 448:413–416.

Morley, J. E., Levine, A. S., Gosnell, B. A., Kneip, J., and Grace, M. 1987. Effect of neuropeptide Y on ingestive behaviors in the rat. *Am. J. Physiol.*, 252:R599–R609.

Morley, J. E., Levine, A. S., Yim, G. K. W., and Lowy, M. T. 1983. Opioid modulation of appetite. *Neurosci. Biobehav. Rev.*, 7:281–305.

Morokoff, P. J., Baum, A., McKinnon, W. R., and Gillilland, R. 1987. Effects of chronic unemployment and acute psychological stress on sexual arousal in men. *Health Psychol.*, 6:545–60.

Morrell, J. I., and Pfaff, D. W. 1978. A neuroendocrine approach to brain function: Localization of sex-steroid concentrating cells in vertebrate brains. *Am. Zool.*, 18:447–460.

Morris, R. G. M., Garrud, P., Rawlins, JNP., and O'Keefe, J. 1982. Place navigation impaired in rats with hippocampal lesions. *Nature*, 297:681–683.

Morris, R., and Nostren-Bertrand, M. 1996. NOS and aggression. *Trends Neurosci.*, 19:277–278.

Mortola, J. F. 1997. From GnRH to SSRIs and beyond: Weighing the options for drug therapy in premenstrual syndrome. *Medscape Womens Health*, 2:3–8.

Moss, H. B., Panzak, G. L., and Tarter, R. E. 1993. Sexual functioning of male anabolic steroid abusers. *Arch. Sex. Behav.*, 22;1–12.

Moss, R. L., and McCann, S. M. 1973. Induction of mating behavior in rats by luteinizing hormone-releasing factor. *Science*, 181:177–179.

Moss, R. L., McCann, S. M., and Dudley, C. A. 1975. Releasing hormones and sexual behavior. *Prog. Brain Res.*, 42:37–46.

Moulton, D. G. 1967. Olfaction in mammals. *Am. Zool.*, 7:421–429.

Mounzih, K., Lu, R., and Chehab, F. F. 1997. Leptin treatment rescues the sterility of genetically obese ob/ob males. *Endocrinology*, 138:1190–1193.

Moyer, K. E. 1968. Kinds of aggression and their physiological basis. *Commun. Behav. Biol.*, 2A:65–87.

Moyer, K. E. 1971. *The Physiology of Hostility.* Markham, Chicago.

Moyer, K. E. 1976. *The Psychobiology of Aggression.* Harper and Row, New York.

Mpitos, G. J., and Davis, W. J. 1973. Learning: Classical and avoidance conditioning in the mollusk, *Pleurobranchea*. *Science*, 180:317–320.

Mrosovsky, N. 1985. Cyclical obesity in hibernators: The search for the adjustable regulator. In J. Hirsch and T. B. Van Itallie (eds.), *Recent Advances in Obesity Research: IV,* pp. 45–56. J. Libbey, London.

Mrosovsky, N. 1988. Seasonal affective disorder, hibernation, and annual cycles in animals: Chipmunks in the sky. *J. Biol. Rhythms,* 3:189–208.

Muehlenkamp, F., Lucion, A., and Vogel, W. H. 1995. Effects of selective serotonin agonists on aggressive behavior in rats. *Pharmacol. Biochem. Behav.*, 50:671–674.

Mulaikal, R. M., Migeon, C. J., and Rock, J. A. 1987. Fertility rates in female patients with congenital adrenal hyperplasia due to 21-hydroxylase deficiency. *N. Engl. J. Med.*, 316:178–182.

Murakami, N., Marumoto, N., Nakahara, K., and Murakami, T. 1997. Daily injections of melatonin entrain circadian activity rhythms of nocturnal rats, but not diurnal chipmunks. *Brain Res.*, 75:240–243.

Murdock, G. P. 1967. *Ethnographic Atlas.* University of Pittsburgh Press, Pittsburgh.

Murphy, B. E. 1997. Antiglucocorticoid therapies in major depression: A review. *Psychoneuroendocrinology*, 22:S125-S132.

Murphy, J. V., and Miller, R. E. 1955. The effect of adrenocorticotrophic hormone (ACTH) on avoidance conditioning in the rat. *J. Comp. Physiol. Psychol.*, 48:47–49.

Murphy, M. R. 1976. Olfactory impairment, olfactory bulb removal and mammalian reproduction. In R. L. Doty (ed.), *Mammalian Olfaction, Reproductive Processes and Behavior,* pp. 95–118. Academic Press, New York.

Murphy, M. R., and Schneider, G. E. 1970. Olfactory bulb removal eliminates mating behavior in the male golden hamster. *Science*, 167:302–304.

Murton, D., and Westwood, N. J. 1980. *Avian Breeding Cycles.* Oxford University Press, New York.

Musselman, D. L. and Nemeroff, C. B. 1996. Depression and endocrine disorders: Focus on the thyroid and adrenal system. *Br. J. Psychiatry, Suppl.*, 1996:S123–128.

Muzzin, P., Eisensmith, R. C., Copeland, K. C., and Woo, S. L. C. 1996. Correction of obesity and diabetes in genetically obese mice by leptin gene therapy. *Proc. Natl. Acad. Sci. U.S.A.*, 93:14804–14808.

Myers, B. M., and Baum, M. J. 1980. Facilitation of copulatory performance in male rats by naloxone: Effects of hypophysectomy, 17 alpha-estradiol, and luteinizing hormone releasing hormone. *Pharmacol. Biochem. Behav.*, 12:365–370.

Myers, K. 1967. Morphological changes in the adrenal glands of wild rabbits. *Nature*, 213:147–150.

Myers, K., Hale, C. S., Mykytowycz, G., and Hughes, R. L. 1971. Effects of varying density and space on sociality and health in animals. In A. Esser (ed.), *Behavior and Environment,* Plenum Press, New York.

Nadler, R. D. 1976. Sexual behavior of captive lowland gorillas. *Arch. Sex. Behav.*, 5:487–502.

Nadler, R. D. 1988. Sexual and reproductive behavior. In J. H. Schwartz (ed.), *Orangutan Biology,* pp. 57–66. Oxford University Press, New York.

Nakahara, K., Murakami, N., Nasu, T., Kuroda, H., and Murakami, T. 1997. Individual pineal cells in chick possess photoreceptive, circadian clock and melatonin-synthesizing capacities *in vitro. Brain Res.*, 774:242–245.

Nakanishi, S., Inove, A., Kita, T., Nakamura, M., Chang, A. C. Y., Cohen, S. N., and Numa, S. 1979. Nucleotide sequence of cloned cDNA for bovine corticotropin-b-lipotropin precursor. *Nature*, 278:423–427.

Nalbandov, A. V. 1976. *Reproductive Physiology of Mammals and Birds.* W. H. Freeman, San Francisco.

Nanda, S. 1990. *Neither Man Nor Woman: The Hijras of India.* Wadsworth Publishing: Belmont, CA.

Napoli-Farris, L., Fratta, W., and Gessa, G. L. 1984. Stimulation of dopamine autoreceptors elicits 'premature ejaculation' in rats. *Pharmacol. Biochem. Behav.*, 20:69–72.

Negus, N. C., and Berger, P. J. 1987. Mammalian reproductive physiology. In H. H. Genoways (ed.), *Current Mammology,* pp. 149–173. Plenum Press, New York.

Nelson, E. E., and Panksepp, J. 1998. Brain substrates of infant-mother attachment: Contributions of opioids, oxytocin, and norepinephrine. *Neurosci. Biobehav. Rev.*, 22:437–452.

Nelson, R. J. 1985. Photoperiod influences reproduction in the prairie vole, Microtus ochrogaster. *Biol. Reprod.*, 33:596–602.

Nelson, R. J. 1987. Photoperiod-nonresponsive morphs: A possible variable in microtine population-density fluctuations. *Am. Nat.*, 130:350–369.

Nelson, R. J. 1997. The use of genetic "knock-out" mice in behavioral endocrinology research. *Horm. Behav.*, 31:188–196.

Nelson, R. J. and Gammie, S. J. In press. Influence of NO on neuroendocrine function and behavior. In L. Ignarro (ed.), *Biology of Nitric Oxide.* Academic Press, New York.

Nelson, R. J., and Demas, G. E. 1996. Seasonal changes in immune function. *Q. Rev. Biol.*, 71:511–548.

Nelson, R. J., and Zucker, I. 1981. Absence of extraocular photoreception in diurnal and nocturnal rodents exposed to direct sunlight. *Comp. Biochem. Physiol.*, 69A:145–148.

Nelson, R. J., Badura, L. L., and Goldman, B. D. 1990. Mechanisms of seasonal cycles of behavior. *Annu. Rev. Psychol.*, 41:81–108.

Nelson, R. J., Demas, G. E., Huang, P., Fishman, M. C., Dawson, V., Dawson, T. M. & Snyder, S. H. 1995. Behavioural abnormalities in male mice lacking neuronal nitric oxide synthase. *Nature*, 378:383–386.

Nelson, R. J., Frank, D., Smale, L., and Willoughby, S. B. 1989. Photoperiod and temperature affect reproductive and nonreproductive functions in male prairie voles (*Microtus ochrogaster*). *Biol. Reprod.*, 40:481–485.

Nelson, R. J., Kriegsfeld, L. J., Dawson, V. L. & Dawson, T. M. 1997. Role of nitric oxide in neuroendocrine regulation of physiology and behavior. *Front. Neuroendocrinol.*, 18: 463–491.

Nelson, R. J., Mason, R. T., Krohmer, R. W., and Crews, D. 1987. Pinealectomy blocks vernal courtship behavior in red-sided garter snakes. *Physiol. Behav.*, 39: 231–233.

Netley, C. 1977. Dichotic listening of callosal agenesis and Turner's syndrome patients. In S. J. Segalowitz and F. A. Gruber (eds.), *Language Development and Neurological Theory,* pp. 133–143. Academic Press, New York.

Netley, C. 1983. Sex chromosome abnormalities and the development of verbal and nonverbal abilities. In C. L. Ludlow and J. A. Cooper (eds.), *Genetic Aspects of Speech and Language Disorders,* pp. 171–195. Academic Press, New York.

Newnham, J. P., Dennett, P. M., Ferron, S. A., Tomlin, S., Legg, C., Bourne, G. L., and Rees, L. H. 1984. A study of the relationship between circulating beta-endorphin-like immunoreactivity and post-partum 'blues.' *Clin. Endocrinol.*, 20:169–177.

Newnham, J. P., Tomlin, S., Ratter, S. J., Bourne, G. L., and Rees, L. H. 1983. Endogenous opiate peptides in pregnancy. *Br. J. Obstet. Gynaecol.,* 90:535–538.

Nicholas, L., Dawkins, K., and Golden, R. N. 1998. Psychoneuroendocrinology of depression. Prolactin. *Psychiatr. Clin. North Am.,* 21:341–358.

Nicholls, T. J., Goldsmith, A. R., and Dawson, A. 1988. Photorefractoriness in birds and comparison with mammals. *Physiol. Rev.,* 68:133–176.

Nielsen, J., and Wohlert, M. 1990. Sex chromosome abnormality found among 34,910 newborn children: Results from a 13-year incidence study in Ahras, Denmark. *Birth Defects Original Articles Series,* 26:209–223.

Nikulina, E. M. 1991. Neural control of predatory aggression in wild and domesticated animals. *Neurosci. Biobehav. Rev.,* 15:545–547.

Nishimori, K., Young, L. J., Guo, Q., Wang, Z., Insel, T. R., and Matzuk, M. M. 1996. Oxytocin is required for nursing, but is not essential for parturition or reproductive behavior. *Proc. Natl. Acad. Sci. U.S.A.,* 93:11699–11704.

Nissen, H. W. 1929. The effects of gonadectomy, vasotomy, and injections of placental and orchic extracts on the sex behavior of the white rat. *Genet. Psychol. Monogr.,* 5:451–547.

Nonacs, R. and Cohen, L. S. 1998. Postpartum mood disorders: Diagnosis and treatment guidelines. *J. Clin. Psychiatry,* 59:S23–40

Norman, A. W., and Litwack, G. 1987. *Hormones.* Academic Press, New York.

Norman, R. L., and Spies, H. G. 1986. Cyclic function in a male macaque: Additional evidence for a lack of sexual differentiation in the physiological mechanisms that regulate the cyclic release of gonadotropin in primates. *Endocrinology,* 118:2608–2610.

Norris, D. O. 1996. *Vertebrate Endocrinology.* (3rd ed.). Academic Press, New York.

Nottebohm, F. 1980a. Brain pathways for vocal learning in birds: A review of the first ten years. In J. M. Sprague and A. N. Epstein (eds.), *Progress in Psychobiology and Physiological Psychology,* Vol. 9, pp. 85–124. Academic Press, New York.

Nottebohm, F. 1980b. Testosterone triggers growth of brain vocal control nuclei in adult female canaries. *Brain Res.,* 189:429–436.

Nottebohm, F. 1981. A brain for all seasons: cyclical anatomical changes in song control nuclei of the canary brain. *Science,* 214:1368–1370.

Nottebohm, F. 1989. From bird song to neurogenesis. *Sci. Am.,* 260:74–79.

Nottebohm, F. 1991. Reassessing the mechanisms and origins of vocal learning in birds. *Trends Neurosci.,* 14:206–211.

Nottebohm, F., Alvarez-Buylla, A., Cynx, J., Kirn, J., Ling, C. Y., Nottebohm, M., Suter, R., Tolles, A., and Williams, H. 1990. Song learning in birds: The relation between perception and production. *Phil. Trans. R. Soc. Lond. [Biol.],* 329:115–124.

Nottebohm, F., and Arnold, A. P. 1976. Sexual dimorphism in vocal control areas of the songbird brain. *Science,* 194:211–213.

Nottebohm, F., Kelly, D. B., and Peton, J. A. 1982. Connections of vocal control nuclei in the canary telencephalon. *J. Comp. Neurol.,* 207:344–357.

Nottebohm, F., Stokes, T. M., and Leonard, C. M. 1976. Central control of song in the canary, Serinus canarius. *J. Comp. Neurol.,* 165:457–486.

Nowak, R. M., and Paradiso, J. L. 1983. *Walker's Mammals of the World.* Johns Hopkins University Press, Baltimore.

Numan, M. 1974. Medial preoptic area and maternal behavior in the female rat. *J. Comp. Physiol. Psychol.,* 87:746–759.

Numan, M. 1988. Neural basis of maternal behavior in the rat. *Psychoneuroendocrinology,* 13:47–62.

Numan, M. 1990. Neural control of maternal behavior. In N. A. Krasnegor and R. S. Bridges (eds.), *Mammalian Parenting,* pp. 231–259. Oxford University Press, Oxford.

Numan, M. 1994. Maternal behavior. In E. Knobil and J. D. Neill (eds.), *The Physiology of Reproduction,* Vol. 2, pp. 221–302. Raven, New York.

Numan, M. and Numan, M. J. 1997. Projection sites of medial preoptic area and ventral bed nucleus of the stria terminalis neurons that express Fos during maternal behavior in female rats. *J. Neuroendocrinol.,* 9:369–384.

Numan, M., and Sheehan, T. P. 1997. Neuroanatomical circuitry for mammalian maternal behavior. *Ann. N. Y. Acad. Sci.,* 807:101–125.

Numan, M., and Numan, M. J. 1994. Expression of fos-like immunoreactivity in the preoptic area of maternally-behaving virgin and postpartum rats. *Behav. Neurosci.,* 108:379–394.

Numan, M., Corodimas, K. P., Numan, M. J., Factor, E. M., and Piers, W. D. 1988. Axon-sparing lesions of the preoptic region and substantia innominata disrupt maternal behavior in rats. *Behav. Neurosci.,* 102:381–396.

Numan, M., Numan, M. J., Marzella, S. R., and Palumbo, A. 1998. Expression of c-fos, fos B, and egr-1 in the medial preoptic area and bed nucleus of the stria terminalis during maternal behavior in rats. *Brain Res.,* 792:348–352.

Nunez, A. A., Siegel, L. I., and Wade, G. N. 1980. Central effects of testosterone on food intake in male rats. *Physiol. Behav.,* 24:469–472.

Nyirenda, M. J., and Seckl, J. R. 1998. Intrauterine events and the programming of adulthood disease: The role of fetal glucocorticoid exposure. *Int. J. Mol. Med.,* 2:607–614.

O'Brien, P. M. S., Craven, D., Selby, S., and Symonds, E. 1979. Treatment of premenstrual syndrome by spironolactone. *Br. J. Obstet. Gynaecol.,* 86:142–147.

O'Carroll, R., Shapiro, C., and Bancroft, J. 1985. Androgens, behaviour and nocturnal erection in hypogonadal men: The effects of varying the replacement doses. *Clin. Endocrinol.,* 23:527–538.

O'Hara, M. W., and Zekoski, E. M. 1988. Postpartum depression: A comprehensive review. In R. Kumar and I. F. Brockington (eds.), *Motherhood and Mental Illness 2: Causes and Consequences,* pp. 17–63. Boston, Wright.

O'Hara, M. W., Schlechte, J. A., Lewis, D. A., and Wright, E. J. 1991. Prospective study of postpartum blues. *Arch. Gen. Psychiatry,* 48:801–806.

O'Malley, B. O. 1989. Did eucaryotic steroid receptors evolve from intracrine gene regulators? *Endocrinology,* 125:1119–1120.

O'Malley, B. W. 1995. Thirty years of steroid hormone action: personal recollections of an investigator. *Steroids,* 60:490–498.

O'Neil, M. F., Means, L. W., Poole, M. C., and Hamm, R. J. 1996. Estrogen affects performance of ovariectomized rats in a two-choice water-escape working memory task. *Psychoneuroendocrinology,* 21:51–65.

Office of Technology Assessment, 1991. *Biological Rhythms: Implications for the Worker* (OTA-BA-463). Government Printing Office, Washington, D.C.

Ogawa, S., Gordan, J. D., Taylor, J., Lubahn, D., Korach, K., and Pfaff, D. W. 1996a. Reproductive functions illustrating direct and indirect effects of genes on behavior. *Horm. Behav.,* 30:487–494.

Ogawa, S., Lubahn, D. B., Korach, K. S., and Pfaff, D. 1995. Behavioral characteristics of transgenic estrogen receptor knockout male mice: Sexual, aggressive, and open-field behaviors. *Endocr. Soc. Abstr.,* 77:133.

Ogawa, S., Lubahn, D. B., Korach, K. S., and Pfaff, D. W. 1997. Behavioral effects of estrogen receptor gene disruption in male mice. *Proc. Natl. Acad. Sci. U.S.A.,* 94:1476–1481.

Ogawa, S., Olazabal, U. E., Parhar, I. S., and Pfaff, D. W. 1994. Effects of intrahypothalamic administration of antisense DNA for progesterone receptor mRNA on reproductive behavior and progesterone receptor immunoreactivity in female rat. *J. Neurosci.,* 14:1766–1774.

Ogawa, S., Taylor, J. A., Lubahn, D. B., Korach, K. S., and Pfaff, D. W. 1996b. Reversal of sex roles in genetic female mice by disruption of estrogen receptor gene. *Neuroendocrinology,* 64:467–470.

Oitzl, M. S., Fluttert, M., and de Kloet, E. R. 1998. Acute blockade of hippocampal glucocorticoid receptors facilitates spatial learning in rats. *Brain Res.,* 797:159–162.

Okuhata, S., and Saito, N. 1987. Synaptic connections of thalamo-cerebral vocal control nuclei of the canary. *Brain Res. Bull.,* 18:35–44.

Oliveras, D., and Novak, M. 1986. A comparison of paternal behavior in the meadow vole, *Microtus pennsylvanicus,* the pine vole, *M. pinetorum,* and the prairie vole, *M. ochrogaster. Anim. Behav.,* 34:519–529.

Olivier, B. and Mos, J. 1992. Rodent models of aggressive behavior and serotonergic drugs. Progress in. *Neuropsychopharmacol. Biol. Psychiatry,* 16:847–870.

Olivier, B., Mos, J.,van Oorschot, R., and Hen, R. 1995. Serotonin receptors and animal models of aggressive behavior. *Pharmacopsychiatry,* 28:80–90.

Olsen, K. L. 1992. Genetic influences on sexual behavior differentiation. In A. A. Gerall, H. Moltz, and I. L. Ward (eds.), *Sexual Differentiation. Handbook of Behavioral Neurobiology,* Vol. 11, pp. 1–40. Plenum, New York.

Olster, D. H., and Blaustein, J. D. 1988. Progesterone facilitation of lordosis in male and female Sprague-Dawley rats following priming with estradiol pulses. *Horm. Behav.,* 22:294–304.

Olton, D. S., and Samuelson, R. J. 1976. Remembrance of places passed: Spatial memory in rats. *J. Exp. Psychol.: Anim. Behav. Processes,* 2:97–116.

Olton, D. S., Walker, J. A., and Gage, F. H. 1978. Hippocampal connections and spatial discriminations. *Brain Res.,* 137:295–308.

Olweus, D. 1983. Testosterone in the development of antisocial behavior in adolescents. In K. T. VanDusen and S. A. Mednick (eds.), *Prospective Studies of Crime and Delinquency,* pp. 475–497. Kluwer-Nijhoff, Boston.

Orchard, J. W. and Best, J. P. 1994. Test violent offenders for anabolic steroid use. *Med. J. Aust.,* 161:232.

Orchinik, M., Licht, P., and Crews, D. 1988. Plasma steroid concentrations change in response to sexual behavior in *Bufo marinus. Horm. Behav.,* 22:338–350.

Orchinik, M., Murray, T. F., and Moore, F. L. 1991. A corticosteroid receptor in neuronal membranes. *Science,* 252:1848–1851.

Oring, L. W., Fivizzani, A. J., and El Halawani, M. E. 1986a. Changes in plasma prolactin associated with laying and hatching in the Spotted Sandpiper. *Auk,* 103:820–822.

Oring, L. W., Fivizzani, A. J., El Halawani, M. E., and Goldsmith, A. 1986b. Seasonal changes in prolactin and luteinizing hormone in the polyandrous Spotted Sandpiper, *Actitis macularia. Gen. Comp. Endocrinol.,* 62:394–403.

Orpen, G., and Fleming, A. S. 1987. Experience with pups sustains maternal responding in postpartum rats. *Physiol. Behav.,* 40:47–54.

Ostermann, K. 1956. Zur Aktivität heimischer Muriden und Gliriden. *Zool. Jahrbuch Abteil. Alle. Zool. Physiol.,* 66:355–375.

Ots, I., and Horak, P. 1996. Great tits Parus major trade health for reproduction. *Proc. R. Soc. Lond. B,* 263:1443–1447.

Owens, K., Peters, P. J., and Bronson, F. H. 1974. Effects of intracranial implants of testosterone propionate on intermale aggression in the castrated male mouse. *Horm. Behav.,* 5:83–92.

Packard, M. G., and Teather, L. A. 1997. Intra-hipppocampal estradiol infusion enhances memoy in ovariectomized rats. *Neuroreport,* 29:3009–3013.

Packard, M. G., Cornell, A. H., and Alexander, G. M. 1997. Rewarding affective properties of intra-nucleus accumbens injections of testosterone. *Behav. Neurosci.,* 111:219–224.

Packard, M. G., Kohlmaier, J. R., and Alexander, G. M. 1996. Post-training intra-hippocampal estradiol injections enhance spatial memory in male rats: Interaction with cholinergic systems. *Behav. Neurosci.,* 110:626–632.

Paglietti, E., Pelligrini-Quarantotti, B., Mereu, G., Gessa, G. 1978. Apomorphine and L-dopa lower ejaculatory threshold in the male rat. *Physiol. Behav.,* 20:559–562.

Pajarinen, J. Laippala, P., Penttila, A., and Karhunen, P. J. 1997. Incidence of disorders of spermatogenesis in middle aged Finnish men, 1981–91: Two necropsy series. *Br. Med. J.,* 314:13–18.

Palfi, S., Ungurean, A., and Vecsei, L. 1997. Basilar artery occlusion associated with anabolic steroid abuse in a17-year-old bodybuilder. *Eur. Neurol.,* 37:190–191.

Palmer, J. D. 1976. *An Introduction to Biological Rhythms.* Academic Press, New York.

Palmer, J. D. 1990. The rhythmic lives of crabs. *Bioscience,* 40:352–357.

Panksepp, J., Herman, B. H., Vilberg, T., Bishop, P., and DeEskinazi, F. G. 1980a. Endogenous opioids and social behavior. *Neurosci. Biobehav. Rev.,* 4:473–487.

Panksepp, J., Meeker, R., and Bean, N. J. 1980b. The neurochemical control of crying. *Pharmacol. Biochem. Behav.,* 12:437–443.

Panksepp, J., Nelson, E., and Bekkedal, M. 1997. Brain systems for the mediation of social separation-distress and social-reward: Evolutionary antecedents and neuropeptide intermediaries. *Ann. N. Y. Acad. Sci.,* 807:78–100.

Panzica, G. C., Viglietti-Panzica, C., and Balthazart, J. 1996. The sexually-dimorphic medial preoptic nucleus of quail: A key brain area mediating steroid action on male sexual behavior. *Front. Neuroendocrinol.,* 17:51–125.

Parlee, M. B. 1980. Positive changes in moods and activation levels during the menstrual cycle in experimentally naive subjects. In A. J. Dan, E. A. Graham, C. P. Beech (eds.), *The Menstrual Cycle,* Vol. 1, pp. 247–263. Springer, New York.

Parlee, M. B. 1982. Changes in moods and activation levels during the menstrual cycle. *Psychol. Women Q.,* 7:119–131.

Parsons, B., MacLusky, N. J., Krieger, M. S., McEwen, B. S., and Pfaff, D. W. 1979. The effects of long-term estrogen exposure on the induction of sexual behavior and measurements of brain estrogen and progestin receptors in the female rat. *Horm. Behav.,* 13:301–313.

Parsons, B., McEwen, B. S., and Pfaff, D. W. 1982. A discontinuous schedule of estradiol treatment is sufficient to activate progesterone-facilitated feminine sexual behavior and to increase cytosol receptors for progestins in the hypothalamus of the rat. *Endocrinology,* 110:613–619.

Parsons, M. W., and Gold, P. E. 1992. Glucose enhancement of memory in elderly humans: An inverted-U dose-response curve. *Neurobiol. Aging,* 13:401–404.

Patchev, V. K., Hayashi, S., Orikasa, C., and Almeida, O. F. X. 1995. Implications of estrogen-dependent brain organization for gender differences in hypothalamo-pituitary-adrenal regulation. *Fed. Am. Soc. Exp. Biol. J.,* 9:419–423.

Payne, A. P., and Swanson, H. H. 1972. The effect of sex hormones on the agonistic behavior of the male golden hamster (*Mesocricetus auratus* Waterhouse). *Physiol. Behav.,* 8:687–691.

Pearlstein, T., Rosen, K., and Stone, A. B. 1997. Mood disorders and menopause. *Endocrinol. Metab. Clin. North Am.,* 26:279–294.

Peck, J. W., and Novin, D. 1971. Evidence that osmoreceptors mediating drinking in rabbits are in the lateral preoptic area. *J. Comp. Physiol. Psychol.,* 74:134–147.

Pedersen, C. A., and Prange, A. J. 1979. Induction of maternal behavior in virgin rats after intracerebroventricular administration of oxytocin. *Proc. Natl. Acad. Sci. U.S.A.,* 76:6661–6665.

Pedersen, C. A., Ascher, J. A., Monroe, Y. L., and Prange, A. J. 1982. Oxytocin induces maternal behavior in virgin female rats. *Science,* 216:648–649.

Pedersen, P. E., and Blass, E. M. 1982. Prenatal and postnatal determinants of the first suckling episode in albino rats. *Dev. Psychobiol.,* 15:349–355.

Pedersen, P. E., Williams, C. L., and Blass, E. M. 1982. Activation and odor conditioning of suckling behavior in 3-day-old albino rats. *J. Exp. Psychol.: Anim. Behav. Processes,* 8:329–341.

Pederson, C. A. 1997. Oxytocin control of maternal behavior: Regulation by sex steroids and offspring stimuli. *Ann. N. Y. Acad. Sci.,* 807:126–145.

Peele, D. B., and Vincent, A. 1989. Strategies for assessing learning and memory, 1978–1987: A comparison of behavioral toxicology, psychopharmacology, and neurobiology. *Neurosci. Biobehav. Rev.,* 13:33–38.

Pelletier, J., and Ortavant, R. 1975. Photoperiodic control of LH release in the ram. *Acta Endocrinol.,* 78:442–450.

Pelleymounter, M. A., Cullen, M. J., Baker, M. B., Hecht, R., Winters, D., Boone, T., and Collins, F. 1995. Effects of the obese gene product on body weight regulation in ob/ob mice. *Science,* 269:540–543.

Pellis, S. M., Field, E. F., Smith, L. K., and Pellis, V. C. 1997. Multiple differences in the play fighting of male and female rats. Implications for the causes and functions of play. *Neurosci. Biobehav. Rev.,* 21:105–20.

Perachio, A. A. 1978. Hypothalamic regulation of behavioural and hormonal aspects of aggression and sexual performance. In D. J. Chivers and J. Herbert (eds.), *Recent Advances in Primatology,* Vol. 1, pp. 549–565. Academic Press, New York.

Perachio, A. A., Alexander, M., and Marr, L. D. 1973. Hormonal and social factors affecting evoked sexual behavior in rhesus monkeys. *Am. J. Phys. Anthropol.,* 38:227–232.

Perachio, A. A., Marr, L. D., and Alexander, M. 1979. Sexual behavior in male rhesus monkeys elicited by electrical stimulation of preoptic and hypothalamic areas. *Brain Res.,* 177:127–144.

Perkins, A., Fitzgerald, J. A., and Moss, G. E. 1995. A comparison of LH secretion and brain estradiol receptors in heterosexual and homosexual rams and female sheep. *Horm. Behav.,* 29:31–41.

Perkins, M. S., Perkins, M. N., and Hitt, J. C. 1980. Effects of stimulus female on sexual behavior of male rats given olfactory tubercle and corticomedial amygdaloid lesions. *Physiol. Behav.,* 25:495–500.

Perras, B., Droste, C., Born, J., Fehm, H. L., and Pietrowsky, R. 1997. Verbal memory after three months of intranasal vasopressin in healthy old humans. *Psychoneuroendocrinology,* 22:387–396.

Perry, P. J., Andersen, K. H., and Yates, W. R. 1990. Illicit anabolic steroid use in athletes. A case series analysis. *Am. J. Sports Med.,* 18:422–428.

Persky, H. Dreisbach, L., Miller, W. R., O'Brien, C. P., Khan, M. A., Lief, H. I., Charney, N., and Straus, D. 1982. The relation of plasma androgen levels to sexual behaviors and attitudes of women. *Psychosom. Med.,* 44:305–319.

Persky, H., O'Brien, C. P., Fine, E., Howard, W. J., Khan, M. A., and Beck, R. W. 1977. The effect of alcohol and smoking on testosterone function and aggression in chronic alcoholics. *Am. J. Psychiatry,* 134:621–625.

Pettersson, F., Fries, H., and Nillius, S. J. 1973. Epidemiology of secondary amenorrhea. I. Incidence and prevalence rates. *Am. J. Obstet. Gynecol.,* 117:80–86.

Pettit, H. O., and Justice, J. B. 1991. Effect of dose on cocaine self-administration and dopamine levels in the nucleus accumbens. *Brain Res.,* 539:94–102.

Pfaff, D. W. 1980. *Estrogens and Brain Function.* Springer-Verlag, New York.

Pfaff, D. W., and Conrad, L. C. A. 1978. Hypothalamic neuroanatomy: Steroid hormone binding and patterns of axonal projections. In G. Bourne (ed.), *International Review of Cytology,* Vol. 54, pp. 245–265. Academic Press, New York.

Pfaff, D. W., and Pfaffmann, C. 1969. Olfactory and hormonal influences on the basal forebrain of the male rat. *Brain Res.,* 15:137–156.

Pfaff, D. W., and Schwartz-Giblin, S. 1988. Cellular mechanisms of female reproductive behaviors. In E. Knobil and J. Neill (eds.), *The Physiology of Reproduction,* pp. 1487–1568. Raven Press, New York.

Pfaff, D. W., Diakow, C., Montgomery, M., Jenkins, F. A. 1978. X-ray cinematographic analysis of lordosis in female rats. *J. Comp. Physiol. Psychol.,* 92:937–941.

Pfaff, D. W., Schwartz-Giblin, S., McCarthy, M. M., and Kow, L.-M. 1994. Cellular and molecular mechanisms of female reproductive behaviors. In E. Knobil and J. Neill (eds.), *The Physiology of Reproduction.* Vol. 2, pp. 107–220. Raven Press, New York.

Pfaus, J. G. 1996. Homologies of animal and human sexual behaviors. *Horm. Behav.,* 30: 187–200.

Pfaus, J. G., and Gorzalka, B. B. 1987. Opioids and sexual behavior. *Neurosci. Biobehav. Rev.* 11:1–34.

Pfaus, J. G., and Heeb, M. M. 1997. Implications of immediate-early gene induction in the brain following sexual stimulation of female and male rodents. *Brain Res. Bull.,* 44:397–407.

Pfaus, J. G., and Phillips, A. G. 1991. Role of dopamine in anticipatory and consummatory aspects of sexual behavior in the male rat. *Behav. Neurosci.,* 105:727–743.

Pfeiffer, C. A. 1935. Origin of functional differences between male and female hypophyses. *Proc. Soc. Exp. Biol. Med.,* 32:603–605.

Pfeiffer, C. A. 1936. Sexual differences of the hypophysis and their determination by the gonads. *Am. J. Anat.,* 58:195–225.

Phoenix, C. H. 1973. Sexual behavior in rhesus monkeys after vasectomy. *Science,* 179:493–494.

Phoenix, C. H. 1974. Effect of dihydrotestosterone on sexual behavior of castrated male rhesus monkeys. *Physiol. Behav.,* 12:1045–1055.

Phoenix, C. H., Goy, R. W., and Resko, J. A. 1968. Psychosexual differentiation as a function of androgenic stimulation. In M. Diamond (ed.), *Perspectives in Reproduction and Sexual Behavior,* pp. 215–246. Indiana University Press, Bloomington, IN.

Phoenix, C. H., Goy, R. W., Gerall, A. A., and Young, W. C. 1959. Organizing action of prenatally administered testosterone propionate on the tissues mediating mating behavior in the female guinea pig. *Endocrinology,* 65:369–382.

Phoenix, C. H., Slob, A. K., and Goy, R. W. 1973. Effects of castration and replacement therapy on sexual behavior of adult male rhesuses. *J. Comp. Physiol. Psychol.,* 81:472–481.

Piazza, P. V., Deroche, V., Deminiere, J. M., Maccari, S., Le Moal, M., and Simon, H. 1993. Corticosterone in the range of stress-induced levels possesses reinforcing properties: implications for sensation-seeking behaviors. *Proc. Natl. Acad. Sci. U. S. A.,* 90: 11738–11742.

Piazza, P. V., Maccari, S., Deminiere, J. M., Le Moal, M., Mormede, P., and Simon, H. 1991. Corticosterone levels determine individual vulnerability to amphetamine self-administration. *Neurobiology,* 88:2088–2092.

Pickard, G. E. 1982. The afferent connections of the suprachiasmatic nucleus of the golden hamster with emphasis on the retinohypothalamic projection. *J. Comp. Neurol.,* 211:65–83.

Pickard, G. E., and Silverman, A. J. 1981. Direct retinal projections to the hypothalamus, piriform cortex and accessory optic nuclei in the golden hamster as demonstrated by a sensitive anterograde horseradish peroxidase technique. *J. Comp. Neurol.,* 196:155–172.

Pierce, J. G. 1988. Gonadotropins: Chemistry and biosynthesis. In E. Knobil and J. D. Neill (eds.), *The Physiology of Reproduction,* pp. 1335–1348. Raven Press, New York.

Pitrosky, B., and Pevet, P. 1997. The photoperiodic response in Syrian hamsters depends upon a melatonin-driven rhythm of sensitivity to melatonin. *Biol. Signals,* 6:264–271.

Pittendrigh, C. S. 1981. Circadian systems: Entrainment. *Handbook of Behavioral Neurobiology,* Vol. 4, pp. 95–124.

Pittendrigh, C. S., and Daan, S. 1976. A functional analysis of circadian pacemakers in nocturnal rodents. IV. Entrainment: Pacemaker as clock. *J. Comp. Physiol.,* 106:291–331.

Platt, J. R. 1964. Strong inference. *Science,* 146:347–353.

Plautz, J. D., Kaneko, M., Hall, J. C., and Kay, S. A. 1997. Independent photoreceptive circadian clocks throughout *Drosophila. Science,* 278:1632–1635.

Pliner, P., and Fleming, A. S. 1983. Food intake, body weight, and sweetness preferences over the menstrual cycle in humans. *Physiol. Behav.,* 30:663–666.

Plotka, E. D., Seal, U. S., Letellier, M. A., Verme, L. J., and Ozoga, J. J. 1984. Early effects of pinealectomy on LH and testosterone secretion in white-tailed deer. *J. Endocrinol.,* 103:1–7.

Plotsky, P. M., Owens, M. J., and Nemeroff, C. B. 1998. Psychoneuroendocrinology of depression. Hypothalamic-pituitary-adrenal axis. *Psychiatr. Clin. North Am.,* 21:293–307.

Poindron, P., and Le Neindre, P. 1980. Endocrine and sensory regulation of maternal behavior in the ewe. *Adv. Study Behav.,* 11:75–119.

Poindron, P., and Levy, F. 1990. Physiological, sensory and experiential determinants of maternal behavior in sheep. In N. A. Krasnegor and R. S. Bridges (eds.). *Mammalian Parenting: Biochemical, Neurobiological, and Behavioral Determinants,* pp. 133–156. Oxford University Press, New York.

Polak, J. M., and Van Noorden, S. 1997. *Introduction to Immunocytochemistry.* Microscopy Handbook Series, 37, Springer-Verlag: New York. 144 pp.

Polo-Kantola, P., Portin, R., Polo, O., Helenius, H., Irjala, K., and Erkkola, R. 1998. The effect of short-term estrogen replacement therapy on cognition: A randomized double-blind, cross-over trial in postmenopausal women. *Obstet. Gynecol.,* 91:459–466.

Pomerantz, S. M. 1990. Apomorphine facilitates male sexual behavior of rhesus monkeys. *Pharmacol. Biochem. Behav.,* 35:659–664.

Pomerantz, S. M., and Goy, R. W. 1983. Proceptive behavior of female rhesus monkeys during tests with tethered males. *Horm. Behav.,* 17:237–248.

Pope, H. G., and Katz, D. L. 1989. Homicide and near-homicide by anabolic steroid users. *J. Clin. Psychiatry,* 51:28–31.

Power, K. L., and Moore, C. L. 1986. Prenatal stress eliminates differential maternal attention to male offspring in Norway rats. *Physiol. Behav.,* 38:667–671.

Powers, J. B., and Winans, S. S. 1975. Vomeronasal organ: Critical role in mediating sexual behavior of the male hamster. *Science,* 187:961–963.

Powers, J. B., Steel, E. A., Hutchison, J. B., Hastings, M. H., Herbert, J., and Walker, A. P. 1989. Photoperiodic influences on sexual behavior in male Syrian hamsters. *J. Biol. Rhythms,* 4:61–78.

Preston, F. S. 1978. The health of female air cabin crews. *J. Occupational Med.,* 20:597–600.

Preston, F. S., Bateman, S. C., Short, R. V., and Wilkinson, R. T. 1973. Effects of flying and/or time changes on menstrual cycle length and on performance in airline stewardesses. *Aerospace Med.,* 44:438–443.

Priestnall, R., and Young, S. 1978. An observational study of caretaking behavior of male and female mice housed together. *Dev. Psychobiol.,* 11:23–30.

Pryce, C. R. 1996. Socialization, hormones, and the regulation of maternal behavior in nonhuman simian primates. *Adv. Study Behav.,* 25:423–473.

Pryce C. R., Döbeli, M., and Martin, R. D. 1993. Effects of sex steroids on maternal motivation in the common marmoset (*Callithrix jacchus*): Development and application of an operant system with maternal reinforcement. *J. Comp. Psychol.,* 107:99–115.

Pucek, M. 1965. Water contents and seasonal changes of the brain weight in shrews. *Acta Theriol.,* 10:353–367.

Purifoy, F. E., and Koopmans, L. H. 1979. Androstenedione, testosterone, and free testosterone concentration in women of various occupations. *Soc. Biol.,* 26:179–188.

Purvis, K., and Haynes, N. B. 1974. Short-term effects of copulation, human chorionic gonadotrophin injection and non–tactile association with a female on testosterone levels in the male rat. *J. Endocrinol.,* 60:429–439.

Purvis, K., Landgren, B., Cekan, Z., and Diczfalusy, E. 1976. Endocrine effects of masturbation in men. *J. Endocrinol.,* 70:439–444.

Quartermain, D. 1976. The influence of drugs on learning and memory. In M. R. Rosenzweig and E. L. Bennett (eds.), *Neural*

*Mechanisms of Learning and Memory*, pp. 508–520. MIT Press, Cambridge, MA.

Quétel, C. 1990. *History of Syphilis*. Johns Hopkins University Press, Baltimore.

Quinlan, D. M., Nelson, R. J., Partin, A. W., Mostwin, J. L., and Walsh, P. C. 1989. The rat as a model for the study of penile erection. *J. Urol.*, 141:656–661.

Racey, P. A., and Skinner, J. D. 1979. Endocrine aspects of sexual mimicry in spotted hyaenas, *Crocuta crocuta*. *J. Zool. (Lond.)*, 187:315–326.

Ragozzino, M. E., Unick, K. E., and Gold, P. E. 1996. Hippocampal acetylcholine release during memory testing in rats: Augmentation by glucose. *Proc. Natl. Acad. Sci. U.S.A.*, 93:4693–4698.

Raisman, G., and Field, P. M. 1973b. Sexual dimorphism in the preoptic area of the rat. *Science*, 173:731–733.

Raisman, G., and Field, P. M. 1973a. Sexual dimorphism in the neurophil of the preoptic area of the rat and its dependence on neonatal androgen. *Brain Res.*, 54:1–29.

Raloff, J. 1994a. The gender benders. *Sci. News*, 145:24–27.

Raloff, J. 1994b. That feminine touch. *Sci. News*, 145:56–59.

Ralph, M. R., and Lehman, M. N. 1991. Transplantation: A new tool in the analysis of the mammalian hypothalamic circadian pacemaker. *Trends Neurosci.*, 14:362–366.

Ralph, M. R., and Menaker, M. 1988. A mutation in the circadian system in the golden hamster. *Science*, 241:1225–1227.

Ralph, M. R., Foster, R. G., Davis, F. C., and Menaker, M. 1990. Transplanted suprachiasmatic nucleus determines circadian period. *Science*, 247:975–978.

Ramenofsky, M. 1984. Agonistic behavior and endogenous plasma hormones in male Japanese quail. *Anim. Behav.*, 32:698–708.

Ramirez, V. D., and McCann, S. M. 1963. Comparisons of the regulation of luteinizing hormone (LH) secretion in immature and adult rats. *Endocrinology*, 72:452–464.

Ramos, C., and Silver, R. 1992. Gonadal hormones determine sex differences in timing of incubation by doves. *Horm. Behav.*, 26:586–601.

Rand, M. N., and Breedlove, S. M. 1987. Ontogeny of functional innervation of bulbocavernosus muscles in male and female rats. Dev. *Brain Res.*, 33:150–152.

Rankin, S. M., and Stay, B. 1985. Ovarian inhibition of juvenile hormone synthesis in the viviparous cockroach, *Diploptera punctata*. *Gen. Comp. Endocrinol.*, 59:230–237.

Rankin, S. M., Palmer, J. O., Yagi, K. J., Scott, G. L., and Tobe, S. S. 1995. Biosynthesis and release of JH during the reproductive cycle of the ring-legged earwig. *Comp. Biochem. Physiol. C*, 110:241–251.

Ranson, E. W. 1982. A developmental analysis of urinary behavior in dogs. Ph.D. Dissertation. University of California, Berkeley.

Ranson, E., and Beach, F. A. 1985. Effects of testosterone on ontogeny of urinary behavior in male and female dogs. *Horm. Behav.*, 19:36–51.

Rasmussen, D. D., Liu, J. H., Wolf, P. L., and Yen, S. S. 1983. Endogenous opioid regulation of gonadotropin-releasing hormone release from the human fetal hypothalamus in vitro. *J. Clin. Endocrinol. Metab.*, 57:881–884.

Reburn, C. J., and Wynne-Edwards, K. E. 1999. Hormonal changes in males of a naturally biparental and a uniparental mammal. *Horm. Behav.* 35:163–167.

Reddy, V. V. R., Naftolin, F., and Ryan, K. J. 1974. Conversion of androstenedione to estrone by neural tissues from fetal and neonatal rat. *Endocrinology*, 94:117–121.

Redican, W. K., and Taub, D. M. 1981. Male parental care in monkeys and apes. In M. E. Lamb (ed.), *The Role of the Father in Child Development*, pp. 345–385. Wiley, New York.

Reed, C. A. 1946. The copulatory behavior of small mammals. *J. Comp. Psychol.*, 39:185–206.

Refinetti, R., and Menaker, M. 1992. Evidence for separate control of estrous and circadian periodicity in the golden hamster. *Behav. Neural Biol.*, 58:27–36.

Reid, R. L., and Yen, S. S. C. 1981. Premenstrual syndrome. *Am. J. Obstet. Gynecol.*, 139:85–97.

Reinisch, J. M. 1974. Fetal hormones, the brain and human sex differences: A heuristic integrative review of the recent literature. *Arch. Sex. Behav.*, 3:51–90.

Reinisch, J. M. 1981. Prenatal exposure to synthetic progestins increases potential for aggression in humans. *Science*, 211:1171–1173.

Reisbick, S., Rosenblatt, J. S., and Mayer, A. D. 1975. Decline of maternal behavior in the virgin and lactating rat. *J. Comp. Physiol. Psychol.*, 89:722–732.

Reiter, R. J. 1970. Endocrine rhythms associated with pineal gland function. In L. W. Hedlund, J. M. Franz, and A. D. Kenny (eds.), *Biological Rhythms and Endocrine Function*, pp. 43–78. Plenum, New York.

Reiter, R. J. 1973. Comparative physiology: Pineal gland. *Annu. Rev. Physiol.*, 35:305–328.

Reiter, R. J. 1973/74. Influence of pinealectomy on the breeding capability of hamsters maintained under natural photoperiod and temperature conditions. *Neuroendocrinology*, 13:366–370.

Reiter, R. J. 1982. *The Pineal and Its Hormones*. Alan R. Liss, New York.

Reiter, R. J. 1998. Melatonin and human reproduction. *Ann. Med.*, 30:103–108.

Rempel-Clower, N. L., Zola, S. M., Squire, L. R., and Amaral, D. G. 1996. Three cases of enduring memory impairment after bilateral damage limited to the hippocampal formation. *J. Neurosci.*, 16:5233–5255.

Resko, J. A., and Roselli, C. E. 1997. Prenatal hormones organize sex differences of the neuroendocrine reproductive system: observations on guinea pigs and nonhuman primates. *Cell. Molec. Neurobiol.*, 17:627–648.

Resko, J. A., Perkins, A., Roselli, C. E., Fitzgerald, J. A., Choate, J. V., and Stormshak, F. 1996. Endocrine correlates of partner preference behavior in rams. *Biol. Reprod.*, 55:120–126.

Reyes, R. J., Zicchi, S., Hamed, H., Chaudary, M. A., and Fentiman, I. S. 1995. Surgical correction of gynaecomastia in bodybuilders. *Br. J. Clin. Pract.*, 49:177–179.

Rhen, T., and Lang, J. W. 1994. Temperature-dependent sex determination in the snapping turtle: Manipulation of the embryonic sex steroid environment. General and Comparative *Endocrinology*, 96:243–254.

Ribble, D. O. 1990. Population and social dynamics of the California mouse (*Peromyscus californicus*). Ph.D. Dissertation, University of California, Berkeley.

Ribble, D. O., and Salvioni, M. 1990. Social organization and nest co-occupancy in *Peromyscus californicus*, a monogamous rodent. *Behav. Ecol. Sociobiol.*, 26: 9–15.

Richards, M. P. M. 1969. Effects of oestrogen and progesterone on nest building in the golden hamster. *Anim. Behav.*, 17:356–361.

Richardson, G. S., and Martin, J. B. 1988. Circadian rhythms in neuroendocrinology and immunology: Influence of aging. *Prog. Neuroendocrinol. Immunol.*, 1:16–20.

Richman, J. A., Raskin, V. D., and Gaines, C. 1991. Gender roles, social support, and postpartum depressive symptomatology: The benefits of caring. *J. Nerv. Ment. Dis.*, 179:139–147.

Richmond, M. E., and Stehn, R. A. 1976. Olfaction and reproductive behavior in microtine rodents. In R. L. Doty (ed.), *Mammalian Olfaction, Reproductive Processes and Behavior*, pp. 197–217. Academic Press, New York.

Richmond, M., and Conaway, C. H. 1969. Induced ovulation and oestrus in *Microtus ochrogaster*. *J. Reprod. Fertil. (Suppl.)*, 6:357–376.

Richter, C. P. 1936. Increased salt appetite in adrenalectomized rats. *Am. J. Physiol.*, 115:155–161.

Richter, C. P. 1968. Inherent twenty-four hour and lunar clocks of a primate: The squirrel monkey. *Commun. Behav. Biol.*, 1:305–332.

Richter, C. P. 1977. Heavy water as a tool for study of the forces that control length of period of the 24-hour clock of the hamster. *Proc. Natl. Acad. Sci. U.S.A.*, 74:1295–1299.

Richter, C. P., Holt, L. E., and Barelare, B. 1938. Nutritional requirements for normal growth and reproduction in rats studied by the self selection method. *Am. J. Physiol.*, 122:734–744.

Riddle, O. 1924/25. Birds without gonads: Their origin, behavior, and bearing on the theory of the internal secretion of the testis. *Br. J. Exp. Biol.*, 2:211–246.

Riddle, O., Bates, R. W., and Lahr, E. L. 1935a. Maternal behavior induced in virgin rats by prolactin. *Proc. Soc. Exp. Biol. Med.*, 32:730–734.

Riddle, O., Bates, R. W., and Lahr, E. L. 1935b. Prolactin induces broodiness in fowl. *Am. J. Physiol.*, 111:352–360.

Ring, J. R. 1944. The estrogen-progesterone induction of sexual receptivity in the spayed female mouse. *Endocrinology*, 34:269–275.

Rissman, E. F. 1991. Frank A. Beach Award. Behavioral endocrinology of the female musk shrew. *Horm. Behav.*, 25:125–127.

Rissman, E. F., and Wingfield, J. C. 1984. Hormonal correlates of polyandry in the spotted sandpiper, Actitis macularia. Gen. Comp. Endocrinol., 56:401–405.

Rissman, E. F., Wersinger, S. R., Taylor, J. A., and Lubahn, D. B. 1997a. Estrogen receptor function as revealed by knockout studies: Neuroendocrine and behavioral aspects. Horm. Behav., 31:232–243.

Rissman, E. F., Early, A. H., Taylor, J. A., Korach, K. S., and Lubahn, D. B. 1997b. Estrogen receptors are essential for female sexual receptivity. Endocrinology, 138:507–510.

Ritter, S., and Taylor, J. S. 1989. Capsaicin abolishes lipoprivic but not glucoprivic feeding in rats. Am. J. Physiol., 256:R1232–1239.

Ritter, S., and Taylor, J. S. 1990. Vagal sensory neurons are required for lipoprivic but not glucoprivic feeding in rats. Am. J. Physiol., 258:R1395–1401.

Ritter, S., Calingasan, N. Y., Hutton, B., and Dinh, T. T. 1992. Cooperation of vagal and central neural systems in monitoring metabolic events controlling feeding behavior. In S. Ritter, R. C. Ritter, and C. D. Barnes (eds.). Neuroanatomy Physiology of Abdominal Vagal Afferents, pp. 240–277. CRC Press, Boca Raton, FL.

Rivest, S., and Rivier, C. 1993. Interleukin-1 beta inhibits the endogenous expression of the early gene c-fos located within the nucleus of LH-RH neurons and interferes with hypothalamic LH-RH release during proestrus in the rat. Brain Res., 613:132–142.

Rivest, S., Deshaies, Y., and Richard, D. 1989. Effects of corticotropin-releasing factor on energy balance in rats are sex dependent. Am. J. Physiol., 257:R1417–R1422.

Rivier, C., and Rivest, S. 1991. Effects of stress on the activity of the hypothalamic-pituitary-gonadal axis: Peripheral and central mechanisms. Biol. Reprod., 45:523–532.

Rivier, C., Rivier, J., and Vale, W. 1986. Stress-induced inhibition of reproductive functions: Role of endogenous corticotropin-releasing factor. Science, 231:607–609.

Robbins, T. W. and Everitt, B. J. 1992. Functions of dopamine in the dorsal and ventral striatum. Sem. Neurosci., 4:119–128.

Roberts, M. H. 1990. Commentary: The properties of cell water relative to the temperature compensation of circadian rhythms. J. Biol. Rhythms, 5:175–176.

Roberts, R. L., Zullo, A., Gustafson, E. A., and Carter, C. S. 1996. Perinatal steroid treatments alter alloparental and affiliative behavior in prairie voles. Horm. Behav., 30:576–582.

Robinson, T. J. 1954. The necessity for progesterone with estrogen for the induction of recurrent estrus in the ovariectomized ewe. Endocrinology, 55:403–408.

Roenneberg, T. and Aschoff, J. 1990a. Annual rhythm of human reproduction: I. Biology, sociology, or both? J. Biol. Rhythms, 5:195–216.

Roenneberg, T., and Aschoff, J. 1990b. Annual rhythm of human reproduction: II. Environmental correlations. J. Biol. Rhythms, 5:217–239.

Rohner-Jeanrenaud, F., Cusin, I., Stainsbury, A., Zakrzewska, K. E., and Jeanrenaud, B. 1996. The loop system between neuropeptide Y and leptin in normal and obese rodents. Horm. Metab. Res., 28:642–648.

Rohwer, S. 1975. The social significance of avian winter plumage variability. Evolution, 29:593–610.

Rohwer, S. 1977. Status signaling in Harris sparrows: Some experiments in deception. Behaviour, 61:107–129.

Rohwer, S., and Rohwer, F. C. 1978. Status signalling in Harris' sparrows: Experimental deceptions achieved. Anim. Behav., 26:1012–1022.

Rohwer, S., and Wingfield, J. C. 1981. A field study of social dominance, plasma levels of luteinizing hormone and steroid hormones in wintering Harris' Sparrows. Z. Tierpsychol., 57:173–183.

Rolls, B. J., and Rolls, E. T. 1982. Thirst. University of Cambridge Press, Cambridge.

Romanes, G. J. 1887. Mental differences between men and women. The Nineteenth Century, 21:654–672.

Romero, L. M., and Wingfield, J. C. 1998. Seasonal changes in adrenal sensitivity alter corticosterone levels in Gambel's white-crowned sparrows (Zonotrichia leucophrys gambelii). Comp. Biochem. Physiol. C., 119:31–36.

Romero, L. M., Ramenofsky, M., and Wingfield, J. C. 1997. Season and migration alters the corticosterone response to capture and handling in an arctic migrant, the white-crowned sparrow (Zonotrichia leucophrys gambelii). Comp. Biochem. Physiol. C., 116:171–177.

Romero, L. M., Soma, K. K., and Wingfield, J. C. 1998b. Hypothalamic-pituitary-adrenal axis changes allow seasonal modulation of corticosterone in a bird. Am. J. Physiol., 274:R1338–1344.

Romero, L. M., Soma, K. K., and Wingfield, J. C. 1998c. The hypothalamus and adrenal regulate modulation of corticosterone release in redpolls (Carduelis flammea): An arctic-breeding song bird. Gen. Comp. Endocrinol., 109:347–355.

Romero, L. M., Soma, K. K., and Wingfield, J. C. 1998d. Changes in pituitary and adrenal sensitivities allow the snow bunting (Plectrophenax nivalis), an arctic-breeding song bird, to modulate corticosterone release seasonally. J. Comp. Physiol. B, 168:353–358.

Romero, L. M., Soma, K. K., O'Reilly, K. M., Suydam, R.,and Wingfield, J. C. 1998a. Hormones and territorial behavior during breeding in snow buntings (Plectrophenax nivalis): An arctic-breeding songbird. Horm. Behav., 33:40–47.

Rose, R. M., Bernstein, I. S., Gordon, T. P., and Lindsley, J. G. 1978. Changes in testosterone and behavior during adolescence in the male rhesus monkey. Psychosom. Med., 40:60–70.

Rose, R. M., Berstein, I. S., and Holaday, J. W. 1971. Plasma testosterone, dominance rank and aggressive behavior in a group of male rhesus monkeys. Nature, 231:366–368.

Roselli, C. E., Abdelgadir, S. E., and Resko, J. A. 1997. Regulation of aromatase gene expression in the adult rat brain. Brain Res. Bull., 44:351–358.

Roselli, C. E., Klosterman, S. A., and Fasasi, T. A. 1996. Sex differences in androgen responsiveness in the rat brain: regional differences in the induction of aromatase activity. Neuroendocrinology, 64:139–145.

Rosenberg, G. D., and Runcorn, S. K. 1975. Conclusions. In G. D. Rosenberg and S. K. Runcorn (eds.), Growth Rhythms and the History of the Earth's Rotation, pp. 535–538. John Wiley and Sons, New York.

Rosenblatt, J. S. 1967. Nonhormonal basis of maternal behavior in the rat. Science, 156:1512–1514.

Rosenblatt, J. S. 1990. Landmarks in the physiological study of maternal behavior with special reference to the rat. In N. A. Krasnegor and R. S. Bridges (eds.), Mammalian Parenting, pp. 40–60. Oxford University Press, Oxford.

Rosenblatt, J. S., and Aronson, L. R. 1958. The decline of sexual behaviour in male cats after castration with special reference to the role of prior sexual experience. Behaviour, 12:285–338.

Rosenblatt, J. S., and Ceus, M. 1998. Estrogen implants in the medial preoptic area stimulate maternal behavior in male rats. Horm. Behav., 33:23–30.

Rosenblatt, J. S., and Siegel, H. I. 1975. Hysterectomy-induced maternal behavior during pregnancy in the rat. J. Comp. Physiol. Psychol., 89:685–700.

Rosenblatt, J. S., Hazelwood, S., and Poole, J. 1996. Maternal behavior in male rats: Effects of medial preoptic area lesions and presence of maternal aggression. Horm. Behav., 30:01–215.

Rosenblatt, J. S., Mayer, A. D., and Siegel, H. I. 1985. Maternal behavior among the nonprimate mammals. In N. T. Adler, D. Pfaff, and R. W. Goy (eds.), Handbook of Behavioral Neurobiology, pp. 229–298. Plenum, New York.

Rosenblatt, J. S., Olufowobi, A., and Siegel, H. I. 1998. Effects of pregnancy hormones on maternal responsiveness, responsiveness to estrogen stimulation of maternal behavior, and the lordosis response to estrogen stimulation. Horm. Behav., 33:104–114.

Rosenblatt, J. S., Siegel, H. I., and Mayer, A. D. 1979. Blood levels of progesterone, estradiol and prolactin in pregnant rats. Adv. Study Behav., 10:225–311.

Rosenfeld, P., Wetmore, J. B., and Levine, S. 1992. Effects of repeated maternal separations on the adrenocortical response to stress of preweanling rats. Physiol. Behav., 52:787–791.

Rosenthal, N. E. 1993. Winter Blues: Seasonal Affective Disorder. Guilford Press, New York.

Rosenthal, N. E., and Wehr, T. A. 1987. Seasonal affective disorders. Psychiatric Ann., 17:670–674.

Rosenthal, N. E., Sack, D. A., Skwerer, R. G., Jacobsen, F. M., and Wehr, T. A. 1988. Phototherapy for seasonal affective disorder. J. Biol. Rhythms, 3:101–120.

Rosenzweig, M. R., and Leiman, A. L. 1989. Physiological Psychology. (2nd ed.). Random House, New York.

Rosenzweig, M. R., Leiman, A. L., and Breedlove, S. M. 1999. Biological Psychology: An Introduction to Behavioral, Cognitive, and Clinical Neuroscience. (2nd ed.). Sinauer Associates, Sunderland, MA.

Ross, S., Denenberg, V. H., Frommer, G. P., and Sawin, P. B. 1959. Genetic, physiological, and behavioral background of reproduction in the rabbit. V. Nonretrieving of neonates. *J. Mammal.*, 40:91–96.

Rothschild, A. J., Langlais, P. J., Schatzberg, A. F., Miller ,M. M., Saloman, M. S., Lerbinger, J. E., Cole, J. O., and Bird, E. D. 1985. The effects of a single acute dose of dexamethasone on monoamine and metabolite levels in rat brain. *Life Sci.*, 36:2491–2501.

Rots, N. Y., du Jong, J., Workel, J. O., Levine, S., Cools, A. R., and De Kloet, E. R. 1996. Neonatal maternally deprived rats have as adults elevated basal pituitary-adrenal activity and enhanced susceptibility to apomorphine. *J. Neuroendocrinol.*, 8:501–506.

Rous, S. N. 1996. *Urology: A Core Textbook,* Blackwell Science Press:Cambridge, MA.

Rowe, F. A., and Smith, W. E. 1972. Effects of peripherally induced anosmia on mating behavior of male mice. *Psychonom. Sci.*, 27:33–34.

Rowlands, I. W., and Weir, B. J. 1984. Mammals: Non-primate euthe-rians. In G. E. Lamming (ed.*)*, *Marshall's Physiology of Reproduction.* Vol. 1, *Reproductive Cycles of Vertebrates*, pp. 455–658. Churchill Livingstone, Edinburgh.

Rowsemitt, C. N. 1986. Seasonal variations in activity rhythms of male voles: Mediation by gonadal hormones. *Physiol. Behav.*, 37:797–803.

Rowsemitt, C. N., Petterborg, L. J., Claypool, L. E., Hoppensteadt, F. C., Negus, N. C., and Berger, J. P. 1982. Photoperiodic induction of diurnal locomotor activity in *Microtus montanus*, the montane vole. *Can. J. Zool.*, 60:2798–2803.

Roy, E. J., Lynn, D. M., and Clark, A. S. 1985. Inhibition of sexual receptivity by anesthesia during estrogen priming. *Brain Res.*, 337:163–166.

Roy-Byrne, P. P., Rubinow, D. R., Hoban, M. C., Grover, G. N., Blank, D. 1987. TSH and prolactin responses to TRH in patients with pre-menstrual syndrome. *Am. J. Psychiatry*, 144:480–484.

Rubin, B. S., and Barfield, R. J. 1983. Progesterone in the ventrome-dial hypothalamus facilitates estrous behavior in ovariectomized, estrogen-primed rats. *Endocrinology*, 113:797–804.

Rubin, R. T., Reinisch, J. M., and Haskett, R. F. 1981. Postnatal gonadal steroid effects on human sexual behavior. *Science*, 211:1318–1324.

Rubinow, D. R., and Schmidt, P. J. 1996. Androgens, brain, and behavior. *Am. J. Psychiatry*, 153:974–984.

Rubinow, D. R., Hoban, M. C., Grover, G. N., Galloway, D. S., Roy-Byrne, R., Andersen, R., and Merriam, G. R. 1988. Changes in plasma hormones across the menstrual cycle in patients with menstrually related mood disorder and in control subjects. *Am. J. Obstet. Gynecol.*, 158:5–11.

Rubinow, D. R., Schmidt, P. J., and Roca, C. A. 1998. Estrogen-sero-tonin interactions: Implications for affective regulation. *Biol. Psychiatry*, 44:839–850.

Ruble, D. N. 1977. Premenstrual symptoms: A reinterpretation. *Science*, 187:291–292.

Ruble, D. N., and Martin, C. L. 1998. Gender development. In W. Damon and N. Eisenberg (eds.). *Handbook of Child Psychology.* Vol. 3. , pp. 933–1016. Wiley, New York.

Ruegg, D., and Rose, H. A. 1991. Biology of *Macropanesthia rhinoc-eros* Saussure (Dictoptera: Balberidae). *Ann. Ent. Soc. Am.*, 84:575–582.

Rusak, B. 1981. *Vertebrate behavioral cycles. Handbook of Behavioral Neurobiology*, Vol. 4, pp. 183–214.

Rusak, B. 1989. The mammalian circadian system: models and physi-ology. *J. Biol. Rhythms*, 4:121–134.

Rusak, B., and Boulos, Z. 1981. Pathways for photic entrainment of mammalian circadian rhythms. *Photochem. Photobiol.*, 34:267–273.

Rushen, J. 1986. Some problems with the physiological concept of "stress". *Aust. Vet. J.*, 63:359–361.

Rutila, J. E., Suri, V., Le, M., So, W. V., Rosbash, M., and Hall, J. C. 1998. CYCLE is a second bHLH-PAS clock protein essential for circadian rhythmicity and transcription of *Drosophila* period and timeless. *Cell*, 93:805–814.

Ryan, C. M., and Williams, T. M. 1993. Effects of insulin-dependent diabetes on learning and memory efficiency in adults. *J. Clin. Exp. Neuropsychol.*, 15:685–700.

Saboureau, M. 1986. Hibernation in the hedgehog: Influence of external and internal factors. In H. C. Heller, X. J. Musacchia, and L. C. H. Wang (eds.), *Living in the Cold: Physiological and Biochemical Adaptations*, pp. 253–263, Elsevier, New York.

Sachar, E. O., Hellman, L., Roffwang, H. Halpern, F., Fukushima, D., and Gallager, T. 1973. Disrupted 24-hour patterns of cortisol

secretion in psychotic depression. *Arch. Gen. Psychiatry*, 28:19–24.

Sachs, B. D. 1995a. Context-sensitive variation in the regulation of erection. In J. Bancroft (ed), *The Pharmacology of Sexual Function Dysfunction*, pp. 97–108. Elsevier Science, Amsterdam.

Sachs, B. D. 1995b. Placing erection in context: The reflexogenic-psychogenic dichotomy reconsidered. *Neurosci. Biobehav. Rev.*, 19:211–224.

Sachs, B. D., Akasofu, K., Citron, J. H., Daniels, S. B., and Natoli, J. H. 1994. Noncontact stimulation from estrous females evokes penile erection in rats. *Physiol. Behav.*, 55:1073–1079.

Sachs, B. D., and Bitran, D. 1990. Spinal block reveals roles for brain and spinal cord in the mediation of reflexive penile erections in rats. *Brain Res.*, 528:99–108.

Sachs, B. D., and Meisel, R. L. 1979. Pubertal development of penile reflexes and copulation in male rats. *Psychoneuroendocrinology*, 4:287–296.

Sachs, B. D., and Meisel, R. L. 1988. The physiology of male sexual behavior. In E. Knobil and J. Neill (eds.), *The Physiology of Reproduction*, pp. 1393–1485. Raven Press, New York.

Sadlier, R. M. F. S. 1969. *The Ecology of Reproduction in Wild and Domestic Mammals,* Methuen, London.

Saenger, P., Levine, L., Wiedemann, E., Schwartz, E., Korth-Schutz, S., Pareira, J., Henig, B., and New, M. 1977. Somatomedin and growth hormone in psychosocial dwarfism. *Paediatr. Paedol. (Suppl)*, 1–33.

Sakai, R. R., Ma, L. Y., He, P. F., and Fluharty, S. J. 1995. Intracerebroventricular administration of angiotensin type 1 (AT1) receptor antisense oligonucleotides attenuate thirst in the rat. *Regul. Pept.*, 59:183–187.

Sakai, R. R., Ma, L-Y., Zhang, D. M., McEwen, B. S., and Fluharty, S. J. 1996. Intracerebroventricular administration of mineralocorti-coid receptor antisense oligonucleotides attenuates adrenal steroid-induced salt appetite in rats. *Neuroendocrinology*, 64:425–529.

Sakuma, Y., and Pfaff, D. W. 1979. Mesencephalic mechanisms for integration of female reproductive behavior in the rat. *Am. J. Physiol.*, 237:R285–R290.

Sakuma, Y., and Pfaff, D. W. 1980. Lh-RH in the mesencephalic cen-tral gray can potentiate lordosis reflex of female rats. *Nature*, 283:566–567.

Saltzman, W., Mendoza, S. P., and Mason, W. A. 1991. Sociophysi-ology of relationships in squirrel monkeys: I. Formation of female dyads. *Physiol. Behav.*, 50:271–280.

Saltzman, W., Schultz-Darken, N. J., and Abbott, D. H. 1996. Behavioural and endocrine predictors of dominance and toler-ance in female common marmosets, *Callithrix jacchus. Anim. Behav.*, 51:657–674.

Samuels, M. H., and Bridges, R. S. 1983. Plasma prolactin concentra-tions in parental male and female rats: Effects of exposure to rat young. *Endocrinology*, 113:1647–1654.

Sanders, D., Warner, P., Backstrom, T., and Bancroft, J. 1983. Mood, sexuality, hormones, and the menstrual cycle: Changes in mood and physical state. *Psychosom. Med.*, 45:487–500.

Santen, F. J., Sofsky, J., Bilic, N., and Lippert, R. 1975. Mechanism of action of narcotics in the production of menstrual dysfunction in women. *Fertil. Steril.*, 26:538–548.

Sapolsky, R. M. 1992a. Neuroendocrinology of the stress-response. In by J. B. Becker, S. M. Breedlove, and D. Crews (eds.). *Behavioral Endocrinology*, pp. 287–324. MIT Press, Cambridge, MA.

Sapolsky, R. M. 1992b. *Stress, the Aging Brain, and the Mechanisms of Neuron Death.* MIT Press, Cambridge, MA.

Sapolsky, R. M. 1994. *Why Zebras Don't Get Ulcers: A Guide to Stress, Stress-Related Diseases, and Coping.* W. H. Freeman, New York.

Sapolsky, R. M., and Meaney, M. J. 1986. Maturation of adrenocorti-cal stress response: Neuroendocrine control mechanisms and the stress hyporesponsive period. *Brain Res. Rev.*, 11:65–76.

Sapolsky, R. M., Krey, L., and McEwen, B. S. 1985. Prolonged gluco-corticoid exposure reduces hippocampal neuron numbeer: Implications for aging. *J. Neurosci.*, 5:1221–1228.

Sar, M., and Stumpf, W. E. 1977. Distribution of androgen target cells in rat forebrain and pituitary after [3H]-dihydrotestosterone administration. *J. Steroid Biochem.*, 8:1131–1135.

Satinoff, E., and Prosser, R. A. 1988. Suprachiasmatic nuclear lesions eliminate circadian rhythms of drinking and activity, but not of body temperature, in male rats. *J. Biol. Rhythms*, 3:1–22.

Saunders, D. S. 1977. *An Introduction to Biological Rhythms.* Wiley, New York.

Sauvage, M. F., Marquet, P., Rousseau, A., Raby, C., Buxeraud, J., and Lachatre, G. 1998. *Toxicol. Appl. Pharmacol.,* 149:127–135.

Savage, A., Ziegler, T. E., and Snowdon, C. T. 1988. Sociosexual development, pair bond formation, and mechanisms of fertility suppression in female cotton-top tamarins (*Saguinus oedipus oedipus*). *Am. J. Primatol.,* 14:345–359.

Savage, M. O., Preece, M. A., Jeffcoate, S. L., Ransley, P. G., Rumsby, G., Mansfield, M. D., and Williams, D. I. 1980. Familial male pseudohermaphroditism due to deficiency of 5α-reductase. *Clin. Endocrinol.,* 12:397–406.

Sawchenko, P. E., and Friedman, M. I. 1979. Sensory functions of the liver: A review. *Am. J. Physiol.,* 236:R5–R20.

Scalia, F., and Winans, S. S. 1976. New perspectives on the morphology of the olfactory system: Olfactory and vomeronasal pathways in mammals. In R. L. Doty (ed.), *Mammalian Olfaction, Reproductive Processes, and Behavior,* pp. 7–28. Academic Press, New York.

Schaal, B., and Marlier, L. 1998. Maternal and paternal perception of individual odor signatures in human amniotic fluid-potential role in early bonding? *Biol. Neonate,* 74:266–273.

Schaal, B., Montagner, H., Hertling, E., Bolzoni, D., Moyse, A., and Quichon, R. 1980. [Olfactory stimulation in the relationship between child and mother.] *Reprod. Nutr. Dev.,* 20:843–858.

Schaefer, G. J. 1988. Opiate antagonists and rewarding brain stimulation. *Neurosci. Biobehav. Rev.,* 12:1–17.

Schanberg, S. M., and Field, T. M. 1987. Sensory deprivation stress and supplemental stimulation in the rat pup and preterm human neonate. *Child Dev.,* 58:1431–1447.

Schanberg, S. M., and Kuhn, C. M. 1985. The biochemical effects of tactile deprivation in neonatal rats. *Perspect. Behav. Med.,* 2:133–148.

Scharff, C., and Nottebohm, F. 1991. A comparative study of the behavioral deficits following lesions of various parts of the zebra finch song system: Implications for vocal learning. *J. Neurosci.,* 11:2896–2913.

Schildkraut, J. M., Batos, E., and Berchuck, A. 1997. Relationship between lifetime ovulatory cycles and overexpression of mutant p53 in epithelial ovarian cancer. *J. Natl. Cancer Inst.,* 89:932–938.

Schindler, G. L. 1979. Testosterone concentration, personality patterns, and occupational choice in women. Ph.D. dissertation, University of Houston.

Schjelderup-Ebbe, T. 1922. Beiträge zür Socialpsychologie des haushuhns. *Z. Psychol.,* 88:225–252.

Schlinger, B. A. 1997. The activity and expression of aromatase in songbirds. *Brain Res. Bull.,* 44:359–364.

Schlinger, B. A., and Arnold, A. P. 1993. Estrogen synthesis in vivo in the adult zebra finch: Additional evidence that circulating estrogens can originate in brain. *Endocrinology,* 133:2610–2616.

Schlinger, B. A., and Callard, G. V. 1990. Aggressive behavior in birds: An experimental model for studies of brain–steroid interactions. *Comp. Biochem. Physiol.,* 97A:307–316.

Schlinger, B. A., Fivizzani, A. J., and Callard, G. V. 1989. Aromatase, 5a- and 5b-reductase in brain, pituitary and skin of the sex-role reversed Wilson's phalarope. *J. Endocrinol.,* 122:573–581.

Schlotts, F. 1988. *The PMS Book.* Ivory Tower Publications, Watertown, MA.

Schmidt, P. J., Nieman, L. K., Danaceau, M. A., Adams, L. F., and Rubinow, D. R. 1998. Differential behavioral effects of gonadal steroids in women with and those without premenstrual syndrome. *N. Engl. J. Med.,* 338:209–216.

Schmidt, P. J., Nieman, L. K., Grover, G. N., Muller, K. L., Merriam, G. R., and Rubinow, D. R. 1991. Lack of effect of induced menses on symptoms in women with premenstrual syndrome. *N. Engl. J. Med.,* 324:1174–1179.

Schneider, J. E., and Wade, G. N. 1987. Body composition, food intake, and brown fat thermogenesis in pregnant Djungarian hamsters. *Am. J. Physiol.,* 253:R314–320.

Schneider, J. E., and Wade, G. N. 1989a. Availability of metabolic fuels controls estrous cyclicity of Syrian hamsters. *Science,* 244:1326–1328.

Schneider, J. E., and Wade, G. N. 1989b. Effects of maternal diet, body weight and body composition on infanticide in Syrian hamsters. *Physiol. Behav.,* 46:815–821.

Schneider, J. E., and Wade, G. N. 1999. Reproductive inhibition in service of energy balance. In K. Wallen and J. E. Schneider (eds.). *Reproduction in Context.* MIT Press, Cambridge, MA.

Schneider, J. E., Goldman, M. D., Tang, S., Bean, B., Ji, H., and Friedman, M. I. 1998. Leptin indirectly affects estrous cycles by increasing metabolic fuel oxidation. *Horm. Behav.,* 33:217–228.

Schneider, M. A., Brotherton, P. L., and Hailes, J. 1977. The effect of exogenous oestrogens on depression in menopausal women. *Med. J. Aust.,* 2:162–163.

Schneider, M. L. 1992a. The effect of mild stress during pregnancy on birth weight and neuromotor maturation in rhesus monkey infants (*Mucaca mulatta*). *Infant Behav. Dev.,* 15:389–403.

Schneider, M. L. 1992b. Prenatal stress exposure alters postnatal behavioral expression under conditions of novelty challenge in rhesus monkey infants. *Dev. Psychobiol.,* 25:529–540.

Schneider, M. L., and Coe, C. L. 1993. Repeated social stress during pregnancy impairs neuromotor development of the primate infant. *Dev. Behav. Pediatr.,* 14:81–87.

Schulz, H., and Lavie, P. 1985. *Ultradian Rhythms in Physiology and Behavior.* Springer-Verlag, Berlin.

Schuurman, T. 1980. Hormonal correlates of agonistic behavior in adult male rats. *Prog. Brain Res.,* 53:415–420.

Schwabl, H., and Kriner, E. 1991. Territorial aggression and song of male European robins (*Erithacus rubecula*) in autumn and spring: Effects of antiandrogen treatment. *Horm. Behav.,* 25:180–194.

Schwagmeyer, P. L. 1979. The Bruce effect: An evaluation of male/female advantages. *Am. Nat.,* 114:932–938.

Schwanzel-Fukuda, M., and Pfaff, D. W. 1989. Origin of luteinizing hormone-releasing hormone neurons. *Nature,* 138:161–164.

Schwanzel-Fukuda, M., Bick, D., and Pfaff, D. W. 1989. Luteinizing hormone-releasing hormone (LHRH)-expressing cells do not migrate normally in an inherited hypogonadal (Kallmann) syndrome. *Mol. Brain Res.,* 6:311–326.

Schwartz, M. W., Figlewicz, D. P., Baskin, D. G., Woods, S. C., and Porte, D. Jr. 1992. Insulin in the brain: a hormonal regulator of energy balance. *Endocr. Rev.,* 13:387–414.

Schwartz, W. J., and Gainer, H. 1977. Suprachiasmatic nucleus: Use of $^{14}$C-labeled deoxyglucose uptake as a functional marker. *Science,* 197:1089–1091.

Schwartz, W. J., Bosis, N. A., and Hedley-Whyte, E. T. 1986. A discrete lesion of ventral hypothalamus and optic chiasm that disturbed the daily temperature rhythm. *J. Neurol.,* 233:1–4.

Scott, J. P., and Fredericson, E. 1951. The causes of fighting in mice and rats. *Physiol. Zool.,* 24:273–309.

Searcy, W. A., and Wingfield, J. C. 1980. The effects of androgen and anti-androgen on dominance and aggressiveness in male red-winged blackbirds. *Horm. Behav.,* 14:126–135.

Sedivy, J. M., and Sharp, P. A. 1989. Positive genetic selection for gene disruption in mammalian cells by homologous recombination. *Proc. Nat. Acad. Sci. U.S.A.,* 86, 227–231.

Seegal, R. F., and Goldman, B. D. 1975. Effects of photoperiod on cyclicity and serum gonadotropins in the Syrian hamster. *Biol. Reprod.,* 12:223–231.

Segreti, J., Gheusi, G., Dantzer, R., Kelley, K. W., and Johnson, R. W. 1997. Defect in interleukin-1beta secretion prevents sickness behavior in C3H/HeJ mice. *Physiol. Behav.,* 61:873–878.

Selye, H. 1936. A syndrome produced by diverse nocuous agents. *Nature,* 138:32–35.

Selye, H. 1937a. Studies on adaptation. *Endocrinology,* 21:169–188.

Selye, H. 1937b. The significance of the adrenals for adaptation. *Science,* 85:247–248.

Selye, H. 1950. *Stress.* Acta, Inc., Montreal.

Selye, H. 1956. *The Stress of Life.* McGraw-Hill, New York.

Serra, G. B. 1983. *The Ovary.* Raven Press, New York.

Severino, S. K., and Moline, M. L. 1989. *Premenstrual Syndrome: A Clinician's Manual.* Guilford, New York.

Shaham, Y. and Stewart, J. 1994. Exposure to mild stress enhances the reinforcing efficacy of intravenous heroin self-administration in rats. *Psychopharmacology,* 114:523–527.

Shaham, Y., and Stewart, J. 1995. Stress reinstates heroin-seeking in drug-free animals: an effect mimicking heroin, not withdrawal. *Psychopharmacology,* 119:334–341.

Shapiro, H. A. 1937. Effect of testosterone propionate on mating. *Nature,* 139:588–589.

Shapiro, L. E., and Insel, T. R. 1990. Infant's response to social separation reflects adult differences in affiliative behavior: A comparative developmental study in prairie and montane voles. *Dev. Psychobiol.,* 23:375–393.

Shapiro, L. E., Austin, D., Ward, S. E., and Dewsbury, D. A. 1986. Familiarity and female mate choice in two species of voles (*Microtus ochrogaster* and *Microtus montanus*). *Anim. Behav.,* 34:90–97.

Shapiro, S., Schlesinger, E. R., and Nesbitt, R. E. L. 1968. *Infant, Perinatal, Maternal, and Childhood Mortality in the United States.* Harvard University Press, Cambridge, MA.

Sharman, G. B. 1970. Reproductive physiology of marsupials. *Science,* 167:1221–1228.

Shashoua, V. E. 1973. Seasonal changes in the learning and activity patterns of goldfish. *Science*, 181:572–574.

Shaywitz, B. A, Shaywitz, S. E., Pugh, K. R., Constable, R. T., Skudlarski, P., Fulbright, R. K., Bronen, R. A., Fletcher, J. M., Shankweller, D. P., Katz, L., and Gore, J. C. 1995. Sex difference in the functional organization of the brain for language. *Nature*, 373:607–609.

Sheridan, P. J. 1978. Localization of androgen- and estrogen-concentrating neurons in the diencephalon and telencephalon of the mouse. *Endocrinology*, 103:1328–1334.

Sheridan, P. J., Hagino, N., and Weaker, F. J. 1982. Androgen-concentrating cells in the periventricular brain of the female rhesus monkey. *J. Comp. Neurol.*, 207:93–98.

Sherman, P. W. 1988. The clitoris debate and the levels of analysis. *Anim. Behav.*, 37:697–698.

Sherwin, B. B. 1988a. Affective changes with estrogen and androgen replacement therapy in surgically menopausal women. *J. Affect. Disord.*, 14:177–187.

Sherwin, B. B. 1988b. A comparative analysis of the role of androgen in human male and female sexual behavior: Behavioral specificity, critical thresholds, and sensitivity. *Psychobiology*, 16:416–425.

Sherwin, B. B. 1996. Estrogen, the brain, and memory. *Menopause*, 3:97–105.

Sherwin, B. B. 1997. Estrogen effects on cognition in menopausal women. *Neurology*, 48:S21–S26.

Sherwin, B. B. 1998. Estrogen and cognitive functioning in women. *Proc. Soc. Exp. Biol. Med.*, 217:17–22.

Sherwin, B. B., and Gelfand, M. M. 1985. Sex steroids and affect in the surgical menopause: A double-blind, cross-over study. *Psychoneuroendocrinology*, 10:325–335.

Sherwin, B. B., and Gelfand, M. M. 1987. The role of androgen in the maintenance of sexual functioning in oophorectomized women. *Psychosom. Med.*, 49:397–409.

Sherwin, B. B., and Suranyi-Cadotte, B. E. 1990. Up-regulatory effect of estrogen on platelet 3H-imipramine binding sites in surgically menopausal women. *Biol. Psychiatry*, 28:339–348.

Sherwin, B. B., Gelfand, M. M., and Brender, W. 1985. Androgen enhances sexual motivation in females: A prospective, crossover study of sex steroid administration in surgical menopause. *Psychosom. Med.*, 47:339–351.

Shibata, S., and Moore, R. Y. 1988. Electrical and metabolic activity of suprachiasmatic nucleus neurons in hamster hypothalamic slices. *Brain Res.*, 438:374–378.

Shide, D. J., and Blass, E. M. 1989. Opioid-like effects of intraoral infusions of corn oil and Polycose on stress reactions in ten-day-old rats. *Behav. Neurosci.*, 103:1168–1175.

Shiota, M., Sudou, M., and Ohshima, M. 1996. Using outdoor exercise to decrease jet lag in airline crewmembers. *Aviation Space Env. Med.*, 67:1155–1160.

Shippenberg, T., and Herz, A. 1987. Motivational properties of opioids. *Pol. J. Pharmacol. Pharmacy*, 39:577–583.

Short, R. V. 1997. The testis: The witness of the mating system, the site of mutation and the engine of desire. *Acta Paediatr., (Suppl)*, 422:3–7.

Shughrue, P. J. 1998. Estrogen action in the estrogen receptor - knockout mouse: Is this due to ER? *Mol. Psychiatry*, 3:299–302.

Shughrue, P. J., Komm, B., and Merchenthaler, I. 1996. The distribution of estrogen receptor mRNA in the rat hypothalamus. *Steroids*, 61:678–681.

Siegel, H. I. 1985. *The Hamster: Reproduction and Behavior*, Plenum Publishing: New York.

Siegel, H. I., and Rosenblatt, J. S. 1975. Hormonal basis of hysterectomy-induced maternal behavior during pregnancy in the rat. *Horm. Behav.*, 6:211–222.

Siegel, H. I., and Rosenblatt, J. S. 1978. Duration of estrogen stimulation and progesterone inhibition of maternal behavior in pregnancy-terminated rats. *Horm. Behav.*, 11:12–19.

Siegel, H. S. 1959. The relation between crowding and weight of adrenal glands in chickens. *Ecology*, 40:494–498.

Siegel, H. S. 1960. Effect of population density on the pituitary-adrenal cortical axis of cockerels. *Poultry Sci.*, 39:500–510.

Silver, R. 1977. *Parental Behavior in Birds*. Dowden, Hutchinson and Ross, Stroudsburg, PA.

Silver, R. 1978. The parental behavior of ring doves. *Am. Sci.*, 66:209–215.

Silver, R., Andrews, H., and Ball, G. F. 1985. Parental care in an ecological perspective: A quantitative analysis of avian subfamilies. *Am. Zool.*, 25:823–840.

Silver, R., O'Connell, M., and Saad, R. 1979. Effect of androgens on the behavior of birds. In C. Beyer (ed.), *Endocrine Control of Sexual Behavior*, pp. 223–278. Raven Press, New York.

Silverin, B. 1980. Effects of long-acting testosterone treatment on free-living pied flycatchers (*Ficedula hypoleuca*) during the breeding period. *Anim. Behav.*, 28:906–912.

Silverin, B. 1990. Testosterone and corticosterone and their relation to territorial and parental behavior in the pied flycatcher. In J. Balthazart (ed.). *Hormones, Brain and Behaviour in Vertebrates*, Vol. 2, pp. 129–142. Karger, Basel.

Silverin, B., and Goldsmith, A. R. 1983. Reproductive endocrinology of free living Pied flycatchers (*Ficedula hypoleuca*): Prolactin and FSH secretion in relation to incubation and clutch size. *J. Zool. (Lond.)*, 200:119–130.

Simerly, R. B., and Swanson, L. W. 1986. The organization of neural inputs to the medial preoptic nucleus of the rat. *J. Comp. Neurol.*, 246:312–342.

Simerly, R. B., Carr, A. M., Zee, M. C., and Lorang, D. 1996. Ovarian steroid regulation of estrogen and progesterone receptor messenger ribonucleic acid in the anteroventral periventricular nucleus of the rat. *J. Neuroendocrinol.*, 8:45–56.

Simpkins, J. W., Green, P. S., Gridley, K. E., Singh, M., de Fiebre, N. C., and Rajakumar, G. 1997. Role of estrogen replacement therapy in memory enhancement and the prevention of neuronal loss associated with Alzheimer's disease. *Am. J. Med.*, 103:19S–25S.

Simpson, J. B., Epstein, A. N., and Camardo, J. S. 1978. The localization of dipsogenic receptors for angiotensin II in the subfornical organ. *J. Comp. Physiol. Psychol.*, 92:581–608.

Sisk, C. L., and Turek, F. W. 1982. Daily melatonin injections mimic the short day-induced increase in negative feedback effects of testosterone on gonadotropin secretion in hamsters. *Biol. Reprod.*, 27:602–608.

Skuse, D. H., James, R. S., Bishop, D. V., Coppin, B., Dalton, P., Aamodt-Leeper, G., Bacarese-Hamilton, M., Creswell, C., McGurk, R., and Jacobs, P. A. 1997. Evidence from Turner's syndrome of an imprinted X-linked locus affecting cognitive function. *Nature*, 387:652–653.

Skuse, D., and Jacobs, P. 1997. Mosaicism in Turner's syndrome: A reply. *Nature*, 390:569.

Skutch, A. F. 1935. Helpers at the nest. *Auk*, 52:257–273.

Skwerer, R. G., Jacobsen, F. M., Duncan, C. C., Kelly, K. A., Sack, D. A., Tamarkin, L., Gaist, P. A., Kasper, S., and Rosenthal, N. E. 1988. Neurobiology of seasonal affective disorder and phototherapy. *J. Biol. Rhythms*, 3:135–154.

Slawski, B. A. and Buntin, J. D. 1995. Preoptic area lesions disrupt prolactin-induced parental feeding behavior in ring doves. *Horm. Behav.*, 29:248–266.

Slimp, J. C., Hart, B. L., and Goy, R. W. 1978. Heterosexual, autosexual and social behavior of adult male rhesus monkeys with medial preoptic–anterior hypothalamic lesions. *Brain Res.*, 142:105–122.

Slob, A. K., Bax, C. M., Hop, W. C., Rowland, D. L., and van der Werff ten Bosch, J. J. 1996. Sexual arousability and the menstrual cycle. *Psychoneuroendocrinology*, 21:545–558.

Slob, A. K., Ernste, M., and van der Werff ten Bosch, J. J. 1991. Menstrual cycle phase and sexual arousability in women. *Arch. Sex. Behav.*, 20:567–577.

Slonaker, J. R. 1924. The effect of copulation, pregnancy, pseudopregnancy, and lactation on the voluntary activity and food consumption of the albino rat. *Am. J. Physiol.*, 71:362–394.

Sloviter, R. S., Valiquette, G., Abrams, G., Ronk, E., Sollas, A., and Paul, L. 1989. Selective loss of hippocampal granule cells following adrenalectomy. *Science*, 243:535–538.

Smale, L., Nelson, R. J., and Zucker, I. 1988. Daylength influences pelage and plasma prolactin concentrations but not reproduction in the prairie vole, *Microtus ochrogaster*. *J. Reprod. Fertil.*, 83:99–106.

Smale, L., Nunes, C., and Holekamp, K. E. 1997. Sexually dimorphic dispersal in mammals: Patterns, causes, and consequences. *Adv. Study Behav.*, 26:181–250.

Smals, A. G. H., Kloppenbort, P. W. C., and Benraad, T. H. 1976. Circannual cycle in plasma testosterone levels in man. *J. Clin. Endocrinol. Metab.*, 42:979–982.

Smith, A. D. 1988. Psychologic factors in the multidisciplinary evaluation and treatment of erectile dysfunction. *Urol. Clin. North Am.*, 15:41–51.

Smith, C. L., Nawaz, Z., and O'Malley, B. W. 1997. Coactivator and corepressor regulation of the agonist/antagonist activity of the mixed antiestrogen, 4-hydroxytamoxifen. *Mol. Endocrinol.*, 11:657–666.

Smith, C., and Lloyd, B. 1978. Maternal behavior and perceived sex of infant: Revisited. *Child Dev.*, 49:1263–1265.

Smith, D. E., Moser, C., Wesson, D. R., Apter, M., Buxton, M. E., Davison, J. V., Orgel, M., and Buffum, J. 1982. A clinical guide to the diagnosis and treatment of heroin-related sexual dysfunction. *J. Psychoactive Drugs*, 14:91–99.

Smith, G. P., Jerome, C., and Gibbs, J. 1981a. Abdominal vagotomy does not block the satiety effect of bombesin in the rat. *Peptides*, 2:409–411.

Smith, G. P., Jerome, C., Pi-Sunyer, F. X., Kissileff, H. R., and Thornton, J. 1981b. The satiety effect of cholecystokinin: A progress report. *Peptides*, 2:57–59.

Smith, G. T., Brenowitz, E. A., Nalls, B., and Wingfield, J. C. 1991. Testosterone changes song control region volume in photostimulated male Gambel's white-crowned sparrows (*Zonotrichia leucophrys gambelii*). Third International Congress of Neuroethology, Montreal, Quebec.

Smith, G. T., Brenowitz, E., and Wingfield, J. 1997b. Roles of photoperiod and testosterone in seasonal plasticity of the avian song control system. *J. Neurobiol.*, 32:426–42.

Smith, G. T., Brenowitz, E., Beecher, M., and Wingfield, J. 1997a. Seasonal changes in testosterone, neural attributes of song control nuclei, and song structure in wild songbirds. *J. Neurosci.*, 17:6001–6010.

Smith, G. T., Brenowitz, E., Wingfield, J., and Baptista, L. 1995. Seasonal changes in song nuclei and song behavior in Gambel's white-crowned sparrows. *J. Neurobiol.*, 28: 114–25.

Smith, R., Cubis, J., Brinsmead, M., Lewin, T., Singh, B., Ownes, P., Chan, E. C., Hall, C., Adler, R., Lovelock, M., Hurt, D., Rowley, M., and Nolan, M. 1990. Mood changes, obstetric experience and alterations in plasma cortisol, beta-endorphin and corticotrophin releasing hormone during pregnancy and the puerperium. *J. Psychosom. Res.*, 34:1941–1947.

Snow, D. W. 1965. The breeding of Audubon's Shearwater (*Puffinus lherminieri*) in the Galapagos. *Auk*, 82:591–597.

Snow, D. W., and Snow, B. K. 1967. The breeding cycle of the swallow-tailed gull *Creagrus furcatus*. *Ibis*, 109:14–24.

Södersten, P. 1973. Estrogen-activated sexual behavior in male rats. *Horm. Behav.*, 4:247–256.

Södersten, P., and Eneroth, P. 1984. Suckling and serum prolactin and LH concentrations in lactating rats. *J. Endocrinol.*, 102:251–256.

Södersten, P., Eneroth, P., and Hansen, S. 1981. Induction of sexual receptivity in ovariectomized rats by pulse administration of oestradiol-17b. *J. Endocrinol.*, 89:55–62.

Sohrabji, F., Nordeen, E. A., and Nordeen, K. W. 1990. Selective impairment of song learning following lesions of a forebrain nucleus in the juvenile zebra finch. *Behav. Neural Biol.*, 53:51–63.

Soma, K. K., Hartman, V. N., Wingfield, J. C., and Brenowitz, E. A. 1999. Seasonal changes in androgen receptor immunoreactivity in the song nucleus HVC of a wild bird. *J. Comp. Neurol.*, 409:224–236.

Soriano, P. 1995. Gene targeting in ES cells. *Annu. Rev. Neurosci.*, 18:1–18.

Soussignan, P., and Koch, P. 1985. Rhythmical stereotypies (leg-swinging) associated with reductions in heart rate in normal school children. *Biol. Psychol.*, 21:161–167.

Southwick, C. H. 1955a. The population dynamics of confined house mice supplied with unlimited food. *Ecology*, 36:212–225.

Southwick, C. H. 1955b. Regulatory mechanisms in house mouse populations: Social behavior affecting litter survival. *Ecology*, 36:627–634.

Stacher, G., Bauer, H., and Steinringer, H. 1978. Cholecystokinin decreases appetite and activation evoked by stimuli arising from the preparation of a meal in man. *Physiol. Behav.*, 23:325–331.

Stanley, B. G., and Leibowitz, S. F. 1985. Neuropeptide Y injected in the paraventricular hypothalamus: A powerful stimulant of feeding behavior. *Proc. Natl. Acad. Sci. U.S.A.*, 82:3940–3943.

Stanton, M. E., and Levine, S. 1990. Inhibition of infant glucocorticoid stress response: Specific role of maternal cues. *Dev. Psychobiol.*, 23:411–426.

Starkman, M., Gebarski, S. S., Berent, S., and Schteingart, D. A. 1992. Hippocampal formation volume, memory dysfunction and cortisol levels in patients with Cushing's syndrome. *Biol. Psychiatry*, 32:756–765.

Staub, N. L., and De Beer, M. 1997. The role of androgens in female vertebrates. *Gen. Comp. Endocrinology*, 108:1–24.

Stearns, E., Winter, J., and Faiman, C. 1973. Effects of coitus on gonadotrophin, prolactin and sex steroid levels in man. *J. Clin. Endocrinol. Metab.*, 37:687–691.

Steeghs, K., Oerlemans, F., and Wieringa, B. 1995. Mice deficient in ubiquitous mitochondrial creatine kinase are viable and fertile. *Biochim. Biophys. Acta*, 1230, 130–138.

Steffens, A. B., Strubbe, J. H., Balkan, B., and Scheurink, A. J. W. 1990. Neuroendocrine mechanisms involved in regulation of body weight, food intake and metabolism. *Neurosci. Biobehav. Rev.*, 14:305–313.

Stein, L. J., and Woods, S. C. 1981. Cholecystokinin and bombesin act independently to decrease food intake in the rat. *Peptides*, 2:431–436.

Steinach, E. 1894. Investigations into the comparative physiology of the male sexual organs, with particular reference to the accessory sexual glands. trans. by M. Clarke. In C. S. Carter (ed.), *Hormones and Sexual Behavior*, pp. 11–30. Stroudsburg, Dowden, Hutchinson and Ross, Incorporated.

Steinach, E. 1910. Geschlechstrieb und echt sekundare Geschlechtsmerkmale als Folge der innersekretorisechen Funcktion der Keimdrusen. II. Uber die Enstehung des Umklammerunsreflexes bei Froschen. *Z. Physiol.*, 24:551–570.

Steinach, E. 1913. Feminierung von Männchen und Maskulierung von Weibchen. *Z. Physiol.*, 27:717–723.

Steinach, E. 1936. Zur Geschichte des mannlichen Sexuall-hormons und seiner Wirkungen beim Saugetier und beim Menschen. *Wien. Klin. Wochenschr.*, 49:161–172.

Steinach, E. 1940. *Sex and Life.* New York, Viking.

Steinberger, A., and Ward, D. N. 1988. Inhibin. In E. Knobil and J. D. Neill (eds.), *The Physiology of Reproduction*, pp. 567–583. Raven Press, New York.

Stephan, F. K., and Zucker, I. 1972. Circadian rhythms in drinking behavior and locomotor activities are eliminated by hypothalamic lesions. *Proc. Natl. Acad. Sci. U.S.A.*, 69:1583–1586.

Stern, J. E., and Armstrong, W. E. 1998. Reorganization of the dendritic trees of oxytocin and vasopressin neurons of the rat supraoptic nucleus during lactation. *J. Neurosci.*, 18:841–853.

Stern, J. M. 1989. Maternal behavior: Sensory, hormonal and neural determinants. In F. R. Bush and S. Levine (eds.), *Psychoendocrinology*, pp. 104–226. Academic Press, San Diego.

Stern, J. M. 1990. Multisensory regulation of maternal behavior and masculine sexual behavior: A revised view. *Neurosci. Biobehav. Rev.*, 14:183–200.

Stern, J. M. 1996. Somatosensation and maternal care in Norway rats. *Adv. Study Behav.*, 25, 243:294.

Stern, J. M. 1997. Offspring-induced nurturance: Animal-human parallels. *Dev. Psychobiol.*, 31:19–37.

Stern, J. M., and Johnson, S. K. 1990. Ventral somatosensory determinants of nursing behavior in Norway rats. I. Effects of variations in the quality and quantity of pup stimuli. *Physiol. Behav.*, 47:993–1011.

Stern, J. M., and Lonstein, J. S. 1996. Nursing behavior in rats is impaired in a small nestbox and with hyperthermic pups. *Dev. Psychobiol.*, 29:101–122.

Stern, J. M., Dix, L., Bellomo, C., and Thramann, C. 1992. Ventral trunk somatosensory determinants of nursing behavior in Norway rats: 2. Role of nipple and surrounding sensations. *Psychobiology*, 20:71–80.

Stern, K., and McClintock, M. K. 1998. Regulation of ovulation by human pheromones. *Nature*, 392:177–179.

Stern, M., and Hildebrandt-Karraker, K. 1989. Sex stereotyping of infants: A review of gender labelling studies. *Sex Roles*, 20:501–522.

Sternberg, D. B., Issacs, K., Gold, P. E., and McGaugh, J. L. 1985. Epinephrine facilitation of appetitive learning: Attenuation with adrenergic receptor antagonists. *Behav. Neural Biol.*, 44:447–453.

Sternberg, D. B., Korol, D., Novack, G., and McGaugh, J. L. 1986. Epinephrine-induced memory facilitation: Attenuation by adrenergic receptor antagonists. *Eur. J. Pharmacol.*, 129:189–193.

Stevens, R., and Goldstein, R. 1981. Effects of neonatal testosterone and estrogen on open-field behavior in rats. *Physiol. Behav.*, 26:551–553.

Stewart, J. 1988. Current themes, theoretical issues, and preoccupations in the study of sexual differentiation and gender-related behaviors. *Psychobiology*, 16:315–320.

Stewart, J., and Cygan, D. 1980. Ovarian hormones act early in development to feminize adult open-field behavior in the rat. *Horm. Behav.*, 14:20–32.

Stockard, C. R., and Papanicolaou, G. N. 1917. The existence of a typical oestrous cycle in the guinea-pig with a study of its histological and physiological changes. *Am. J. Anat.*, 22:225–283.

Stone, C. P. 1922. The congenital sexual behavior of the young male albino rat. *J. Comp. Psychol.*, 2:95–153.

Stone, C. P. 1923. Further study of the sensory functions in the activation of sexual behavior in the young male albino rat. *J. Comp. Psychol.,* 3:469–473.

Stone, C. P. 1924. The awakening of copulatory behavior in the male albino rat. *Am. J. Physiol.,* 68:407–428.

Stone, C. P. 1925. Preliminary note on the maternal behavior of rats living in parabiosis. *Endocrinology,* 9:505–512.

Stone, C. P. 1927. The retention of copulatory ability in male rats following castration. *Am. J. Physiol.,* 7:369–387.

Stone, C. P. 1938a. Loss and restoration of copulatory activity in adult male rats following castration and subsequent injections of testosterone propionate. *Endocrinology,* 23:529.

Stone, C. P. 1938b. Activation of impotent male rats by injections of testosterone propionate. *J. Comp. Psychol.,* 25:445–450.

Stone, C. P. 1938c. Effects of cortical destruction on reproductive behavior and maze learning in albino rats. *J. Comp. Psychol.,* 26:217–236.

Stone, C. P. 1939. Copulatory activity in adult male rats following castration and injections of testosterone propionate. *Endocrinology,* 24:165–174.

Stone, C. P., and Commins, W. D. 1936. The effect of castration at various ages upon the learning ability of male albino rats: II. Relearning after an interval of one year. *J. Genet. Psychol.,* 48:20–28.

Stone, C. P., Barker, R. G., and Tomlin, M. I. 1935. Sexual drive in potent and impotent male rats as measured by the Columbia obstruction apparatus. *J. Genet. Psychol.,* 47:33–48.

Stopa, E. G., Johnson, J. K., Friedman, D. I., Ryer, H. I., Reidy, J., Kuo-LeBlanc, V., and Albers, H. E. 1995. Neuropeptide Y receptor distribution and regulation in the suprachiasmatic nucleus of the Syrian hamster (*Mesocricetus auratus*). *Peptide Res.,* 8:95–100.

Storey, A. E., Courage, C., and Wynne-Edwards, K. 1997. Of mice and men: Why is there variation in the social cues that trigger mammalian paternal care? Paper presented at the Animal Behaviour Society meeting, June 1999, College Park, MD.

Stratakis, C. A. and Chrousos, G. P. 1995. Neuroendocrinology and pathophysiology of the stress system. *Ann. N. Y. Acad. Sci.,* 771:1–18.

Strauss, R. H., Liggett, M. T., and Lanese, R. R. 1985. Anabolic steroid use and perceived effects in ten weight-trained women athletes. *J. A. M. A.,* 253:2871–2873.

Stricker, E. M. 1968. Some physiological and motivational properties of the hypovolemic stimulus for thirst. *Physiol. Behav.,* 3:379–385.

Stricker, E. M. 1978. The renin-angiotensin system and thirst: Some unanswered questions. *Fed. Proc.,* 37:2704–2710.

Stricker, E. M. 1984. Biological bases of hunger and satiety: Therapeutic implications. *Nutr. Rev.,* 42:333–340.

Stricker, E. M., and Verbalis, J. G. 1988. Hormones and behavior: The biology of thirst and sodium appetite. *Am. Sci.,* 76:261–267.

Stricker, E. M., and Verbalis, J. G. 1990a. Control of appetite and satiety: Insight from biologic and behavioral studies. *Nutr. Rev.,* 48:49–56.

Stricker, E. M., and Verbalis, J. G. 1990b. Sodium appetite. In E. M. Stricker (ed.), *Handbook of Behavioral Neurobiology,* Vol. 10, pp. 387–419. Plenum, New York.

Stricker, E. M., and Verbalis, J. G. 1991. Caloric and noncaloric controls of food intake. *Brain Res. Bull.,* 27:299–303.

Stricker, E. M., Cooper, P. H., Marshall, J. F., and Zigmond, M. J. 1979. Acute homeostatic imbalances reinstate sensorimotor dysfunctions in rats with lateral hypothalamic lesions. *J. Comp. Physiol. Psychol.,* 93:512–521.

Stricker, E. M., Hosutt, J. A., and Verbalis, J. G. 1987. Neurohypophyseal secretion in hypovolemic rats: Inverse relation to sodium appetite. *Am. J. Physiol.,* 252:R889–R896.

Stricker, E. M., Rowland, N., Saller, C. F., and Friedman, M. I. 1977. Homeostasis during hypoglycemia: Central control of adrenal secretion and peripheral control of feeding. *Science,*196:79–81.

Strobel, A., Issad, T., Camoin, L., Ozata, M., and Strosberg, A. D. 1998. A leptin missense mutation associated with hypogonadism and morbid obesity. *Nat. Genet.,* 18:213–215.

Strubbe, J. H., Steffens, A. B., and De Ruiter, L. 1977. Plasma insulin and the time pattern of feeding in the rat. *Physiol. Behav.,* 18:81–86.

Su, T. P., Pagliaro, M., Schmidt, P. J., Pickar, D., Wolkowitz, O., and Rubinow, D. R. 1993. Neuropsychiatric effects of anabolic steroids in male normal volunteers. *J. A. M. A.,* 269:2760–2764.

Suchecki, D., Mozaffarian, D., Gross, G., Rosenfeld, P., and Levine, S. 1993. Effects of maternal deprivation on the ACTH stress response in the infant rat. *Neuroendocrinology,* 57:204–212.

Suomi, S. J. 1977. Adult male-infant interactions among monkeys living in nuclear families. *Child Dev.,* 48:1215–1270.

Suomi, S. J. 1991. Early stress and adult emotional reactivity in rhesus monkeys. *Ciba Found. Symp.,* 156:171–183.

Susman, J. L. 1996. Postpartum depressive disorders. *J. Fam. Pract.,* 43:S17–24.

Svare, B. 1983. *Hormones and Aggressive Behavior.* Plenum, New York.

Svare, B. 1990. Maternal aggression: Hormonal, genetic, and developmental determinants. In N. A. Krasnegor and R. S. Bridges (eds.), *Mammalian Parenting,* pp. 118–132. Oxford University Press, Oxford.

Svare, B., and Gandelman, R. 1976. Postpartum aggression in mice: Experiential and environmental factors. *Horm. Behav.,* 7:407–416.

Svare, B., Mann, M. A., Broida, J., and Michael, S. 1982. Maternal aggression exhibited by hypophysectomized parturient mice. *Horm. Behav.,* 16:455–461.

Svare, B., Miele, J., and Kinsley, C. 1986. Mice: Progesterone stimulates aggression in pregnancy-terminated females. *Horm. Behav.,* 20:194–200.

Swaab, D. F., and Fliers, E. A. 1985. A sexually dimorphic nucleus in the human brain. *Science,* 228:1112–1114.

Swaab, D. F., and Hofman, M. A. 1984. Sexual differentiation of the human brain: A historical perspective. *Prog. Brain Res.,* 61:361–374.

Swann, J., and Fiber, J. M. 1997. Sex differences in function of a pheromonally stimulated pathway: role of steroids and the main olfactory system. *Brain Res. Bull.,* 44:409–413.

Sweeney, B. M. 1976. Evidence that membranes are components of circadian oscillators. In J. W. Hastings and H. G. Schweiger (eds.), *Molecular Basis of Circadian Rhythms,* pp. 267–281. Abakon Verlagsgesellschaft, Berlin.

Sweeney, T., Donovan, A., Karsch, F. J., Roche, J. F., and O'Callaghan, D. 1997. Influence of previous photoperiodic exposure on the reproductive response to a specific photoperiod signal in ewes. *Biol. Reprod.,* 56:916–920.

Szymusiak, R., and Satinoff, E. 1982. Acute thermoregulatory effects of unilateral electrolytic lesions of the medial and lateral preoptic area in rats. *Physiol. Behav.,* 28:161–170.

Taibell, A. 1928. Risveglio artificiale di istinti tipicamenta feminili nei maschi di faluni uccelli. *Atti. Soc. Nat. Mat. Modena,* 59:93–102.

Takahashi, J. S. 1991. Circadian rhythms: From gene expression to behavior. *Curr. Opinion Neurobiol.,* 1:556–561.

Takahashi, J. S. 1992. Circadian clock genes are ticking. *Science,* 258:238–240.

Takahashi, J. S. 1993. Circadian-clock regulation of gene expression. *Curr. Opinion Genet. Devel.,* 3:301–309.

Takahashi, J. S., and Menaker, M. 1980. Interaction of estradiol and progesterone: Effects on circadian locomotor rhythms in female golden hamsters. *Am. J. Physiol.,* 239:R497–R504.

Takahashi, J. S., Kondo, H., Yoshimura, M., and Ochi, Y. 1974. Thyrotropin responses to TRH in depressive illness: Relation to clinical subtypes and prolonged duration of depressive episode. *Folia Psychiatrica Neurol. Japonica,* 28:355–365.

Takahashi, J. S., Kornhauser, J. M., Koumenis, C., and Eskin, A. 1993. Molecular approaches to understanding circadian oscillations. *Annu. Rev. Physiol.,* 55:729–753.

Takahashi, J. S., Murakami, N., and Nikaido, S. S. 1989. The avian pineal, a vertebrate model system of the circadian oscillator: Cellular regulation of circadian rhythms by light, second messengers, and macromolecular synthesis. *Rec. Prog. Horm. Res.,* 45:279–352.

Takahashi, J. S., Pinto, L. H., and Vitaterna, M. H. 1994. Forward and reverse genetic approaches to behavior in the mouse. *Science,* 264, 1724–1733.

Takahashi, L. K. 1998. Prenatal stress: Consequences of glucocorticoids on hippocampal development and function. *Int. J. Dev. Neurosci.,* 16:199–207.

Tamarkin, L., Hutchison, J. S., and Goldman, B. D. 1976. Regulation of serum gonadotropins by photoperiod and testicular hormone in the Syrian hamster. *Endocrinology,* 99:1528–1533.

Tanagho, E. A., Lue, T. F., and McClure, R. D. 1988. *Contemporary Management of Impotence Infertility,* Williams & Wilkins, Baltimore.

Tanner, J. M. 1962. *Growth at Adolescence.* Blackwell, Oxford.

Tartaglia, L. A., Dembski, M., Weng, X., Deng, N., Culpepper, J., Devos, R., Richards, G. J., Campfield, L. A., Clark, F. T., Deeds, J., Muir, C., Sanker, S., Moriarty, A., Moore, K. J., Smutko, J. S.,

Mays, G. G., Woolf, E. A., Monroe, C. A., and Tepper, R. I. 1995. Identification and expression cloning of a leptin receptor, OB-R. *Cell,* 83:1263–1271.

Tate-Ostroff B. and Bridges, R. S. 1985. Plasma prolactin levels in parental male rats: effects of increased pup stimuli. *Horm. Behav.,* 19:220–226.

Taylor, J. W. 1979. The timing of menstruation-related symptoms assessed by a daily symptoms rating scale. *Acta Psychiatrica Scand.,* 60:87–105.

Taylor, W. N., and Black, A. B. 1987. Pervasive anabolic steroid use among health club athletes. *Ann. Sports Med.,* 3:155–159.

Taymans, S. E., DeVries, A. C., DeVries, DeVries, M. B., Nelson, R. J., Friedman, T. C., Castro, M., Detera-Wadleigh, S., Carter, C. S., and Chrousos, G. P. 1997. The hypothalamic-pituitary-adrenal axis of prairie voles (*Microtus ochrogaster*): Evidence for target tissue glucocorticoid resistance. *Gen. Comp. Endocrinol.,* 106:48–61.

Tegelman, R., Carlström, K., and Pousette, A. 1988. Hormone levels in male ice hockey players during a 26-hour cup tournament. *Int. J. Androl.,* 11:361–368.

Telner, J., Lepore, F., and Guillemot, J. P. 1979. Effects of seratonin content on pain sensitivity in the rat. *Pharmacol. Biochem. Behav.,*10: 657–661.

Tepper, B. J., and Friedman, M. I. 1991. Altered acceptability of and preference for sugar solutions by diabetic rats is normalized by high-fat diet. *Appetite,* 16:25–38.

Terkel, J., and Rosenblatt, J. S. 1968. Maternal behavior induced by maternal blood plasma injected into virgin rats. *J. Comp. Physiol. Psychol.,* 65:479–482.

Terkel, J., and Rosenblatt, J. S. 1972. Humoral factors underlying maternal behavior at parturition. *J. Comp. Physiol. Psychol.,* 80:365–371.

Terman, M. 1988. On the question of mechanism in phototherapy for seasonal affective disorder: Considerations for clinical efficacy and epidemiology. *J. Biol. Rhythms,* 3:155–172.

Teyler, T. J. and Discenna, P. 1984. Long-term potentiation as a candidate mnemonic device. *Brain Res.,* 319:15–28.

Thase, M. E. 1989. Comparison between seasonal affective disorder and other forms of recurrent depression. In N. E. Rosenthal and M. C. Blehar (eds.), *Seasonal Affective Disorders and Phototherapy,* pp. 64–78. Guilford Press, New York.

Thiessen, D. D., and Rodgers, D. A. 1961. Population density and endocrine function. *Psychol. Bull.,* 58:441–451.

Thomas, J. A., and Birney, E. C. 1979. Parental care and mating system of the prairie vole, *Microtus ochrogaster. Behav. Ecol. Sociobiol.,* 5:171–186.

Thomas, S. A., and Palmiter, R. D. 1997. Impaired maternal behavior in mice lacking norepinephrine and epinephrine. *Cell,* 91:583–592.

Thompson, C. I. 1980. *Controls of Eating.* Jamaica, New York, Spectrum.

Thompson, C. W., and Moore, M. C. 1992. Behavioral and hormonal correlates of alternative reproductive strategies in a polygynous lizard: tests of the relative plasticity and challenge hypotheses. *Horm. Behav.,* 26:568–585.

Thompson, C., Stinson, D., and Smith, A. 1990. Seasonal affective disorder and season-dependent abnormalities of melatonin suppression of light. *Lancet,* 336:703–706.

Thompson, D. A., Welle, S. L., Lilavivat, U., Pericaud, L., and Campbell, R. G. 1982. Opiate receptor blockade in man reduces 2-Deoxy-D-glucose induced food intake, but not hunger, thirst, and hypothermia. *Life Sci.,* 31:847–852.

Thrun, L. A., Dahl, G. E., Evans, N. P., and Karsch, F. J. 1997. Effect of thyroidectomy on maintenance of seasonal reproductive suppression in the ewe. *Biol. Reprod.,* 56:1035–1040.

Thys-Jacobs, S. and Alvir, M. J. 1995. Calcium-regulating hormones across the menstrual cycle: Evidence of a secondary hyperparathyroidism in women with PMS. *J. Clin. Endocrinol. Metab.,* 80:2227–2232.

Thys-Jacobs, S., Starkey, P., Bernstein, D., and Tian, J. 1998. Calcium carbonate and the premenstrual syndrome: Effects on premenstrual and menstrual symptoms. Premenstrual Syndrome Study Group. *Am. J. Obstet. Gynecol.,* 179:444–452.

Tian, M., Broxmeyer, H. E., Fan, Y., Lai, Z., Zhang, S., Aronica, S., Cooper, S., Bigsby, R. M., Steinmetz, R., Engle, S. J., Mestek, A., Pollock, J. D., Lehman, M. N., Jansen, H. T., Ying, M., Stambrook, P. J., Tischfield, J. A., and Yu, L. 1997. Altered hematopoiesis, behavior, and sexual function in μ-opioid receptor-deficient mice. *J. Exp. Med.,* 185:1517–1522.

Tiemstra, J. D. and Patel, K. 1998. Hormonal therapy in the management of premenstrual syndrome. *J. Am. Fam. Pract.,* 11:378–381.

Tinbergen, N. 1935. The behavior of the red-necked Phalarope in spring. *Ardea,* 24:1–42.

Tinbergen, N. 1951. *The Study of Instinct.* Oxford University Press, Oxford.

Toates, F. 1995. *Stress: Conceptual Biological Aspects.* Wiley: New York.

Tonegawa, S. 1995. Mammalian learning and memory studied by gene targeting. *Ann. N. Y. Acad. Sci.,* 758, 213–217.

Toran-Allerand, C. D. 1984. On the genesis of sexual differentiation of the central nervous system: Morphogenetic consequences of steroidal exposure and possible role of a-fetoprotein. In G. J. DeVries, J. P. C. DeBruin, H. B. M. Uylings, M. A. Corner (eds.), *Sex Differences in the Brain,* pp. 63–98. Elsevier, Amsterdam.

Tosini, G., and Menaker, M. 1998. The clock in the mouse retina: Melatonin synthesis and photoreceptor degeneration. *Brain Res.,* 789:221–228.

Toyoda, F., Tanaka, S., Matsuda, K., and Kikuyama, S. 1994. Hormonal control of response to and secretion of sex attractants in Japanese newts. *Physiol. Behav.,* 55:569–576.

Tramontin, A. D., and Brenowitz, E. A. 2000. Seasonal plasticity in the adult brain. *Trends in Neurosci.,* 23:251–258.

Trivers, R. L. 1972. Parental investment and sexual selection. In B. G. Campbell (ed.), *Sexual Selection and the Descent of Man.* 1871–1971, pp. 136–179. Aldine, Chicago.

Trobec, R. J., and Oring, L. W. 1972. Effects of testosterone propionate implantation on lek behavior of sharp-tailed grouse. *Am. Midland Nat.,* 87:531–536.

Truman, J. W. 1992. The eclosion hormone system of insects. *Progr. Brain Res.,* 92:361–374.

Trumbo, S. T. 1996. Parental care in invertebrates. *Adv. Study Behav.,* 25:3–51.

Trumbo, S. T. 1997. Juvenile hormone-mediated reproduction in burying beetles: From behavior to physiology. *Arch. Ins. Biochem. Physiol.,* 35:479–490.

Trumbo, S. T., Borst, D. W., and Robinson, G. E. 1995. Rapid elevation of juvenile hormone titer during behavioral assessment of the breeding resource by the burying beetle, *Nicrophorus orbicollis. J. Insect Physiol.,* 41:535–543.

Tsai, C. 1925. The relative strength of sex and hunger motives in the albino rat. *J. Comp. Psychol.,* 5:407.

Tsai, C. C., and Yen, S. S. 1971. Acute effects of intravenous infusion of 17-beta estradiol on gonadotropin release in pre- and postmenopausal women. *J. Clin. Endocrinol. Metab.,* 32:766–771.

Tserotas, K., and Merino, G. 1998. Andropause and the aging male. *Arch. Androl.,* 40:87–93.

Turek, F. W., and Campbell, C. S. 1979. Photoperiodic regulation of neuroendocrine-gonadal activity. *Biol. Reprod.,* 20:32–50.

Turek, F. W., Elliott, J. A., Alvis, J. D., and Menaker, M. 1975. The interaction of castration and photoperiod in the regulation of hypophyseal and serum gonadotropin levels in male golden hamsters. *Endocrinology,* 96:854–860.

Turner, B. N., Perrin, M. R., and Iverson, S. L. 1975. Winter coexistence of voles in spruce forest: Relevance of seasonal changes in aggression. *Can. J. Zool.,* 53:1004–1011.

Turner, C. D., and Bagnara, J. T. 1971. *General Endocrinology.* Saunders, Philadelphia.

Tuttle, W. W., and Dykshorn, S. 1928. The effect of castration and ovariectomy on spontaneous activity and ability to learn. *Proc. Soc. Exp. Biol. Med.,* 25:569–570.

Twiggs, D. G., Popolow, H. B., and Gerall, A. A. 1978. Medial preoptic lesions and male sexual behavior: Age and environmental interactions. *Science,* 200:1414–1415.

Tyler, S. J. 1972. The behaviour and social organization of the New Forest ponies. *Anim. Behav. Monogr.,* 5:87–196.

Tyndale-Biscoe, H., and Renfree, M. 1987. *Reproductive Physiology of Marsupials.* Cambridge University Press, Cambridge.

Tyrrell, C. L., and Cree, A. 1998. Relationships between corticosterone concentration and season, time of day and confinement in a wild reptile *(Tuatara, Sphenodon punctatus). Gen. Comp. Endocrinol.,* 110:97–108.

Udry, J. R., and Morris, N. M. 1968. Distribution of coitus in the menstrual cycle. *Nature,* 220:593–595.

Uhrich, J. 1938. The social hierarchy in albino mice. *J. Comp. Psychol.,* 23:373–413.

Uno, H., Tarara, R., Else, J. G., Suleman, M. A., and Sapolsky, R. M. 1989. Hippocampal damage associated with prolonged and fatal stress in primates. *J. Neurosci.,* 9:1705–1711.

Ursin, H., Baade, E., and Levine, S. 1978. *Psychobiology of Stress: A Study of Coping Men.* Academic Press: London.

Ussher, J. 1989. *The Psychology of the Female Body.* Routledge, New York.

Valenstein, E. S., and Young, W. C. 1955. An experiential factor influencing the effectiveness of testosterone proprionate in eliciting sexual behavior in male guinea pigs. *Endocrinology,* 56:173–185.

Valenstein, E. S., Kakolewski, J. V., and Cox, V. C. 1967. Sex differences in taste preference for glucose and saccharine solutions. *Science,* 156:942–943.

Van de Kar, L. D., Richardson-Morton, K. D., and Rittenhouse, P. A. 1991. Stress: Neuroendocrine and pharmacological mechanisms. In G. Jasmin and M. Cantin (eds.). *Stress Revisited: Neuroendocrinology of Stress. Methods and Achievements in Experimental Pathology,* Vol 14:133–173. Karger, Basel.

van der Lee, S., and Boot, L. M. 1955. Spontaneous pseudopregnancy in mice. *Acta Physiol. Pharmacol. Neer.,* 4:442–443.

Van Dis, H., and Larsson, K. 1971. Induction of sexual arousal in the castrated male rat by intracranial stimulation. *Physiol. Behav.,* 6:85–86.

van Furth, W. R., Wolterink, G., and van Ree, J. M. 1995. Regulation of masculine sexual behavior: Involvement of brain opioids and dopamine. *Brain Res. Rev.,* 21:162–184.

Van Goozen, S. H., Wiegant, V. M., Endert, E., Helmond, F. A., and Van de Poll, N. E. 1997. Psychoendocrinological assessment of the menstrual cycle: the relationship between hormones, sexuality, and mood. *Arch. of Sex. Behav.,* 26:359–382.

Van Leeuwen, F. W., Caffe, A. R., and DeVries, G. J. 1985. Vasopressin cells in the bed nucleus of the stria terminalis of the rat: Sex differences and the influence of androgens. *Brain Res.,* 325:391–394.

Van Oers, H. J., de Kloet, E. R., Whelan, T., and Levine, S. 1998. Maternal deprivation effect on the infant's neural stress markers is reversed by tactile stimulation and feeding but not by suppressing corticosterone. *J. Neurosci.,* 18:10171–10179.

van Tienhoven, A. 1983. *Reproductive Physiology of Vertebrates.* Cornell University Press, Ithaca.

Vancassel, M., Foraste, M., Strambi, A., and Strambi, C. 1984. Normal and experimentally induced changes in hormonal hemolymph titres during parental behavior of the earwig, *Labidura riparia. Gen. Comp. Endocrinol.,* 56:444–456.

Vandenbergh, J. G. 1967. Effect of the presence of a male on the sexual maturation of female mice. *Endocrinology,* 81:345–349.

Vandenbergh, J. G. 1969. Endocrine coordination in monkeys: Male sexual responses to the female. *Physiol. Behav.,* 4:261–264.

Vandenbergh, J. G. 1983. Pheromonal regulation of puberty. In J. G. Vandenbergh (ed.), *Pheromones and Reproduction in Mammals,* pp. 95–112. Academic Press, New York.

Vandenbergh, J. G. 1994. Pheromones. In E. Knobil and J. D. Neill (eds.). *The Physiology of Reproduction.* (2nd ed.), pp. 343–359. Raven Press, New York.

Veldhuis, J. D., Evans, W. S., Demers, L. M., Thorner, M. O., Wakat, D., and Rogol, A. D. 1985. Altered neuroendocrine regulation of gonadotropin secretion in women distance runners. *J. Clin. Endocrinol. Metab.,* 61:557–563.

Velle, W. 1987. Sex differences in sensory functions. *Perspect. Biol. Med.,* 30: 490–522.

Vergnes, M., Depaulis, A., and Boehrer, A. 1986. Parachlorophenylalanine-induced seratonin depletion increases offensive but not defensive aggression in male rats. *Physiol. Behav.,* 36(4):653–658.

Vermeulen, A., Rubens, R., and Verdonck, L. 1972. Testosterone secretion and metabolism in male senescence. *J. Clin. Endocrinol. Metab.,* 34:730–735.

Viau, V., and Meaney, M. J. 1991. Variations in the hypothalamic-pituitary-adrenal response to stress during the estrous cycle of the adult rat. *J. Neurosci.,* 12:2503–2511.

Virgin, C. E., and Sapolsky, R. M. 1997. Styles of male social behavior and their endocrine correlates among low-ranking baboons. *Am. J. Primatol.,* 42:25–39.

vom Saal, F. S. 1979. Prenatal exposure to androgen influences morphology and aggressive behavior of male and female mice. *Horm. Behav.,* 12:1–11.

vom Saal, F. S., and Bronson, F. H. 1980. Variation in length of the estrous cycle in mice due to former uterine proximity to male fetuses. *Biol. Reprod.,* 22:777–780.

vom Saal, F. S., and Finch, C. E. 1988. Reproductive senescence: Phenomena and mechanisms in mammals and selected vertebrates. In E. Knobil and J. Neill (eds.), *Physiology of Reproduction,* pp. 2351– 2413. Raven Press, New York.

Waber, D. 1976. Sex differences in cognition: A function of maturation rate. *Science,* 192:572–574.

Wada, J. A. 1976. *Sex differences in brain asymmetry.* International Neuropsychological Society, Toronto.

Wada, J. A., Clarke, R. A., and Hamm, A. 1975. Cerebral hemisphere asymmetry in humans. Cortical speech zones in 100 adult and 100 infant brains. *Arch. Neurol.,* 32:239–246.

Wade, G. N. 1972. Gonadal hormones and behavioral regulation of body weight. *Physiol. Behav.,* 8:523–534.

Wade, G. N. 1976. Sex hormones, regulatory behaviors and body weight. *Adv. Study Behav.,* 6:201–279.

Wade, G. N. 1986. Sex steroids and energy balance: Sites and mechanisms of action. *Ann. N. Y. Acad. Sci.,* 474:389–399.

Wade, G. N., and Gray, J. M. 1978. Cytoplasmic 17β-[3H]estradiol binding in rat adipose tissues. *Endocrinology,* 103:1695–1701.

Wade, G. N., and Gray, J. M. 1979. Gonadal effects on food intake and adiposity: A metabolic hypothesis. *Physiol. Behav.,* 22:583–593.

Wade, G. N., and Zucker, I. 1970. Modulation of food intake and locomotor activity in female rats by diencephalic hormone implants. *J. Comp. Physiol. Psychol.,* 72:328–336.

Wade, G. N., Jennings, G., and Trayhurn, P. 1986. Energy balance and brown adipose tissue thermogenesis during pregnancy in Syrian hamsters. *Am. J. Physiol.,* 250:R845–R850.

Wade, G. N., Lempicki, R. L., Panicker, A. K., Frisbee, R. M., and Blaustein, J. D. 1997. Leptin facilitates and inhibits sexual behavior in female hamsters. *Am. J. Physiol.,* 272:R1354–R1358.

Wade, J., and Arnold, A. P. 1996. Functional testicular tissue does not masculinize development of the zebra finch song system. *Proc. Natl. Acad. Sci. U.S.A.,* 93:5264–5268.

Wahlstrom, G. 1965. *Circadian Clocks.* North-Holland, Amsterdam.

Walker, W. A., and Feder, H. H. 1977. Inhibitory and facilitory effects of various anti-estrogens on the induction of female sexual behavior by estradiol benzoate in guinea pigs. *Brain Res.,* 134:455–465.

Walker, W. A., and Feder, H. H. 1979. The comparative potency of various steroids to complete the priming process for lordosis in guinea pigs. *Horm. Behav.,* 12:299–308.

Wallen, K. 1990. Desire and ability: Hormones and the regulation of female sexual behavior. *Neurosci. Biobehav. Rev.,* 14:233–241.

Wallen, K., and Goy, R. W. 1977. Effects of estradiol benzoate, estrone, and propionates of testosterone or dihydrotestosterone on sexual and related behaviors of ovariectomized rhesus monkeys. *Horm. Behav.,* 9:228–248.

Wallen, K., Winston, L. A., Gaventa, S., Davis-DaSilva, M., and Collins, D.C. 1984. Periovulatory changes in female sexual behavior in group-living rhesus monkeys. *Horm. Behav.,* 18:431–450.

Wang, C., and Swerdloff, R. S. 1997. Androgen replacement therapy. *Ann. Med.,* 29:365–370.

Wang, G. H. 1923. The relation between 'spontaneous' activity and oestrous cycle in the white rat. *Comp. Psychol. Monogr.,* 2:1–27.

Wang, G. H. 1924. The changes in the amount of daily food-intake of the albino rat during pregnancy and lactation. *Am. J. Physiol.,* 71:735–741.

Wang, Z., and Young, L. J. 1997. Ontogeny of oxytocin and vasopressin receptor binding in the lateral septum in prairie and montane voles. *Brain Res.: Dev. Brain Res.,* 104:191–195.

Ward, I. L. 1984. The prenatal stress syndrome: Current status. *Psychoneuroendocrinology,* 9:3–11.

Ward, I. L. 1992. Sexual behavior: The product of perinatal hormonal and prepubertal social factors. In *Sexual Differentiation,* Vol. 11 of *Handbook of Behavioral Neurobiology,* edited by A. A. Gerall, H. Moltz, and I. L. Ward, Plenum Press: New York.

Ward, I. L., and Reed, J. 1985. Prenatal stress and prepubertal social rearing conditions interact to determine sexual behavior in male rats. *Behav. Neurosci.,* 99:301–309.

Ward, I. L., and Stehm, K. E. 1991. Prenatal stress feminizes juvenile play patterns in male rats. *Physiol. Behav.,* 50:601–605.

Ward, I. L., and Weisz, J. 1980. Maternal stress alters plasma testosterone in fetal males. *Science,* 207:328–329.

Ward, I. L., Ward, O. B., French, J. A., Hendricks, S. E., Mehan, D., and Winn, R. J. 1996. Prenatal alcohol and stress interact to attenuate ejaculatory behavior, but not serum testosterone or LH in adult male rats. *Behav. Neurosci.,* 110:1469–1477.

Ward, I. L., Ward, O. B., Winn, R. J., and Bielawski, D. 1994. Male and female sexual behavior potential of male rats prenatally exposed to the influence of alcohol, stress, or both factors. *Behav. Neurosci.,* 108:1188–1195.

Ward, O. B., Wexler, A. M., Carlucci, J. R., Eckert, M. A., and Ward, I. L. 1996. Critical periods of sensitivity of sexually dimorphic spinal nuclei to prenatal testosterone exposure in female rats. *Horm. Behav.,* 30:407–415.

Ward, P. 1965. Seasonal changes in the sex ratio of Quelea quelea. *Ibis,* 107:397–399.

Warden, C. J., Jenkins, T. N., and Warner, L. H. 1935. *Comparative Psychology: A Comprehensive Treatise: Principles and Methods.* Vol. 1. Ronald Press: New York, NY.

Warner, L. H. 1927. A study of sex behavior in the white rat by means of the obstruction method. *Comp. Psychol. Monogr.,* 4:1–68.

Warren, M. P., and Shortle, B. 1990. Endocrine correlates of human parenting. In N. A. Krasnegor and R. S. Bridges (eds.), *Mammalian Parenting,* pp. 209–230. Oxford University Press, Oxford.

Warren, S. G., and Juraska, J. M. 1997. Spatial and nonspatial learning across the rat estrous cycle. *Behav. Neurosci.,* 111:259–266.

Warren, S. G., Humphreys, A. G., Juraska, J. M., and Greenough, W. T. 1995. LTP varies across the estrous cycle: Enhanced synaptic plasticity in proestrus rats. *Brain Res.,* 703:26–30.

Watanabe, Y., Gould, E., and McEwen, B. S. 1992. Stress induces atrophy of apical dendrites of hippocampal CA3 pyramidal neurons. *Brain Res.,* 588:341–345.

Waterhouse, J., Reilly, T., and Atkinson, G. 1998. Melatonin and jet lag. *Br. J. Sports Med.,* 32:98–99.

Watson, J. S. 1969. Operant conditioning of visual fixation in infants under visual and auditory reinforcement. *Dev. Psychol.,* 1:508–516.

Watson, J. T., and Adkins-Regan, E. 1989. Testosterone implanted in the preoptic area of male Japanese quail must be aromatized to activate copulation. *Horm. Behav.,* 23:432–447.

Wayne, N. L., Malpaux, B., and Karsch, F. J. 1988. How does melatonin code for day length in the ewe: Duration of nocturnal melatonin release or coincidence of melatonin with a light-entrained sensitive period. *Biol. Reprod.,* 39:66–75.

Weatherford, S. C., Laughton, W. B., Salabarria, J., Danho, W., Tilley, J. W., Netterville, L. A., Schwartz, G. J., and Moran, T. H. 1993. CCK satiety is differentially mediated by high- and low-affinity CCK receptors in mice and rats. *Am. J. Physiol.,* 264:R244–R249.

Weaver, D. R., Provencio, I., Carlson, L. L., and Reppert, S. M. 1991. Melatonin receptors and signal transduction in photorefractory Siberian hamsters (*Phodopus sungorus*). *Endocrinology,* 128:1086–1092.

Weaver, D. R., Rivkees, S. A., and Reppert, S. M. 1989. Localization and characterization of melatonin receptors in rodent brain by in vitro autoradiography. *J. Neurosci.,* 9:2581–2590.

Wehr, T. A. 1998. Effect of seasonal changes in daylength on human neuroendocrine functions. *Horm. Res.,* 49:118–124.

Wehr, T. A., Wirz-Justice, A., Goodwin, F. K., Duncan, W., and Gillin, J. C. 1979. Phase advance of the circadian sleep-wake cycle as an antidepressant. *Science,* 206:710–713.

Weigle, D. S., Bukowski, T. R., Foster, D.C., Holderman, S., Kramer, J. M., Lasser, G., Lofton-Day, C. E., Prunkard, D. E., Raymond, C., and Kuijper, J. L. 1995. Recombinant ob protein reduces feeding and body weight in the ob/ob mouse. *J. Clin. Inv.,* 96:2065–2070.

Weil-Malharbe, H., Axelrod, J., and Tomchick, R. 1959. Blood-brain barrier for adrenaline. *Science,* 129:1226–1228.

Weinstock, M. 1997. Does prenatal stress impair coping and regulation of hypothalmic-pituitary-adrenal axis. *Neurosci. Biobehav. Rev.,* 21:1–10.

Weisinger, R. S., Considine, P., Denton, D. A., Leksell, L, McKinley, M. J., Mouw, D. R., Muller, A. F., and Tarjan, E. 1982. Role of sodium concentration of the cerebrospinal fluid in the salt appetite of sheep. *Am. J. Physiol.,* 242:R51–R63.

Weiss, J. M. 1968. Effects of coping response on stress. *J. Comp. Physiol. Psychol.,* 65:251–260.

Weiss, J. M. 1972. Biological factors in stress and disease. *Sci. Am.,* 226:104–113.

Weller, A., and Blass, E. M. 1988. Behavioral evidence for cholecystokinin-opiate interactions in neonatal rats. *Am. J. Physiol.,* 255:R901–907.

Weller, A., and Blass, E. M. 1990. Cholecystokinin conditioning in rats: Ontogenesis determinants. *Behav. Neurosci.,* 104:199–206.

Welsh, T. H., Kemper-Green, C. N., and Livingston, K. N. 1999. Stress and reproduction. In E. Knobil and J. D. Neill (eds.). *Encyclopedia of Reproduction,* pp. 662–674. Academic Press, San Diego.

Werren, J. H., Gross, M. R., and Shine, R. 1980. Paternity and the evolution of male parental care. *J. Theor. Biol.,* 82:619–631.

West, S. D., and Dublin, H. T. 1984. Behavioral strategies of small mammals under winter conditions: Solitary or social? *Bull. Carnegie Museum Nat. Hist.,* 10:293–300.

Wever, R. A. 1989. Light effects on human circadian rhythms: A review of recent Andechs experiments. *J. Biol. Rhythms,* 4:161–185.

Wever, R. A., Polasek, J., and Wildgruber, C. M. 1983. Bright light affects human circadian rhythms. *Pflugers Arch.,* 396:85–87.

Whalen, R. E., and Johnson, F. 1987. Individual differences in the attack behavior of male mice: A function of attack stimulus and hormonal state. *Horm. Behav.,* 21:223–233.

White, G. F., Katz, J., and Scarborough, K. E. 1992. The impact of professional football games upon violent assaults on women. *Violence Victims,* 7:157–171.

Whitfield-Rucker, M., and Cassone, V. 1996. Melatonin binding in the house sparrow song control system: sexual dimorphism and the effect of photoperiod. *Horm. Behav.,* 30:528–37.

Whitten, W. K. 1956a. The effect of removal of the olfactory bulbs on the gonads of mice. *J. Endocrinol.,* 14:160–163.

Whitten, W. K. 1956b. Modification of the oestrus cycle of the mouse by external stimuli associated with the male. *J. Endocrinol.,* 13:399–404.

Whitten, W. K. 1957. Effect of exteroceptive factors on the oestrus cycle of mice. *Nature,* 180:1456–1457.

Whittenberger, J. R., and Tilson, R. L. 1980. The evolution of monogamy: Hypotheses and evidence. *Annu. Rev. Ecol. Syst.,* 11:197–232.

Widdowson, E. 1951. Mental contentment and physical growth. *Lancet,* (13 June), 1316–1328.

Widowski, T. M., Porter, T. A., Ziegler, T. E., and Snowdon, C. T. 1992. The stimulatory effect of males on the initiation, but not the maintenance of ovarian cycling in cotton-top tamarins (*Saguinus oedipus*). *Am. J. Primatol.,* 26:97–108.

Wiesner, B. P., and Mirskaia, L. 1930. *Q. J. Exp. Physiol.,* 20:273–294.

Wiesner, B. P., and Sheard, N. M. 1933. *Maternal Behavior in Rats.* Oliver and Boyd, London.

Wilkins, L., and Richter, C. P. 1940. A great craving for salt by a child with cortico-adrenal insufficiency. *J. A. M. A.,* 114:866–868.

Williams, C. L. 1996. Short-term but not long-term estradiol replacement improvs radial arm maze performance of young and aging rats. *Soc. Neurosci. Abstr.,* 22:1164.

Williams, C. L., and Meck, W. H. 1991. The organizational effects of gonadal steroids on sexually dimorphic spatial ability. *Psychoneuroendocrinology,* 16:155–176.

Williams, C. L., Barnett, A. M., Meck, W. H. 1990. Organizational effects of early gonadal secretions on sexual differentiation in spatial memory. *Behav. Neurosci.,* 104:84–97.

Williams, J. R., Catania, K. C., and Carter, C. S. 1992. Development of partner preferences in female prairie voles (*Microtus ochrogaster*): The role of social and sexual experience. *Horm. Behav.,* 26:339–349.

Williams, J. R., Insel, T. R., Harbaugh, C. R., and Carter, C. S. 1994. Oxytocin centrally administered facilitates formation of a partner preference in female prairie voles (*Microtus ochrogaster*). *J. Neuroendocrinol.,* 6:247–250.

Wilson, A. P., and Vessey, S. H. 1968. Behavior of free-ranging castrated rhesus monkeys. *Folia Primatol.,* 9:1–14.

Wilson, E. O. 1975. *Sociobiology.* Belknap Press of Harvard University Press, Cambridge, MA.

Wilson, J. D., George, F. W., and Griffin, J. E. 1981. The hormonal control of sexual development. *Science,* 211:1278–1284.

Wilson, J. R., Adler, N., and LeBoeuf, B. 1965. The effects of intromission frequency on successful pregnancy in the female rat. *Proc. Natl. Acad. Sci. U.S.A.,* 53:1392–1395.

Winans, S. S., and Powers, J. B. 1974. Neonatal and two-stage olfactory bulbectomy: Effects on male hamster sexual behavior. *Behav. Biol.,* 10:461–471.

Wingfield, J. C. 1988. Changes in reproductive function of free-living birds in direct response to environmental perturbations. In M. H. Stetson (ed.), *Processing of Environmental Information in Vertebrates,* pp. 121–148. Springer-Verlag, Berlin.

Wingfield, J. C., and Farner, D. S. 1980. Control of seasonal reproduction in temperate-zone birds. *Prog. Reprod. Biol.,* 5:62–101.

Wingfield, J. C., and Moore, M. C. 1987. Hormonal, social, and environmental factors in the reproductive biology of free-living male birds. In D. Crews (ed.), *Psychobiology of Reproductive Behavior,* pp. 148–175. Prentice Hall, Englewood Cliffs, NJ.

Wingfield, J. C., and Wada, M. 1989. Changes in plasma levels of testosterone during male–male interactions in the song sparrow, Melospiza melodia: Time course and specificity of response. *J. Comp. Physiol. A,* 166:189–194.

Wingfield, J. C., Ball, G. F., Dufty, A. M., Hegner, R. E., and Ramenofsky, M. 1987. Testosterone and aggression in birds. *Am. Sci.,* 75:602–608.

Wingfield, J. C., Deviche, P., Sharbaugh, S., Astheimer, L. B., Holberton, R., Suydam, R., and Hunt, K. 1994. Seasonal-changes of the adrenocortical responses to stress in redpolls, *Acanthis flammea*, in Alaska. *J. Exp. Zool.*, 270:372–380.

Wingfield, J. C., Hegner, R. E., Dufty, A. M., and Ball, G. F. 1990. The "challenge hypothesis": Theoretical implications for patterns of testosterone secretion, mating systems, and breeding strategies. *Am. Nat.*, 136:829–846.

Wingfield, J. C., Jacobs, J., and Hillgarth, N. 1997. Ecological constraints and the evolution of hormone-behavior interrelationships. *Ann. N. Y. Acad. Sci.*, 807:22–41.

Wingfield, J. C., Whaling, C. S., and Marler, P. 1994. Communication in vertebrate aggression and reproduction: The role of hormones. In E. Knobil and J. D. Neill (eds.), *The Physiology of Reproduction* (2nd ed.), pp. 303–342. Raven Press, New York.

Winslow, J. T., Hastings, N., Carter, C. S., Harbaugh, C. R., and Insel, T. R. 1993. A role for central vasopressin in pair bonding monogamous prairie voles. *Nature*, 365:545–548.

Wirz-Justice, A., Bucheli, C., Graw, P., Kielholz, P., Fisch, H. U., and Woggon, B. 1986. Light treatment of seasonal affective disorder in Switzerland. *Acta Psychiatrica Scand.*, 74:193–204.

Wirz-Justice, A., Cajochen, C., and Nussbaum, P. 1997. A schizophrenic patient with an arrhythmic circadian rest-activity cycle. *Psychiatry Res.*, 14:83–90.

Wise, D. A., and Pryor, T. L. 1977. Effects of ergocornine and prolactin on aggression in the postpartum golden hamster. *Horm. Behav.*, 8:30–39.

Wise, R. A. 1996. Neurobiology of addiction. *Curr. Opin. Neurobiol.*, 6:243–251.

Wise, R. A., and Rompre, P. P. 1989. Brain dopamine and reward. *Annu. Rev. Psychol.*, 40: 191–225.

Wisniewski, A. B. 1998. Sexually-dimorphic patterns of cortical asymmetry, and the role for sex steroid hormones in determining cortical patterns of lateralization. *Psychoneuroendocrinology*, 23:519–547.

Witkin, H. A., Mednick, S. A., Schulsinger, F., Bakkestrom, E., Christiansen, K. O., Goodenough, D. R., Hirschhorn, K., Lundsteen, C., Owens, D. R., Philip, J. et al., 1976. Criminality in XYY and XXY men. *Science*, 193:547–555.

Wolff, E., and Wolff, E. 1951. The effects of castration on bird embryos. *J. Exp. Zool.*, 116:59–97.

Wolff, J. O. 1985. Behavior. In R. H. Tamarkin (ed.). *Biology of New World* Microtus. American Society of Mammalogists, Shippensberg, PA.

Wolters, C. A., Yu, S. L., Hagen, J. W., and Kail, R. 1996. Short-term memory and strategy use in children with insulin-dependent diabetes mellitus. *J. Consult. Clin. Psychol.*, 64:1397–1405.

Wong, M., and Moss, R. L. 1992. Long-term and short-term electrophysiological effects of estrogen on the synaptic properties of hippocampal CA1 neurons. *J. Neurosci.*, 12:3217–3225.

Wong, M., Thompson, T. L., and Moss, R. L. 1996. Nongenomic actions of estrogen in the brain: physiological significance and cellular mechanisms. *Crit. Rev. Neurobiol.*, 10:189–203.

Wood, D. L., Sheps, S. G., Elveback, L. R., and Schirder, A. 1984. Cold pressor test as a predictor of hypertension. *Hypertension*, 6:301–306.

Wood, G. E., and Shors, T. J. 1998. Stress facilitates classical conditioning in males, but impairs classical conditioning in females through activational effects of ovarian hormones. *Proc. Natl. Acad. Sci. U.S.A.*, 95:4066–4071.

Wood, R. I. 1997. Thinking about networks in the control of male hamster sexual behavior. *Horm. Behav.*, 32:40–45.

Woods, S. C., and Porte, D. 1983. The role of insulin as a satiety factor in the central nervous system. *Adv. Metab. Disord.*, 10:457–468.

Woods, S. C., Chavez, M., Park, C. R., Riedy, C., Kaiyala, K., Richardson, R. D., Figlewicz, D. P., Schwartz, M. W., Porte, D. Jr, and Seeley, R. J. 1996. The evaluation of insulin as a metabolic signal influencing behavior via the brain. *Neurosci. Biobehav. Rev.*, 20:139–144.

Woods, S. C., Figlewicz, D. P., Madden, L., Porte, D., Sipols, A. J., and Seeley, R. J. 1998. NPY and food intake: Discrepancies in the model. *Regul. Pept.*, 75:403–408.

Woods, S. C., Lotter, E. C., McKay, L. D., and Porte, D. 1979. Chronic intracerebroventricular infusion of insulin reduces food intake and body weight of baboons. *Nature*, 282:503–505.

Woods, S. C., West, D. B., Stein, L. J., McKay, L. D., Lotter, E. C., Porte, S. G., Kenney, N. J., and Porte, D., Jr. 1981. Peptides and the control of meal size. *Diabetologia*, 20:305–313.

Woodside, B., and Leon, M. 1980. Thermoendocrine influences on maternal nesting behavior in rats. *J. Comp. Physiol. Psychol.*, 94:41–60.

Woodside, B., Pelchat, R., and Leon, M. 1980. Acute elevation of the heat load of mother rats curtails maternal nest bouts. *J. Comp. Physiol. Psychol.*, 94:61–68.

Woolley, C. S. 1998. Estrogen-mediated structural and functional synaptic plasticity in the female rat hippocampus. *Horm. Behav.*, 34:140–148.

Woolley, C. S., Gould, E., and McEwen, B. S. 1990b. Naturally occurring fluctuations in the dendritic spine density in adult hippocampal neurons. *J. Neurosci.*, 10:4035–4039.

Woolley, C. S., Gould, E., and McEwen, B. S. 1990a. Exposure to excess glucocorticoids alters dendritic morphology of adult hippocampal pyramidal neurons. *Brain Res.*, 531:225–231.

Worrall, G. J., Chaulk, P. C., and Moulton, N. 1996. Cognitive function and glycosylated hemoglobin in older patients with type II diabetes. *J. Diabetes Complications*, 10:320—24.

Worthy, K., Haresign, W., Dodson, S., McLeod, B. J., Foxcroft, G. R., and Haynes, N. B. 1985. Evidence that the onset of the breeding season in the ewe may be independent of decreasing plasma prolactin concentrations. *J. Reprod. Fertil.*, 75:237–246.

Wu, F. C. 1997. Endocrine aspects of anabolic steroids. *Clin. Chem.*, 43:1289–1292.

Wurtman, J. J., Wurtman, R. J., Mark, S., Tsay, R., Gilbert, W., and Growdon, J. 1985. D-Fenfluramine selectively suppresses carbohydrate snacking by obese subjects. *Int. J. Eat. Disord.*, 4:89–99.

Wurtman, R. J. 1975. The effects of light on man and other animals. *Annu. Rev. Physiol.*, 37:467–83.

Wurtman, R. J., and Wurtman, J. J. 1989. Carbohydrates and Depression. *Sci. Am.*, 68:68–75.

Wuttke, W., Arnold, P., Becker, D., Creutzfeldt, O., Langenstein, S., and Tirsch, W. 1975. Circulating hormones, EEG and performance in psychological tests of women with and without oral contraceptives. *Psychoneuroendocrinology*, 1:141–151.

Wynne-Edwards, K. E. 1998. Evolution of parental care in *Phodopus*: Conflict between adaptations for survival and adaptations for rapid reproduction. *Am. Zool.*, 38:238–250

Wynne-Edwards, K. E., Terranova, P. F., and Lisk, R. D. 1987. Cyclic Djungarian hamsters, Phodopus campbelli, lack the progesterone surge normally associated with ovulation and behavioral receptivity. *Endocrinology*, 120:1308–1316.

Wynne-Edwards, V. C. 1965. Self-regulating systems in populations of animals. *Science*, 147:1543–1548.

Wysocki, C. J. 1979. Neurobehavioral evidence for the involvement of the vomeronasal system in mammalian reproduction. *Neurosci. Biobehav. Rev.*, 3:301–341.

Wysocki, C. J., and Lepri, J. J. 1991. Consequences of removing the vomeronasal organ. *J. Steroid Biochem. Mol. Biol.*,39:661–669.

Wysocki, C. J., Katz, Y., and Bernhard, R. 1983. Male vomeronasal organ mediates female-induced testosterone surges in mice. *Biol. Reprod.*, 28:917–922.

Xiao, E., and Ferin, M. 1997. Stress-related disturbances of the menstrual cycle. *Ann. Med.*, 29:215–219.

Yalcinkaya, T. M., Siiteri, P. K., Vigne, J. L., Licht, P., Pavgi, S., Frank, L. G., and Glickman, S. E. 1993. A mechanism for virilization of female spotted hyenas in utero. *Science*, 25;260:1929–1931.

Yamanouchi, K. 1980. Inhibitory and facilitatory neural mechanisms involved in the regulation of lordosis behavior in female rats: effects of dual cuts in the preoptic area and hypothalamus. *Physiol. Behav.*, 25:721–725.

Yamanouchi, K., and Arai, Y. 1980. Inhibitory and facilitory neural mechanisms involved in the regulation of lordosis behavior in female rats: Effects of dual cuts in the preoptic area and hypothalamus. *Physiol. Behav.*, 25:721–725.

Yang, L. Y., and Clemens, L. G. 1996. Relation of intromissions to the female's postejaculatory refractory period in rats. *Physiol. Behav.*, 60:1505–1511.

Yarbrough, W. G., Quarmby, V. E., Simental, J. A., Joseph, D. R., Sar, M., Lubahn, D. B., Olsen, K. L., French, F. S., and Wilson, E. M. 1990. A single base mutation in the androgen receptor gene causes insensitivity in the testicular feminized rat. *J. Biol. Chem.*, 265:8893–8900.

Yaskin, V. A. 1984. Seasonal changes in brain morphology in small mammals. In J. F. Merrit (ed.), *Winter Ecology of Small Mammals*, pp. 183–189. Special Publication of the Carnegie Museum of Natural History, No. 10.

Yehuda, R., Giller, E. L., and Mason, J. W. 1993. Psychoneuroendocrine assessment of posttraumatic stress disorder: Current progress and new directions. *Prog. Neuropsychopharmacol. Biol. Psychiatry*, 17:541–550.

Yehuda, R., Kahana, B., Binder-Brynes, K., Southwick, S. M., Mason, J. W., and Giller, E. L. 1995. Low urinary cortisol excretion in Holocaust survivors with posttraumatic stress disorder. *Am. J. Psychiatry,* 152:982–986.

Yellon, S. M., Hutchison, J. S., and Goldman, B. D. 1989. Sexual differentiation of the steroid feedback mechanism regulating follicle-stimulating hormone secretion in the Syrian hamster. *Biol. Reprod.,* 41:7–14.

Yen, S. S. C., and Jaffe, R. B. 1991. *Reproductive Endocrinology.* (3rd ed.). Saunders, San Francisco,

Yen, S. S., Morales, A. J., and Khorram, O. 1995. Replacement of DHEA in aging men and women. Potential remedial effects. *Ann. N. Y. Acad. Sci. ,* 774:128–142.

Yerkes, R. M., and Dodson, J. D. 1908. The relation of strength of stimulus to rapidity of habit formation. *J. Comp. Neurol. Psychol.,* 18:458–482.

Yerkes, R. M., and Elder, J. H. 1936. Oestrus, receptivity, and mating in chimpanzee. *Comp. Psychol. Monogr.,* 13:1–39.

Yesalis, C. E., Barsukiewicz, C. K., Kopstein, A. N., and Bahrke, M. S. 1997. Trends in anabolic-androgenic steroid use among adolescents. *Arch. Pediatr. Adolesc. Med.,* 151:1197–1206.

Yirmiya, R., Avitsur, R., Donchin, O., and Cohen, E. 1995. Interleukin-1 inhibits sexual behavior in female but not in male rats. *Brain Behav. Immunity,* 9:220–233.

Yogman, M. W. 1990. Male parental behavior in humans and nonhuman primates. In N. A. Krasnegor and R. S. Bridges (eds.), *Mammalian Parenting,* pp. 461–481. Oxford University Press, Oxford.

Yokosuka, M., Xu, B., Pu, S., Kalra, P. S., and Kalra, S. P. 1998. Neural substrates for leptin and neuropeptide Y (NPY) interaction: Hypothalamic sites associated with inhibition of NPY-induced food intake. *Physiol. Behav.,* 64:331–338.

Yonkers, K. A. 1997. Antidepressants in the treatment of premenstrual dysphoric disorder. *J. Clin. Psychiatry,* 58:4–10.

Young, E. and Korszun, A. 1998. Psychoneuroendocrinology of depression. Hypothalamic-pituitary-gonadal axis. *Psychiatry Clin. North Am.,* 21:309–323.

Young, I. M. 1990. *Justice and the Politics of Difference.* Princeton University Press, Princeton.

Young, L. J., Winslow, J. T., Wang, Z., Gingrich, B., Guo, Q., Matzuk, M. M., and Insel, T. R. 1997. Gene targeting approaches to neuroendocrinology: Oxytocin, maternal behavior, and affiliation. *Horm. Behav.,* 31:221–231.

Young, W. C. 1937. The vaginal smear picture, sexual receptivity, and the time of ovulation in the guinea pig. *Anat. Rec.,* 67:305–539.

Young, W. C. 1961. The hormones and mating behavior. In W. C. Young (ed.), *Sex and Internal Secretions,* Vol. 2, pp. 1173–1239. Williams & Wilkins, Baltimore.

Young, W. C., and Plough, H. H. 1926. On the sterilization of *Drosophila* by high temperature. *Biol. Bull.,* 51:189–198.

Young, W. C., Dempsey, E. W., and Myers, H. I. 1935. Cyclic reproductive behavior in the female guinea pig. *J. Comp. Psychol.,* 19:313–335.

Young, W. C., Dempsey, E. W., Hagquist, C. W., and Boling, J. L. 1939. Sexual behavior and sexual receptivity in the female guinea pig. *J. Comp. Psychol.,* 27:49–68.

Young, W. C., Dempsey, E. W., Myers, H. I., and Hagquist, C. W. 1938. The ovarian condition and sexual behavior in the female guinea pig. *Am. J. Anat.,* 63:457–487.

Youngstrom, T. G., Weiss, M. L., and Nunez, A. A. 1987. A retinal projection to the paraventricular nuclei of the hypothalamus in the Syrian hamster (*Mesocricetus auratus*). *Brain Res. Bull.,* 19:747–750.

Youthed, G. J., and Moran, R. C. 1969. The lunar day activity rhythm of myrmeleontid larvae. *J. Insect Physiol.,* 15:1259–1271.

Zahavi, A., and Zahavi, A. 1997. *The Handicap Principle.* Oxford University Press: New York.

Zamorano, P. L., Mahesh, V. B., DeSevilla, L. M., horich, L. P., Bhat, G. K., and Brann, D. W. 1997. Expression and localization of the leptin receptor in endocrine and neuroendocrine tissues of the rat. *Neuroendocrinology,* 65:223–228.

Zarrow, M. X., Denenberg, V. H., and Anderson, C. O. 1965. Rabbit: Frequency of suckling in the pup. *Science,* 150:1835–1836.

Zarrow, M. X., Farooq, A., Denenberg, V. H., Sawin, P. B., and Ross, S. 1963. Maternal behaviour in the rabbit: Endocrine control of maternal-nest building. *J. Reprod. Fertil.,* 6:375–383.

Zarrow, M. X., Gandelman, R., and Denenberg, V. H. 1971. Prolactin: Is it an essential hormone for maternal behavior in the mammal? *Horm. Behav.,* 2:343–354.

Zehr, J. L., Maestripieri, D., and Wallen, K. 1998. Estradiol increases female sexual initiation independent of male responsiveness in rhesus monkeys. *Horm. Behav.,* 33:95–103.

Zhang, S. D., and Odenwald, W. F. 1995. Misexpression of the white (*w*) gene triggers male-male courtship in Drosophila. *Proc. Natl. Acad. Sci. U.S.A.,* 92:5525–5529.

Zhang, S., McGaugh, J. L., Juler, R. G., and Introini-Collison, I. B. 1987. Naloxone and [Met5]-enkephalin effects on retention: Attenuation by adrenal denervation. *Eur. J. Pharmacol.,* 138:37–44.

Zhang, Y., Proenca, R., Maffei, M., Barone, M., Leopold, L., and Friedman, J. M. 1994. Positional cloning of the mouse obese gene and its human homologue. *Nature,* 372: 425–432.

Zigmond, M. J., Abercrombie, E. D., Berger, T. W., Grace, A. A., and Stricker, E. M. 1991. Compensations after lesions of central dopaminergic neurons: Some clinical and basic implications. *Trends Neurosci.,* 13:290–296.

Zimmerberg, B., Brunelli, S. A., and Hofer, M. A. 1994. Reduction of rat pup ultrasonic vocalizations by the neuroactive steroid allopregnanolone. *Pharmacol. Biochem. Behav.,* 47:735–738.

Zimmerman, N. H., and Menaker, M. 1979. The pineal gland: The pacemaker within the circadian system of the house sparrow. *Proc. Natl. Acad. Sci. U.S.A.,* 76:999–1003.

Zinn, A. R. 1993. Turner Syndrome: The case of the missing sex chromosome. *Trends Genet.,* 9(3):90–93.

Zucker, I. 1966. Facilitory and inhibitory effects of progesterone on sexual responses of spayed guinea pigs. *J. Comp. Physiol. Psychol.,* 62:376–381.

Zucker, I. 1968. Biphasic effects of progesterone on sexual receptivity in the female guinea pig. *J. Comp. Physiol. Psychol.,* 65, 472–478.

Zucker, I. 1969. Hormonal determinants of sex differences in saccharine preferences, food intake, and body weight. *Physiol. Behav.,* 4:595–602.

Zucker, I. 1980. Light, behavior, and biologic rhythms. In D. T. Krieger and J. C. Hughes (eds.), *Neuroendocrinology,* pp. 93–101. Sinauer Associates, Sunderland, MA.

Zucker, I. 1988a. Neuroendocrine substrates of circannual rhythms. In D. J. Kupfer, T. H. Monk, and J. D. Barchas (eds.), *Biological Rhythms and Mental Disorders,* pp. 219–251. Guilford Press, New York.

Zucker, I. 1988b. Seasonal affective disorders: Animal models Non fingo. *J. Biol. Rhythms,* 3:209–223.

Zucker, I., and Licht, P. 1983. Circannual and seasonal variations in plasma luteinizing hormone levels of ovariectomized ground squirrels (*Spermophilus lateralis*). *Biol. Reprod.,* 28:178–85.

Zucker, I., Cramer, C. P., and Bittman, E. L. 1980. Regulation by the pituitary gland of circadian rhythms in the hamster. *J. Endocrinol.,* 85:17–25.

Zucker, I., Lee, T. M., and Dark, J. 1991. The suprachiasmatic nucleus and annual rhythms in mammals. In D.C. Klein, S. M. Reppert, and R. Y. Moore (eds.), *The Suprachiasmatic Nucleus: The Mind's Clock,* pp. 246–260. Elsevier, New York.

Zucker, I., Wade, G. N., and Ziegler, R. 1972. Sexual and hormonal influences on eating, taste preferences, and body weight of hamsters. *Physiol. Behav.,* 8:101–111.

Zucker, K. J. 1996. Commentary on Diamond's "Prenatal predisposition and the clinical management of some pediatric conditions. *J. Sex Marital Ther.,* 22:148– 160.

Zweibel, L. J., Hardin, P. E., Liu, X., Hall, J. C., and Rosbash, M. 1991. A post-transcriptional mechanism contributes to circadian cycling of a per-galactosidase fusion protein. *Proc. Natl. Acad. Sci. U.S.A.,* 88:3882–3886.

Zweifel, J. E. and O'Brian, W. H. 1997. A meta-analysis of the effect of hormone replacement therapy upon depressed mood. *Psychoneuroendocrinology,* 22:189–212.

# Illustration Credits

# Index

# About the Book

**Editor:** Peter Farley
**Production Editors:** Kerry Falvey, Paula Noonan
**Copy Editor:** Norma Roche
**Production Manager:** Christopher Small
**Book Production:** Wendy Beck, Janice Holabird
**Book and Cover Design:** Wendy Beck
**Cover Manufacturer:** Henry N. Sawyer Company, Inc.
**Book Manufacturer:** Courier Companies, Inc.

# Peptide and protein hormones

| Hormone | Abbreviation | Source | Major biological action |
|---|---|---|---|
| ***Ovaries*** | | | |
| Relaxin | | Corpora lutea | Permits relaxation of various ligaments during parturition |
| Inhibin (Folliculostatin) | | Follicles | Inhibits FSH secretion |
| ***Pancreas*** | | | |
| Glucagon | | $\alpha$-cells | Glycogenolysis in liver |
| Insulin | | $\beta$-cells | Glucose uptake from blood; glycogen storage in liver |
| Somatostatin | | $\delta$-cells | Inhibits insulin and glucagon secretion |
| Pancreatic polypeptide | PP | Peripheral cells of pancreatic islets | Effects on gut in pharmacological doses |
| ***Pituitary*** | | | |
| Adrenocorticotropic hormone | ACTH | Anterior pituitary | Stimulates synthesis and release of glucocorticoids |
| Vasopressin (Antidiuretic hormone) | ADH or AVP | Posterior pituitary | Increases water reabsorption in kidney |
| $\beta$-endorphin | | Intermediate lobe of pituitary | Analgesic actions |
| Follicle-stimulating hormone | FSH | Anterior pituitary | Stimulates development of ovarian follicles and secretion of estrogens; stimulates spermatogenesis |
| Growth hormone | GH | Anterior pituitary | Mediates somatic cell growth |
| Lipotropin | LPH | Anterior pituitary | Fat mobilization; precursor of opioids |
| Luteinizing hormone | LH | Anterior pituitary | Stimulates Leydig cell development and testosterone production in males; stimulates corpora lutea development and production of progesterone in females |
| Melanocyte-stimulating hormone | MSH | Anterior pituitary | Affects memory; affects skin color in amphibians |
| Oxytocin | | Posterior pituitary | Stimulates milk letdown and uterine contractions during birth |
| Prolactin | PRL | Anterior pituitary | Many actions relating to reproduction, water balance, etc. |
| Thyroid-stimulating hormone (Thyrotropin) | TSH | Anterior pituitary | Stimulates thyroid hormone secretion |
| ***Placenta*** | | | |
| Chorionic gonadotropin | CG | Placenta | LH-like functions; maintains progesterone production during pregnancy |
| Chorionic somatomammotropin (Placental lactogen) | CS (PL) | Placenta | Acts like PRL and GH |
| ***Testes*** | | | |
| Müllerian inhibitory hormone | MIH | Fetal Sertoli cells of testes | Mediates regression of Müllerian duct system |
| Inhibin (Folliculostatin) | | Seminiferous tubules (and ovaries) | Controls FSH secretion |
| ***Thyroid/Parathyroid*** | | | |
| Calcitonin | CT | C-cells of thyroid | Lowers serum $Ca^{2+}$ levels |
| Parathyroid hormone | PTH | Parathyroid gland | Stimulates bone resorption; increases serum $Ca^{2+}$ levels |
| Thyroxine (Tetraiodothyronine) | $T_4$ | Follicular cells | Increases oxidation rates in tissue |
| Triiodothyronine | $T_3$ | Follicular cells | Increases oxidation rates in tissue |